Primer on the Metabolic Bone Diseases and Disorders of Mineral Metabolism

Second Edition

**An Official Publication of the
American Society for Bone and Mineral Research**

Primer on the Metabolic Bone Diseases and Disorders of Mineral Metabolism

Second Edition

Editor

Murray J. Favus, M.D.
Department of Medicine
University of Chicago
Chicago, Illinois

Associate Editors

Sylvia Christakos, Ph.D.
Departments of Biochemistry
and Molecular Biology
University of Medicine and Dentistry
of New Jersey
New Jersey Medical School
Newark, New Jersey

Michael Kleerekoper, M.D.
Bone and Mineral Division
Henry Ford Hospital
Detroit, Michigan

Elizabeth Shane, M.D.
Department of Medicine
College of Physicians and Surgeons
Columbia University
New York, New York

Robert F. Gagel, M.D.
Endocrine Section
M.D. Anderson Cancer Center
Houston, Texas

Craig B. Langman, M.D.
Division of Nephrology
Children's Memorial Hospital
Northwestern University
Chicago, Illinois

Andrew F. Stewart, M.D.
Departments of Endocrinology
West Haven V.A. Medical Center
West Haven, Connecticut, and
Yale University School of Medicine
New Haven, Connecticut

Michael P. Whyte, M.D.
Metabolic Research Unit
Shriners Hospital for Crippled Children
and Departments of Medicine and
Pediatrics
Washington University School of Medicine
St. Louis, Missouri

Raven Press 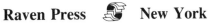 New York

Raven Press, Ltd., 1185 Avenue of the Americas, New York, New York 10036

Made in the United States of America

Library of Congress Cataloging-in-Publication Data

Primer on the metabolic bone diseases and disorders of mineral
    metabolism / [edited by] Murray J. Favus.—2nd ed.
        p.   cm.
    Includes bibliographical references and index.
    ISBN 0-7817-0083-3
    1. Bone—Metabolism—Disorders.   2. Mineral metabolism—
Disorders.   I. Favus, Murray J.
    [DNLM: 1. Bone Diseases, Metabolic.   2. Bone and Bones—
metabolism.   3. Minerals—metabolism.   WE 250 P953 1993]
RC930.P75   1993
616.7′16—dc20
DNLM/DLC
for Library of Congress   93-14940
                                                                  CIP

The material contained in this volume was submitted as previously unpublished material, except in the instances in which credit has been given to the source from which some of the illustrative material was derived.

Great care has been taken to maintain the accuracy of the information contained in the volume. However, neither Raven Press nor the editors and Merck can be held responsible for errors or for any consequences arising from the use of the information contained herein.

Materials appearing in this book prepared by individuals as part of their official duties as U.S. Government employees are not covered by the above-mentioned copyright.

9   8   7   6   5   4   3   2   1

Contents

Section I: Anatomy and Biology of Bone Matrix and Cellular Elements

**Section II: Calcium, Magnesium, Phosphorus Homeostasis and Physiology
and Biochemistry of Calcium Regulating Hormones**

Section X: Nephrolithiasis

Section XI: Appendix

Contributors

John S. Adams, M.D.
Dennis L. Andress, M.D.
Louis V. Avioli, M.D.
Roland Baron, D.D.S., Ph.D
David J. Baylink, M.D.
Daniel D. Bikle, M.D., Ph.D.
John P. Bilezikian, M.D.
Arthur E. Broadus, M.D., Ph.D.
William J. Burtis, M.D., Ph.D.
Ernesto Canalis, M.D.
Thomas O. Carpenter, M.D.
Russell W. Chesney, M.D.
Sylvia Christakos, Ph.D.
Thomas L. Clemens, Ph.D.
Jack W. Coburn, M.D.
Fredric L. Coe, M.D.
Gilbert J. Cote, Ph.D.
Leonard J. Deftos, M.D.
Pierre D. Delmas, M.D., Ph.D.
Marc K. Drezner, M.D.
Howard Duncan, M.D.
Murray J. Favus, M.D.
Robert F. Gagel, M.D.
Susan C. Galbraith, M.D.
Harry K. Genant, M.D.
Francis H. Glorieux, M.D., Ph.D.
William G. Goodman, M.D.
Theodore J. Hahn, M.D.
John G. Haddad, Jr., M.D.
Hunter Heath III, M.D.
Helen L. Henry, Ph.D.
Keith A. Hruska, M.D.
Karl L. Insogna, M.D.
Jeffrey A. Jackson, M.D.
Thomas P. Jacobs, M.D.
C. Conrad Johnston, Jr., M.D.
Kastytis Karvelis, M.D.
Sundeep Khosla, M.D.
Michael Kleerekoper, M.D.
Gordon L. Klein, M.D., M.P.H.
Sambasiva R. Kottamassu, M.D.

Henry M. Kronenberg, M.D.
Craig B. Langman, M.D.
Jacob Lemann, Jr., M.D.
Michael A. Levine, M.D.
Uri A. Liberman, M.D., Ph.D
Robert Lindsay, Ph.D., M.B.Ch.B,
  F.R.C.P.
Lawrence E. Mallette, M.D., Ph.D.
Stephen J. Marx, M.D.
Malachi J. McKenna, M.D., F.A.C.P.
L. Joseph Melton III, M.D.
Gregory R. Mundy, M.D.
Robert A. Nissenson, Ph.D.
Anthony W. Norman, Ph.D.
Michael E. Norman, M.D.
A. Michael Parfitt, M.D.
Joan H. Parks, M.S.
Anthony A. Portale, M.D.
Andrew K. Poznanski, M.D.
J. Edward Puzas, Ph.D.
L. Darryl Quarles, M.D.
Jorge A. Ramirez, M.D.
D. Sudhaker Rao, M.B.B.S.
Robert R. Recker, M.D.
Gideon A. Rodan, M.D., Ph.D.
Felice Rolnick, M.D.
Robert K. Rude, M.D.
Isidro B. Salusky, M.D.
Gino V. Segre, M.D.
Elizabeth Shane, M.D.
Louis M. Sherwood, M.D.
Ethel S. Siris, M.D.
Eduardo Slatopolsky, M.D.
Andrew F. Stewart, M.D.
Gordon J. Strewler, M.D.
Jozsef Szabo, M.D.
Steven L. Teitelbaum, M.D.
John D. Termine, Ph.D.
David C. Wang, M.D.
Robert S. Weinstein, M.D.
Michael P. Whyte, M.D.

The American Society for Bone and Mineral Research

The American Society for Bone and Mineral Research (ASBMR) was founded in 1977 to bring together the increasing number of clinical and experimental scientists involved in the investigation of bone and mineral metabolism. Since then the Society has experienced remarkable growth in its membership, and its annual meetings have become the premier event for exchange of new knowledge in this developing field. From its inception the Society has emphasized support and encouragement of its young members, whose contributions are recognized at the meeting. More than three years ago the Society started publishing the Journal of Bone and Mineral Research, which provides on a continuing basis an additional focus for the burgeoning interest in this field of inquiry and application.

Our areas of interest cross many disciplines—both basic and clinical—and, as is frequently the case with newly evolving disciplines, it has received relatively sparse coverage in the formal curricula of many of our schools. The Society has therefore taken the initiative to provide an up-to-date presentation of the principles and the tools applied to the diagnosis, investigation, and therapy of metabolic bone disorders. We wish to thank our members, who have generously devoted their time to put together this excellent Primer, which we hope will help students and practitioners in the health sciences and will attract new devotees to this field.

John G. Haddad, Jr., M.D.
Gideon A. Rodan, M.D., Ph.D.
Past Presidents, ASBMR

Preface to the First Edition

Our understanding of the scientific basis for clinical bone and mineral disorders has grown rapidly since the founding of the American Society for Bone and Mineral Research (ASBMR) in 1977. The number of basic scientists and clinicians involved in either research or patient care in bone and mineral metabolism has grown dramatically, attracting the interest of medical students, house officers, and practitioners. While textbooks of Medicine, Pediatrics, Endocrinology, Nephrology, Radiology, and Orthopedic Surgery devote chapters or sections to metabolic bone disease, none provide a comprehensive description of the clinical manifestations of the diseases and the basic science necessary to understand pathophysiology. Three years ago the Education Committee of the ASBMR undertook the task of creating a comprehensive educational source, and this *Primer* is the result of our efforts.

The primary purpose of the *Primer* is to provide a comprehensive, yet concise description of the clinical manifestations, pathophysiology, diagnostic approaches and therapeutics of diseases that come under the rubric of 'bone and mineral disorders'.

The organization of the *Primer* into twelve sections reflects the several basic science and clinical disciplines that contribute to the field. The first three sections contain the basic science core material that provides the underpinning of our understanding of normal bone and mineral structure and biology. Section I contains a thorough description of the gross anatomy and ultrastructure of bone, the physiology of skeletal growth, development and remodeling, the biochemistry of the bone matrix and the unique structural features and functions of the cellular elements of bone. Section II provides a dynamic view of the biologic importance of the major elements of bone (usually referred to as the minerals) and their body distribution and balance, including the processes of accumulation and elimination across epithelial barriers in the intestine and kidney. Section III focuses on the details of the synthesis, secretion, metabolism and biologic actions of the key hormones (parathyroid hormone, vitamin D and calcitonin) that regulate skeletal growth and re-modeling, calcium homeostasis and the assimilation of minerals to support these processes.

The clinical portion of the *Primer* begins with the eleven chapters in Section IV. Laboratory assays, radiographic and imaging techniques and bone histomorphometry used to evaluate patients suspected of having bone or mineral disorders are described. Section V contains 26 chapters which describe the many clinical entities that may present to the clinician with disordered levels of serum minerals including hyper- and hypo- calcemia, -phosphatemia and -magnesemia. Chapters in Section VI describe the several genetic and acquired causes of the classic metabolic bone diseases of rickets, osteomalacia and osteoporosis and the many presentations of renal osteodys-trophy.

Section VII contains the genetic and developmental disorders that primarily affect bone. These conditions may present in infancy, childhood, or adulthood as abnormal radiographs, fractures, growth retardation or skeletal pain. Section VIII includes vascular, tumoral and degenerative processes that may cause bone pain, skeletal deformity and fracture. Section IX is devoted solely to Paget's disease of bone, a common and important entiry with many presentations.

Diseases characterized by pathologic calcification of soft tissue are presented in Section X, and Section XI contains the metabolic disorders in which pathologic crystalization is selective for the urinary tract.

Section XII is the Appendix, composed of seven subsections containing information useful to the practitioner, including growth charts, ossification center tables, normal values for commonly used biochemical analyses, instructions on how to conduct and interpret dynamic tests of calcio-tropic hormone secretion, recommended daily mineral and vitamin D intake for all ages and a drug formulary.

The full credit for any educational benefit that the *Primer* may offer goes to the many scientists and clinicians who have captured their knowledge and experience on the pages of their chapters. The high quality of their contributions and their cooperation are deeply appreciated. I am also deeply indebted to the seven Associate Editors of the *Primer*: Sylvia Christakos, Robert Gagel, Michael Kleerekoper, Craig Langman, Elizabeth Shane, Andrew Stewart and Michael Whyte for their hard work and devotion to the project. Their ability to enlist the participation of over seventy authors, continued enthusiasm and critical editing served to forge the *Primer* into its final form. I also express my deepest appreciation to the presidents of ASBMR who held office during the development of the *Primer*—Norman Bell, Gideon Rodan, John Haddad and Armen Tashjian. They were most generous in devoting time and effort to find the resources necessary to bring the *Primer* to publication.

I would also express my sincere appreciation to the people at Byrd Press for their guidance and assistance in the preparation and publication of the *Primer*. Finally, I would like to gratefully acknowledge Shirley Hohl, ASBMR Executive Secretary, and John Hohl for their much valued assistance in preparing the *Primer* for publication and distribution.

Murray J. Favus, M.D.
The University of Chicago
Pritzker School of Medicine

Preface to the Second Edition of the *Primer*

Like many other branches of medicine, the field of bone and mineral metabolism continues to undergo rapid transformation through the application of molecular biology and recombinant DNA technology. Just 3 years ago, as the first edition of the *Primer* was being published, many bone proteins, cytokines, and growth factors were in short supply. Today, clinical investigators are given sufficient quantities of these and other new agents to test their potency in altering human bone formation and remodeling. The same technology is making progress toward understanding genetic disorders at the molecular level, as with X-linked hypophosphatemic rickets. The molecular basis for common diseases such as primary hyperparathyroidism is also becoming unraveled, and a further understanding of the links between abnormal calcium metabolism and cancer has been advanced by the cloning of the parathyroid hormone-related peptide (PTHrP).

The explosion of the new knowledge must be integrated into our present understanding of the pathogenesis and treatment of bone and mineral disorders. Thus, several chapters from the first edition have undergone extensive rewriting, and new chapters have been added to maintain the editorial goal of maintaining the *Primer* as a comprehensive yet concise source of knowledge of the field. Readers of the first edition will feel comfortable with the format of the second edition, as we have retained the basic 11-part framework. New chapters have been added to the basic science sections such as the one devoted to PTHrP, and others have been added to the clinical sections, such as the radiographic essentials of osteoporosis. Because of the ever-expanding interest in osteoporosis, a section on bone densitometry has been added to the Appendix.

Murray J. Favus, M.D.

Acknowledgments

The credit for any success the *Primer* may enjoy belongs to the members of ASBMR, whose chapters are filled with the very best of their scientific knowledge and teaching skills. Their commitment to excellence in writing and their outstanding cooperation deserves my most sincere appreciation. I also acknowledge the many members of the Society who have made suggestions and offered their participation to improve this edition. As with the first edition, the associate editors—Sylvia Christakos, Robert F. Gagel, Michael Kleerekoper, Craig B. Langman, Elizabeth Shane, Andrew F. Stewart, and Michael P. Whyte—deserve special recognition for their devotion to the *Primer*. They join me in acknowledging the excellent cooperation and well-organized effort led by Jasna Markovac and her staff at Raven Press.

SECTION I

Anatomy and Biology of Bone Matrix and Cellular Elements

1. Anatomy and Ultrastructure of Bone

Roland Baron, D.D.S., Ph.D.

*Departments of Orthopaedics and Cell Biology, Yale University, School of
Medicine, New Haven, Connecticut*

Bone is a specialized connective tissue that makes up, together with cartilage, the skeletal system. These tissues serve three functions: (1) *mechanical:* support and site of muscle attachment for locomotion; 2) *protective:* for vital organs and bone marrow; and 3) *metabolic:* reserve of ions for the entire organism, especially *calcium and phosphate.* (Serum calcium homeostasis is essential to life.)

In bone, as in all connective tissues, the fundamental constituents are the *cells* and the *extracellular matrix.* The latter is particularly abundant in this tissue and is composed of collagen fibers and noncollagenous proteins. The matrix of bone, as well as the matrices of cartilage and the tissues forming the teeth, however, has the unique ability to become *calcified.*

BONE AS AN ORGAN: MACROSCOPIC ORGANIZATION

Anatomically, one can distinguish two types of bones in the skeleton, flat bones (skull bones, scapula, mandible, and ileum) and long bones (tibia, femur, and humerus), which derive from two distinct types of histogenesis [intramembranous and endochondral, respectively (see ''Bone Histogenesis and Growth'')], although the development and growth of long bones actually involve both types.

The external examination of a long bone shows two wider extremities (epiphysis), a more or less cylindrical tube in the middle (midshaft or diaphysis) and a progressive passage from one to the other (metaphysis). In a growing long bone, the epiphysis and the metaphysis are separated by a layer of cartilage, the *epiphyseal cartilage* (also called *growth plate*); cells proliferate the matrix later calcifies. This layer of proliferative cells and expanding cartilage matrix is responsible for the longitudinal growth of bones and becomes entirely calcified and remodeled by the end of the growth period (see ''Bone Histogenesis and Growth''). The external part of the bones is formed by a thick and dense layer of calcified tissue, the cortex *(compact bone)* which, in the diaphysis, encloses the medullary cavity where the hematopoietic bone marrow is housed. Toward the metaphysis and the epiphysis, the cortex becomes progressively thinner and the internal space is filled with a network of thin, calcified trabeculae, the *cancellous bone* also named spongy or *trabecular bone.* The spaces enclosed by these thin trabeculae are also filled with hematopoietic bone marrow and are in continuity with the medullary cavity of the diaphysis. The bone surfaces at the extremities that take part in the articular joint are covered with a layer of articular cartilage that does not calcify.

There are consequently two bone surfaces, where the bone is in contact with the soft tissues: an external surface *(periosteal surface)* and an internal surface *(endosteal surface).* These surfaces are lined with osteogenic cells organized in layers: the *periosteum* and the *endosteum,* respectively. Cortical and trabecular bone are constituted of the same cells and the same matrix elements, but there are structural and functional differences. The structural differences are essentially quantitative: 80–90% of the volume of compact bone is calcified vs. 15–25% in the trabecular bone (the remaining volume is occupied by bone marrow, blood vessels, and connective tissue); but 70–85% of the interface with soft tissues is at the endosteal bone surface. The functional differences are a consequence of these structural differences and vice versa: *the cortical bone fulfills mainly the mechanical and protective function* and *the trabecular bone the metabolic function.*

BONE AS A TISSUE

Microscopic Organization

Bone Matrix and Mineral

Bone is formed by *collagen fibers* (type I, 90% of total proteins), usually oriented in a preferential direction, and noncollagenous proteins. Spindle- or plate-shaped crystals of *hydroxyapatite* $[Ca_{10}(PO_4)_6(OH)_2]$ are found on the collagen fibers, within them, and in the ground substance. They are generally oriented in the same preferential direction as the collagen fibers. The ground substance is essentially composed of *glycoproteins and proteoglycans.* These highly anionic complexes have a high ion-binding capacity and are thought to play an important part in the calcification process and the fixation of hydroxyapatite crystals to the collagen fibers.

Numerous noncollagenous proteins present in bone matrix have recently been purified and sequenced (see Chapter 4), but their role is only partially characterized. Most of these proteins are synthesized by bone-forming cells, but not all; a number of plasma proteins are preferentially absorbed by the bone matrix, such as α_2-HS-glycoprotein that is synthesized in the liver.

The preferential orientation of the collagen fibers alternates in adult bone from layer to layer giving to this bone a typical *lamellar* structure, best seen under polarized light or in electron microscopy. This organization of fibers allows the highest density of collagen per unit volume of tissue. These lamellae can be parallel to each other if deposited along a flat surface (trabecular bone and periosteum) or concentric if deposited on the surface of a channel centered on a blood vessel *(Haversian System).* However, when bone is formed very rapidly (during histogenesis, fracture healing, tumors, or some metabolic bone diseases), there is no preferential organization of the collagen fibers. They are then found in more or less randomly oriented bundles: this type of bone is called *woven bone,* as opposed to the *lamellar bone* (for a description of the woven bone, see "Bone Histogenesis and Growth").

Cellular Organizations Within the Bone Matrix: Osteocytes

The calcified bone matrix is not metabolically inert, and cells *(osteocytes)* are found embedded deep within the bone in small osteocytic lacunae (25,000/mm³ of bone) (Fig. 1). They were originally bone-forming cells *(osteoblasts)* that have been trapped into their own production of bone matrix, which later became calcified. These cells have numerous and long cell processes rich in microfilaments that are in contact with cell processes from other osteocytes (frequent *gap junctions*), or with processes from the cells lining the bone surface (osteoblasts or flat lining cells in the endosteum or periosteum). These processes are organized during the formation of the matrix and before its calcification; they form a network of thin *canaliculi* permeating the entire bone matrix.

There is a space comprised between the osteocyte's plasma membrane and the bone matrix itself, both in the lacunae and in the canaliculi, the *periosteocytic space,* filled with extracellular fluid, the *Bone ECF.*

The physiological significance of this system is more readily demonstrated by some numbers: The total bone surface area of the canaliculae and lacunae is of the order of 1,000–5,000 m² in an adult human (140 m² for lung capillaries); the volume of Bone ECF is 1.0–1.5 L, and the surface calcium contained on bone mineral crystals is of the order of 5–20 g, which would account for a significant percentage of the total exchangeable bone calcium. The fact that the calcium concentration in the Bone ECF (0.5 mmol/L) is lower than the plasma (1.5 mmol/L) suggests that there is a constant flow of calcium ions out of the bone.

The morphology of these osteocytes varies according to their age and functional activity. Being derived from osteoblasts, a young osteocyte conserves most of the ultrastructural characteristics of this cell except that there is a decrease in the volume of the cell and in the importance of the organelles involved in protein synthesis (rough endoplasmic reticulum, Golgi). An older osteocyte, located deeper within the calcified bone, shows an accentuation of this trend and, in addition, an accumulation of glycogen in its cytoplasm. These cells have been shown to be able to synthesize new bone matrix at the surface of the osteocytic lacunae, which can subsequently calcify. Although they are classically considered able to resorb calcified bone from the same surface, this point has recently been disputed. The *fate* of the osteocytes is to be *phagocytized* and *digested,* together with the other components of bone, during osteoclastic bone resorption. These cells may also play a role in locally activating bone turnover.

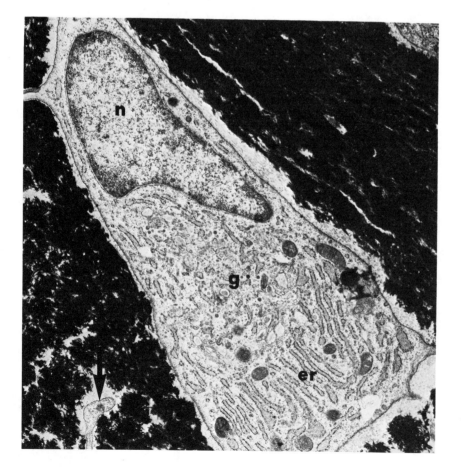

FIG. 1. Osteocyte: Electron microscopy of an osteocyte embedded in calcified bone matrix (black, hydroxyapatite crystals). The cell has a basal nucleus *(n),* a large Golgi complex *(g),* and a relatively well-developed endoplasmic reticulum *(er).* Cytoplasmic extensions can be seen in the matrix *(arrow)* in their canaliculi. Approximate magnification 5,000 ×.

The Bone Surface

Most of the bone tissue turnover occurs at the bone surfaces mainly at the endosteal surface (i.e., at the interface with bone marrow). This surface is morphologically heterogeneous, and this heterogeneity reflects the various specific cellular activities involved in remodeling and turnover.

The Osteoblast and Bone Formation

The osteoblast is the bone lining cell responsible for the production of the matrix constituents (collagen and ground substance) (Fig. 2). It originates from a local mesenchymal stem cell (bone marrow stromal stem cell or connective tissue mesenchymal stem cell). These precursors, upon the right stimulation, undergo proliferation and differentiate into preosteoblasts and then mature osteoblasts. Osteoblasts never appear or function individually, but are always found in clusters of cuboidal cells along the bone surface (~ 100–400 cells per bone-forming site). At the *light microscope level* the osteoblast is characterized by a round nucleus at the base of the cell (opposite to the bone surface), a strongly basophilic cytoplasm, and a prominent Golgi complex located between the nucleus and the apex of the cell. Osteoblasts are always found lining a layer of bone matrix that they are producing and is not yet calcified *(osteoid tissue)*. The presence of the osteoid is due to a time lag between matrix formation and its subsequent calcification (Osteoid Maturation Period ~ 10 days). Behind the osteoblast are usually found one or two layers of cells, activated mesenchymal cells and preosteoblasts. At the *ultrastructural level*, the osteoblast is characterized by: 1) the presence of an extremely well-

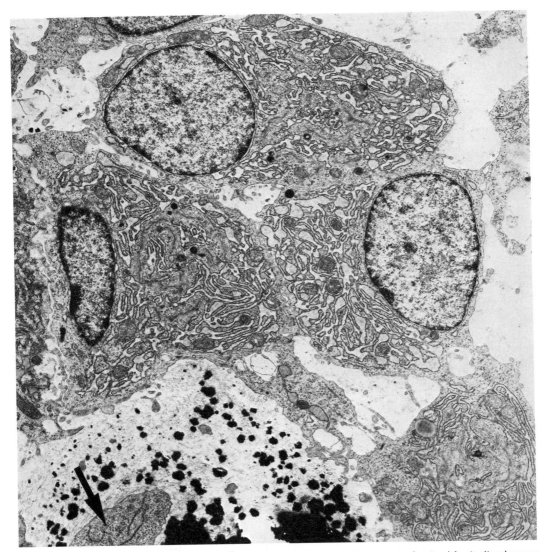

FIG. 2. Osteoblasts and osteoid tissue: Electron microscopy of a group of osteoblasts *(top)* covering a layer of mineralizing osteoid tissue *(bottom)* with a newly embedded osteocyte *(arrow)*. Basal nuclei, prominent Golgi, and endoplasmic reticulum and characteristics of active osteoblasts. Approximate magnification 3,000 ×.

developed rough endoplasmic reticulum with dilated cisternae and a dense granular content, and 2) the presence of a large circular Golgi complex comprising multiple Golgi stacks. Cytoplasmic processes on the secreting side of the cell extend deep into the osteoid matrix and are in contact with the osteocyte processes in their canaliculi. Junctional complexes (gap junctions) are often found between the osteoblasts. The plasma membrane of the *osteoblast is characteristically rich in alkaline phosphatase* (serum alkaline phosphatase is used as an index of bone formation) and has been shown to have receptors for para-

thyroid hormone, but not for calcitonin; osteoblasts also express receptors for estrogens and vitamin D_3 in their nuclei. Toward the end of the secreting period the osteoblasts will become either a flat lining cell or an osteocyte.

The Osteoclast and Bone Resorption

The osteoclast is the bone lining cell responsible for bone resorption (Figs. 3 and 4).

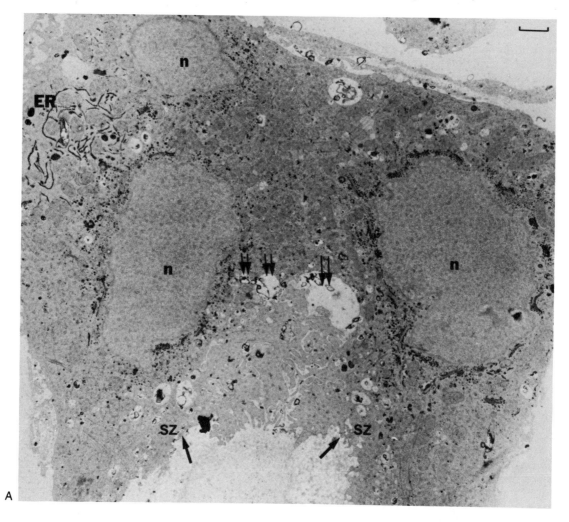

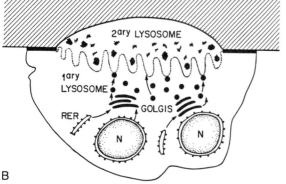

OSTEOCLAST

FIG. 3. Osteoclast. **A:** Section of an osteoclast reacted for the lysosomal enzyme arylsulfatase. The osteoclast contains multiple nuclei *(n)*, an endoplasmic reticulum where lysosomal enzymes are synthesized *(ER)*, and prominent Golgi stacks around each nucleus. The cell is attached to bone matrix *(bottom)* and forms a separate compartment underneath itself, limited by the sealing zone *(SZ, single arrows)*. The plasma membrane of the cell facing this compartment is extensively folded and forms the ruffled border, with pockets of extracellular space between the folds *(double arrows)*. Multiple small vesicles transporting enzymes toward the bone matrix can be seen in the cytoplasm. Approximate magnification 9,000 ×. **B:** Schematic representation of enzyme secretion polarity in osteoclasts. (From Baron R., et al., *J. Cell Biol.,* 101:2210–2222, 1985.)

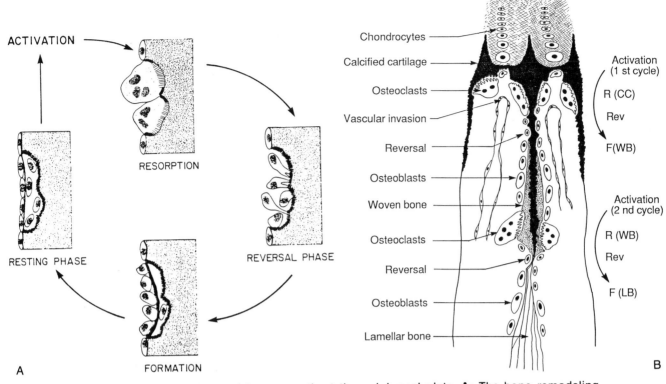

FIG. 4. Bone remodeling and bone growth at the epiphyseal plate. **A:** The bone remodeling sequence as it occurs in trabecular bone (the same principles apply to Haversian remodeling). (See text for full explanation.) **B:** Schematic representation of the cellular events occurring at the growth plate in long bones. *R*, resorption; *Rev*, reversal; *F*, formation; *CC*, calcified cartilage; *WB*, woven bone; *LB*, lamellar bone (see text for full explanation).

Morphology. The osteoclast is a *giant multinucleated cell* (4–20 nuclei) usually found in contact with a calcified bone surface and within a lacuna *(Howship's lacunae),* which is the result of its own resorptive activity. It is possible to find up to four or five osteoclasts in the same resorptive site, but there usually are only one or two per site. Under the *light microscope,* the nuclei appear as variable within the same cell: either round and euchromatic or very irregular in contour and heterochromatic, possibly reflecting the asynchronous fusion of mononuclear precursors. The cytoplasm is "foamy" with many vacuoles. The contact zone with the bone is characterized by the presence of a *ruffled border* and dense patches on each side of it known as the *sealing zone.*

Characteristic ultrastructural features of this cell are the abundance of Golgi complexes characteristically disposed around each nucleus, mitochondria, and transport vesicles loaded with lysosomal enzymes. The most prominent feature of the osteoclast is, however, the existence of deep foldings of the plasma membrane in the area facing the bone matrix: they form the *ruffled border* that is surrounded by a ring of contractile proteins serving to attach the cell to the bone surface and sealing off the subosteoclastic bone resorbing compartment *(sealing zone).* The attachment of the cell to the matrix is performed via integrin receptors, binding to specific sequences in matrix proteins. The plasma membrane in the ruffled border area contains proteins otherwise present at the limiting membrane of lysosomes and related organelles, and a specific type of electrogenic proton ATPase involved in acidification. The basolateral plasma membrane of the osteoclast is highly and specifically enriched in (Na^+,K^+)ATPase (sodium pumps), $HCO3^-/Cl^-$ exchangers, and Na^+/H^+ exchangers.

Mechanisms of Bone Resorption. *Lysosomal enzymes* are actively synthesized by the osteoclast and are found in the endoplasmic reticulum, Golgi, and many transport vesicles; these lysosomal enzymes are secreted, via the ruffled border, into the extracellular bone resorbing compartment; these enzymes reach a high enough extracellular concentration because this compartment is sealed off. The transport and targeting of these enzymes for secretion at the apical pole of the osteoclast involves *mannose-6-phosphate receptors.* Furthermore, the cell secretes nonlysosomal enzymes such as collagenase.

The *osteoclast acidifies* the extracellular compartment by secreting protons across the ruffled-border membrane (proton pumps). Recent evidence would suggest the presence of an electrogenic proton-pump ATPase, related to but different from the kidney tubule acidifying cells. The protons are provided to the pumps by the enzyme *carbonic anhydrase,* highly concentrated in the cytosol of this cell, and ATP and CO_2 are provided by the mitochondriae. The basolateral membrane activity exchanges bicarbonate for chloride, thereby avoiding an alkalinization of the cytosol. The basolateral sodium pumps might be involved in secondary active transport of calcium and/or protons in association with Na^+, Ca^+ exchanger and/or Na^+, H^+ antiport. This cell could therefore function similarly to kidney tubule or gastric parietal cells, which also acidify a lumen.

The extracellular bone resorbing compartment is therefore the functional equivalent of a secondary lysosome with 1) a low pH, 2) lysosomal enzymes, and 3) the substrate. The *low pH* dissolves the crystals, exposing the matrix. *The enzymes,* now at optimal pH, degrade the matrix components; the residues from this extracellular digestion are either internalized, or transported across the cell (transcytosis) and released at the basolateral domain, or else released during periods of relapse of the sealing zone, possibly induced by a calcium sensor in response to the rise via extracellular calcium in the bone resorbing compartment.

Chronologically, the crystals are mobilized by digestion of their link to collagen (noncollagenous proteins) and dissolved by the acid environment. The residual collagen fibers are digested by either the activation of latent collagenase and the action of cathepsins at low pH.

Clinically, this explains why: 1) bone resorption helps to maintain calcium and Pi levels in the plasma, and 2) hydroxyproline and N-terminal collagen peptides concentration in the urine are used as an indirect measurement of bone resorption in humans (collagen type I is highly enriched in hydroxyproline and pyridoxiline links).

Origin and Fate of the Osteoclast. It is the work of Walker on osteopetrotic mice that established the hematogenous origin of the osteoclast. Cells of the mononuclear–phagocyte lineage are the most likely candidates to differentiate into osteoclasts. However, the differentiation into osteoclasts may occur at the promonocyte stage, but monocytes and macrophages, already committed to their own lineage, might still be able to form osteoclasts under the right circumstances.

Recent work has suggested that, despite its mononuclear phagocytic origin, the osteoclast membrane is devoid of F_c and C_3 receptors, as well as of several other macrophage markers; it is, however, rich in nonspecific esterase and synthesizes lysozyme as mononuclear phagocytes. Monoclonal antibodies have been produced that recognize osteoclasts and do not see the macrophage. Receptors for calcitonin, but not for parathyroid hormone, are present on the osteoclast membrane, and estrogen, but not vitamin D receptors, has been found in these cells.

BONE REMODELING

The activity of the bone cells previously described and formed along the surfaces of bone, mainly the *endosteal* surface, results in *bone remodeling* the process by which bone grows and is *turned over.* Bone formation and bone resorption do not, however, occur along the bone surface at random; they are part of the turnover mechanism replacing old bone by new bone. *In the normal adult skeleton, bone formation occurs only where bone resorption has previously occurred.* The sequence of events at the remodeling site is therefore *Activation-Resorption-For-mation* (ARF sequence). During the intermediate phase between resorption and formation (Reversal Phase), some macrophage-like uncharacterized mononuclear cells are observed in the remodeling focus, and a *cement line,* marking the limit of resorption and "cementing" together the old and the new bone, is formed.

BONE HISTOGENESIS AND GROWTH

There are two types of histogenesis of bone: the *intramembranous ossification* (flat bones) and the *endochondral ossification* (long bones). The essential difference between them is the presence or absence of a cartilaginous phase.

Intramembranous Ossification

In intramembranous ossification, a group of mesenchymal cells within a highly vascularized area of the embryonic connective tissue undergoes division and differentiates *directly* into preosteoblasts and then osteoblasts. These cells will synthesize a bone matrix with the following characteristics: 1) the collagen fibers are not preferentially oriented but appear as *irregular bundles,* 2) the osteocytes are large and extremely numerous, and 3) calcification is delayed and does not proceed in an orderly fashion but as irregularly distributed patches. This type of bone is called *woven bone.* At the periphery, mesenchymal cells keep differentiating and follow the same steps. Blood vessels are incorporated between the woven bone trabeculae and will form the hematopoietic *bone marrow.* Later, this woven bone is remodeled, following the ARF sequence, and progressively replaced by mature *lamellar bone.*

Endochondral Ossification

Formation of a Cartilage Model

Mesenchymal cells will undergo division and differentiate into *prechondroblasts* and then *chondroblasts.* These cells will secrete the cartilaginous matrix. Like the osteoblasts, the chondroblasts will progressively be embedded within their own matrix production and are then called *chondrocytes,* lying within lacunae. But, *unlike the osteocytes,* they will continue to proliferate for some time, this being allowed in part by the gel-like consistency of cartilage. At the periphery of this cartilage (*perichondrium*), the mesenchymal cells will continue to proliferate and differentiate. This is called the *appositional growth.* Another type of growth is observed in the cartilage by synthesis of new matrix between the chondrocytes (*interstitial growth*). In the growth plate, the cells appear in regular columns called the *isogeneous groups.* Later on, the chondrocytes will enlarge progressively and become *hypertrophic* and die (see below).

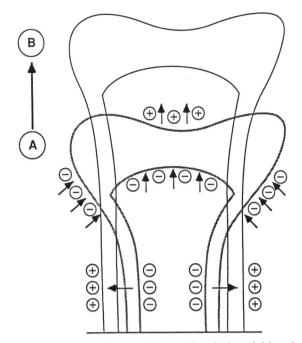

FIG. 5. Resorption (−) and formation (+) activities during the longitudinal growth of bones: During the growth from A to B, the cortex in the diaphysis must be resorbed inside and reformed outside *(bottom)*. The growth plate moves upward (see Fig. 4B), and the wider parts of the bone must be reshaped into a diaphysis. (From Jee WSS: The skeletal tissues. In: Weiss L (ed) *Histology, Cell and Tissue Biology.* Elsevier Biomedical, New York, pp 200–255, 1983.)

Vascular Invasion and Longitudinal Growth (Remodeling)

The embryonic cartilage is avascular. During its early development, a ring of woven bone is formed by intramembranous ossification in the future midshaft area under the perichondrum (which is then a periosteum). Just after the calcification of this woven bone, blood vessels (preceded by osteoclasts) will penetrate this bone and the cartilage with the blood supply that will form the hematopoietic bone marrow.

The *growth plate* in a growing long bone, shows, from the epiphyseal area to the diaphyseal area, the following cellular events (Fig. 5). *A proliferative zone* is where the chondroblasts are dividing actively, forming isogenous

groups, and actively synthesizing the matrix. These cells become progressively larger, enlarging their lacunae in the *hypertrophic zone.* Lower in the epiphyseal plate, the matrix of the longitudinal cartilage septa selectively calcifies *(zone of provisional calcification).* The chondrocytes become highly vacuolated and then die. Once calcified, the cartilage matrix is resorbed by *osteoclasts,* followed by blood vessels in the *zone of invasion.* However, these osteoclasts resorb only partially the calcified longitudinal septa. After resorption, *osteoblasts* differentiate and form a layer of woven bone on top of the cartilaginous remnants of the longitudinal septa. *This is therefore the first ARF sequence remodeling the cartilage and replacing it by woven bone.* The trabeculae that are formed are called the *primary spongiosa.* Still lower in the growth plate, this woven bone will be subjected to *further remodeling* (ARF sequence), replacing the woven bone and the cartilaginous remnants with lamellar bone, reaching the mature state of trabecular bone called *secondary spongiosa* (Fig. 4B).

Growth in Diameter and Shape Modification (Modeling)

Growth in the diameter of the shaft is the result of the deposition of new *membranous bone* beneath the periosteum that will continue throughout its life. In this case, resorption does not immediately precede formation. The midshaft is narrower than the metaphysis, and the growth of a long bone will progressively destroy the lower part of the metaphysis and transform it into a diaphysis. This is done through continuous resorption by osteoclasts beneath the periosteum.

SELECTED REFERENCES

1. Jee WSS: The skeletal tissues. In: Weiss L (ed) *Histology, Cell and Tissue Biology.* Elsevier Biomedical, New York, pp 200–255, 1983
2. Nijweide P, Burger EH, Feyen JHM: Cells of bone: Proliferation, differentiation and hormonal regulation. *Physiol Rev* 66:855–886, 1986
3. Baron R, Chakraborty M, Chatterjee D, Horne W, Lomri A, Ravesloot J-H: Biology of the osteoclast. In: Mundy GR and Martin TJ (eds) *Physiology and Pharmacology of Bone.* Springer Verlag, New York, 1993 (in press)
4. Suda T, Takahashi N, Martin TJ: Modulation of osteoclast differentiation. *Endocrine Rev* 13:66–80, 1992

2. Molecular Defects of Bone Development

Steven L. Teitelbaum, M.D.

*Department of Pathology and Laboratory Medicine, Jewish Hospital at
Washington University Medical Center, St. Louis, Missouri*

Molecular biology continues to profoundly impact skeletal research . As such, it is now possible to precisely identify genetic alterations of well-characterized clinical disorders. This combination of molecular and clinical information has afforded unforeseen insights into the function in bone homeostasis, of proteins coded by the mutated gene's normal counterpart. Most importantly, due to direct targeting of underlying genetic defects or their molecular consequences, we are entering an era in which therapy of previously untreatable diseases is becoming a reality. This chapter focuses on four genetic disorders of the skeleton, each of which has provided major insights into the role played by the wild type gene in bone matrix development.

OSTEOPETROSIS

The osteopetroses are that family of congenital diseases falling under the rubric, "marble bone disease." Increased skeletal mass due to dysfunctional osteoclasts' failure to resorb bone normally is the commonality of this group. Although there are exceptions, the phenotype of human osteopetrosis may be subdivided into the infantile malignant form (Albers–Schoenberg disease) inherited as an autosomal recessive and the so-called benign, autosomal dominant form. Patients with benign osteopetrosis can expect a relatively normal life. Before the advent of marrow transplantation (1), the recessive form was invariably fatal within the first decade.

Regardless of genotype, the osteopetroses are characterized by a strikingly radiopaque skeleton, with loss of distinction between cortex and marrow space. Although intramembranous bone accumulates, the pathological hallmark of all forms of the disease is the persistence of "cartilaginous bars" deep within metaphyseal and diaphyseal bone. These islands of devitalized cartilage surrounded by bone represent the residue of nonresorbed primary spongiosa, a component of endochondral ossification (2).

Osteopetrosis provides an example of a rare disorder yielding major insights into the normal function of a cell, in this case, the osteoclast. The pioneering work in this arena came from Donald Walker (3) who, exploiting the numerous animal models of the disease, showed that specific strains of osteopetrotic mice could be cured by parabiosis to normal litter mates or by transplantation of normal spleen or marrow cells. These observations established that a hematogenous factor is responsible for osteoclast development. Proof that the osteoclast is, in fact, of hematopoietic origin derived from an experiment in nature in which a osteopetrotic girl was cured by marrow transplanted from her brother (1). In this instance,

the posttransplant osteoclasts contained the male chromosome delineating the cells' marrow derivation. Subsequent efforts in which osteoclasts were generated *in vitro* from pure populations of mononuclear phagocyte precursors confirmed the ontogenetic relationship of these cells (4).

This information, coupled with an understanding of the means by which osteoclasts degrade bone (5), prompted appreciation of the fact that the osteopetrosis phenotype represents a variety of pathogenetic mechanisms. Reflecting the osteoclast's relationship to monocyte–macrophages, the *op/op* osteopetrotic mouse, which lacks osteoclasts, fails for example, to express the macrophage-specific growth factor M-CSF (CSF-1) (6). The defect has been localized to a point mutation in the coding region of the M-CSF gene (7).

We now know that acidification of the cell-bone interface is an essential step in osteoclast-mediated bone resorption (8). Such acidification is derived from protons generated under the influence of carbonic anhydrase. One would expect, therefore, that defects in osteoclast-mediated acidification would manifest themselves clinically as deficient bone resorption. In fact, renal tubular acidosis is known to occur in osteopetrotic patients, and at least one affected family is lacking in carbonic anhydrase II (9). This observation, taken with the capacity of carbonic anhydrase inhibitors to block bone resorption, suggests that the skeletal lesion in these patients reflects their inability to normally produce intracellular protons.

Generation of intraosteoclastic protons is followed by their transport into the isolated resorptive microenvironment at the cell-bone interface. Acidification of this extracellular third compartment to a pH approximating 4.0–4.5 is under the aegis of a vacuolar proton pump (H^+-ATPase) similar to that expressed by the intercalated cell of the renal tubule (8). It appears, in fact, that the osteoclast is the major mammalian proton-transporting cell. Given the above, one would expect defective expression of the osteoclast proton pump to manifest itself clinically as retarded bone resorption. Indeed, marrow-generated osteoclast-like cells derived from a patient with a sclerosing skeletal disorder known as craniometaphyseal dysplasia fails to degrade bone and to express the resorptive proton pump (10).

An elegant experiment yielding unexpected results recently provided major insights into osteoclast biology and the pathogenesis of osteopetrosis. In this circumstance the cellular protooncogene, c-src, was disrupted in mice that are surprisingly osteopetrotic (11). The src(−) mice generate numerous osteoclasts, but the cells cannot form a ruffled membrane which is their resorptive organelle. The defect in osteoclast function in src(−) mice appears to be a manifestation of failure to express the src gene product by osteoclasts per se, and is not related to an accessory cell defect.

The precise role the src gene product plays in osteoclastic bone resorption is not yet in hand, but the tyrosine kinase may participate in intracellular signaling via extracellular stimuli. It is known that the integrin receptor $\alpha_v\beta_3$ modulates osteoclastic bone resorption *in vitro* (12) and that an $\alpha_v\beta_3$ ligand translocates a c-src substrate from an intracellular location to the plasma membrane. Most importantly, the c-src gene product is physically associated with $\alpha_v\beta_3$, further indicating that the protooncogene functions in osteoclasts by transmitting critical signals from bone matrix to the resorptive cell.

Thus, defective expression of c-src or M-CSF results in the osteopetrotic phenotype. Given, however, that c-src is fundamental to differentiated osteoclast function and M-CSF is a cytokine critical to osteoclast precursor maturation, one would expect distinct histological manifestations of the two genetic defects. In fact, the src(−) mutant contains abundant, yet ineffective osteoclasts (11), whereas the M-CSF–deficient mouse fails to generate the cells in normal numbers (13). Because the defect in src(−) mice lies not in their ability to generate osteoclasts but in the capacity of the cells to resorb bone, the animals are rescued by transplantation of normal osteoclast precursors. In contrast, M-CSF–deficient animals are incapable of inducing osteoclast precursor differentiation and thus, in this case, transplantation is ineffective. Rescue of these animals, as would be expected, requires M-CSF administration (14) (Fig. 1).

OSTEOGENESIS IMPERFECTA

Osteogenesis imperfecta (brittle bone disease) is a genetic disorder of the skeleton resulting in bone fragility. Although the disease is often fatal *in utero,* those who survive fall into a spectrum of skeletal dysfunction ranging from little or no deformity to relentless crippling associated with hundreds of fractures. The clinical manifestations of the disease mirror the degree of osteopenia. In general, cortical bone is more diminished than is trabecular, consistent with the unique structural instability experienced by these patients.

For reasons unknown, remodeling is typically brisk in osteogenesis imperfecta (15), and virtually the entire endosteal surface is covered by an osteoid seam lined, in turn, by cuboidal, "active-appearing" osteoblasts. In keeping with a rapid rate of matrix synthesis, peritrabecular marrow fibrosis and woven bone formation—hallmarks of accelerated remodeling—are often prominent. Finally, the histological impression of brisk remodeling is confirmed by kinetic histomorphometry using double tetracycline labeling (15). It is important to realize that the accelerated rate of bone formation characterizing this disease is not the result of increased matrix synthesis by each osteoblast, but a reflection of recruiting large numbers of osteoblasts into the osteogenic process.

The phenotypes of osteogenesis imperfecta are generally categorized into four groups, depending upon severity

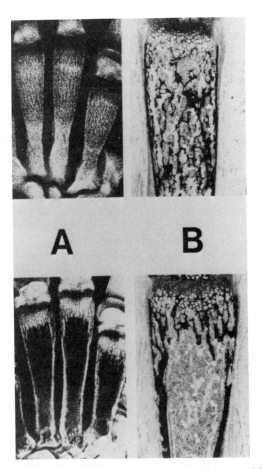

FIG. 1. Influence of 14 days treatment with recombinant human M-CSF on metacarpal bones of *op/op* mouse. *Upper panels* are untreated and *lower panels* are treated. **A:** Note increased density of bone in untreated animals and its resolution with M-CSF. **B:** Histologically, the increased density is due to abundant skeletal tissue throughout the medullary space that markedly diminishes with treatment. (From Felix R, Cecchini MG, Fleish H: Macrophage colony stimulating factor restores *in vivo* bone resorption in the *op/op* osteopetrotic mouse. *Endocrinology* 127:2592–2594, 1990.)

and associated hallmarks such as dentinogenesis imperfecta, blue sclerae, and deafness (16). Although these guidelines are helpful, one must keep in mind that the clinical manifestations of osteogenesis imperfecta are, in reality, a continuum.

Studies of cultured skin fibroblasts have established osteogenesis imperfecta as a family of inherited diseases, with virtually all patients having mutations of one of two genes encoding type I procollagen (17,18). Type I collagen consists of two $\alpha_1(1)$ and one $\alpha_2(1)$ chains arranged in a triple helix that is the functional form of the molecule. Formation of the triple helix depends on the presence of a glycine residue in every third position, and the structure is stabilized by other components such as hydroxyproline.

The molecular defects in osteogenesis imperfecta, although almost always involving type I collagen, are varied. More than 70 such mutations are known. There are, however, two general categories of defects, those that retard collagen production and those leading to structural defects in the collagen molecule. The former, namely synthetic abnormalities, are generally associated with the milder forms of the disease. These patients typically produce about one-half the normal amount of type I collagen. It is this deficiency in collagen mass that leads to increased scleral transparency and the high frequency of blue sclerae in patients with mild osteogenesis imperfecta. Other mechanisms have been described, but the paucity of collagen most often reflects the steady-state levels of mRNA transcripts of the $\alpha_1(1)$ gene. Although a precise association has not been established, the decrease in the volume of lamellar bone surrounding each osteocyte often found in patients with osteogenesis imperfecta is probably a pathological manifestation of reduced bone collagen synthesis by individual osteoblasts (19).

The more severe forms of osteogenesis imperfecta are generally due to mutations leading to instability of the collagen helix. These mutations most often involve substitution of bulkier amino acids for specific glycines leading to structurally abnormal chains that either are incapable of forming a triple helical structure or fail to package into normal fibrils. In the case of defective triple helix formation, the unfolded procollagen chains are degraded intra-cellularly by a process termed procollagen suicide (17). Mutations that permit development of the triple helix, albeit abnormally structured, are often characterized by dendritic or thin fibrils. This molecular event is pathologically mirrored by the thin bone collagen fibers that may be found in patients with osteogenesis imperfecta (20) (Fig. 2).

HYPOPHOSPHATASIA

The alkaline phosphatases are a family of enzymes expressed on the plasma membrane (ectoenzymes) of cells, including osteoblasts, whose role in promoting skeletal mineralization was established by the rare genetic disease, hypophosphatasia. The disorder—whether appearing in the perinatal, infantile, childhood, or adult phase—is always attended by osteomalacia and, in affected children, endochondral calcification is invariably abnormal (rickets) (21). The clinical consequences of hypophosphatasia are generally severe and often fatal, but relatives of those with the adult form may be comparatively asymptomatic despite histological evidence of defective bone mineralization (22,23).

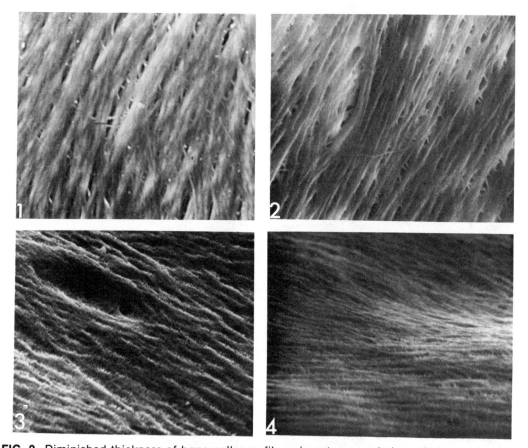

FIG. 2. Diminished thickness of bone collagen fibers in osteogenesis imperfecta as viewed by scanning electron microscopy (2200 ×). *Panel 1* is from a normal patient, and *panels 2–4* are derived from three patients with osteogenesis imperfecta. The mean thickness of collagen in each affected patient is <50% normal. (From Teitelbaum SL, Kraft WJ, Lang R, Avioli LV: Bone collagen aggregation abnormalities in osteogenesis imperfecta. *Calcif Tissue Res* 17:75–79, 1974.)

The primary defect in all forms of hypophosphatasia is failure to adequately express tissue nonspecific alkaline phosphatase (TNSALP), the isoform found in bone and cartilage. In fact, the hypophosphatasia and TNSALP genes are closely linked on chromosome 1p36. The molecular pathogenesis of the disease in ~50% of patients exhibiting the entire clinical spectrum of hypophosphatasia involves a variety of point mutations in the TNSALP gene locus (24). Moreover, in at least some patients, the disease is not a reflection of global osteoblast dysfunction, as other cellular proteins are normally produced.

Although the precise role alkaline phosphatase plays in bone mineralization is not yet in hand, the fact that hypophosphatasia is always attended by osteomalacia establishes that the enzyme is critical to the calcification process. Specifically, bone alkaline phosphatase, whether measured histologically or biochemically, is almost invariably reduced in patients with the disease.

The details by which hypophosphatasia retards skeletal mineralization are still unknown, but the most reasonable scenario involves inorganic pyrophosphate (PPi) metabolism. Because the enzyme catalyzes the conversion of PPi to inorganic phosphate and AMP, when TNSALP is deficient, PPi accumulates in extracellular tissues. Here, PPi is believed to inhibit formation of hydroxylapatite, the major component of the inorganic phase of bone. On the other hand, extraskeletal calcification often suggests that the mineralizing activities of alkaline phosphatase may be limited to the skeleton.

VITAMIN D DEPENDENCY RICKETS II

Vitamin D dependency rickets (VDDR II) is an autosomal recessive disorder of the vitamin D receptor manifest clinically as resistance to exogenous $1,25(OH)_2D_3$. In fact, probably reflecting attendant secondary hyperparathyroidism, the circulating $1,25(OH)_2D_3$ levels in affected patients are generally extremely high (25).

Because of insights gained into its molecular pathogenesis, this disorder, although rare, has served as an experiment in nature elucidating the biology of vitamin D receptor. Simply put, $1,25(OH)_2D_3$ effects gene transcription by binding to its intracellular receptor. The unoccupied receptor is believed to reside in the cytoplasm or nucleus. Upon occupancy of the cytoplasmic receptor by $1,25(OH)_2D_3$, it translocates to the nucleus. The ligand-receptor complex in association with other proteins interacts with vitamin D response elements in the promotor regions of target genes. The occupied receptor in this context serves as a transcription factor, ultimately enhancing or suppressing gene expression.

Although VDDR II always reflects abnormalities of vitamin D receptor structure or function, a variety of mech-

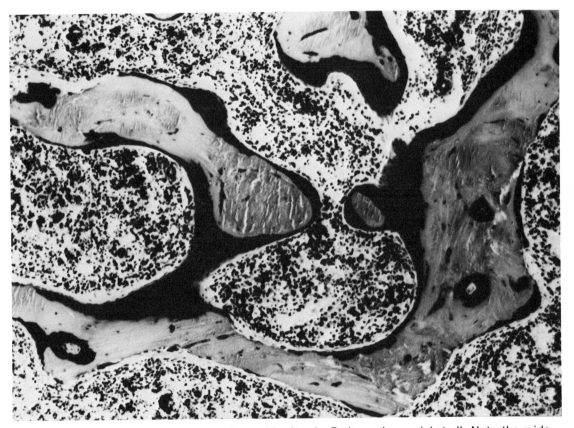

FIG. 3. Bone biopsy taken from patient with vitamin D dependency rickets II. Note the wide osteoid seams (dark staining material) indicative of severe osteomalacia (undecalcified, Goldner stain). (Courtesy of Dr. Francis H. Glorieux and Rose Travers, Montreal Shriners Hospital.)

anistic defects have been identified. For example, patients may 1) fail to adequately express the vitamin D receptor (26); 2) the receptor may be adequately expressed, but $1,25(OH)_2D_3$ binding may be deficient (27); or 3) the receptor within the cytoplasm may normally bind $1,25(OH)_2D_3$, but the ligand-receptor complex may not translocate to the nucleus (26). Failure to extract occupied receptors from the nucleus probably reflects their diminished affinity for vitamin D response elements in the promotor regions of target genes and the consequent inability of such receptors to promote transcription. In the latter circumstance, mutations exist in the "zinc-finger" region of the receptor, the structure by which it binds to DNA (28).

Because $1,25(OH)_2D_3$ is fundamental to osteoblast and osteoclast differentiation and hence skeletal mineralization and resorption, both components of bone remodeling are often disturbed in states of vitamin D resistance. Although histological material is available from only a few patients with the disorder, in those circumstances in which skeletal tissue has been examined, one encounters severe osteomalacia (Fig. 3) and rickets. Due to attendant secondary hyperparathyroidism reflecting resistance to the calcemic effects of $1,25(OH)_2D_3$ on intestine and bone, the skeletal manifestations of parathyroid hormone excess, namely osteitis fibrosa, may be particularly prominent (29,30). The presence of abundant osteoclasts in this lesion underscores the redundancy of factors promoting osteoclast differentiation and the reality that abundant parathyroid hormone may compensate in this regard for inability to respond to, or deficient, $1,25(OH)_2D_3$.

The phenotype of VDDR II establishes the central role vitamin D plays in skeletal mineralization and cell differentiation. Vitamin D receptors are virtually ubiquitous and known to promote maturation not only of bone cells, but also those derived from numerous other tissues as well. In fact, the blunting of intestinal absorption of calcium attending vitamin D deficiency or resistance probably represents retarded maturation of intestinal mucosa. As pertains to a particularly striking feature of VDDR II, namely total alopecia, hair sheath cells from normal patients respond to $1,25(OH)_2D_3$, whereas the same cells from those affected with the disease fail to do so (31). Similarly, $1,25(OH)_2D_3$ targets directly to osteoblasts and plays a central role in gene regulation as the cells differentiate. In so doing, the steroid promotes the capacity of osteoblasts to mineralize matrix (32). Thus, while circulating levels of calcium and phosphorous are often suppressed in VDDR II, the pathogenesis of the underlying osteomalacia probably reflects failure of $1,25(OH)_2D_3$ to differentiate osteoblasts into the bone mineralizing phenotype.

REFERENCES

1. Coccia PF, Krivit W, Cervenka J, Clawson CC, Kersey JH, Kim TH, Nesbit ME, Ramsay NKC, Warkentin PI, Teitelbaum SL, Kahn AJ, Brown DM: Successful bone marrow transplantation for infantile malignant osteopetrosis. *N Engl J Med* 302: 701–708, 1980
2. Shapiro F, Glimcher MJ, Holtrop ME, Tashjian AH, Brickley-

Parsons D, Kenzora JE: Human osteopetrosis. A histological, ultrastructural, and biochemical study. *J Bone Joint Surg* 62A: 384–399, 1980
3. Walker DG: Experimental osteopetrosis. *Clin Orthop Rel Res* 97:158–174, 1973
4. Alvarez JI, Teitelbaum SL, Blair HC, Greenfield EM, Athanasou NA, Ross FP: Generation of avian cells resembling osteoclasts from mononuclear phagocytes. *Endocrinology* 128: 2324–2335, 1991
5. Blair HC, Schlesinger PH, Ross FP, Teitelbaum SL: Recent advances toward understanding osteoclast physiology. *Clin Orthop Rel Res* 1993 (in press)
6. Wiktor-Jedrzejczak W, Ahmed A, Szczylik C, Skelly PR: Hematological characterization of congenital osteopetrosis in op/op mouse. Possible mechanism for abnormal macrophage differentiation. *J Exp Med* 156:1516–1527, 1982
7. Yoshida H, Hayashi SI, Kunisada T, Ogawa M, Nishikawa S, Okamura H, Sudo T, Schultz LD, Nishikawa SI: The murine mutation osteopetrosis is in the coding region of the macrophage colony stimulating factor gene. *Nature* 345:442–444, 1990
8. Blair HC, Teitelbaum SL, Ghiselli R, Gluck S: Osteoclastic bone resorption by a polarized vacuolar proton pump. *Science* 245: 855–857, 1989
9. Sly WS, Hewett-Emmett D, Whyte MP, Yu Y-S L, Tashian RE: Carbonic anhydrase II deficiency identified as the primary defect in the autosomal recessive syndrome of osteopetrosis with renal tubular acidosis and cerebral calcification. *Proc Natl Acad Sci USA* 80:2752–2756, 1983
10. Yamamoto T, Kurihara N, Yamaoka K, Ozono K, Okada M, Yamamoto K, Matsumoto S, Michigami T, Ono J, Okada S: Bone marrow-derived osteoclast-like cells from a patient with craniometaphyseal dysplasia lack expression of osteoclast-reactive vacuolar proton pump. *J Clin Invest* 91:362–367, 1993
11. Soriano P, Montgomery C, Geske R, Bradley A: Targeted disruption of the c-src proto-oncogene leads to osteopetrosis in mice. *Cell* 64:693–702, 1991
12. Ross FP, Alvarez JI, Chappel J, Sander D, Butler WT, Farach-Carson MC, Mintz KA, Robey PG, Teitelbaum SL, Cheresh DA: Interactions between the bone matrix proteins osteopontin and bone sialoprotein and the osteoclast integrin $\alpha_v\beta_3$ potentiate bone resorption. *J Biol Chem* 1993 (in press).
13. Marks SC, Seifert MF, McGuire JL: Congenitally osteopetrotic (op/op) mice are not cured by transplants of spleen or bone marrow cells from normal littermates. *Metab Bone Dis Rel Res* 5: 183–186, 1984
14. Felix R, Cecchini MG, Fleisch H: Macrophage colony stimulating factor restores *in vivo* bone resorption in the *op/op* osteopetrotic mouse. *Endocrinology* 127:2592–2594, 1990
15. Jett S, Ramser JR, Frost HM, Villanueva AR: Bone turnover and osteogenesis imperfecta. *Arch Pathol* 81:112–116, 1966
16. Sillence DO, Senn A, Danks DM: Genetic heterogeneity in osteogenesis imperfecta. *J Med Genet* 16:101–116, 1979
17. Kuivaniemi H, Tromp G, Prockop DJ: Mutations in collagen genes: Causes of rare and some common diseases in humans. *FASEB J* 5:2052–2060, 1991
18. Byers PH, Steiner RD: Osteogenesis imperfecta. *Annu Rev Med* 43:269–282, 1992
19. Falvo KA, Bullough PG: Osteogenesis imperfecta: A histometric analysis. *J Bone Joint Surg* 55A:275–286, 1973
20. Teitelbaum SL, Kraft WJ, Lang R, Avioli LV: Bone collagen aggregation abnormalities in osteogenesis imperfecta. *Calcif Tissue Res* 17:75–79, 1974
21. Caswell AM, Whyte MP, Russell RGG: Hypophosphatasia and the extracellular metabolism of inorganic pyrophosphate: Clinical and laboratory aspects. *Crit Rev Clin Lab Sci* 28:175–232, 1991
22. Weinstein RS, Whyte MP: Heterogeneity of adult hypophosphatasia. Report of severe and mild cases. *Arch Intern Med* 141: 727–731, 1981
23. Fallon MD, Teitelbaum SL, Weinstein RS, Goldfischer S, Brown DM, Whyte MP: Hypophosphatasia: Clinicopathologic comparison of the infantile, childhood, and adult forms. *Medicine* 63:12–24, 1984
24. Henthorn PS, Raducha M, Fedde KN, Lafferty MA, Whyte MP:

Different missense mutations at the tissue-nonspecific alkaline phosphatase gene locus in autosomal recessively inherited forms of mild and severe hypophosphatasia. *Proc Natl Acad Sci USA* 89:9924–9928, 1992

25. Bell NH: Vitamin D-dependent rickets type II. *Calcif Tissue Int* 31:89–91, 1980
26. Liberman UA, Eil C, Marx SJ: Resistance to 1,25-dihydroxyvitamin D. Association with heterogeneous defects in cultured skin fibroblasts. *J Clin Invest* 71:192–200, 1983
27. Pike JW, Dokoh S, Haussler MR, Liberman UA, Marx SJ, Eil C: Vitamin D₃-resistant fibroblasts have immunoassayable 1,25-dihydroxyvitamin D₃ receptors. *Science* 224:879–881, 1984
28. Hughes MR, Malloy PJ, Kieback DG, Kesterson RA, Pike JW, Feldman D, O'Malley BW: Point mutations in the human vitamin D receptor gene associated with hypocalcemic rickets. *Science* 242:1702–1705, 1988
29. Brooks MH, Bell NH, Love L, Stern PH, Orfei E, Queener SF,

Hamstra AJ, DeLuca HF: Vitamin-D-dependent rickets type II. Resistance of target organs to 1,25-dihydroxyvitamin D. *N Engl J Med* 298:996–999, 1978
30. Zerwekh JE, Glass K, Jowsey J, Pak CYC: An unique form of osteomalacia associated with end organ refractoriness to 1,25-dihydroxyvitamin D and apparent defective synthesis of 25-hydroxyvitamin D. *J Clin Endocrinol Metab* 49:171, 1979
31. Arase S, Sadamoto Y, Kuwana R, Nakanishi H, Fujie K, Takeda K, Takeda E: The effect of 1,25-dihydroxyvitamin D₃ on the growth and differentiation of cultured human outer root sheath cells from normal subjects and patients with vitamin D-dependent rickets type II with alopecia. *J Dermatol Sci* 2:353–360, 1991
32. Lian J, Stewart C, Puchasz E, Mackowiak S, Shalhoub V, Collart D, Zambetti G, Stein G: Structure of the rat osteocalcin gene and regulation of vitamin D-dependent expression. *Proc Natl Acad Sci USA* 86:1143–1147, 1989

3. The Osteoblast

J. Edward Puzas, Ph.D.

Department of Orthopaedics, University of Rochester School of Medicine, Rochester, New York

Bone forming cells, by definition, are the cells responsible for the production of true bone. For the purposes of this discussion we will define bone as that tissue formed by the deposition of mineral ions within a collagenous framework. The mineral must be in the form of hydroxyapatite and the collagen must be type I collagen. Although this definition seems self-evident, it does exclude a number of mineralized tissues, which through the years, have been grouped with true bone. Some examples of such mineralizing nonbone tissues are dentin and enamel in teeth, calcifying cartilage in the developing growth plate of long bones, virtually any organ in pathological calcification states, arterial and aortic walls. There are, however, some forms of ectopic or heterotopic bone that do fit the criteria of true bone. These forms of bone frequently occur after orthopaedic surgery or in rare metabolic disease states. A discussion of this type of pathological bone or related calcification syndromes is found in Section IX. The reader is also referred to review articles on the topic (1,2).

The term "bone forming cell" can be equated with the term "osteoblast." That is, wherever there is authentic bone being formed, there must be present a population of osteoblasts. The remainder of this chapter is organized into three categories: (1) the histological and metabolic characteristics of osteoblasts, 2) the process by which osteoblasts form bone, and 3) the factors and hormones that control osteoblast function.

HISTOLOGICAL AND METABOLIC CHARACTERISTICS OF OSTEOBLASTS

The histological characteristics of an osteoblast reflect the fact that it is a very metabolically active cell. The orientation of organelles is polarized and is shown in Fig. 1. Most frequently, there is an extensive network of rough endoplasmic reticulum clustered in the cytosol nearest the bone surface. This material stains deeply with basophilic stains and is most pronounced in cells that are actively forming bone. As it is in any cell, the granular-appearing membrane organelles that form the rough endoplasmic reticulum are due to the presence of a large number of ribosomes associated with mRNA. The numbers of these structures are closely associated with the protein synthetic and secretory activity of cells. As will be discussed, the osteoblast is actively producing collagen for the extracellular matrix and would normally be expected to have an extensive rough endoplasmic reticulum.

The nucleus is usually found in the cytosol at the opposite end of the cell. The nuclear material is similar to other eukaryotic cells and remains in a diffuse uncondensed state during interphase. There are usually present one to three nucleoli. A mature functioning osteoblast does not divide. That is, the mitotic forms of prophase, metaphase, anaphase, and telophase do not appear in osteoblasts. If ever such structures are observed, by convention, the cell must be considered a progenitor form of an osteoblast or an osteoblast that has reverted back to a more progenitor or primitive state.

Positioned between the nucleus and rough endoplasmic reticulum is an intricate Golgi apparatus. This structure is present because of the large of amount of type I collagen that is secreted from these cells. Normally the Golgi apparatus does not stain intensely and as such appears as a clear zone in the middle of the cell.

Another characteristic that can be demonstrated histochemically is the presence of a substantial amount of the enzyme, alkaline phosphatase. Bone-specific alkaline phosphatase has been localized to the plasma membrane of osteoblasts, and although it is known to be present in

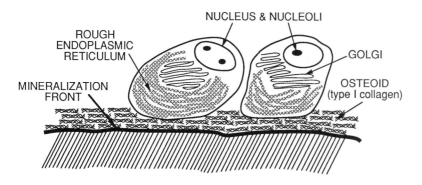

FIG. 1. Osteoblast orientation. Diagrammatic display of the orientation of the major cell organelles of an active osteoblast. These cells usually reside on actively forming bone surfaces. There is a copious amount of rough endoplasmic reticulum near the bone surface. This rough endoplasmic reticulum is separated from the eccentric nucleus by a large and active Golgi complex. The mineralization front is the edge of advancing calcification. The maturing collagen between the cell and the mineralization front is known as an osteoid seam.

large amounts, its true function has not yet been identified. Speculations as to its role in mineralization have been published since 1923 (3), and it is clear that alkaline phosphatase activity correlates with bone formation, but whether it is a causative agent for the calcification process has not been convincingly shown. Other theories regarding a role for alkaline phosphatase have centered around regulation of cell proliferation, and phosphate transport (4).

OSTEOBLAST LINEAGE

Three forms of the osteoblast cell lineage are recognized. They are progenitor osteoblasts (preosteoblasts), mature osteoblasts, and osteocytes. From a phylogenetic point of view, it is known that osteoblasts arise from cells in the condensing mesenchyme and as such are one form of connective tissue. Because mesenchymal cells can give rise to a number of tissue types, it is not until a cell is committed to the osteoblast lineage that it can be histologically differentiated as a bone forming cell. All three cell phenotypes are illustrated in Fig. 2.

Preosteoblast

A committed progenitor cell destined to become an osteoblast has a number of distinguishing features. First, these cells are physically near bone forming surfaces. That is, they are usually present where active mature osteoblasts are synthesizing bone. Their appearance is that of an elongated cell with an elongated nucleus. Most often they are found in a stratum type of configuration a few cell layers distant from the active osteoblasts (Fig. 2). Second, they have the capacity to divide. Frequently mitotic characters can be found in these cells. Third, these cells usually stain less intensely for alkaline phosphatase, and there is no evidence of a developed rough endoplasmic reticulum. That is, they have not yet acquired many of the differentiated characteristics of mature osteoblasts.

Osteoblast

A mature osteoblast is derived from a preosteoblast and expresses all of the differentiated functions required to synthesize bone. The change from preosteoblast to osteoblast is not a quantal process. There is a gradient of differentiation that becomes fully expressed when the mature form of the cell reaches the bone surface. Once the osteoblast has reached the surface its function is to synthesize and secrete collagen and ultimately to mineralize it. Usually, active osteoblasts are found within a matrix that they themselves have synthesized. It is within this matrix at the mineralization front that the process of hydroxyapatite crystal growth occurs. The mineralization front is the advancing edge of calcification and is usually 5–50 μm away from the osteoblast surface. The area between the osteoblast and the mineralizing front is often referred to as an "osteoid seam." The depth and character of the osteoid seam can be diagnostic for some forms of bone disease (such as osteomalacia and rickets) (Figs. 1 and 2).

Osteocyte

An osteocyte is an osteoblast that has become encased in calcified bone. During the process of bone formation,

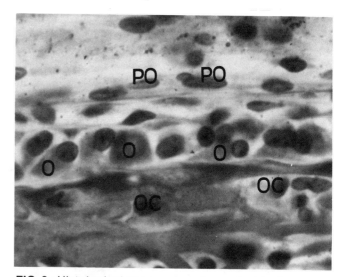

FIG. 2. Histological appearance of preosteoblasts, osteoblasts, and osteocytes. Elongated cells with elongated nuclei that are adjacent to osteoblasts are preosteoblasts (osteoprogenitor cells). They are indicated by the letters "PO." Plump, basophilic cells lining the bone surface are osteoblasts. They are indicated by the letter "O." Cells that have become embedded in osteoid are known as osteocytes. They are indicated by the letters "OC."

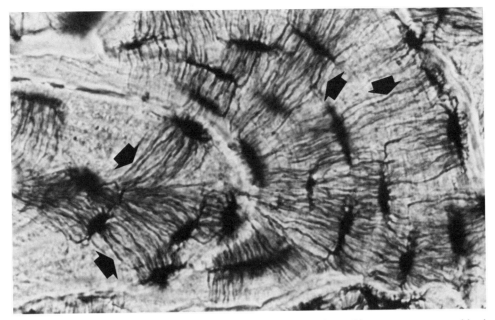

FIG. 3. Photomicrograph of mature bone. This unstained section of bone was prepared by hand grinding a fragment of adult bone until it became translucent. The osteocytes form concentric layers around a central nutrient vessel. The canaliculi of the osteocytes (indicated by *arrows*) form a fine network of tubules through which diffusion of solutes and gases can occur. The canaliculi may also form a communication network between the cells.

the osteoblast determines its own fate by calcifying itself into a lacunae (Fig. 2). Approximately 10–20% of osteoblasts eventually become osteocytes and, although it can be said that not all osteoblasts survive as osteocytes, it is true that all osteocytes had their origin from osteoblasts. At the point of total encasement the metabolic activity of the cell dramatically decreases due to the lack of nutrient diffusion. The only source of nutrients and gas exchange to which the osteocyte has access is that which can occur through small canals known as canaliculi. These canaliculi are actually the remnants of cellular processes that extended from the osteoblast during bone mineralization. The canaliculi form an extensive array of connecting tubules, and it has been speculated that these tubules form a communication as well as nutrient network. Figure 3 is a photomicrograph of mature bone in which a number of osteocytes are visible. The numerous fine tubular connections between the osteocytes are known as canaliculi.

PROGRESSION OF CELLS THROUGH THE OSTEOBLAST LINEAGE

Many of the most enlightening studies demonstrating the origin and fate of preosteoblasts, osteoblasts, and osteocytes were performed a number of years ago (5,6). These works utilized timed radiolabeled thymidine exposure to monitor the progression of a cell through the osteoblast lineage. In principle, the method called for injection of a single dose of high specific activity tritium-labeled thymidine into a series of experimental animals. Because thymidine is incorporated only into newly forming DNA, the bone cells that were labeled immediately after the in-

jection were preosteoblasts in the process of cell division. There was no label in osteoblasts or osteocytes. A few days after the injection the cells that contained the radioactive label were the osteoblasts and after a few weeks the cells with the label were the osteocytes. Because it is known that osteoblasts and osteocytes do not divide it was evident that the label that appeared in these cells originated in the preosteoblasts. Thus, the initial cells to be labeled had progressed through the maturation process and their progression was monitored by visualizing the labeled DNA. In fact, the lifetime and differentiation time for osteoblasts could be calculated with these and other techniques, and it was shown that mature osteoblast appearance required not more than a few days and that they were active for up to 12 weeks before progressing into osteocytes (7,8).

PROCESSES BY WHICH OSTEOBLASTS FORM BONE

There are a number of sequential steps in the formation of bone. They are 1) synthesis and intracellular processing of type I collagen; 2) secretion and extracellular processing of the collagen; 3) the formation of microfibrils, fibrils, and ultimately fibers from the collagen; and 4) maturation of the collagen matrix with subsequent nucleation and growth of hydroxyapatite crystals. All of these functions are under the control of the osteoblast, with the eventual product being a fully calcified bone consisting by weight of 35% organic matrix and 65% inorganic crystalline material.

Type I Collagen Synthesis

Type I collagen is the most abundant form of collagen and is found in highest concentrations in skin, bone, and tendons. It is by far the major collagenous component of bone and is believed to be the only form necessary for true intramembranous bone formation. There are at present 13 types of collagen that have been identified (9). Clearly, it is beyond the scope of this work to discuss the nature and role of all of these molecules and therefore the reader is referred to other publications (10).

Type I collagen formed by osteoblasts is synthesized like all other proteins in a cell. Messenger RNA translation is accomplished with ribosomal activity and all of the cofactors, tRNAs, and energy requirements normally associated with protein synthesis. Of the three protein chains that comprise a type I collagen molecule, two are identical and they are termed "α_1" chains. The second chain type has a different amino acid composition and is termed an "α_2" chain. The short-hand configuration for type I collagen is, therefore, $[\alpha_1]_2 [\alpha_2]_1$. The chemistry of collagen synthesis, chain registration, helix formation, and fibril formation are discussed in Chapter 4.

One of the major and yet poorly understood areas of collagen metabolism in bone formation is the so-called "maturation of the osteoid matrix." This maturation of the collagen fibers must occur before the matrix is competent to support mineralization. The best way to illustrate this point is to describe the process of bone formation at a remodeling site. From the point of view of collagen synthesis and its mineralization, there are three distinct stages during formation. In the first stage, collagen is deposited at a rapid rate and an ever-thickening osteoid seam is produced. In the second stage, the rate of mineralization increases to match the rate of collagen synthesis, and the osteoid seam width remains constant. In the third stage, the rate of collagen synthesis decreases and mineralization continues until the osteoid seam disappears. These three processes are diagramatically demonstrated in Fig. 4. The maturation of the collagen matrix is ex-

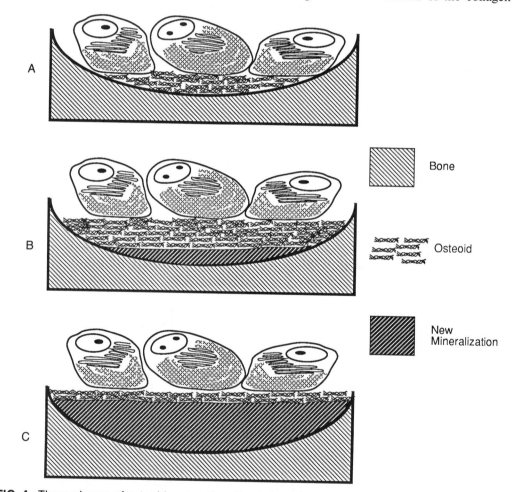

Bone

Osteoid

New Mineralization

FIG. 4. Three phases of osteoid maturation. Depiction of the phenomenon of osteoid maturation during the mineralization process. **A:** Active osteoblasts synthesizing a collagen matrix. Matrix synthesis proceeds without corresponding mineralization and consequently the osteoid seam thickness increases. **B:** The onset of mineralization. The mineralization rate matches the osteoid synthetic rate thereby maintaining a constant seam thickness. **C:** A decreasing rate of osteoid synthesis with a constant rate of mineralization. The seam will then eventually disappear. This sequential process is due to an obligator maturation that must occur in the newly synthesized osteoid. The mechanism of the maturation is not known.

pressed as the ratio of the mineralization rate (μm/day) to the osteoid seam width (μm). Thus, the maturation of the collagen has a unit of time (days). This ratio has become known as the "mineralization lag time." Mineralization lag time describes the length of time it takes for the osteoid matrix to acquire the characteristics necessary to support mineralization. The mineralization lag time is on the order of 5–10 days in adults and its magnitude can sometimes be diagnostic for metabolic bone disease. Biochemically the mineralization lag time remains undefined. Some theories support a role for cross-linking of collagen in the osteoid, others support the removal of a mineralization inhibitor (see below). Whatever the actual mechanism of osteoid maturation, it is apparent that newly deposited collagen cannot provide a substrate for normal mineralization until it has "matured."

Mineralization

Mineralization of the collagen substructure is another unique function of the osteoblast. Although not all of the details of this process are known many important pieces of data have been established. For example, the mineral in mature fully calcified bone is mostly in the form of carbonated hydroxyapatite crystals. These crystals are needle-shaped and rod-like and have a diameter of 30–50 Å and a length of up to 600 Ås. It has been suggested that they lie linearly along the collagen fibrils and in some instances may penetrate some of the larger fibers. The actual process of mineral precipitation, however, remains obscure. In fact there are a number of paradoxical observations that have been made in trying to examine the process of calcification experimentally. For example, it appears that once the hydroxyapatite has been formed further growth of the crystal can occur in the absence of cell activity. In other words, under physiological conditions, the extracellular fluid is supersaturated with regard to calcium and phosphate when in the presence of hydroxyapatite. If crystal growth were not somehow mediated, the entire blood and extracellular fluid would be depleted of calcium and phosphate at the expense of hydroxyapatite formation. This finding was one of the major pieces of evidence for proposing an ionic barrier between bone and blood and is the reason why devitalized bone will support mineralization if implanted in tissue fluids or bathed in physiological solutions of calcium and phosphate. Therefore, the continuing processes of mineralization appear to be controlled at both the initiation stages as well as the deposition stages of hydroxyapatite formation.

Measurements of Bone Formation

Although we may not understand all of the physical and chemical processes of osteoid maturation and mineralization, it has been possible to define and measure many parameters of bone formation. An entire histological discipline has grown up around the methods needed to make these accurate measurements of skeletal activity. The sampling sites, embedding and sectioning techniques,

TABLE 1. *Parameters of bone formation under the control of osteoblasts*

Bone mass (% microscopic area that is cancellous bone)	22.8
Osteoid volume (volume of uncalcified osteoid as compared with bone mm³/cm³)	4.4
Osteroid surface (% bone surface covered by osteoid)	7.5
Osteoid seam width (μm)	11.5
Mineral apposition rate (μm/day)	0.5
Trabecular diameter (mean diameter of trabeculae in cancellous bone, μm)	283.0
Bone-osteoblast interface (% of bone surface in direct contact with osteoblasts)	3.8

staining and quantification, and a number of other variables must be considered when measuring formation (and resorption) rates. Table 1 is brief list of some of the normal values that have been obtained from human bone. Typically, over 50 different measurements (or calculations from measurements) can be made from a bone section, and with these measurements an accurate picture of the metabolic activity of osteoblasts can be obtained. A detailed discussion of bone histomorphometry with excellent histological and morphometrical examples has recently been published (11) and the reader is referred to this work and Chapter 25.

FACTORS AND HORMONES THAT CONTROL OSTEOBLAST FUNCTION

This area is one of the most active and important topics being investigated in bone research today. It is in this arena where molecular biological, immunological, and biochemical techniques have merged to attempt to understand not only the disease processes, but also the normal processes of bone metabolism. It is probably from these lines of research that new therapies will emerge for diseases such as osteoporosis.

For many years it was believed that the two most important bone target hormones were parathyroid hormone (PTH) and 1,25-dihydroxyvitamin D$_3$. Both of these hormones were known to be responsible for increasing the level of calcium in the blood, PTH by virtue of its stimulatory action on bone resorption and 1,25-dihydroxyvitamin D$_3$ by virtue of its stimulatory action on intestinal calcium transport. The direct effects of these hormones on osteoblasts were, at best at this stage of our knowledge, controversial. It was assumed that if calcium were needed to maintain blood levels then the effects of PTH and 1,25-dihydroxyvitamin D$_3$ on osteoblasts would be, if anything, to hinder new bone formation. For these reasons, only sporadic reports of the direct effects of these hormones on osteoblasts appeared. However, in general, the tone of these reports supported an anabolic role for both hormones, a conclusion that was inconsistent with their role in mineral homeostasis.

In osteoblasts, PTH was shown to mediate ion and amino acid transport, stimulate cAMP, regulate collagen synthesis, and bind to a specific receptor (12–16). 1,25-Dihydroxyvitamin D_3 was also shown to stimulate matrix and alkaline phosphatase synthesis, production of bone-specific proteins, and bind to a receptor (17–20). The question was raised as to why hormones responsible for elevating serum calcium levels would have such marked and diverse effects on bone forming cells. Many theories were put forward to explain some of these phenomena but it was not until new cell isolation techniques were developed and the interest in bone growth factors was stimulated that a clearer picture became evident. It now appears that the osteoblast may be the central cell through which bone resorption as well as bone formation is mediated. Many of the initial effects observed on osteoblasts (such as calcium flux changes, cAMP elevation, and phospholipase C activation) may have been reflections of a signaling system that controls all of the cells in bone.

These theories gained widespread support when it was shown that a number of bone resorbing agents (such as PTH and lymphokines) had no direct effect on isolated osteoclasts. It was not until isolated osteoclasts were mixed with isolated osteoblasts that the bone resorbing effects of these agents were restored. To document further the observation, it was shown that culture medium that was recovered from isolated osteoblasts exposed to bone resorbing agents was also stimulatory for isolated osteoclasts. These results supported the hypothesis that the osteoblast releases a soluble factor after exposure to agents such as PTH and then this factor stimulates osteoclastic bone resorption. In other words, hormonal regulation of bone resorption occurs by an osteoblast-mediated mechanism (21). An active search for the molecule(s) responsible for this effect is currently underway.

Regulation of the bone forming activity of osteoblasts has also been an active area of investigation. Other sections in this primer have documented these regulations in more detail, and the reader is referred to them for an in-depth analysis. Briefly, however, it now appears that at least 10–15 local factors have been isolated that participate in controlling all aspects of osteoblast function. Many of these factors have been isolated from bone matrix itself. Table 2 lists some of the molecules.

Of interest in this scheme of regulation is that the factors that influence osteoblast activity were probably deposited in bone by the osteoblasts themselves. In addition to the processes of collagen synthesis and mineralization, these cells also produce and sequester growth factors into the bone matrix. The reason for this was not entirely clear. However, as our knowledge has evolved, it has become apparent that there is a very tight coupling between bone resorption and bone formation. In the processes of remodeling in the adult skeleton almost all osteoclastic activity is followed by osteoblastic activity. Excavated resorption lacunae are refilled by waves of formation. That this sequence is locally regulated in a spatial and temporal way provides one of the key observations in determining the mechanism of resorption/formation coupling (22). The general current belief is that osteoclasts release the sequestered growth factors during the process of resorption. The factors then diffuse a short distance and stimulate mesenchymal cells to proliferate and ultimately differentiate into preosteoblasts and osteoblasts. These cells then reform the bone replacing not only the collagen and mineral but also the growth factors. This is one of the mechanisms by which the skeleton attempts to preserve its bone mass. Obviously, interference with the resorption/formation coupling can lead to inappropriate regulation of bone mass and in fact both too little (osteoporosis) and too much (osteopetrosis) bone have been documented in resorption/formation coupling diseases.

CONCLUSIONS

Over the years we have come to understand many of the mechanisms by which bone is formed. Such studies, by necessity, have focused on the osteoblast. The important features of this cell are the following:

1. Osteoblasts arise from osteoprogenitor cells of mesenchymal origin and are the source of the terminally differentiated osteocyte.
2. Osteoblasts have the ability to synthesize type I collagen and regulate its mineralization into a specific crystalline form.
3. Osteoblasts are autocrine regulatory cells. They can synthesize and deposit growth factors in bone matrix which, when released by bone resorption processes, restimulate further osteoblastic activity.
4. Osteoblasts mediate the systemic signals for the recruitment and activity of osteoclasts.

TABLE 2. *Growth factor activity produced by bone or isolated from bone matrix*

Transforming growth factor β 1, 2, and 3
Bone morphogenetic proteins 1 through 7
Insulin-like growth factors I and II
Platelet-derived growth factor
Acidic and basic fibroblast growth factor

There are currently a number of less well-defined factors undergoing investigation. These new factors may contribute unique molecules to this list or they may demonstrate some degree of homology with known molecules.

REFERENCES

1. Sawyer JR, Myers MA, Rosier RN, Puzas JE: Heterotopic ossification: clinical and cellular aspects. *Calcif Tissue Int* 49: 208–215, 1991
2. O'Conner JM: *Soft Tissue Ossification*. Springer-Verlag, New York, 1983
3. Robison R: The possible significance of hexosephosphoric esters in ossification. *Biochem J* 17:286–293, 1923
4. Puzas JE: Phosphotyrosine phosphatase activity in bone cells: An old enzyme with a new function. *Adv Prot Phosphatases* 3: 237–256, 1986
5. Tonna EA, Cronkite EP: The periosteum: Autoradiographic studies on cellular proliferation and transformation utilizing tritiated thymidine. *Clin Orth Rel Res* 30:218–232, 1963
6. Tonna EA, Cronkite EP: An autoradiographic study of periosteal cell proliferation with tritiated thymidine. *Lab Invest* 11: 455–461, 1962

7. Kimmel DB, Jee WSS: Bone cell kinetics during longitudinal bone growth in the rat. *Calc Tissue Int* 32:123–133, 1980
8. Tran VPT, Vignery A, Baron R: Cellular kinetics of the bone remodeling sequence in the rat. *Anat Rec* 202:445–451, 1982
9. Burgeson RE, Nimni ME: Collagen types. Molecular structure and tissue distribution. *Clin Orthop* 282:250–272, 1992
10. Mayne R, Burgeson RE (eds): *Structure and Function of Collagen Types.* Academic Press, New York, 1987
11. Malluche HH, Faugere M-C: *Atlas of Mineralized Bone Histology.* Karger, New York, 1986
12. Donahue HJ, Fryer MJ, Eriksen EF, Heath H: Differential effects of parathyroid hormone and its analogs on cytosolic calcium ion and cAMP levels in cultured rat osteoblast-like cells. *J Biol Chem* 263:13522–13527, 1988
13. Rosenbusch JP, Nichols G Jr: Parathyroid hormone effects on amino acid transport into bone cells. *Endocrinology* 81:553–557, 1967
14. Lomri A, Marie PJ: Effect of parathyroid hormone and forskolin on cytoskeletal protein synthesis in cultured mouse osteoblastic cells. *Biochim Biophys Acta* 970:333–342, 1988
15. Kream BE, Rowe D, Smith MD, Maher V, Majeska R: Hormonal regulation of collagen synthesis in a clonal rat osteosarcoma cell line. *Endocrinology* 119:1922–1928, 1986
16. Hesch RD, Brabant G, Rittinghaus EF, Atkinson MJ, Harms H: Pulsatile secretion of parathyroid hormone and its action on a type I and type II PTH receptor: A hypothesis for understanding osteoporosis. *Calcif Tissue Int* 42:341–344, 1988
17. Harrison JR, Clark NB: Avian medullary bone in organ culture: Effects of vitamin D metabolites on collagen synthesis. *Calcif Tissue Int* 39:35–43, 1986
18. Fritsch J, Grosse B, Lieberherr M, Balsan S: 1,25-Dihydroxyvitamin D is required for growth-independent expression of alkaline phosphatase in cultured rat osteoblasts. *Calcif Tissue Int* 37:639–645, 1985
19. Price PA, Baukol SA: 1,25-Dihydroxyvitamin D increases synthesis of the vitamin K dependent bone protein by osteosarcoma cells. *J Biol Chem* 255:11660–11663, 1980
20. McDonnell DP, Pike JW, O'Malley BW: The vitamin D receptor: A primitive steroid receptor related to thyroid hormone receptor. *J Steroid Biochem* 30:41–46, 1988
21. Chambers RJ, McSheehy PMJ, Thomson BM, Fuller K: The effect of calcium regulating hormones and prostaglandins on bone resorption by osteoclasts disaggregated from neonatal rabbit bones. *Endocrinology* 116:234–239, 1985
22. Parfitt AM: Bone remodeling: Relationship to the amount and structure of bone and the pathogenesis and prevention of fractures. In: Riggs BL, Melton LJ (eds) *Osteoporosis: Etiology, Diagnosis and Management.* Raven Press, New York, pp 45–93

4. Bone Matrix Proteins and the Mineralization Process

John D. Termine, Ph.D.

Lilly Research Laboratories, Eli Lilly and Company, Indianapolis, Indiana

Bone comprises the largest proportion of the body's connective tissue mass. As such, it consists of extracellular connective tissue proteins and the cells that first make and then maintain them. Unlike other connective tissues, the bone matrix is physiologically mineralized with tiny crystallites of a basic, carbonate-containing calcium phosphate called hydroxyapatite. In this regard, the bone mineral most closely resembles a geological mineral crystalline form called dahlite. Further, the bone matrix is unique along the classical connective tissues in that it is constantly regenerated throughout life as a consequence of bone turnover.

COLLAGEN

Some 85–90% of the total bone protein consists of type I collagen fibers. This is the most abundant form of collagen found in the body and is widely distributed in connective tissue. Bone contains little, if any, of the other forms of collagen and differs from most other connective tissues in this regard. The bone collagen fibers are highly insoluble because of their many covalent intra- and intermolecular cross-links, the type and pattern of which differs from that in soft connective tissues (1). The basic building block of the bone matrix fiber network is the type I collagen molecule, which is a triple-helical, coiled coil (supercoil) containing two identical $\alpha_1(I)$ chains and a structurally similar but genetically different $\alpha_2(I)$ chain. The collagen coil is created because every third residue in each chain's helical domain (~1000 amino acids or 300 nm in length) is glycine. This amino acid has no bulky side chain and affords a convenient folding element for the molecule. Collagen chains also contain a high proportion of proline, a ring amino acid, most of which immediately follows glycine. The gly-X-Y repeating triplet (where X is often proline) makes the collagen structure unique in biology (2).

In the matrix, individual collagen molecules are packed end to end with a short space (gap) between them. The molecule are packed laterally in a one-quarter stagger array so that each molecule is offset from its neighbor by approximately one-fourth of its length. This three-dimensional arrangement constitutes the fiber structure found in the bone extracellular space. Further, all the information necessary to fold into native molecules (see below) and then pack into fibrous protein resides in the primary sequence of the individual collagen chain.

The genes for the $\alpha_1(I)$ and $\alpha_2(I)$ chains of collagen are found on chromosomes 17 and 7, respectively (3). Each gene consists of multiple small expressing regions (called exons) that code for protein, interspersed by larger, noncoding DNA regions (introns). The messenger RNA for each collagen chain codes a biosynthesized precursor procollagen chain ~160,000 Da in size. Following removal of a short (~20 residue) leader sequence, the procollagen chains consist of a central, 100,000 Da final cleaved form with propeptide extensions attached at both the amino and carboxy termini of ~25,000 and 35,000 Da, respectively [for the α_1(I) chain]. The carboxy-terminal propeptide facilitates molecular folding of the trimeric procollagen molecule, which is secreted in an unprocessed form. Either concomitant with or subsequent to secretion from the cell, the procollagen peptide extensions are removed as fiber formation occurs (4). These propeptide extensions seem to assist in fibril formation and eventually become entrapped in the final matrix of bone (5). The propeptide extensions of type I collagen can also escape to serum where they have proved to be useful markers of bone formation (6). The preponderance of propeptide type I collagen extensions found in serum come from bone turnover. The propeptide extensions of type III collagen are often measured (along with those of type I) to correct for nonbone collagen synthesis (6). Such propeptide extension measurements have correlated significantly with direct histomorphometric measurements of bone formation (7).

Several posttranslational modifications of collagen occur during its biosynthesis and secretion. Specific amino-terminal and carboxy-terminal peptidases cleave the peptide extensions from the procollagen molecule. Intracellular modifications include hydroxylation of some proline and lysine residues, and addition of galactose to certain hydroxylysines and serine phosphorylation. Extracellular modifications (following fibril formation) include complexation with noncollagen proteins (see below) and cross-link formation. Intra- and intermolecular covalent cross-links are formed by lysyl oxidase action on collagen lysine and/or hydroxylysine residues (8,9). In bone, multiple cross-linking sites combine extracellularly to form pyridinium ring structures (the pyridinolines) tying several collagen monomer molecules together within the formed collagen fiber, thereby rendering it completely insoluble (10). These pyridinium cross-links are only released on degradation of the mineralized collagen fibrils during bone resorption. Measurement of these ring cross-link structures in urine have proved to be excellent measures of bone resorption (11).

NONCOLLAGEN PROTEIN

Noncollagenous proteins (NCPs) comprise 10–15% of the total bone protein content. Approximately one-fourth of the bone NCP is exogenously derived, being adsorbed or entrapped in the bone matrix space (12). This fraction is largely composed of serum-derived proteins that are acidic in character and that become bound to the hydroxyapatite mineral of bone. Some of these proteins may be advantageous to the tissue. For example, trapped growth factors [e.g., platelet-derived growth factor (PDGF)] could easily contribute to the regeneration of bone on injury (12). Other proteins such as serum albumin may merely be present adventitiously.

On a mole to mole basis, however, it can be calculated that the bone cell synthesizes and secretes as many molecules of NCP as it does of collagen. Remember, triple helical collagen has a molecular weight of over 300,000,

whereas most bone NCPs are approximately one-tenth that in size. Thus, a considerable portion, roughly half, of the osteoblast's matrix-directed biosynthetic activities are devoted to NCP molecules. These can be broken down into four general groups of protein products: 1) cell attachment proteins; 2) proteoglycans; 3) γ-carboxylated (gla) proteins; and 4) growth-related proteins. These classifications are often overlapping, and most of the physiological roles for individual bone protein constituents remain undefined at present (Table 1).

All connective tissue cells interact with their extracellular environment in response to chemical stimuli that direct and/or coordinate specific cell functions, such as proliferation, migration, and differentiation. These particular interactions involve cell attachment and spreading via transient, focal adhesions to extracellular macromolecules. This is done via the integrin family of cell surface receptors that transduce signals to the cytoskeleton (13). Bone cells synthesize four proteins that affect cell attachment; fibronectin (FN), thrombospondin (TSP), osteopontin (OP), and bone sialoprotein (BSP) (14,15). Three of these—TSP, OP, and BSP—are strong binders of ionic calcium and are found in the mineralized bone extracellular space (14,16). One, OP, is a reasonably well-phosphorylated phosphoprotein that, like FN and TSP, is found in bone and nonbone tissue systems (17). Osteopontin is found in many tissues other than bone, whereas BSP is almost exclusively found in the skeleton (18). Both OP and BSP are known to anchor osteoclasts to the bone extracellular space in cell regions called clear zones (19,20). Specific extracellular matrix receptors called integrins bind to these molecules allowing the osteoclasts to first form ruffled borders and then resorb bone (21).

Proteoglycans are macromolecules that contain acidic polysaccharide side chains (glycosaminoglycans) attached to a central core protein. In bone, two types of glycosaminoglycan are found: chondroitin sulfate (the predominant form), a polymer of sulfated N-acetylgalactosamine and glucuronic acid, and heparin sulfate, a polymer of sulfated N-acetylglucosamine and glucuronic acid. The bone cell heparin sulfate proteoglycan product is membrane-associated and, as for all connective tissues, probably facilitates interaction of the osteoblast with extracellular macromolecules (some of which are cell attachment proteins such as FN or TSP) and heparin-binding growth factors (22,23).

Chondroitin sulfate in bone is attached to three separate core proteins (23). One of these, presumed to be pericellular in locale, is ~300,000 Da in size (resultant proteoglycan ~600–800 kDa) and resembles a proteoglycan product synthesized by fibroblasts called versican (24). Its role is not yet understood, but it may be important in maintaining the integrity of the environment immediately outside of the cell membrane space. The vast bulk of the glycosaminoglycans of bone are attached to two small ($\approx$40 kDa) proteoglycan core proteins that are similar but separate gene products (16). These are called PG-I (which has two attached 50,000 Da chondroitin sulfate chains) and PG-II (having one attached chain), based on their relative electrophoretic migration on sodium dodecyl sulfate gels (16). PG-I (biglycan) is more abundant in developing (i.e., fetal

TABLE 1. *Principal bone cell noncollagen products secreted to the bone matrix*

Name	Approximate size	Potential function
Thrombospondin	450,000 (trimer)	Cell attachment
Fibronectin	440,000 (dimer)	Cell attachment, spreading
Biglycan (proteoglycan I)	170,000 (monomer)	Unknown
Decorin (proteoglycan II)	120,000 (monomer)	Collagen fibrillogenesis
Bone sialoprotein	75,000 (monomer)	Cell attachment, others unknown
Osteopontin	50,000 (monomer)	Cell attachment, spreading
Osteonectin	35,000 (monomer)	Ca^{2+}, mineral binding; others unknown
Matrix gla protein	9,000 (monomer)	Unknown
Osteocalcin	6,000 (monomer)	Ca^{2+} binding, bone turnover

or young) than in adult bone, whereas PG-II (decorin) is found in all stages of bone development. Decorin is distributed predominantly in the extracellular matrix space of connective tissues, whereas biglycan tends to be found in pericellular locales (25). A similar developmental distribution for these two proteoglycans is found in other connective tissues (22). PG-II has been called decorin because it binds to collagen fibrils and has been implicated in the regulation of collagen fibrillogenesis (26). Although the exact physiological functions of the small proteoglycans have not been definitively elucidated, they are generally assumed to be important for the integrity of most connective tissue matrices. One function might rise from their ability to bind and inactivate the transforming growth factor-β (TGF-β) family in the extracellular space (27). By this property, decorin and biglycan can influence cell proliferation and differentiation in a variety of connective tissues, including bone.

Vitamin K-dependent γ-carboxylation occurs on two bone NCPs, osteocalcin (bone gla-protein) and matrix-gla-protein (MGP). The production of dicarboxylic glutamyl (gla) residues also occurs in blood-clotting proteins where enhanced calcium-binding to gla side chains is important to the bioactivity of these molecules. Osteocalcin (~6 kDa in size) appears to be a bone-specific gla-containing protein, whereas MGP (~9 kDa) is found in cartilage and bone (28). The synthesis of osteocalcin in bone is greatly stimulated by 1,25(OH)$_2$ vitamin D$_3$, and this protein is now thought to be involved as a signal in the bone turnover cascade (29). BGP (osteocalcin) and MGP are partially homologous structurally (28), but it is as yet unclear as to how they may function physiologically either together or separately in bone tissue. Nevertheless, osteocalcin measurements in serum have proved valuable as markers of bone turnover in metabolic disease states (30).

A number of proteins in bone appear to be associated with the life cycle and function of the osteoblast. These proteins may be growth factors, such as TGF-β1–5 and insulin-like growth factors, osteoblast secretion products that can stimulate osteoblast cell growth in an autocrine and/or paracrine fashion (31,32). Thus, the growth potential of a bone cell may result from its own genetic framework and involve transcription of both known growth factors and their receptors in the same cell population.

Other bone cell products may be associated with the growth and/or differentiation of the osteoblast in an indirect or as yet undefined fashion. One of the hallmarks of the osteoblast phenotype is the synthesis of high levels of alkaline phosphatase (33). This enzyme is first found on the osteoblast plasmalemma, and some of this becomes cleaved from the cell surface and adsorbed within the mineralized bone matrix space. The function of alkaline phosphatase in bone cell biology has been the matter of much speculation, but remains undefined to the present day.

The most abundant NCP produced by bone cells is osteonectin, a phosphorylated glycoprotein accounting for ~2% of the total protein of developing bone in most animal species. The protein has high affinity for binding ionic calcium and physiological hydroxyapatite (34). It also binds to collagen (34) and thrombospondin (35). Osteonectin protein is found in platelets (36) and in nonbone tissues that are rapidly proliferating, remodeling, or undergoing profound changes in tissue architecture (37,38). Thus, the protein is associated with growing tissue, and in nonbone systems (but not in bone itself), its transcription and synthesis appear to be shut down or absent under steady-state conditions. Osteonectin biosynthesis is upregulated again in nonbone systems during wound repair and in some conditions of cell culture. Its function(s) in bone may be multiple, being potentially associated with osteoblast growth and/or proliferation, as well as with matrix mineralization (see below). Osteonectin can bind and inactivate the B-chain forms of PDGF (PDGF-BB and PDGF-AB) (39). Because PDGF is a potent regulator of the cell cycle, osteonectin could, by this binding, affect cell proliferation and growth in a variety of tissues. In some specialized tissues, such as forming capillaries, osteonectin alters endothelial cell shape and thus seems to influence blood vessel formation (40).

MINERALIZATION

Two mechanisms for bone mineralization have been described, one predominant in both calcified cartilage and primitive woven bone, the other in lamellar bone. Calcified cartilage and woven bone seem to mineralize via matrix vesicles (41), membrane-bound bodies that exocytose from the plasma membrane and migrate to the loose extracellular matrix space. The lipid-rich inner membrane of these vesicles becomes the nidus for hydroxyapatite crystal formation and, eventually, crystallization proceeds to the point of obliteration of the vesicle membrane producing a spherulite of clustered, tiny (50A

× 200A × 400A) crystals. These spherulites conglomerate until a continuous mineralized mass is achieved throughout the matrix space. In this context, the matrix vesicle is on a "suicide" mission and its "death" leads to mineral encrustation. The driving force for this mineral cascade, once initiated, seems to be the mineral crystals themselves that are first associated with the matrix vesicle membrane. The rate of mineralization in both woven and (see below) lamellar bone seems to depend on the presence of inhibitor molecules (e.g., pyrophosphate and acidic NCPs), which in solution seem to regulate the kinetics of the mineralization process (42). Thus, in this type of calcification, the cell buds off organelles capable of mineral accumulation and then synthesizes proteins that can control the rate at which crystallization proceeds.

The extracellular matrix in nonfetal and more abundant lamellar bone is tightly packed with well-aligned collagen fibrils that are "decorated" with complexed NCPs (e.g., proteoglycan and osteonectin). Either because there simply is insufficient space for them or for developmental reasons, matrix vesicles are rarely (if ever) seen in lamellar bone. Instead, mineralization proceeds in association with the heteropolymeric (collagen-NCP complex) matrix fibrils themselves. Somewhat more mineral appears associated with aligned gap regions (or "hole" zones) of the fibers (three-dimensional channels resulting from the spaces between longitudinally associated collagen monomers), which have more room for inorganic ions that the rest of the fibril structure. Other loci for the bone mineral appears to be between the collagen fibrils in a brick and mortar fashion (43). It is unknown whether the driving force for mineralization is the bone collagen itself or its associated NCPs. Purified collagen appears to be a poor initiator of crystal deposition and may serve a merely mechanical role in this regard. The extent of mineralization in the bone matrix space appears limited by the volume of bone occupied by its insoluble organic fibrous protein content alone. Decreased mineralization seems to occur under conditions of mineral ion deprivation, such as osteomalacia, and is fully reversible or increasing the pool of ions available for this purpose.

REFERENCES

1. Eyre DR, Dickson IR, Van Ness K: Collagen cross-linking in human bone and articular cartilage. *Biochem J* 252:495–500, 1988
2. Miller EJ: Recent information on the chemistry of the collagens. In: Butler WT (ed) *The chemistry and biology of mineralized tissues.* Ebsco Media, Birmingham, pp 80–93, 1985
3. Myers JC, Emanuel BS: Chromosomal localization of human collagen genes. *Collagen Relat Res* 7:149–159, 1987
4. Fleischmajer R, Perlish JS, Olsen BR: Amino and carboxyl propeptides in bone collagen fibrils during embryogenesis. *Cell Tissue Res* 247:105–109, 1987
5. Fisher LW, Gehron Robey P, Tuross N, Otsuka A, Tepen DA, Esch FS, Shimasaki S, Termine JD: The M_r 24,000 phosphoprotein from developing bone is the NH_2-terminal propeptide of the α1 chain of type I collagen. *J Biol Chem* 262:13457–13463, 1987
6. Krane SM, Munoz AJ, Harris ED: Urinary polypeptides related to collagen synthesis. *J Clin Invest* 49:716–720, 1970
7. Parfitt AM, Simon LS, Villanueva AR, Krane SM: Procollagen type I carboxy-terminal extension peptide in serum as a marker of collagen biosynthesis in bone. Correlation with iliac bone formation rates and comparison with total alkaline phosphatase. *J Bone Min Res* 2:427–436, 1987
8. Yamauichi M, Katz EP, Mechanic GL: Intermolecular cross-linking and stereospecific molecular packing in type I collagen fibrils of the periodontal ligament. *Biochemistry* 25:4907–4913, 1986
9. Robins SP, Duncan A: Pyridinium cross-links of bone collagen and location in peptides isolated from rat femur. *Biochim Biophys Acta* 914:233–239, 1987
10. Eyre DR, Dickson IR, Van Ness K: Collagen cross-linking in human bone and articular cartilage. Age-related changes in the content of mature hydroxypyridinium residues. *Biochem J* 252:495–500, 1988
11. Uebelhart D, Gineyts E, Chapuy M-C, Delmas PD: Urinary excretion of pyridinium cross-links; a new marker of bone resorption in metabolic bone disease. *Bone Min* 8:87–96, 1990
12. Termine JD: Non-collagen proteins in bone. In: Evered D, Harnett S (eds) *Cell and Molecular Biology of Vertebrate Hard Tissues, Ciba Foundation Symposium 136.* John Wiley and Sons, Chichester, pp 178–190, 1988
13. Ruoslahti E, Pierschbacher MD: New perspectives in cell adhesion: RGD and integrins. *Science* 238:491–497, 1987
14. Gehron Robey P, Young MF, Fisher LW, McClain TD: Thrombospondin is an osteoblast-derived component of mineralized extracellular matrix. *J Cell Biol* 108:719–727, 1988
15. Somerman MJ, Fisher LW, Foster RA, Sauk JJ: Human bone sialoprotein I and II enhance fibroblast attachment *in vitro.* *Calcif Tissue Int* 43:50–53, 1988
16. Fisher LW, Hawkins GR, Tuross N, Termine JD: Purification and partial characterization of small proteoglycans I and II, bone sialoproteins I and II and osteonectin from the mineral compartment of developing human bone. *J Biol Chem* 262:9702–9708, 1987
17. Mark MP, Prince CW, Gay S, Austin RL, Butler WT: 44kDal bone phosphoprotein (osteopontin) antigenicity at ectopic sites in newborn rats: kidney and nervous tissues. *Cell Tiss Res* 251:23–30, 1988
18. Gehron Robey P, Bianco P, Termine JD: The cellular biology and molecular biochemistry of bone formation. In: Coe FL, Favus MJ (eds) *Disorders of Bone and Mineral Metabolism.* Raven Press, New York, pp 241–263, 1992
19. Reinholt FP, Hultenby K, Oldberg A, Heinegard D: Osteopontin—A possible anchor osteoclasts to bone. *Proc Natl Acad Sci USA* 87:4473–4475, 1990
20. Bianco P, Fisher LW, Young MF, Termine JD, Gehron Robey P: Expression of bone sialoprotein (BSP) in developing human tissues. *Calcif Tissue Int* 49:421–426, 1991
21. Zambonin-Zallone A, Teti A, Grano M, et al.: Immunocytochemical distribution of extracellular matrix receptors in human osteoclasts; a β3 integrin is co-localized with vinculin and talin in the podosomes of osteoclastoma giant cells. *Exp Cell Res* 182:645–652, 1989
22. Hook M, Woods A, Johansson S, Kjellen L, Couchman Jr: Functions of proteoglycans at the cell surface. In: Evered E, Whelan J (eds) *Functions of the Proteoglycans, Ciba Foundation Symposium 124.* John Wiley and Sons, Chichester, pp 143–156, 1986
23. Beresford JN, Fedarko NS, Fisher LW, Midura RJ, Yanagishita M, Termine JD, Gehron Robey P: Analysis of the proteoglycans synthesized by human bone cells *in vitro.* *J Biol Chem* 262:17164–17172, 1987
24. Krusius T, Gehlsen KR, Ruoslahti E: A fibroblast chondroitin sulfate proteoglycan core protein contains lectin-like and growth factor-like sequences. *J Biol Chem* 262:13120–13125, 1987
25. Bianco P, Fisher LW, Young MF, Termine JD, Gehron Robey P: Expression and localization of the two small proteoglycans biglycan and decorin in developing human skeletal and nonskeletal tissues. *J Histochem Cytochem* 38:1549–1563, 1990
26. Ruoslahti E: Structure and biology of proteoglycans. *Ann Rev Cell Biol* 4:229–255, 1988
27. Okuda S, Languino LR, Ruoslahti E, Border WA: Elevated expression of transforming growth factor-β and proteoglycan production in experimental glomerulonephritis. *J Clin Invest* 86:453–462, 1990

28. Price PA: Vitamin K-dependent bone proteins. In: Cohn DV, Martin TJ, Meunier PJ (eds) *Calcium Regulation and Bone Metabolism: Basic and Clinical Aspects, vol 9.* Elsevier Science Publishers, Amsterdam, pp 419–425, 1987

29. Glowacki J, Lian JB: Impaired recruitment of osteoclast progenitors by osteocalcin-deficient bone implants. In: Butler WT (ed) *The Chemistry and Biology of Mineralized Tissues.* Ebsco Media, Birmingham, pp 164–169, 1985

30. Price PA, Parthemore JG, Deftos LJ: New biochemical marker for bone metabolism. *J Clin Invest* 66:878–883, 1980

31. Gehron Robey P, Young MF, Flanders KC, Roche NS, Kondaiah P, Reddi AH, Termine JD, Sporn MB, Roberts AB: Osteoblasts synthesize and respond to TGF-beta *in vitro. J Cell Biol* 105:457–463, 1987

32. Canalis E, McCarthy T, Centrella M: Isolation and characterization of insulin-like growth factor I (somatomedin C) from cultures of fetal rat calvariae. *Endocrinology* 122:22–27, 1988

33. Rodan GA, Heath JK, Yoon K, Noda M, Rodan SB: Diversity of the osteoblast phenotype. In: Evered D, Harnett S (eds) *Cell and Molecular Biology of Vertebrate Hard Tissues, Ciba Foundation Symposium 136.* John Wiley and Sons, Chichester, pp 78–85, 1988

34. Termine JD, Kleinman HK, Whitson SW, Conn KM, McGarvey ML, Martin GR: Osteonectin, a bone-specific protein linking mineral to collagen. *Cell* 26:99–105, 1981

35. Clezardin P, Malaval L, Ehrensperger AS, Delmas P, Dechavanne M, McGregor JL: Complex formation of human thrombospondin with osteonectin. *Eur J Biochem* 175:275–284, 1988

36. Stenner DD, Tracy RP, Riggs BL, Mann KG: Human platelets contain and secrete osteonectin, a major protein of mineralized bone. *Proc Natl Acad Sci USA* 83:6892–6896, 1986

37. Holland PWH, Harper SJ, McVey JH, Hogan BLM: *In vivo* expression of mRNA for the Ca^{+2}-binding protein SPARC (osteonectin) revealed by *in situ* hybridization. *J Cell Biol* 105:473–482, 1987

38. Wewer UM, Albrechtsen R, Fisher LW, Young MF, Termine JD: Osteonectin/SPARC/BM-40 in human decidua and carcinoma, tissues characterized by de novo formation of basement membrane. *Am J Pathol* 132:345–355, 1988

39. Raines EW, Lane TF, Iruela-Arispe ML, Ross R, Sage EH: The extracellular protein SPARC interacts with platelet-derived growth factor (PDGF)-AB and -BB and inhibits the binding of PDGF to its receptors. *Proc Natl Acad Sci USA* 89:1281–1285, 1992

40. Lane TF, Iruela-Arispe ML, Sage EH: Regulation of gene expression by SPARC during angiogenesis *in vitro. J Biol Chem* 267:16736–16745, 1992

41. Bonucci E: The locus of initial calcification in cartilage and bone. *Clin Orthop Rel Res* 78:108–139, 1971

42. Termine JD, Eanes ED, Conn KM: Phosphoprotein modulation of apatite crystallization. *Calcif Tiss Int* 31:247–251, 1980

43. Weiner S, Traub W: Organization of hydroxyapatite crystals within collagen fibrils. *FEBS Lett* 206:262–266, 1986

5. Bone Resorbing Cells

Gregory R. Mundy, M.D.

Department of Medicine and Endocrinology, University of Texas Health Science Center, San Antonio, Texas

The major and possibly sole bone resorbing cell is the osteoclast. Other cells, however, have been linked to bone resorption. These include osteocytes, monocytes, tumor cells, and osteoblasts. Osteocytic bone resorption, also called "osteocytic osteolysis," was first described over 30 years ago by histologists examining light microscopy sections. It was thought that osteocytic osteolysis was due to expansion of the osteocyte lacunae in which osteocytes are embedded in bone. However, more recent observations with scanning electron microscopy make it unlikely that osteolysis by osteocytes occurs (1). Use of scanning electron microscopy shows that bone resorption is characterized by easily discernible degradative changes in the bone matrix. These are not observed around osteocytes. Boyde and coworkers consider apparent osteolysis by osteocytes an artifact of observations made in bone that is rapidly turning over (fetal or woven bone). From time to time, other cells have also been linked to bone resorption. Monocytes and macrophages have been shown to degrade devitalized bone (2,3). These observations strengthen the notion that monocytes and osteoclasts have a common precursor, a concept that in light of subsequent data appears likely to be true. However, there are no resorption pits associated with monocytes or macrophages when they lie against bone surfaces, and it is unlikely that they have a major role in bone degradation. Similarly, tumor cells have also been shown to resorb devitalized bone by causing release of previously incorporated calcium (4). Again, resorption pits are not found around tumor cells, even *in vivo* (5). Recent suggestions have been made that osteoblasts may act as helper cells in the process of osteoclastic resorption by preparing the bone surface for later attack by osteoclastic enzymes, although there is still little direct evidence to support this theory.

Although osteoclasts are clearly the major bone resorbing cells, osteoclast activity may be modulated by other cells such as osteoblasts and immune cells.

OSTEOCLAST MORPHOLOGY

Osteoclasts have been studied extensively using light microscopy, transmission electron microscopy, and scanning electron microscopy. They are unique and highly specialized cells. They are localized on endosteal bone surfaces, in Haversian systems, and also occasionally on periosteal surfaces. They are not commonly seen on normal bone surfaces, but are found frequently at sites of actively remodeling bones, such as the metaphyses of growing bones or in pathological circumstances, such as adjacent to collections of tumor cells. They are large multinucleated cells, varying in size up to 100 nuclei in diameter in pathologic states and containing, on average, 10–20 nuclei. The number of nuclei in osteoclasts are related to the species, more being seen in the cat and fewer in the mouse. The nuclei are centrally placed and usually contain 1–2 nucleoli. Osteoclasts have primary lysosomes, numerous and pleomorphic mitochondria, and a specific area of the cell membrane that abuts to the bone surface known as the ruffled border. This area of the cell membrane is comprised of folds and invaginations that allow intimate contact with the bone surface. This is the site at which resorption of bone occurs and the resorption bay (also known as the Howship's lacuna) is formed. Some workers have considered the confined and circumscribed space between the ruffled border and the bone surface is equivalent to a secondary lysosome (6). The ruffled border is surrounded by a clear zone that appears free of organelles, but in fact contains actin filaments and appears to anchor the ruffled border area to the bone surface undergoing resorption.

CRITERIA FOR DEFINITION OF THE OSTEOCLAST

Some of the morphologic features of the osteoclast have been used as criteria for identification. These include multinuclearity, pleomorphic mitochondria, and presence of the ruffled border adjacent to areas of resorbed bone. These criteria have received much attention in recent years as investigators have attempted to isolate osteoclasts in vitro and distinguish them from other cells. Osteoclasts are difficult to distinguish from macrophage polykaryons, which are related cells with a similar lineage. Some of the features of the osteoclast that aid in the distinction from macrophage polykaryons include the capacity to resorb bone, capacity to form a ruffled border, contraction of the cytoplasm on exposure to calcitonin, cross-reactivity with osteoclast-specific monoclonal antibodies (although it has not been convincingly shown that any current antibodies are absolutely specific for the osteoclast), appropriate responses to calciotropic hormones, and absence of the Fc receptor. The presence of tartrate-resistant acid phosphatase is a helpful marker, but not useful for distinguishing human osteoclasts from macrophage polykaryons. Responsivity to osteotropic hormones also has been used as a criterion for identification of osteoclasts. Osteoclast stimulating agents [including parathyroid hormone (PTH), interleukin-1, tumor necrosis factor (TNF), transforming growth factor-α (TGF-α), and 1,25-dihydroxyvitamin D] activate osteoclasts. Inhibitors of osteoclast activity include calcitonin, γ-interferon, and transforming growth factor-β (TGF-β). However, the effects of some of these factors are not specific for osteoclasts. For example, 1,25-dihydroxyvitamin D promotes not only the fusion of osteoclasts, but also enhances the fusion of macrophages to form polykaryons (7). Moreover, some of these factors are species-specific. For example, calcitonin may not cause contraction of avian osteoclast cytoplasmic membranes. Recent evidence suggests that macrophages can be induced to form multinucleated cells, form resorption pits, and respond to calcitonin. A reasonable compromise is to denote cells as functional osteoclasts if they form resorption pits, are multinucleated, and respond to calcitonin, although recognizing that some authentic osteoclasts are not multinucleated, do not form resorption pits, and do not respond to calcitonin.

MOLECULAR MECHANISMS OF BONE RESORPTION

Osteoclasts resorb bone by the production of proteolytic enzymes and hydrogen ions in the localized environment under the ruffled border of the cell. Hydrogen ions are generated in the cell by the enzyme carbonic anhydrase type II. They are then pumped across the ruffled border by a proton pump, apparently similar but not identical to the proton pump in the intercalated cells of the kidney (8). Lysosomal enzymes are also released by the osteoclast, and the hydrogen ions produced by the proton pump provide an optimal environment for these proteolytic enzymes to degrade the bone matrix.

The osteoclast is a motile cell. It resorbs bone to form a lacuna and then moves across the bone surface to resorb a separate area of bone. The tracks of its path can often be followed (1). Periods of locomotion are not associated with resorption. When the cell stops moving, it usually starts resorbing bone.

Some diseases are due to disturbances in the molecular mechanisms responsible for bone resorption. For example, it has recently been shown that there is an unusual form of inherited osteopetrosis in children in which there is a deficiency of the carbonic anhydrase type II isoenzyme (9). The osteoclasts in this disease are incompetent, bone is not resorbed and the bone marrow cavity is not formed. Children with this disease also have renal tubular acidosis, due to a similar enzyme defect in renal tubular cell leading to impairment of hydrogen ion secretion.

Several other processes may be involved in the complex process of osteoclastic bone resorption. Some workers have suggested that the surface of the bone is prepared for the osteoclast by the actions of collagenase released by bone lining cells or osteoblasts. The osteoclasts then produce acid and lysosomal enzymes that complete the process. Because osteoblasts have the capacity to produce enzymes that could activate latent collagenase, such as plasminogen activator, such a mechanism is possible. However, studies with scanning electron microscopy show that osteoclasts do not require osteoblast preparation of the bone surface for resorption to occur, and isolated osteoclasts can resorb bone surfaces without the support of any other cells.

Data have been found to suggest that oxygen-derived free radicals are involved in the resorption of bone by osteoclasts (10). Many degradative processes by phagocytic cells are associated with radical production, and bone resorption seems another. The use of radical generating systems in vivo and in vitro show that enzymes that deplete tissues of radicals, such as superoxide dismutase, block osteoclastic bone resorption stimulated by PTH or interleukin-1. Staining reactions with nitroblue tetrazolium show that radical generation occurs within osteoclasts. Radicals could be involved in the degradation of bone under the ruffled border. However, the demonstration that radical generation is associated with new osteoclast formation suggests that radicals also have a cellular effect on the formation of osteoclasts.

The active resorbing osteoclast is a highly polarized cell. The ruffled border is the highly specialized area of the osteoclast cell membrane that lies adjacent to the bone surface. Recent data has shown that the attachment of the osteoclast to the bone surface is an essential requirement for resorption to occur. This attachment process involves, at least in part, cell membrane-bound proteins called integrins. Integrins attach to specific proteins in the bone matrix. One of the integrins important for osteoclast function is the vitronectin receptor (11). Antibodies to this receptor preferentially recognize osteoclasts. Attachment to bone matrix proteins involves specific Arg-Gly-Asp (RGD) amino acid sequences in the bone matrix proteins, and synthetic peptides are being developed that compete with osteoclast integrins for binding to these proteins, preventing osteoclasts attaching to the bone surface and thereby inhibiting bone resorption.

Recent observations have shown that a specific tyrosine kinase is required for osteoclasts to form resorption pits. The protooncogene src is a ubiquitous intracellular tyrosine kinase that is membrane-bound and has been linked to function of the cytoskeleton. In experiments in which the src gene was deleted from mice by targeted disruption in embryonic stem cells, it has been possible to breed mice that do not have the capacity to express src. In these mice, it was found unexpectedly that the mice have osteopetrosis, the bone disease characterized by nonfunctioning osteoclasts (12). More detailed examination of these mice has shown that multinucleated cells form on bone surfaces in src-deficient animals, but these multinucleated cells cannot form ruffled borders and resorb bone (13). These results indicate that this intracellular tyrosine kinase is essential for normal bone resorption and suggest a potential therapeutic target for the development of new inhibitors of bone resorption.

FORMATION AND ACTIVATION OF OSTEOCLASTS

Osteoclasts arise from hematopoietic mononuclear cells in the bone marrow (7). Mononuclear osteoclast precursors can circulate in the blood. At endosteal bone surfaces the precursors proliferate, fuse to form multinucleated cells, form ruffled borders, and resorb bone. The cell of origin for the osteoclast in the bone marrow is still debated. The weight of evidence suggests it is a pluripotent stem cell that has the capacity in response to appropriate stimuli to differentiate into a granulocyte, monocyte, or osteoclast. The most likely stem cell is a colony-forming unit for the granulocyte-macrophage series (CFU-GM).

It was shown over 10 years ago that osteoclasts formed by fusion of precursors at the bone surface. These precursors circulated in the blood as mononuclear cells.(14,15).

LESSONS FROM OSTEOPETROSIS

Osteopetrosis is the bone disorder characterized by impaired osteoclast function. It is clearly a heterogeneous disorder. There are a number of different variants in rodents that have now been well-described, as well as a number of different forms that occur in humans. Although a rare disease, this is a very informative condition for osteoclast biologists. Because specific molecular and genetic defects have been found in some types of osteopetrosis, studies of variants of this disorder have characterized some of the molecular mechanisms responsible for osteoclastic bone resorption. For example, in one rare variant seen in humans, there is deficient expression of the osteoclast enzyme carbonic anhydrase type II, which is responsible for osteoclast proton production (9). Because proton production is necessary for normal bone resorption, patients with abnormalities in expression of this enzyme have impaired bone resorption and subsequent osteopetrosis. In several of the murine models of osteopetrosis, it has been possible to identify genes that are essential for osteoclast function. For example, in one naturally occurring animal model of osteopetrosis, the op/op murine variant, there is impaired production of colony stimulating factor-1 (CSF-1) by stromal cells in the osteoclast microenvironment (16). As a consequence, osteoclasts fail to form and bone is not resorbed. This model shows that, during the neonatal period in mice, production of normal CSF-1 is required for normal osteoclast formation. In another recently described murine variant, tumor biologists experimenting with specific disruption of the src protooncogene have shown that this protooncogene, which encodes an intracellular tyrosine kinase, is required for normal osteoclastic bone resorption (12). However, the defect is different from that seen in the op/op variant of osteopetrosis. In src-deficient mice, osteoclasts form, but they do not become polarized and are incapable of forming ruffled borders and resorbing bone. Unlike the op/op variant, the defect in src deficiency is not in the microenvironment of the osteoclast, but rather in the mature osteoclast itself.

TECHNIQUES FOR STUDYING OSTEOCLASTS

Osteoclasts are very inaccessible cells, and so direct studies on these cells have been difficult to perform. For these reasons, detailed information on their behavior has not been available until recently, when isolation techniques have been developed for studying them in vitro. Techniques are now available for studying isolated preformed osteoclasts obtained from chicks, rodents, and baboons and for studying the formation of osteoclasts from marrow precursors (7,17). These techniques are providing a tremendous boon to advances in this area of bone cell biology, for they allow the determination of the modes of actions of factors that stimulate and inhibit bone resorption.

REGULATION OF OSTEOCLAST ACTIVITY

Osteoclasts lie on bone surfaces in a bed of elliptical or fusiform spindle-shaped cells called lining cells, which are probably members of the osteoblast lineage. When exposed to a bone resorbing agent, the first response is that these lining cells retract and the osteoclasts insinuate an arm into the retracted area, a ruffled border forms, and bone is resorbed at the exposed surface (1). The molecular mechanisms by which these complicated processes are controlled are unknown. Why lining cells retract as specific sites and how the osteoclast is activated is still not clear. It appears most likely that the osteoclast is activated by a soluble signal released from the lining cell (18,19).

Many hormones and factors have not been shown to stimulate osteoclast activity. Their mechanisms of action differ. Osteoclastic resorption may be stimulated by factors that enhance proliferation of osteoclast progenitors, which cause differentiation of committed precursors into mature cells or activation of the mature multinucleated cell to resorb bone (20). Similarly, osteoclasts could be inhibited by agents that block proliferation of precursors, which inhibit differentiation or fusion, or which inactivate the mature multinucleated resorbing cell. Current evidence indicates that most factors that stimulate or inhibit osteoclasts act on at least two of these steps. Regulation of osteoclast formation is shown diagrammatically in Fig. 1.

Systemic Hormones

The systemic hormones parathyroid hormone, 1,25-dihydroxyvitamin D, and calcitonin all influence osteoclast activity.

Parathyroid Hormone

Parathyroid hormone stimulates differentiation of committed progenitors to fuse to form mature multinucleated osteoclasts. It also activates preformed osteoclasts to resorb bone. The activation of osteoclasts is indirect, probably mediated through cells in the osteoblast lineage such as the lining cells (19). The mechanisms by which osteoblasts send the second signal to the multinucleated osteoclasts in response to PTH is not known.

1,25-Dihydroxyvitamin D

1,25-Dihydroxyvitamin D is a potent stimulator of osteoclastic bone resorption. Like PTH, it stimulates osteo-

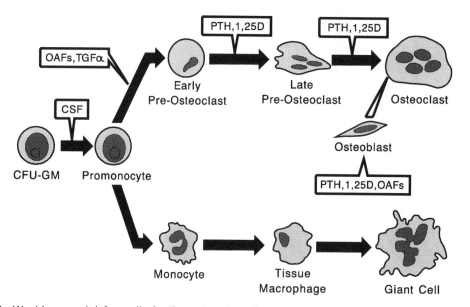

FIG. 1. Working model for cells in the osteoclast lineage and the sites of actions of various factors. The osteoclast most likely arises from a hematopoietic precursor it shares with the formed elements of the blood (CFU-GM). Early cells in the osteoclast lineage such as CFU-GM are pluripotent (i.e., they can differentiate along the granulocyte-macrophage lineage or the osteoclast lineage) and have high proliferative capacity. As these cells become further committed to the osteoclast lineage, they gradually lose proliferative potential. Factors such as TGF-α, the CSFs, and the osteoclast activating factors (immune cell products such as interleukin-1 and TNF) act as regulatory growth factors on these mononuclear osteoclast precursors. As the mononuclear cells proceed down the osteoclast lineage, they become further differentiated and eventually fuse to form immature osteoclasts. Systemic hormones such as PTH and 1,25-dihydroxyvitamin D stimulate the differentiation process. In the presence of bone, the mature osteoclast becomes polarized, forms a ruffled border, and with appropriate stimulation begins to resorb bone. Osteoclast activating factors and the systemic hormones such as PTH and 1,25-dihydroxyvitamin D can also act on the mature osteoclast (probably indirectly via other cells) to stimulate resorption.

clast progenitors to differentiate and fuse (7). It has a similar effect on macrophage polykaryons that are not osteoclasts. It also activates mature preformed osteoclasts, possibly by a similar mechanism to that of PTH. 1,25-Dihydroxyvitamin D also has other effects on bone resorption that are indirect. It is a potent immunoregulatory molecule (21). It inhibits T-cell proliferation and the production of the cytokine interleukin-2. Under some circumstances, it can enhance interleukin-1 production from cells with monocyte characteristics. Thus, the overall effects of 1,25-dihydroxyvitamin D on bone resorption are multiple and complex.

Calcitonin

Calcitonin is a polypeptide hormone that is a potent inhibitor of osteoclastic bone resorption, but its effects are only transient. Osteoclasts escape from the inhibitory effects of calcitonin following continued exposure (22). Thus, patients treated for hypercalcemia with calcitonin will respond for only a limited period of time before hypercalcemia recurs (usually 48–72 hr). Even in Pagetic patients, the beneficial effects of calcitonin may eventually be lost with continued treatment. Calcitonin causes cytoplasmic contraction of the osteoclast cell membrane, which has been correlated with its capacity to inhibit bone resorption (23). It also causes the dissolution of mature osteoclasts into mononuclear cells. However, it also inhibits osteoclast formation, inhibiting both proliferation of the progenitors and inhibiting differentiation of the committed precursors. The effects of calcitonin on osteoclasts are mediated by cAMP.

Local Hormones

Local hormones may be more important than systemic hormones for the initiation of physiologic bone resorption and the normal bone remodeling sequence. Because bone remodeling occurs in discrete and distinct packets throughout the skeleton, it seems probable that the cellular events are controlled by factors generated in the microenvironment of bone. Recently, a number of potent local stimulators and inhibitors of osteoclast activity have been identified.

Interleukin-1

There are two interleukin-1 molecules: interleukin-1α and β. Their effects on bone appear to be the same and are mediated through the same receptor. Interleukin-1 is released by activated monocytes, but also by other types of cells, including osteoblasts and tumor cells. It is a potent stimulator of osteoclasts. It works at all phases in the formation and activation of osteoclasts. It stimulates proliferation of the progenitors and differentiation of committed precursors into mature cells (24). It also activates the mature multinucleated osteoclast indirectly through another cell (possibly a bone lining cell) (25).

Interleukin-1 also stimulates osteoclastic bone resorption when infused in vivo and causes a substantial increase in the plasma calcium (26,27). At least part of its effects may be mediated via prostaglandin generation. It has recently been implicated as a potential mediator of bone resorption and increased bone turnover in osteoporosis (28). It may be responsible for the increase in bone resorption seen in some malignancies, as well as the localized bone resorption associated with collections of chronic inflammatory cells in diseases such as rheumatoid arthritis.

Lymphotoxin and Tumor Necrosis Factor

Lymphotoxin and TNF are molecules that are related functionally to interleukin-1. Many of their biological properties overlap with those of interleukin-1. They share the same receptor with each other, which is distinct from that of interleukin-1. Their effects on bone are synergistic with interleukin-1. Lymphotoxin is released by activated T-lymphocytes and TNF by activated macrophages. TNF is one of the mediators of the systemic effects of endotoxic shock. It also causes wasting (cachexia) and suppresses erythropoiesis or red blood cell formation. Lymphotoxin and TNF stimulate proliferation of osteoclast progenitors, cause fusion of committed precursors to form multinucleated cells, and activate multinucleated cells (through cells in the osteoblast lineage) to resorb bone (29–31). Lymphotoxin may be an important mediator of bone resorption in myeloma (32). Lymphotoxin and TNF causes osteoclastic bone resorption and hypercalcemia when infused or injected in vivo (30,32,33).

Colony Stimulating Factor-1

The growth regulatory factor CSF-1, which was once thought to be specific for the monocyte-macrophage lineage, has recently been shown to be required for normal osteoclast formation in rodents during the neonatal period. In the op/op variant of osteopetrosis, there is impaired production of CSF-1, and the consequence is osteopetrosis due to decreased normal osteoclast formation. The disease can be cured by treatment with CSF-1 (34). CSF-1 is produced by stromal cells in the osteoclast microenvironment. Presumably cells in the osteoclast lineage contain the CSF-1 receptor (a receptor tyrosine kinase), and this is the mechanism by which CSF-1 mediates osteoclast formation.

Osteoclastpoietic Factor

Because the osteoclast shares a common precursor with the formed elements of the blood, and CFU-GM are precursors for the osteoclast, it has long been wondered if there is a lineage specific growth regulatory factor for osteoclast formation. There have been two reports suggesting that such a factor may exist (35,36). Tumors that are associated with hypercalcemia often also cause leukocytosis due to production of various CSFs. In human and murine tumors associated with the hypercalcemia-leuko-cytosis syndrome, in addition to CSFs, these tumors have been shown to produce a 17 kDa peptide that stimulates osteoclast formation. Complete purification and cloning of this factor are awaited with interest.

γ-Interferon

γ-Interferon is a multifunctional lymphokine produced by activated T-lymphocytes. In contrast to the other immune cell products, it inhibits osteoclastic bone resorption (37,38). Its major effect appears to be to inhibit differentiation of committed precursors to mature cells (39). It also has effects on osteoclast precursor proliferation, but is less potent. Unlike calcitonin, it does not cause cytoplasmic contraction of isolated osteoclasts.

Transforming Growth Factor-β

TGF-β is a multifunctional polypeptide that is produced by immune cells, but is also released from the bone matrix during resorption. TGF-β has unique effects on osteoclasts. In most systems, it inhibits osteoclast formation by inhibiting both proliferation and differentiation of osteoclast precursors (24,40). In addition, it directly inhibits the activity of mature osteoclasts by decreasing superoxide production and inhibits accumulation of tartrate-resistant acid phosphatase in osteoclasts. Because TGF-β has a powerful effect on osteoblasts (stimulates proliferation and synthesis of differentiated proteins, increases mineralized bone formation) (41), it may be a pivotal factor in the bone remodeling process. For example, it could be released during this resorption process and then be available as a natural endogenous inhibitor of continued osteoclast activity. At the same time, working in conjunction with other bone factors, it may lead to osteoblast stimulation and the eventual formation of new bone. However, the effects of TNF-β are complex and may differ in different species. In one system, neonatal mouse calvariae, it stimulates prostaglandin generation that in turn leads to bone resorption, which is the opposite effect to that seen in the rat or human systems (42).

Other Factors

There are a number of other factors whose precise role in physiological and pathological bone resorption are still to be delineated.

Vitamin A

Vitamin A is the only fully characterized factor that has a direct stimulatory effect on osteoclasts (43). Vitamin A excess eventually leads to increased bone resorption in vivo and hypercalcemia. It is unknown if the effects of vitamin A on osteoclasts have physiological significance.

Transforming Growth Factor-α

Transforming growth factor-α, like the related compound epidermal growth factor, is a powerful stimulator of osteoclastic bone resorption (42,44–46). Transforming growth factor-α is produced by many tumors and is likely involved in increased bone resorption associated with cancer. It is probably produced normally during embryonic life. It stimulates the proliferation of osteoclast progenitors and probably also acts on nonmature multinucleated cells. Its actions on osteoclasts are comparable to those of the CSFs on other hematopoietic cells (47). The effects of TGF-α on bone cells are mediated through the receptor, although it is more potent than the epidermal growth factor on bone resorption. Injections or infusions of TGF-α increase the plasma calcium in vivo (33).

Neutral Phosphate

Neutral phosphate inhibits osteoclast activity in organ cultures (48). The precise mode of action is not clear. Phosphate is a useful form of therapy in patients with increased bone resorption and diseases such as cancer or primary hyperparathyroidism, although it may have other effects in addition to those of inhibiting bone resorption such as impairment of calcium absorption from the gut.

Pharmacologic Agents

A number of pharmacologic agents have been used as inhibitors of bone resorption and are useful therapies in patients with diseases such as malignancy associated with hypercalcemia. These include plicamycin (mithramycin), gallium nitrate, and the bisphosphonates (20). All of these agents inhibit osteoclastic activity, although their mechanism of action is unknown. In the case of the cytotoxic drugs plicamycin and gallium nitrate, it is possible that their actions are mediated through cytotoxic effects on osteoclasts or inhibition of proliferation of the osteoclast progenitors.

Prostaglandins

Prostaglandins have complex and multiple effects on osteoclasts depending on the species. Prostaglandins have been linked to the hypercalcemia and increased bone resorption associated with malignancy and chronic inflammation (49). However, the effects of prostaglandins are confusing. Prostaglandins of the E series stimulate osteoclastic bone resorption in organ culture. Moreover, some bone resorbing factors, and particularly growth factors, appear to mediate their effects through the production of prostaglandins in mouse bones. Prostaglandins inhibit the formation of human osteoclasts and cause cytoplasmic contraction of isolated osteoclasts in much the same way as calcitonin. However, prostaglandins stimulate the formation of mouse multinucleated osteoclasts from marrow progenitors. The overall significance of prostaglandin depends on the species studied. Their overall effects on bone resorption in man are still a mystery.

Leukotrienes

Leukotrienes, like prostaglandins, are arachidonic acid metabolites that have been linked to osteoclastic bone resorption (50). They are produced by the metabolism of arachidonic acid by a 5-lipoxygenase enzyme. Several of these leukotrienes have been shown to activate osteoclasts *in vitro,* and may be related to the bone resorption seen in giant cell tumors of bone. These arachidonic acid metabolites have different effects on osteoclasts to prostaglandins of the E series, which stimulate osteoclastic bone resorption in organ culture, and cause transient inhibition of the activity of isolated osteoclasts. In contrast, the leukotrienes stimulate osteoclastic bone resorption in organ culture, but also enhance the capacity of isolated osteoclasts to form resorption pits.

Thyroid Hormones

The thyroid hormones thyroxine and triiodothyronine stimulate osteoclastic bone resorption in organ cultures (51). Some patients with hyperthyroidism have increased bone loss, increased osteoclast activity, and hypercalcemia. Thyroid hormones act directly on osteoclastic bone resorption but their precise mode of action is unknown.

Glucocorticoids

Glucocorticoids inhibit osteoclast formation *in vitro* and inhibit osteoclastic bone resorption in organ cultures. Their efficacy depends on the stimulus to bone resorption. They are less effective in inhibiting bone resorption stimulated by PTH than they are in inhibiting bone resorption stimulated by cytokines such as interleukin-1 (52).

In vivo, glucocorticoid administration is associated with increased bone resorption. This is an indirect effect, and is due to the effects of glucocorticoids to inhibit calcium absorption from the gut. As a consequence, parathyroid gland activity is stimulated and secondary hyperparathyroidism leads to a generalized increase in osteoclastic bone resorption.

Estrogens and Androgens

Estrogen lack is associated with increased osteoclastic bone resorption in the 10 years following menopause (53). The mechanisms are not clear. Separate reports have suggested estrogens may affect osteoclasts directly (54), but in addition estrogens may mediate their effects on osteoclasts indirectly by suppressing the production of bone resorbing cytokines such as interleukin-1 and interleukin-6 (55–57). These notions suggested estrogen withdrawal, e.g., at menopause, then leads to enhanced bone resorption.

REFERENCES

1. Jones SJ, Boyde A, Ali NN, Maconnachie E: A review of bone cell substratum interactions. *Scanning* 7:5–24, 1985
2. Mundy GR, Altman AJ, Gondek M, Bandelin JG: Direct resorption of bone by human monocytes. *Science* 196:1109–1111, 1977
3. Kahn AJ, Stewart CC, Teitelbaum SL: Contact-mediated bone resorption by human monocytes in vitro. *Science* 199:988–990, 1978
4. Eilon G, Mundy GR: Direct resorption of bone by human breast cancer cells in vitro. *Nature* 276:726–728, 1978
5. Boyde A, Maconnachie E, Reid SA, Delling G, Mundy GR: Scanning electron microscopy in bone pathology: Review of methods. Potential and application. *Scanning Elec Micros* IV: 1537–1554, 1986
6. Baron R, Vignery A, Horowitz M: Lymphocytes, macrophages and the regulation of bone remodeling. In: Peck WA (ed) *Bone and Mineral Research,* vol II. Elsevier, New York, pp 175–242, 1983
7. Roodman GD, Ibbotson KJ, MacDonald BR, Kuehl TJ, Mundy GR: 1,25(OH)2 vitamin D3 causes formation of multinucleated cells with osteoclast characteristics in cultures of primate marrow. *Proc Natl Acad Sci USA* 82:8213–8217, 1985
8. Blair HC, Teitelbaum SL, Ghiselli R, Gluck S: Osteoclastic bone resorption by a polarized vacuolar proton pump. *Science* 245: 855–857, 1989
9. Sly WS, Whyte MP, Sundaram V, et al.: Carbonic anhydrase II deficiency in 12 families with the autosomal recessive syndrome of osteopetrosis with renal tubular acidosis and cerebral calcification. *N Engl J Med* 313:139–145, 1985
10. Garrett IR, Boyce BF, Oreffo ROC, Bonewald L, Poser P, Mundey GR: Oxygen-derived free radicals stimulate osteoclastic bone resorption in rodent bone in vitro and in vivo. *J Clin Invest* 85:632–639, 1990
11. Davies J, Warwick J, Totty N, Philip R, Helfrich M, Horton M: The osteoclast functional antigen, implicated in the regulation of bone resorption, is biochemically related to the vitronectin receptor. *J Cell Biol* 109:1817–1826, 1989
12. Soriano P, Montgomery C, Geske R, Bradley A: Targeted disruption of the c-src proto-oncogene leads to osteopetrosis in mice. *Cell* 64:693–702, 1991
13. Boyce BF, Byars J, McWilliams S, et al.: Histological and electron microprobe studies of mineralization in aluminum-related osteomalacia. *J Clin Pathol* 45:502–508, 1992
14. Kahn AJ, Simmons DJ: Investigation of the cell lineage in bone using a chimera of chick and quail enbryonic tissue. *Nature* 258: 325–327, 1975
15. Walker DG: Control of bone resorption by hematopoietic tissue. The induction and reversal of congenital osteopetrosis in mice through the use of bone marrow mononuclear phagocytes. *J Exp Med* 156:1604–1614, 1975
16. Wiktor-Jedrzejczak W, Urbanowska E, Aukerman SL, et al.: Correction by CSF-1 of defects in the osteopetrotic op/op mouse suggests local, developmental, and humoral requirements for this growth factor. *Exp Hematol* 19:1049–1054, 1991
17. Zambonin Zallone A, Teti A, Primavera MV: Isolated osteoclasts in primary culture: First observations on structure and survival in cultured media. *Anat Embryol* 165:405–413, 1982
18. Rodan GA, Martin TJ: Role of osteoblasts in hormonal control of bone resorption—A hypothesis. *Calcif Tiss Int* 33:349–351, 1981
19. McSheehy PMJ, Chambers TJ: Osteoblastic cells mediate osteoclastic responsiveness to parathyroid hormone. *Endocrinology* 118:824–828, 1986
20. Mundy GR, Roodman GD: Osteoclast ontogeny and function. In: Peck W (ed) *Bone and Mineral Research,* vol V. Elsevier, New York, pp 209–280, 1987
21. Tsoukas CD, Provvedini DM, Manolagas SC: 1,25-Dihydroxyvitamin D3: A novel immunoregulatory hormone. *Science* 224: 1438–1440, 1984
22. Wener JA, Gorton SJ, Raisz LG: Escape from inhibition of resorption in cultures of fetal bone treated with calcitonin and parathyroid hormone. *Endocrinology* 90:752–759, 1972

23. Chambers TJ, Magnus CJ: Calcitonin alters the behavior of isolated osteoclasts. *J Pathol* 136:27–40, 1982

24. Pfeilschifter JP, Seyedin S, Mundy GR: Transformed growth factor β inhibits bone resorption in fetal rat long bone cultures. *J Clin Invest* 82:680–685, 1988

25. Thomson BM, Saklatvala J, Chambers TJ: Osteoblasts mediate interleukin-1 stimulation of bone resorption by rat osteoclasts. *J Exp Med* 164:104–112, 1986

26. Sabatini M, Boyce B, Aufdemorte T, Bonewald L, Mundy GR: Infusions of recombinant human interleukin-1α and β cause hypercalcemia in normal mice. *Proc Natl Acad Sci* 85:5235–5239, 1988

27. Boyce BF, Aufdemorte TB, Garrett IR, Yates AJP, Mundy GR: Effects of interleukin-1 on bone turnover in normal mice. *Endocrinology* 123:1142–1150, 1989

28. Pacifici R, Rifas L, McCracken R, et al.: Ovarian steroid treatment blocks a postmenopausal increase in blood monocyte interleukin-1 release. *Proc Natl Acad Sci USA* 86:2398–2402, 1989

29. Bertolini DR, Nedwin GE, Bringman TS, Mundy GR: Stimulation of bone resorption and inhibition of bone formation in vitro by human tumour necrosis factors. *Nature* 319:516–518, 1986

30. Johnson RA, Boyce BF, Mundy GR, Roodman GD: Tumors producing human TNF induce hypercalcemia and osteoclastic bone resorption in nude mice. *Endocrinology* 124:1424–1427, 1989

31. Thomson BM, Mundy GR, Chambers TJ: Tumor necrosis factors alpha and beta induce osteoblastic cells to stimulate osteoclastic bone resorption. *J Immunol* 138:775–779, 1987

32. Garrett IR, Durie BGM, Nedwin GE, et al.: Production of the bone resorbing cytokine lymphotoxin by cultured human myeloma cells. *N Engl J Med* 317:526–532, 1987

33. Tashjian AH Jr, Voelkel EF, Lazzaro M, et al.: Tumor necrosis factor-alpha (cachectin) stimulates bone resorption in mouse calvaria via a prostaglandin-mediated mechanism. *Endocrinology* 120:2029–2036, 1987

34. Felix R, Cecchini MG, Fleiscih H: Macrophage colony stimulating factor restore in vivo bone resorption in the op/op osteopetrotic mouse. *Endocrinology* 127:2592–2594, 1990

35. Lee MY, Eyre DR, Osborne WRA: Isolation of a murine osteoclast colony-stimulating factor. *Proc Natl Acad Sci USA* 88:8500–8504, 1991

36. Yoneda T, Kato I, Bonewald LF, Chisoku H, Burgess WH, Mundy GR: A novel osteoclastpoietic peptide: Purification and characterization. *J Bone Min Res* 6(suppl):454, 1991

37. Gowen M, Mundy GR: Actions of recombinant interleukin-1, interleukin-2 and interferon gamma on bone resorption in vitro. *J Immunol* 136:2478–2482, 1986

38. Gowen M, Nedwin G, Mundy GR: Preferential inhibition of cytokine stimulated bone resorption by recombinant interferon gamma. *J Bone Min Res* 1:469–474, 1986

39. Takahashi N, Mundy GR, Kuehl TJ, Roodman GD: Osteoclast like formation in fetal and newborn long term baboon marrow cultures is more sensitive to 1,25-dihydroxyvitamin D3 than adult long term marrow cultures. *J Bone Min Res* 2:311–317, 1987

40. Chenu C, Pfeilschifter J, Mundy GR, Roodman GD: Transforming growth factor β inhibits formation of osteoclast-like cells in long-term human marrow cultures. *Proc Natl Acad Sci USA* 85:5683–5687, 1988

41. Noda M, Camilliere JJ: In vivo stimulation of bone formation by transforming growth factor-beta. *Endocrinology* 124:2991–2994, 1989

42. Tashjian AH Jr, Voelkel EF, Lloyd W, et al.: Actions of growth factors on plasma calcium. Epidermal growth factor and human transforming growth factor-alpha cause elevation of plasma calcium in mice. *J Clin Invest* 78:1405–1409, 1986

43. Fell HB, Mellanby E: The effect of hypervitaminosis A on embryonic limb bones cultured in vitro. *J Physiol* 116:320–349, 1952

44. Ibbotson KJ, D'Souza SM, Smith DD, Carpenter G, Mundy GR: EGF receptor antiserum inhibits bone resorbing activity produced by a rat Leydig cell tumor associated with the humoral hypercalcemia of malignancy. *Endocrinology* 116:469–471, 1985

45. Ibbotson KJ, Harrod J, Gowen M: Human recombinant transforming growth factor alpha stimulates bone resorption and inhibits formation in vitro. *Proc Natl Acad Sci USA* 83:2228–2232, 1986

46. Stern PH, Krieger NS, Nissenson RA, et al.: Human transforming growth factor alpha stimulates bone resorption in vitro. *J Clin Invest* 76:2016–2020, 1985

47. Takahashi N, MacDonald BR, Hon J, Winkler ME, Derynck R, Mundy GR, Roodman GD: Recombinant human transforming growth factor alpha stimulates the formation of osteoclast-like cells in long term human marrow cultures. *J Clin Invest* 78:894–898, 1986

48. Raisz LG, Niemann I: Effect of phosphate, calcium and magnesium on bone resorption and hormonal responses in tissue culture. *Endocrinology* 85:446–452, 1969

49. Tashjian AH, Voelkel EF, Levine L, et al.: Evidence that the bone resorption-stimulating factor produced by mouse fibrosarcoma cells is prostaglandin E2: A new model for the hypercalcemia of cancer. *J Exp Med* 136:1329–1343, 1972

50. Gallwitz WE, Mundy GR, Lee CH, et al.: 5-Lipoxygenase metabolites of a stromal cell line (1433) activate osteoclasts and giant cells from human giant cell tumors of bone. *J Biol Chem* 1993 (in press)

51. Mundy GR, Shapiro JL, Bandelin JG, Canalis EM, Raisz LG: Direct stimulation of bone resorption by thyroid hormones. *J Clin Invest* 58:529–534, 1976

52. Mundy GR, Rick ME, Turcotte R, Kowalski MA: Pathogenesis of hypercalcemia in lymphosarcoma cell leukemia. Role of an osteoclast activating factor-like substance and mechanism of action for glucocorticoid therapy. *Am J Med* 65:600–606, 1978

53. Lindsay R, Hart DM, Forrest C, et al.: Prevention of spinal osteoporosis in oophorectomised women. *Lancet* 2:1151–1153, 1980

54. Oursler MJ, Osdoby P, Pyfferoen J, Riggs BL, Spelsberg TC: Avian osteoclasts as estrogen target cells. *Proc Natl Acad Sci USA* 88:6613–6617, 1991

55. Pacifici R, Rifas L, McCracken R, et al.: Ovarian steroid treatment blocks a postmenopausal increase in blood monocyte interleukin-1 release. *Proc Natl Acad Sci USA* 86:2398–2402, 1989

56. Jilka RL, Hangoc G, Girasole G, et al.: Increased osteoclast development after estrogen loss: mediation by interleukin-6. *Science* 257:88–91, 1992

57. Girasole G, Jilka RL, Passeri G, et al.: 17-Beta-estradiol inhibits interleukin-6 production by bone marrow-derived stromal cells and osteoblasts in vitro—A potential mechanism for the antiosteoporotic effect of estrogens. *J Clin Invest* 89:883–891, 1992

6. Regulation of Bone Remodeling

Ernesto Canalis, M.D.

*Departments of Research, Medicine, and Orthopedics, Saint Francis
Hospital and Medical Center, Hartford, Connecticut, and University of
Connecticut School of Medicine, Farmington, Connecticut*

Bone remodeling is a complex process involving a number of cellular functions directed toward the coordinated resorption and formation of new bone. Bone remodeling is regulated by systemic hormones and by local factors, which affect cells of the osteoclast or osteoblast lineage and exert their effects on: 1) the replication of undifferentiated cells, 2) the recruitment of cells, and 3) the differentiated function of cells. The endproduct of remodeling is the maintenance of a mineralized bone matrix, and the major organic component of this matrix is collagen. Bone metabolism is regulated by polypeptide, steroid, and thyroid hormones, as well as by local factors that play a direct and important role in bone remodeling (Table 1) (1,2). The local factors are synthesized by skeletal cells and include growth factors and prostaglandins. Growth factors are polypeptides that regulate the replication and differentiated function of cells. Growth factors have effects on cells of the same class (autocrine factors) or other cells within the tissue (paracrine factors). Prostaglandins are currently the only known local regulators of bone remodeling that do not have a polypeptide structure. The existence of local factors is not unique to the skeletal system, because nonskeletal tissues also synthesize and respond to autocrine growth factors. Growth factors are also present in the circulation and may act as systemic regulators of skeletal and nonskeletal metabolism, but the locally produced factor has a more direct and possibly important function in cell growth. Circulating hormones may act on skeletal cells either directly or indirectly, modulating the synthesis, activation, receptor binding, and binding proteins of a local growth factor, which in turn stimulates or inhibits bone formation or bone resorption (Fig. 1). It is likely that hormones are important in the targeting of growth factors to tissues expressing specific hormonal receptors. Growth factors may play a critical role in the coupling of bone formation to bone resorption and possibly in pathophysiological processes.

HORMONAL REGULATION OF BONE REMODELING

Bone metabolism is regulated by a variety of systemic hormones that act on bone forming and bone resorbing cells (Fig. 2).

Polypeptide Hormones

Parathyroid Hormone and Calcitonin

Parathyroid hormone (PTH) is a polypeptide with a molecular weight (MW) of 9,500. PTH stimulates bone resorption, although the effect is not direct because the osteoclast does not have PTH receptors, and the presence of osteoblasts or osteoblast-derived factors is necessary to observe its resorptive action. PTH has complex effects on bone formation, and it can stimulate and inhibit bone collagen or matrix synthesis. Continuous treatment with PTH results in an inhibition of bone formation in vitro. This effect is due to a direct inhibition of bone collagen synthesis by PTH occurring at the transcriptional level. In contrast, intermittent treatment with PTH results in a stimulation of bone collagen synthesis and bone formation (3). The anabolic effect of PTH appears to be mediated at least in part by an increased synthesis of insulin-like growth factor (IGF) I. This stimulation of skeletal IGF I synthesis is due to an increase in cAMP, and other inducers of cAMP mimic the effect of PTH on IGF I production (4). PTH also has a mitogenic effect on bone, although the exact cells affected have not been clearly characterized. The dual role of PTH stimulating bone resorption and bone formation should not be a surprise, because these processes are coupled, and it is possible that specific growth factors, such as IGF I, are important in the coupling of bone formation and bone resorption.

Calcitonin (CT), a 32 amino acid polypeptide with a MW of 3,000 is known to inhibit bone resorption but it does not modify bone formation. Most of the CT actions have been observed at a relatively high dose, and this peptide may be more important as a pharmacological than physiological hormone.

Insulin

Insulin is a polypeptide with a MW of 6,000 synthesized by the β-cells of the pancreas. Insulin does not regulate bone resorption, but it causes a marked stimulation of bone matrix synthesis and cartilage formation, making it among the most important systemic hormones modulating normal skeletal growth. In addition, insulin is necessary for normal bone mineralization, and individuals and experimental animals with untreated diabetes mellitus have impaired skeletal growth and mineralization. Insulin has direct stimulatory effects on skeletal tissue, but it also increases IGF I production by the liver; therefore, some of its in vivo effects might be mediated by IGF I. Insulin stimulates bone matrix synthesis, but at physiological concentrations it does not alter bone cell replication. The stimulatory effect of insulin on matrix synthesis is due to its actions on the differentiated function of the osteoblast rather than an increase in the number of collagen-producing cells (5). Proinsulin is 100-fold less potent than insulin in stimulating bone collagen synthesis, and C-peptide

TABLE 1. *Hormonal and local regulators of bone remodeling*

Hormones
  Polypeptide hormones
    Parathyroid hormone
    Calcitonin
    Insulin
    Growth hormone
  Steroid hormones
    1,25-Dihydroxyvitamin D_3
    Glucocorticoids
    Sex steroids
  Thyroid hormones
Local Factors
  "Classic" polypeptide growth factors
    Insulin-like growth factors
    Transforming growth factor-β family of peptides
    Fibroblast growth factors or heparin binding growth factors
    Platelet-derived growth factor
  Cytokines from the immune and hematological systems
    Interleukins
    Tumor necrosis factor
    Colony-stimulating factors
  Other factors
    Prostaglandins

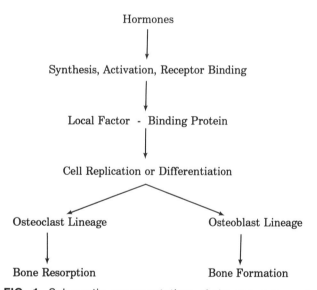

FIG. 1. Schematic representation of the regulation of bone remodeling by hormones and local factors.

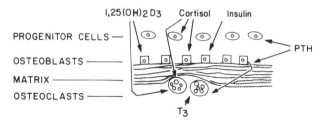

FIG. 2. Regulation of bone formation and bone resorption by hormones.

does not modify this process. The actions of insulin and IGF I are somewhat different because, in addition to the effects on osteoblast differentiated function, IGF increases the number of bone matrix synthesizing cells.

Growth Hormone

Growth hormone (GH), a pituitary polypeptide with a MW of 21,000, does not have direct effects on bone resorption, and its direct actions on bone formation have remained controversial. GH causes a small stimulation of IGF I by skeletal cells and through this local factor GH may regulate bone formation. The direct effect of GH on bone formation may be limited because bone cells may express only a low level of GH receptors. Less controversial is the stimulatory effect of GH on bone formation *in vivo*, because GH appears necessary for the maintenance of normal bone mass.

Steroids

Vitamin D

1,25-Dihydroxyvitamin D_3 [$1,25(OH)_2D_3$], a hormone synthesized primarily but not exclusively by the kidney, has similar functions to PTH. $1,25\text{-}(OH)_2D_3$ stimulates bone resorption and has complex effects on bone formation (6). Whereas $1,25(OH)_2D_3$ is necessary for normal growth and bone mineralization, it does not stimulate bone formation directly. $1,25\text{-}(OH)_2D_3$ enhances the synthesis of osteocalcin (bone Gla protein), a peptide known to be exclusively synthesized by the osteoblast, indicating that $1,25(OH)_2D_3$ has direct stimulatory effects on this cell. Although osteocalcin has been postulated to play a function in osteoclast recruitment and on bone formation, its exact role in bone remodeling is not known (7). The complex effects of $1,25(OH)_2D_3$ on bone formation may be related to a variety of actions of this steroid. $1,25\text{-}(OH)_2D_3$ directly inhibits bone collagen synthesis, but increases the binding of IGF I to its receptor in cells of the osteoblastic lineage, and stimulates the synthesis of selected IGF binding proteins that may modify IGF actions and concentrations (8).

Glucocorticoids

Glucocorticoids are steroid hormones that have marked effects on bone and mineral metabolism. Glucocorticoids stimulate bone resorption *in vivo*, possibly because they decrease calcium absorption with a subsequent increase in PTH. For the most part glucocorticoids have direct inhibitory effects on bone resorption and collagen degradation (9). The actions of glucocorticoids on bone formation are complex (10). After short-term treatment at physiological concentrations, they stimulate bone collagen synthesis, possibly by increasing the binding of IGF I to its receptor. In contrast, their long-term effect on bone collagen synthesis is inhibitory probably due to a marked decrease in preosteoblastic cell replication. This results in a severe depletion of osteoblasts available to synthesize bone matrix and could play a role in the pathogenesis of steroid-induced osteoporosis. Glucocorticoids inhibit the synthesis of IGF I by bone cells and this may in part explain their inhibitory effects on bone formation.

Sex Steroids

Estrogens and androgens are important in the skeletal maturation of growing individuals and in the prevention of bone loss. Estrogen receptors are expressed at a low level by bone cells; consequently, it is difficult to demonstrate direct effects of estrogens on bone formation or bone resorption. *In vivo*, estrogens decrease bone resorption and by doing so they prevent bone loss, but their actions may be indirect (11). Estrogens have been shown to decrease the synthesis of cytokines, such as interleukin-6, which are present in the bone microenvironment and play a role in the stimulation of bone resorption (12). The inhibition of their synthesis may be important in the mechanism of action of estrogen decreasing bone resorption.

Thyroid Hormones

Thyroid hormones are necessary for normal growth and development, acting primarily on cartilage formation, in conjunction with IGF I. In contrast to their important role on cartilage and linear growth, thyroid hormones do not stimulate bone matrix synthesis or cell replication. They do, however, stimulate bone resorption. This effect has clinical consequences. Hyperthyroid patients may have hypercalcemia, and postmenopausal patients on chronic thyroid suppression may be prone to develop osteopenia (13,14).

LOCAL REGULATION OF BONE REMODELING

Bone is a rich source of growth factors with important actions in the regulation of bone formation and bone resorption (Fig. 3). Frequently, these local factors are synthesized by skeletal cells, although selected factors are derived from cells of the immune or hematological system and as such are present in the bone microenvironment.

"Classic" Polypeptide Growth Factors

Insulin-Like Growth Factors

Insulin-like growth factors are growth hormone-dependent polypeptides with a MW of 7,600 (15). Two IGFs have been characterized, IGF I and IGF II. These peptides are synthesized by multiple tissues, including bone, and have similar biological properties although IGF I is 4 to 7 times more potent than IGF II (16). Under some conditions IGF may act as systemic agent; however, local IGFs have a direct and probably more significant effect on tissue growth. IGF I is one of the more thoroughly studied growth factors, and using biochemical and histomorphometric analysis, it was shown to enhance bone collagen and matrix synthesis and to stimulate the replication of cells of the osteoblast lineage. The IGF I effect on matrix synthesis is only in part dependent on an increased number of cells, and IGF I directly modulates the differentiated function of the osteoblast. IGF I also decreases bone collagen degradation. Because of its significant effects on bone cell function, it is likely that IGF I plays a fundamental role in the process of bone formation and in the maintenance of bone mass.

The synthesis and binding of IGF I to its bone cell receptor is regulated by hormones and by local factors, which are likely to modify the availability and effects of IGF I. PTH, as well as other agents that stimulate cAMP in bone cells, are the major stimulators of IGF I synthesis (4). Glucocorticoids inhibit skeletal IGF I synthesis, and this may be important in the mechanism of glucocorticoid action decreasing bone formation and possibly bone mass (17). Local factors like prostaglandin E_2 also enhance IGF I synthesis and IGF I and II binding to bone cells. β_2-microglobulin, a polypeptide found in serum and on the surface of almost all mammalian cells, has similar stimulatory effects on bone formation as IGF I and II probably due to an increase in the binding of IGF to its osteoblast receptor. Bone cells also secrete IGF binding proteins (IGFBPs). So far, six IGFBPs have been identified and termed IGFBP-1–6, and unstimulated bone cells synthesize all of them except for IGFBP 1 (18). The precise role of the IGFBPs is not understood; they may prolong the half-life of IGF, neutralize or enhance its biological activity, or be involved in the transport of IGF to its target cells. The regulation of IGFBP synthesis in bone cells is complex, and studies are not complete at this time. Selected IGFBPs are under cAMP and others under IGF I and II control, suggesting the existence of local feedback mechanisms to prevent overexposure of bone cells to IGF.

Transforming Growth Factor-β Family

Transforming growth factors are polypeptides that were initially defined by their ability to induce nonneoplastic

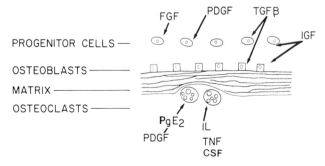

FIG. 3. Regulation of bone formation and bone resorption by growth factors and cytokines.

indicator cells (surface-adherent, density-dependent growth-regulated fibroblasts) to form anchorage-independent colonies in soft agar suspension cultures. This process was considered linked to neoplastic transformation, because tumor-derived cells can form colonies spontaneously. However, it is now known that transforming growth factor-β (TGF-β) plays multiple functions in the regulation of normal cell metabolism. TGF-β is a polypeptide with a MW of 25,000 and is synthesized by many tissues, including bone. Three forms of TGF-β, which seem to have similar biological activities, are present in bone: TGF-β_1, TGF-β_2, and TGF-β_3. TGF-β stimulates the replication of precursor cells of the osteoblast lineage, and it also has a direct stimulatory effect on bone collagen synthesis (19). Therefore, TGF-β modulates bone matrix synthesis by various mechanisms, including an increase in the number of cells capable of expressing the osteoblast phenotype, as well as direct actions on the differentiated function of the osteoblast. TGF-β also decreases bone resorption. Hormones capable of inducing bone resorption, such as PTH, increase the release of active TGF-β from bone, and the available TGF-β could be instrumental in suppressing further bone resorption and initiating the bone forming phase of remodeling (20).

There are a number of additional polypeptides, which share amino acid sequence with TGF-β. These include various bone morphogenetic proteins or osteoinductive factors (21). Bone morphogenetic proteins induce the formation of normal endochondral bone formation and some have similar activities to those of TGF-β. Because of their ability to increase the formation of new bone, bone morphogenetic proteins may be important in the treatment of fractures.

Fibroblast Growth Factors

Acidic and basic fibroblast growth factors (FGFs) or heparin binding growth factors 1 and 2 are polypeptides with an approximate MW of 17,000 (22). Initially, these two factors were obtained from the central nervous system, but recent studies have shown that acidic and basic FGF are synthesized by a variety of normal and malignant tissues. FGFs are angiogenic factors considered important for neovascularization and wound healing. Bone contains acidic and basic FGF, and both factors stimulate bone cell replication, which results in an increased bone cell population capable of synthesizing bone collagen (23). Thus, bones treated with FGF synthesize a higher amount of collagenous matrix because they contain a greater number of collagen-synthesizing cells, but not because of a direct effect of FGF on the differentiated function of the osteoblast. The stimulatory effects of FGFs on neovascularization, in association with those on bone cell replication, suggest that they are important in the process of healing and bone repair; particularly, because they are not secreted cell products and their release could occur after cell injury or death. Neither acidic nor basic FGF modify bone resorption or matrix degradation.

Platelet-Derived Growth Factor

Platelet-derived growth factor (PDGF), a polypeptide with a MW of 30,000, was initially isolated from blood platelets and was considered important in the early phases of wound repair (24). Normal and neoplastic tissues also synthesize PDGF, indicating that it may act as a systemic or local regulator of tissue growth. PDGF is a dimer of the products of two genes, PDGF A and B, so that mature peptides can exist as a PDGF AA or BB homodimer or as a PDGF AB heterodimer. PDGF AB and BB are the predominant isoforms present in the systemic circulation, whereas PDGF AA is secreted by normal bone cells. In contrast, osteosarcoma cells express both PDGF genes and have the potential to synthesize all the PDGF isoforms. PDGF stimulates bone resorption and bone cell replication (25). This suggests that it may be important in bone remodeling or repair, probably in association with other factors, but PDGF does not stimulate bone collagen synthesis by direct actions on the differentiated function of the osteoblast.

Cytokines from the Immune and Hematological Systems

A number of cytokines with important effects on the immune and hematological system also act on skeletal cells. It is believed they act directly on bone cells either because they are derived from marrow cells and are present in the bone microenvironment or because they are synthesized by bone cells. The cytokines include interleukin (IL)-1, IL-6, macrophage and granulocyte/macrophage colony stimulating factors, and tumor necrosis factor (TNF). These factors have important effects on bone remodeling and stimulate bone resorption either directly or by enhancing the recruitment of osteoclasts, the bone resorbing cells.

IL-1 exists in two forms: IL-1α and IL-1β. They have partial amino acid homology and similar biological activities. IL-1 has complex effects on bone remodeling, and it stimulates bone resorption and bone cell replication. IL-1 seems relevant in the mechanism of hypercalcemia of certain hematological malignancies, and increased IL-1 levels were reported in selected cases of osteoporosis (26). IL-1 increases the synthesis of IL-6, which increases bone resorption probably through the recruitment of cells of the osteoclast lineage. The synthesis of IL-6 is diminished by estrogens, and the phenomenon could explain the decrease in bone resorption observed after estrogen therapy (12). TNF-α or cachectin, is a cytokine known for its cytostatic, cytolytic, and antiviral actions. However, TNF-α is also important in a variety of normal cellular responses, and, in contrast to its growth inhibitory properties on tumor cells, it stimulates the growth of nontransformed cells. TNF-α stimulates bone resorption and bone cell replication, and the cells that replicate under the influence of TNF differentiate and synthesize bone collagen (27). Colony-stimulating factors play a role in the maturation of osteoclasts, and granulocyte/macrophage–colony-stimulating factor secretion is stimulated by PTH.

In summary, bone remodeling is a complex process regulated by systemic hormones and local factors. Hormones regulate the synthesis, activation, effects, and binding proteins of the local factors, which have a direct action on cellular metabolism, and modify the replication or differentiated function of cells of the osteoblast or osteoclast lineage. It is possible that the role of the hormones is to provide tissue specificity for a given growth factor, because most of these factors are synthesized by a variety of skeletal and nonskeletal systems. Bone-associated factors may play a role in the maintenance of normal bone remodeling, have a function in wound and fracture healing, or play a role in the pathogenesis of specific bone disease and hypercalcemia.

REFERENCES

1. Canalis E: The hormonal and local regulation of bone formation. *Endocr Rev* 4:62–77, 1983
2. Canalis E, McCarthy TL, Centrella M: Growth factors and cytokines in bone cell metabolism. *Annu Rev Med* 42:17–24, 1991
3. Canalis E, Centrella M, Burch W, McCarthy TL: Insulin-like growth factor I mediates selective anabolic effects of parathyroid hormone in bone cultures. *J Clin Invest* 83:60–65, 1989
4. McCarthy TL, Centrella M, Canalis E: Cyclic AMP induces insulin-like growth factor I synthesis in osteoblast-enriched cultures. *J Biol Chem* 265:15353–15356, 1990
5. Canalis E: Effect of insulin-like growth factor I on DNA and protein synthesis in cultured rat calvaria. *J Clin Invest* 66:709–719, 1980
6. DeLuca HF: Vitamin D revisited. *Clin Endocrinol Metab* 9:1–26, 1980
7. Lian JB, Coutts M, Canalis E: Studies of hormonal regulation of osteocalcin synthesis in cultured fetal rat calvariae. *J Biol Chem* 260:8706–8710, 1985
8. Canalis E, Centrella M, McCarthy TL: The role of insulin-like growth factors in bone remodeling and bone metabolism: basic and clinical aspects. In: *Excerpta Medica, vol 11*. Elsevier, Amsterdam, pp 258–265, 1992
9. Raisz LG, Trummel CL, Wener JA, Simmons H: Effect of glucocorticoids on bone resorption in tissue cultures. *Endocrinology* 90:961–967, 1972
10. Canalis E: Effects of glucocorticoids on type I collagen synthesis, alkaline phosphatase activity, and deoxyribonucleic acid content in cultured rat calvariae. *Endocrinology* 112:931–939, 1983
11. Caputo C, Meadows D, Raisz LG: Failure of estrogens and androgens to inhibit bone resorption in tissue cultures. *Endocrinology* 98:1065–1068, 1976
12. Jilka RL, Hangoc G, Girasole G, Passeri G, Williams DC, Abrams JS, Boyce B, Broxmeyer H, Manolagas SC: Increased osteoclast development after estrogen loss: Mediation by interleukin-6. *Science* 257:88–91, 1992
13. Mundy GR, Shapiro JL, Bandelin JG, Canalis EM, Raisz LG: Direct stimulation of bone resorption by thyroid hormones. *J Clin Invest* 58:529–534, 1976
14. Baran DT, Braverman LE: Thyroid hormones and bone mass (editorial). *J Clin Endocrinol Metab* 72:1182–1183, 1991
15. Daughaday WH, Rotwein P: Insulin-like growth factors I and II. Peptide, messenger ribonucleic acid and gene structures, serum, and tissue concentrations. *Endocr Rev* 10:68–91, 1989
16. McCarthy TL, Centrella M, Canalis E: Regulatory effects of insulin-like growth factor I and II on bone collagen synthesis in rat calvarial cultures. *Endocrinology* 124:301–309, 1989
17. McCarthy TL, Centrella M, Canalis E: Cortisol inhibits the synthesis of insulin-like growth factor I in skeletal cells. *Endocrinology* 126:1569–1575, 1990
18. Shimasaki S, Gao L, Shimonaka M, Ling N: Isolation and molecular cloning of insulin-like growth factor-binding protein-6. *Mol Endocrinol* 5:938–948, 1991
19. Centrella M, McCarthy T, Canalis E: Transforming growth factor beta is a bifunctional regulator of replication and collagen synthesis in osteoblast-enriched cell cultures from fetal rat bone. *J Biol Chem* 262:2869–2874, 1987
20. Pfeilschifter J, Seyedin SM, Mundy GR: Transforming growth factor beta inhibits bone resorption in fetal rat long bone cultures. *J Clin Invest* 82:680–685, 1988
21. Wozney JM, Rosen V, Celeste AJ, Mitsock LM, Whitters MJ, Kriz RW, Hewick RM, Wang EA: Novel regulators of bone formation: molecular clones and activities. *Science* 242:1528–1534, 1988
22. Burgess WH, Wehlman T, Firesel R, Johnson WV, Maciag T: Multiple forms of endothelial cell growth factor. *J Biol Chem* 260:11389–11392, 1985
23. Canalis E, Centrella M, McCarthy T: Effects of basic fibroblast growth factor on bone formation in vitro. *J Clin Invest* 81:1572–1577, 1988
24. Heldin CH, Westermark B: PDGF-like growth factors in autocrine stimulation of growth. *J Cell Physiol* 5:31–34, 1987
25. Canalis E, McCarthy TL, Centrella M: Effects of platelet-derived growth factor on bone formation in vitro. *J Cell Physiol* 140:530–537, 1989
26. Dewhirst FE, Stashenko PP, Mole JE, Tsurumachi T: Purification and partial sequence of human osteoclast activating factor, identity with interleukin-1. *J Immunol* 135:2562–2568, 1985
27. Bertolini DR, Nedwin GE, Bringman TS, Smith DD, Mundy GR: Stimulation of bone resorption and inhibition of bone formation in vitro by human tumor necrosis factors. *Nature* 319:516–518, 1986

Calcium, Magnesium, Phosphorus Homeostasis and Physiology and Biochemistry of Calcium Regulating Hormones

7. Physiological Functions of Calcium, Magnesium, and Phosphorus and Mineral Ion Balance

Arthur E. Broadus, M.D., Ph.D.

Departments of Internal Medicine and Physiology, Yale University School of Medicine, New Haven, Connecticut

Life began in a primordial sea rich in potassium and magnesium and poor in sodium and calcium, and it is felt that the present composition of intracellular fluids, rich in potassium and magnesium and poor in sodium and calcium, reflects this ancient heritage (1). With time, geological changes altered the composition of the seas to one rich in sodium and calcium, and primitive organisms adapted to this altered milieu by developing ion pumps in order to maintain the asymmetry of the concentrations of monovalent and divalent cations across their plasma membranes. Indeed, the evolution of these pumps and channels may be viewed as one of the most fundamental developments in cell biology. The maintenance of the transmembrane potassium/sodium and magnesium/calcium ratios is critically important in the control of cell excitation and the regulation of many aspects of intracellular metabolism. In general, more active tissues such as nerve, liver, and muscle have a higher ratio of potassium/sodium and magnesium/calcium than inactive tissues, such as skin and erythrocytes. In addition, more active tissues have a higher phosphorus content than inactive tissues, in keeping with the role of phosphate esters in cellular energy metabolism.

CALCIUM

An adult human contains approximately 1,000 g of calcium (2). Some 99% of this calcium is in the skeleton in the form of hydroxyapatite, and 1% is contained in the extracellular fluids and soft tissues. About 1% of the skeletal content of calcium is freely exchangeable with the extracellular fluids. Although small as a percentage of skeletal content, this exchangeable pool is approximately equal to the total content of calcium in the extracellular fluids and soft tissues, and serves as an important buffer or storehouse of calcium. The extracellular concentration of calcium ions (Ca^{2+}) is in the range of 10^{-3} M, whereas the concentration of Ca^{2+} in the cytosol is $\sim 10^{-6}$ M.

Calcium plays two predominant physiological roles in the organism. In bone, calcium salts provide the structural integrity of the skeleton. In the extracellular fluids and in the cytosol, the concentration of calcium ions is critically important in the maintenance and control of a number of biochemical processes, and the concentrations of Ca^{2+} in both compartments are maintained with great constancy.

PHOSPHORUS

An adult contains approximately 600 g of phosphorus. Some 85% of this phosphorus is present in crystalline form in the skeleton and plays a structural role. About 15% is present in the extracellular fluids, largely in the form of inorganic phosphate ions, and in soft tissues, almost totally in the form of phosphate esters. Intracellular phosphate esters and phosphorylated intermediates are involved in a number of important biochemical processes, including the generation and transfer of cellular energy. Intracellular and extracellular concentrations of phosphorus (as the phosphate divalent anion) are $\sim 1 \times 10^{-4}$ and 2×10^{-4} M, respectively, and these concentrations are less rigidly maintained than are those of calcium and magnesium.

MAGNESIUM

An adult contains approximately 25 g or 2,000 mEq of magnesium. About two-thirds is present in the skeleton and one-third in soft tissues. The magnesium in bone is not an integral part of the hydroxyapatite lattice structure but appears to be located on the crystal surface. Only a minor fraction of the magnesium in bone is freely exchangeable with extracellular magnesium. Magnesium is the most abundant intracellular divalent cation, and cellular magnesium is important as a cofactor for a number of enzymatic reactions and in the regulation of neuromuscular excitability. Approximately 1% of total body magnesium is contained in the extracellular compartment, and its concentration in plasma does not provide a reliable index of either total body or soft tissue magnesium content. The concentration of magnesium ions (Mg^{2+}) is $\sim 5 \times 10^{-4}$ M in the cytosol, as well as in the extracellular fluids, and its concentration in both compartments is rigidly maintained.

EXTRACELLULAR MINERAL METABOLISM

Calcium

There are three definable fractions of calcium in serum: ionized calcium ($\sim 50\%$), protein-bound calcium ($\sim 40\%$), and calcium that is complexed, mostly to citrate and phosphate ions ($\sim 10\%$) (3). Both the complexed and ionized fractions are ultrafilterable, so that $\sim 60\%$ of the total calcium in serum crosses semipermeable membranes. About 90% of the protein-bound calcium is bound to albumin and the remainder to globulins. Alterations in the serum albumin concentration can have a major influence on the measured total serum calcium concentration. At pH 7.4, each g/dL of albumin binds 0.8 mg/dL of calcium, and this simple relationship can be used to mentally "correct" the total serum calcium concentration when circulating albumin is abnormal (e.g., given measured albumin and calcium concentrations of 2.0 and 7.4 mg/dL, respectively, the "corrected" serum calcium concentration at an albumin concentration of 4.0 g/dL is 9.0 mg/dL). Calcium is bound largely to the carboxyl groups in albumin, and this binding is highly pH-dependent. Acute acidosis decreases binding and increases ionized calcium, and acute alkalosis increases binding with a consequent decrease in ionized calcium. These changes are not reflected in the total serum calcium concentration and can only be appreciated by actual measurement of ionized serum calcium at the ambient pH. Calcium concentrations are typically recorded in mg/dL (mg%); these concentrations can be converted to molar units simply by dividing by 4 (e.g., 10 mg/dL converts to 2.5 mM).

It is the ionized fraction of calcium (Ca^{2+}) that is physiologically important and that is rigidly maintained by the combined effects of parathyroid hormone (PTH) and 1,25-dihydroxyvitamin D [1,25(OH)$_2$D]. Examples of the physiological functions of extracellular Ca^{2+} include 1) serving as a cofactor in the coagulation cascade (e.g., for factors VII, IX, X, and prothrombin), 2) maintenance of the normal mineral ion product required for skeletal mineralization, and 3) contributing stability to plasma membranes by binding to phospholipids in the lipid bilayer and also regulating the permeability of plasma membranes to sodium ions. A reduction in ionized calcium increases sodium permeability and enhances the excitability of all excitable tissues; an increase in ionized calcium has the opposite effect.

Phosphorus

Serum inorganic phosphate also exists as three fractions: ionized, protein-bound, and complexed. Protein binding is relatively insignificant for phosphate, representing some 10% of the total, but ~35% is complexed to sodium, calcium, and magnesium. Thus, ~90% of the inorganic phosphate in serum is ultrafilterable. The major ionic species of phosphate in serum at pH 7.4 is the divalent anion (HPO_4^{2-}).

In contrast to calcium, the serum phosphorus concentration varies quite widely and is influenced by age, sex, diet, pH, and a variety of hormones. An adequate serum phosphate concentration is important in maintaining a sufficient ion product for normal mineralization.

Magnesium

About 55% of serum magnesium is ionized, with 30% being protein-bound and 15% complexed. The protein-bound fraction interacts with the carboxyl groups of albumin and is influenced by pH in a fashion analogous to that of calcium. It is the ionized fraction of magnesium that is physiologically important (e.g., to plasma membrane excitability). The extracellular concentration of ionized magnesium is tightly controlled by the tubular maximum or threshold for magnesium in the nephron (4).

CELLULAR MINERAL METABOLISM

A detailed summary of the numerous metabolic functions of calcium, magnesium, and phosphorus within cells is beyond the scope of this syllabus. This section attempts simply to highlight briefly some of the important roles of these ions in cellular physiology.

Calcium

The control of cellular calcium homeostasis is complex, and the regulation of the concentration of the calcium ion in the cytosol is as rigidly maintained as is its concentration in extracellular fluids (5,6). Cells are bathed in extracellular fluids containing ~10^{-3} M Ca^{2+}. The concentration of Ca^{2+} in the cytoplasm is ~10^{-6}M, or one one-thousandth that in extracellular fluids. Cytosolic calcium is to some extent buffered by binding to other cytoplasmic constituents, and certain cells contain a specific calcium binding protein, which may serve as a buffer and/or a calcium transport protein within the cytosol. The mitochondria and microsomes contain 90–99% of the intracellular calcium, bound largely to organic and inorganic phosphates. The calcium content of these organelles is sufficient to replenish cytosolic calcium some 500 times.

The low Ca^{2+} concentration in the cytosol is maintained by three pump-leak transport systems: an external system located in the plasma membrane and two internal systems located in the microsomal membrane and the inner mitochondrial membrane, respectively. Calcium diffuses into the cytosol across these three membranes. Each of the three pumps is oriented in a direction of calcium egress from the cytosol; each requires energy, and each shares a high affinity for calcium (K_m ~10^{-6} M).

The importance of these three calcium transport systems in regulating cellular calcium metabolism varies considerably from cell to cell, depending on the function of a particular cell type. Several examples serve to illustrate how the details of cellular calcium homeostasis have been adapted to subserve the specific physiological function of a given cell type.

Calcium ion is the coupling factor linking excitation and contraction in all forms of skeletal and cardiac muscle (5). In striated muscle, the microsomes are extensively developed as the sarcoplasmic reticulum, which serves as the principle storehouse of intracellular calcium in muscle and is the most highly developed calcium transport system known. Depolarization of the plasma membrane is accompanied by the entry of a small amount of extracellular calcium into the cell, and this acts as a trigger to release large quantities of calcium stored in the sarcoplasmic reticulum. The abrupt increase in cytosolic calcium interacts with troponin, a specific calcium-binding protein, leading to a conformational change and the actin-myosin interaction that constitutes muscle contraction. The reticulum vesicles are capable of reaccumulating the large quantity of cytosolic calcium with the extreme speed required by the relaxation process.

In most mammalian cells other than muscle, the principle internal calcium pump-leak system is that of the inner mitochondrial membrane. In a number of cells, calcium serves as a second messenger, mediating the effects of membrane signals on the release of secretory products (e.g., neurotransmitters, exocrine secretions such as amylase, and endocrine secretions such as insulin and aldosterone) (5). The calcium messenger system involves a flow of information along several pathways: 1) a calmodulin pathway and 2) a C-kinase pathway. It is now recognized that in many cells several branches of the calcium messenger system and the cAMP messenger system are intimately related, and these systems are integrated in such a way that the net cellular response to a given stimulus is determined by a complex interplay between these systems (5).

Phosphorus

The transport of phosphate ions across the plasma membrane and the membranes of intracellular organelles proceeds passively but is determined by the movement of cations, mostly calcium. The phosphate content in mitochondria is high, where it is largely in the form of calcium salts. The cytoplasmic concentration of free phosphate ions is estimated to be quite low, and the remaining portion of intracellular phosphate is either bound or in the form of organic phosphate esters. These phosphate esters play a variety of critically important roles in cellular metabolism: purine nucleotides provide the cell with stored energy; phosphorylated intermediates are concerned with energy conservation and transfer; phospholipids are major constituents of cell membranes, and the phosphorylation of proteins is an important means of regulating their function.

Magnesium

Magnesium is the most abundant intracellular divalent cation and is the second most abundant intracellular cation after potassium. Approximately 60% of cellular magnesium is contained in the mitochondria, and it is estimated that only 5–10% of intracellular magnesium exists as free ions in the cytoplasm. The transport mechanisms responsible for maintaining the asymmetric distribution of magnesium in intracellular compartments are less well studied than the corresponding calcium transport systems, but it is clear that the cellular metabolism of calcium and magnesium is regulated independently. Magnesium is an essential cofactor in the function of a wide variety of key enzymes, including essentially all enzymes concerned with the transfer of phosphate groups, all reactions that require ATP, and each of the steps concerned with the replication, transcription, and translation of genetic information.

MINERAL ION BALANCE AND MECHANISMS FOR MAINTAINING SYSTEMIC MINERAL HOMEOSTASIS

Mineral ion metabolism at the cellular and organ level and the regulation of these processes by PTH and $1,25(OH)_2D$ are described in detail in other chapters in this primer. The information herein attempts to integrate these processes at the level of the intact organism and describes the fine set of checks and balances that regulate mineral homeostasis in vivo.

The term mineral ion balance refers to the state of mineral homeostasis in the organism vis-à-vis the environment. In zero balance, mineral intake and accretion exactly match mineral losses; in positive balance, mineral intake and accretion exceed mineral losses, and in negative balance, mineral losses exceed mineral intake and accretion. A growing child is in positive mineral balance, whereas an immobilized patient is in negative mineral balance. Formal balance studies are a relic of the past and are no longer performed, but the concept of balance is central to even a cursory understanding of systemic mineral ion homeostasis. Figure 1 is a schematic representation of calcium, phosphorus, and magnesium metabolism in a normal adult who is in zero mineral ion balance and who is consuming an average Western diet.

The total extracellular pool of calcium is ~900 mg. This pool is in dynamic equilibrium with calcium entering and exiting via the intestine, bone, and renal tubule. In zero balance, bone resorption and formation are equivalent, and the net quantity of calcium absorbed by the intestine, ~175 mg/day, is quantitatively excreted into the urine. Therefore, under normal circumstances net calcium absorption provides a surplus of calcium that considerably exceeds systemic requirements. At middle age and beyond, normal adults lose ~1% of their skeletons yearly; this is the equivalent of a calcium loss of ~25 mg/day.

The extracellular pool of orthophosphate is ~550 mg (Fig. 1). This pool is in dynamic equilibrium with phosphorus entry and exit via the intestine, bone, kidney, and soft tissues (not depicted in the figure). In zero balance, fractional net phosphorus absorption is about two-thirds of phosphorus intake; this amount represents a vast excess over systemic requirements and is quantitatively excreted into the urine.

The extracellular pool of magnesium is ~250 mg and is in bidirectional equilibrium with magnesium fluxes across the intestine, kidney, bone, and soft tissues (Fig. 1). In zero balance, the magnesium derived from net intestinal absorption, ~100 mg/day, represents a systemic surplus and is quantitatively excreted.

The key points made in the preceding paragraphs are basically two: 1) normally, hormonal and/or intrinsic mechanisms of mineral ion absorption in the intestine provide the organism with a mineral supply that exceeds systemic mineral needs by a considerable measure, and 2) the renal tubule plays the dominant quantitative role in maintaining normal mineral homeostasis. Within this framework, minor fluctuations in systemic requirements are easily met by the surfeit of normal mineral absorption and do not require hormonal adjustments.

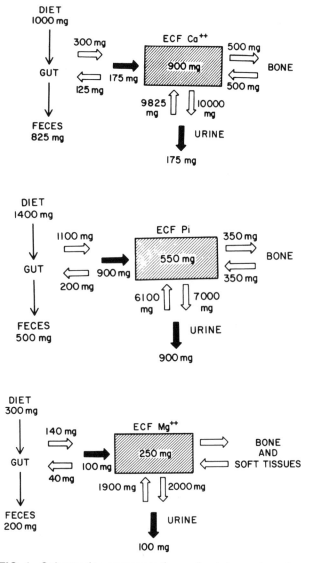

FIG. 1. Schematic representations of calcium, phosphorus, and magnesium fluxes in a normal adult in zero mineral ion balance. The *open arrows* denote unidirectional mineral fluxes, and the *solid arrows* denote net fluxes. (From Stewart AF, Broadus AE: Mineral metabolism. In: Felig P, Baxter JD, Broadus AE, Frohman LA (eds) *Endocrinology and Metabolism,* 2nd ed. McGraw-Hill, New York, 1987.)

Systemic Calcium Homeostasis and Maintenance of a Normal Serum Calcium Concentration

The parathyroid chief cell is exquisitively sensitive to the ionized serum calcium concentration and is capable of responding to changes in this concentration so small that they are unmeasurable by human hands. The integrated actions of PTH on distal tubular calcium reabsorption, bone resorption, and 1,25(OH)$_2$D-mediated intestinal calcium absorption are responsible for the fine regulation of the serum ionized calcium concentration. The precision of this integrated control is such that in a normal individual serum ionized calcium probably fluc-

tuates by no more than 0.1 mg/dL in either direction from its normal setpoint value throughout the day. Distal tubular calcium reabsorption and osteoclastic bone resorption are the major control points in minute-to-minute serum calcium homeostasis; of these two processes, the effect of PTH on the distal tubule is quantitatively the most important. Together, these effects constitute a classical "short-loop" feedback system on the parathyroid chief cell. Adjustments in the rate of intestinal calcium absorption via the PTH-1,25(OH)$_2$D axis require approximately 24–48 hr to become maximal. This axis represents a classical "long-loop" feedback system.

An abrupt reduction in dietary calcium intake to <100 mg/day or the administration of 80 mg of furosemide daily to a normal individual represent moderate hypocalcemic challenges; in each case, the initial deficit of calcium is in the range of 100–150 mg/day. A series of adjustments occurs, leading to a new steady state by 48 hr. A moderate increase in the secretion rate of PTH results in 1) increased calcium reabsorption from the distal tubule, 2) increased mobilization of calcium and phosphorus from bone, and 3) increased synthesis of 1,25(OH)$_2$D, which participates with PTH in bone resorption and increases the efficiency of calcium and phosphorus absorption in the intestine. The increased circulating concentration of PTH resets the renal tubular phosphate threshold/glomerular filtration rate (TmP/GFR) at a lower level so that the increased amount of phosphorus mobilized from bone and absorbed from the intestine in quantitatively excreted into the urine. In the new steady state, serum calcium has returned to normal, serum phosphorus is unchanged or slightly reduced, and a state of mild secondary hyperparathyroidism and efficient intestinal mineral absorption exists. At this point, the initial requirement for calcium mobilization from the skeleton is largely replaced by the enhanced absorption of calcium in the intestine.

The systemic mechanisms for the prevention of hypercalcemia consist largely of a reversal of the sequence just described, namely, an inhibition of PTH and 1,25(OH)$_2$D synthesis, with a reduction in calcium mobilization from bone, absorption from the intestine, and reclamation from the distal renal tubule. Whether the putative effects of calcitonin are of pathophysiological importance in humans remains unclear. The bottleneck in the defense against hypercalcemia is the limited capacity of the kidneys to excrete calcium. In theory, normal kidneys can excrete a calcium load of 1,000 mg or more/day. In practice, calcium excretion rates in this range are rarely seen. Limitations in the theoretical ability of the kidney to combat hypercalcemia include 1) the fact that abnormalities in distal tubular reabsorption are actually involved in the genesis of hypercalcemia in a number of conditions (e.g., primary hyperparathyroidism); 2) the fact that a degree of renal impairment frequently accompanies many hypercalcemic conditions; and 3) the fact that an increased calcium concentration inhibits the ability of the renal tubule to conserve water, which may lead to a vicious cycle of dehydration, prerenal azotemia, and worsening hypercalcemia. One or more of these limitations can usually be demonstrated in any given patient with hypercalcemia.

A patient with advanced breast carcinoma metastatic

to bone represents a severe hypercalcemic challenge. In such a patient, calcium is mobilized from bone by local osteolytic mechanisms; parathyroid function and $1,25(OH)_2D$ synthesis are appropriately suppressed, and the normal mechanisms of bone resorption, intestinal calcium absorption, and distal tubular calcium reabsorption are virtually eliminated. Initially, these adjustments may lead to a compensated steady state in which ~800–1,000 mg/day of mobilized calcium is excreted, with a serum calcium that is high-normal or only slightly elevated. With advancing disease or, as often occurs, with immobilization resulting from the basic disease process or an intercurrent illness, the quantity of mobilized calcium overwhelms the renal capacity for calcium excretion, and the spiral of hypercalcemia, dehydration, azotemia, and worsening hypercalcemia begins. In this circumstance, the serum calcium may climb from 10.5 to 15 mg/dL within 48 hr.

Systemic Phosphorus Homeostasis and Maintenance of a Normal Serum Phosphorus Concentration

The kidney plays the dominant role in systemic phosphorus homeostasis and maintains the serum phosphorus concentration at a value very close to the tubular phosphorus threshold or TmP/GFR. Because of the normal efficiency and lack of fine regulation of phosphorus absorption in the intestine, only in unusual circumstances (e.g., prolonged use of phosphate-binding antacids) is the systemic supply of phosphorus a limiting factor in phosphorus homeostasis. Thus, most disorders associated with chronic hypophosphatemia and/or phosphorus depletion in humans result from either intrinsic (e.g., familial hypophosphatemic rickets) or extrinsic (e.g., primary hyperparathyroidism) alterations in TmP/GFR. Similarly, most conditions of chronic hyperphosphatemia result from intrinsic (e.g., renal impairment) or extrinsic (e.g., hypoparathyroidism) abnormalities in the renal threshold for phosphorus. Acute hypophosphatemia most commonly results from the flux of extracellular phosphate ions into soft tissues.

The sequence of events initiated in the face of a hypophosphatemic challenge include: 1) stimulation of $1,25(OH)_2D$ synthesis in the kidney, 2) enhanced mobilization of phosphorus and calcium from bone, and 3) hypophosphatemia-induced increase in TmP/GFR (the exact mechanism of which is unknown). The increased circulating concentration of $1,25(OH)_2D$ leads to increases in phosphorus and calcium absorption in the intestine and provides an additional stimulus to phosphorus and calcium mobilization from bone. The increased flow of calcium from bone and the intestine results in an inhibition of PTH secretion, which diverts the systemic flow of calcium into the urine and further increases TmP/GFR. The net result of this sequence of adjustments is a return of the serum phosphorus concentration to normal without change in the serum calcium concentration.

The defense against hyperphosphatemia consists largely of a reversal of the sequence of adjustments just described. The principal humoral factor that combats hyp-

erphosphatemia is PTH. An acute rise in the serum phosphorus concentration produces a transient fall in the concentration of serum-ionized calcium and a stimulation of PTH secretion, which reduces TmP/GFR and leads to a readjustment in serum phosphorus and calcium concentrations. A prolonged rise in the serum phosphorus concentration results in 1) an intrinsic downward adjustment in TmP/GFR that is independent of PTH and 2) a persistent increase in PTH secretion that can ultimately lead to chief cell hyperplasia. If hyperphosphatemia is prolonged and severe (e.g., as occurs in chronic renal insufficiency), the degree of secondary hyperparathyroidism is sufficient to lead to the typical findings of parathyroid bone disease.

Systemic Magnesium Homeostasis and Maintenance of a Normal Serum Magnesium Concentration

The understanding of systemic magnesium homeostasis remains at a relatively primitive state. Unlike calcium and phosphorus, there appears to be no important systemic or hormonal regulation of the magnesium concentration in the extracellular fluids. Instead, maintenance of the serum magnesium concentration seems to result from the combined fluxes of magnesium at the levels of the intestine, kidney, intracellular fluids, and perhaps the skeleton. The kidney is primarily responsible for the regulation of the serum magnesium concentration.

The fractional absorption of magnesium is ~30%. In conditions of dietary magnesium excess a smaller proportion may be absorbed, and in conditions of dietary magnesium deficiency a higher proportion may be absorbed. The cellular mechanisms mediating magnesium absorption in the small intestine are poorly defined but would appear to consist of both passive and facilitated (but not active) elements. These elements do not seem to be sensitive to PTH, calcitonin, or $1,25(OH)_2D$. Thus, the net quantity of magnesium absorbed appears to be primarily a function of magnesium intake.

Of the ~2,000 mg of magnesium filtered per day, 96% is reabsorbed along the nephron and some 4% is excreted in the urine (fractional magnesium excretion). The mechanisms of magnesium reabsorption along the nephron at a cellular level are poorly understood, but, as is the case for calcium and phosphorus, it is possible to define a renal magnesium threshold or tubular maximum for magnesium (TmMg). The TmMg represents the net effects of magnesium reabsorption at different sites along the nephron. The TmMg is ~1.4 mg/dL when expressed as a function of the ultrafilterable serum magnesium concentration or 2.0 mg/dL when expressed as a function of the total serum magnesium concentration (4). The tubular maximum functions essentially as a setpoint for reabsorption, such that magnesium filtered at a concentration above the TmMg is excreted and that filtered at a concentration beneath the TmMg is retained. As in the intestine, renal tubular magnesium handling does not appear to be regulated by systemic or hormonal mechanisms in any important way.

In summary, systemic magnesium homeostasis does not appear to be hormonally regulated and therefore reflects largely the quantitative interplay of net magnesium absorption in the intestine and the fractional excretion of magnesium by the kidney. The fractional excretion of magnesium functions as a Tm-limited process and is primarily responsible for maintaining the serum magnesium concentration within rather narrow limits. The fine regulation of the serum magnesium concentration in the absence of hormonal controls provides an excellent example of the biological power of a Tm-limited transport process.

REFERENCES

1. Rasmussen H, Bordier P: *The Physiologic and Cellular Basis of Metabolic Bone Disease.* Williams & Wilkins, Baltimore, 1974

2. Krane SM: Calcium, phosphate and magnesium. In: Rasmussen H (ed) *International Encyclopedia of Pharmacology and Therapeutics, vol 1.* Pergamon Press, London, pp 19–59, 1970
3. Marshall RW: Plasma fractions. In: Nordin BEC (ed) *Calcium, Phosphate and Magnesium Metabolism.* Churchill Livingstone, London, pp 162–185, 1976
4. Rude RK, Singer FR: Magnesium deficiency and excess. *Ann Rev Med* 32:245–253, 1981
5. Rasmussen H, Rasmussen J: Calcium as intracellular messenger: From simplicity to complexity. *Curr Top Cell Regul* 31:1–109, 1990
6. Borle AB: Control, modulation and regulation of cell calcium. *Rev Physiol Biochem Pharmacol* 90:13–153, 1981
7. Stewart AF, Broadus AE: Mineral metabolism. In: Felig P, Baxter JD, Broadus AE, Frohman LA (eds) *Endocrinology and Metabolism, 2nd ed.* McGraw-Hill, New York, pp 1317–1453, 1987 (Much of the material in the present summary was drawn from this chapter.)

8. Intestinal Absorption of Calcium, Magnesium, and Phosphorus

Jacob Lemann, Jr., M.D.

Nephrology Division, Medical College of Wisconsin, Milwaukee, Wisconsin

Intestinal absorption of calcium (Ca), magnesium (Mg), and phosphorus (P) [phosphate (PO_4)] determines the supply of these minerals to meet the needs of increasing body mass, especially bone mineralization, during growth and the ongoing needs related to tissue turnover and bone remodeling in adults. The quantities of Ca, Mg, and PO_4 that are absorbed by the intestine are determined by the availability of these minerals in the diet and by the capacity of the intestine to absorb them. In general, intestinal mineral absorption represents the sum of two transport processes: saturable transcellular absorption that is physiologically regulated and nonsaturable paracellular absorption that is dependent on mineral concentration within the lumen of the gut.

Serum concentrations, urinary concentrations, and urinary excretion rates of Ca, Mg, or PO_4 are easily and routinely measured in the evaluation and care of patients with disorders of mineral metabolism and bone. However, quantitation of intestinal absorption of Ca, Mg, and PO_4 is difficult and has generally been assessed only in a research setting. Several techniques are available.

Metabolic balance: Subjects are fed constant diets and duplicate diets are analyzed for Ca, Mg, and PO_4. The subjects must be adapted to the diet for 7–10 days, especially if the quantity of Ca, Mg, or PO_4 in the diet differs significantly from a given subject's customary intake. In addition, because defecation occurs at irregular intervals, the subjects are continuously fed a measured quantity of a nonabsorbable marker that can be easily and reliably quantitated in the feces to verify achievement of the steady-state and to assign a time interval to the stool collections. Polyethylene glycol (PEG), chromium sesquioxide, or small segments of radiopaque tubing are often used as markers. Following the adaptation period, feces are collected during a balance period of at least 6 days duration and analyzed for Ca, Mg, and PO_4. Dietary intake minus average daily fecal excretion during the balance period provides an estimate of net intestinal absorption of Ca, Mg, or PO_4.

Absorption from a single meal following intestinal washout: After overnight fasting, subjects undergo intestinal lavage over a period of 4 hr with a solution that does not cause either net intestinal absorption or secretion of water and electrolytes. Four hours following completion of lavage, they are fed a meal together with a known amount of the nonabsorbable marker PEG. A duplicate meal is analyzed for Ca, Mg, and PO_4. Twelve hours after the meal intestinal lavage is repeated by 3 hr. The rectal effluent is collected and, together with any stool passed after ingestion of the meal, analyzed for Ca, Mg, PO_4, and PEG. Intake in the meal minus effluent excretion, corrected for the recovery of PEG, provides an estimate of net intestinal absorption of Ca, Mg, or PO_4. The study can be repeated on a separate day when the subjects ingest only PEG without food to measure the quantities of Ca, Mg, or PO_4 secreted into the intestine. Total intestinal Ca, Mg, or PO_4 absorption (true absorption) can then be calculated as the sum of net absorption from the meal plus the quantity appearing in the effluent during fasting.

Both the balance method and the intestinal washout method provide estimates of actual net mineral input to the body from the intestine.

Absorption of isotopic minerals: A measured quantity of ^{47}Ca is administered orally. The fraction of the dose absorbed can be estimated either by external counting of radioisotope in the arm at a fixed time after dosing, by counting of isotope in serial blood samples and expressing fractional absorption as percentage of dose/liter plasma when counts peak, or by collecting and counting isotope excreted in the feces over 4–6 days after dosing and subtracting isotope excreted from the dose. Alternatively and more precisely, a measured quantity of ^{45}Ca can be administered intravenously together with the oral dose of ^{47}Ca. Ca absorption can then be estimated from the ratio of isotope concentrations or specific activities in serum or urine, or the absorption rate can be estimated by compartmental kinetic analysis using multiple serum samples collected over 4–6 hr after dosing. The stable isotopes ^{42}Ca and ^{44}Ca have also been used with measurement by mass spectrometry. Absorption of isotopic Mg and PO_4 have not been studied because ^{28}Mg has a half-life of only 21 hr and because of the unacceptably intense β-emission of ^{32}P.

Segmental intestinal absorption: Subjects fast overnight and a triple-lumen tube is passed to the duodenum, jejunum, ileum, or colon. Perfusate containing Ca, Mg, and PO_4 together with a nonabsorbable marker is instilled via the proximal lumen and aspirated at a constant rate from both the middle lumen, where mixing of the perfusate with intestinal contents has been completed, and from the distal lumen. The length of the intestinal study segment between the middle and distal lumens is usually 30 cm. Absorption of Ca, Mg, or PO_4 can then be estimated by the change in mineral concentration in the fluid aspirated distally relative to that aspirated at the end of the mixing segment, taking into account the simultaneous change in PEG concentration as a measure of perfusate absorption.

Indirect assessment of intestinal mineral absorption: After overnight fasting and collection of control urine and blood specimens, subjects are given 25 mmol Ca (1,000 mg) orally. Two subsequent 2-hr urines are collected together with blood samples 1 and 3 hr after the load. Fasting $U_{Ca}V$/glomerular filtration rate (GFR) is normally <0.035 mmol/L GFR (<0.13 mg/100 ml GFR) and among subjects exhibiting normal rates of intestinal Ca absorption the increment in $U_{Ca}V$/GFR following the load is <0.05 mmol/L GFR (<0.2 mg/100 ml GFR). Greater increases in $U_{Ca}V$/GFR after the oral Ca load provide evidence for increased intestinal Ca absorption.

CALCIUM

The relationship between net intestinal Ca absorption/day (dietary Ca intake/day minus fecal Ca excretion/day) and dietary Ca intake/day, derived from metabolic balance studies of healthy adults, is illustrated in Fig. 1. On the average, net intestinal Ca absorption is less than zero (e.g., fecal Ca excretion/day exceeds dietary Ca intake/day) when dietary Ca intake/day is <5 mmol/day (<200 mg/day). Thus, on the average, healthy adults require daily Ca intakes >10 or more mmol/day (>400 mg/day) to maintain Ca balance, taking into account both the inability of the normal kidney to excrete urine that is essentially free of Ca (unlike Na, Mg, or PO_4) and ongoing minor skin losses of Ca. As dietary Ca intake/day rises

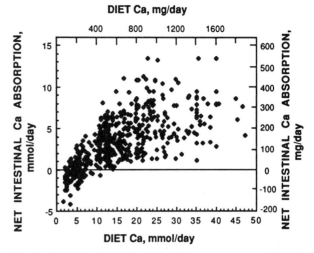

FIG. 1. Net intestinal Ca absorption as measured by the metabolic balance method in relation to dietary Ca intake among healthy adults.

from minimal intakes of 3–5 mmol/day (120–200 mg/day), net intestinal Ca absorption/day increases, but in progressively decreasing quantity such that when Ca intake exceeds about 25 mmol/day (1,000 mg/day) net intestinal Ca absorption tends, on the average, to plateau at an average value of ~7.5 mmol/day (300 mg/day). The curvilinear relationship between net intestinal Ca absorption and dietary Ca intake reflects the sum of two absorptive mechanisms: active, saturable absorption and passive absorption dependent on the concentration gradient between intestinal lumen and blood. The wide variation of net intestinal Ca absorption among healthy adults at any given level of dietary intake that is seen in Fig. 1, especially when dietary Ca intake exceeds 15–20 mmol/day (600–800 mg/day), is presumed to reflect primarily variation in active Ca absorption between subjects.

Currently, 1,25-dihydroxyvitamin D [1,25(OH)$_2$D or calcitriol] is the only recognized hormonal stimulus of active intestinal Ca absorption that occurs principally in the duodenum and jejunum. Figure 2 shows the average rela-

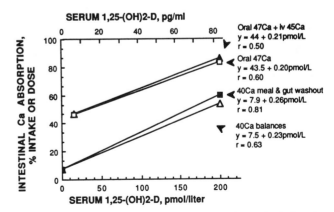

FIG. 2. Average relationships between intestinal Ca absorption as a percentage of intake and serum 1,25(OH)$_2$D concentrations.

tionships between dietary Ca absorption and serum $1,25(OH)_2D$ concentrations, when absorption is measured by the balance technique, by postmeal intestinal washout, and by two isotopic methods. Ca absorption is expressed as a percentage of dietary or meal intake or isotope administered. Dietary Ca intake during the balance studies averaged 22 mmol/day (880 mg/day) and Ca intake in the washout studies was 7.55 mmol/meal (302 mg/meal), equivalent to 22.6 mmol/day (906 mg/day) in three meals. As shown in Fig. 2, the slopes of fractional Ca absorption as a function of serum $1,25(OH)_2D$ are nearly identical for all of the techniques of measurement of Ca absorption and the average magnitude of these slopes [~0.2% Ca absorbed/pmol $1,25(OH)_2D$/L or ~0.5% Ca absorbed/pg $1,25(OH)_2D$/mL] documents the critical dependence of Ca absorption on prevailing serum $1,25(OH)_2D$ in human beings. Moreover, the data for the balance studies and the intestinal washout studies, which reflect actual input of Ca to the body, indicate that in the absence of $1,25(OH)_2D$ only ~7% of a normal Ca intake is absorbed.

The interaction of dietary Ca intake and prevailing serum $1,25(OH)_2D$ concentrations as determinants of net intestinal Ca absorption is depicted in Fig. 3. When dietary Ca intake is very low, 4 mmol/day (160 mg/day), net intestinal Ca absorption reaches a maximum of ~3 mmol/day (120 mg/day), even when serum $1,25(OH)_2D$ levels are higher than the upper limit of the normal range (>135 pmol/l or >56 pg/mL). By contrast, when dietary Ca intake is normal, 20 mmol/day (800 mg/day), net intestinal Ca absorption may exceed 10 mmol/day (400 mg/day), a value at the upper limit of the wide normal range shown in Fig. 1, when serum $1,25(OH)_2D$ levels average 120 pmol/L (50 pg/ml), a concentration that is within the upper limit of the normal range. Thus, reduced net intestinal Ca absorption occurs when either dietary Ca intake is limited,

TABLE 1. *Causes of reduced and increased intestinal Ca absorption*

Reduced Ca absorption	Increased Ca absorption
$1,25(OH)_2$ deficiency 　Vitamin D deficiency 　Vitamin D-dependent rickets, type I (25-OH-D-1-α-hydroxylase deficiency) Chronic kidney disease Hypoparathyroidism $1,25(OH)_2D$ resistance 　Vitamin D-dependent rickets, type II [absent or abnormal receptors for $1,25(OH)_2D$ or in postreceptor events mediating hormone action] Intestinal disease	Increased $1,25(OH)_2D$ 　During growth 　Hyperparathyroidism 　Sarcoid and other granulomas [extrarenal $1,25(OH)_2D$ synthesis] Idiopathic hypercalciuria [may also include increased sensitivity to $1,25(OH)_2D$ or enhanced absorption by a vitamin D-independent mechanism]

when serum $1,25(OH)_2D$ concentrations are low or when the intestine is unresponsive to this hormone. Increased intestinal Ca absorption occurs when serum $1,25(OH)_2D$ concentrations are high or, possibly, even only high-normal because of the effect of $1,25(OH)_2D$ to upregulate its own receptor. Very high Ca intakes also increase absorption, but such an increase in passive Ca absorption is accompanied by suppression of serum $1,25(OH)_2D$, which would tend to blunt the increase in absorption. The major disorders reducing or enhancing intestinal Ca absorption are listed in Table 1.

MAGNESIUM

The relationship between net intestinal Mg absorption/day (dietary Mg intake/day minus fecal Mg excretion/day) and dietary Mg intake/day, derived from metabolic balance studies of healthy adults, is illustrated in Fig. 4. Net

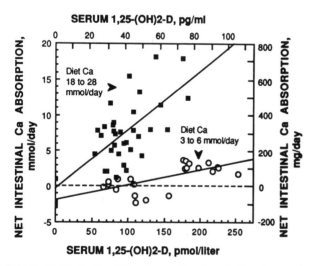

FIG. 3. Net intestinal Ca absorption in relation to serum $1,25(OH)_2D$ concentrations among subjects fed normal Ca diets [*solid symbols;* net intestinal Ca absorption, mmol/day = $-0.4 + 0.082$ serum $1,25(OH)_2D$, pmol/L; $r = 0.71$] or low Ca diets [*open symbols;* net intestinal Ca absorption, mmol/day = $-2.0 + 0.021$ serum $1,25(OH)_2D$, pmol/L; $r = 0.56$].

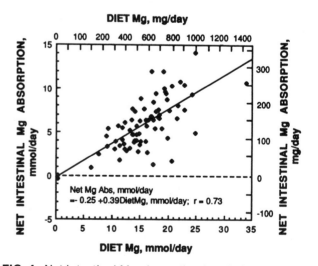

FIG. 4. Net intestinal Mg absorption in relation to dietary Mg intake among healthy adults.

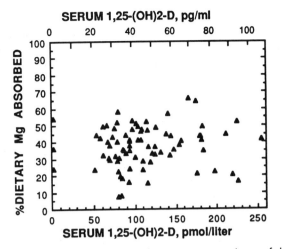

FIG. 5. Lack of a relationship between percentage of diet Mg absorbed ([diet Mg] − [fecal Mg]*100/[diet Mg]) and serum 1,25(OH)$_2$D in adults.

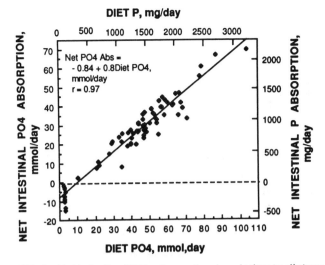

FIG. 6. Net intestinal PO$_4$ absorption in relation to dietary PO$_4$ intake among healthy adults.

intestinal Mg absorption is directly related to dietary Mg intake, on the average ~35–40% being absorbed when dietary Mg intake is in the normal range for adults of 7–30 mmol/day (168–720 mg/day). Because Mg is a constituent of all cells and normal diets contain foods of cellular origin, dietary Mg intake is generally proportional to total caloric intake, thus ensuring adequate intestinal Mg absorption. The data in Fig. 4 also include observations from studies of Mg balance using synthetic diets that are nearly Mg-free. Net intestinal Mg absorption is less than zero [e.g., fecal Mg excretion/day exceeds dietary Mg intake/ day only when dietary Mg intake is <2 mmol/day (48 mg/ day)]. The variation in net intestinal Mg absorption among healthy subjects at any given normal level of dietary Mg intake appears to be related to other constituents of the diet, such as PO$_4$, that complex Mg within the intestinal lumen and limit absorption. In contrast to Ca absorption, Mg absorption is not increased as serum 1,25(OH)$_2$D concentrations vary from undetectable to high among adults (Fig. 5). Dietary Mg intakes exceeding 35 mmol/day (840 mg/day) seldom occur spontaneously. Additional oral Mg is often taken as a cathartic Mg(OH)$_2$ or Mg-citrate, and whereas a small fraction of this Mg may be absorbed, such an effect is apt to lead to hypermagnesemia only in the presence of significant reductions in kidney function. Thus, Mg-containing laxatives and antacids should not be given to patients with kidney disease. Reduced intestinal Mg absorption occurs with diffuse intestinal diseases causing malabsorption or as a consequence of laxative abuse.

PHOSPHATE

Intestinal PO$_4$ absorption, like the absorption of Ca, is dependent on both passive PO$_4$ transport related to the lumenal [PO$_4$] prevailing after a meal and on active PO$_4$ transport that is stimulated by 1,25(OH)$_2$D. The relationship between net intestinal PO$_4$ absorption/day (dietary PO$_4$ intake/day minus fecal PO$_4$ excretion/day) and dietary PO$_4$ intake/day, derived from metabolic balance

studies in healthy adults, is shown in Fig. 6. As for Mg absorption in relation to dietary Mg intake, PO$_4$ absorption is directly related to dietary PO$_4$ intake. Because PO$_4$ is a major constituent of all cells, dietary PO$_4$ intake seldom is <20 mmol/day (<620 mg P/day) among healthy adults. Based on studies using synthetic diets providing only 2–3 mmol PO$_4$/day (62–93 mg P/day), there is net intestinal secretion of PO$_4$ when dietary PO$_4$ intake is <10 mmol/day (<310 mg P/day), fecal PO$_4$ excretion exceeding dietary PO$_4$ intake. When dietary PO$_4$ intake varies over the usual normal range of 25–60 mmol/day (775–1,860 mg P/day), 60–80% of dietary PO$_4$ is absorbed. Higher oral PO$_4$ intakes seldom occur spontaneously.

Intestinal PO$_4$ absorption is reduced in vitamin D-deficiency and the administration of 1,25(OH)$_2$D to patients with chronic renal failure who lack this hormone stimulates jejunal PO$_4$ absorption. However, experimental elevations of serum 1,25(OH)$_2$D in healthy subjects does not further stimulate jejunal PO$_4$ absorption significantly and, as shown in Fig. 7, fractional PO$_4$ absorption estimated

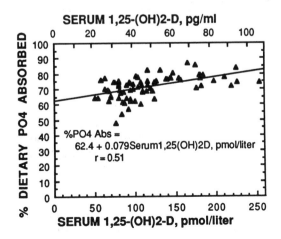

FIG. 7. Relationship between percentage dietary PO$_4$ absorbed ([diet PO$_4$] − [fecal PO$_4$]*100/[diet PO$_4$]) and serum 1,25(OH)$_2$D concentrations in adults.

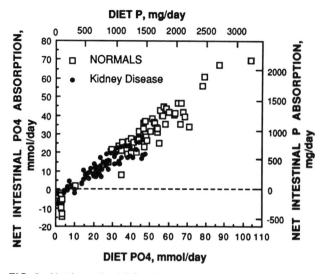

FIG. 8. Net intestinal PO_4 absorption in relation to dietary PO_4 intake among patients with chronic kidney disease ($C_{creatinine}$ 3–50 ml/min; *solid circles*) and healthy adults *(open squares).*

by the balance technique increases only slightly, although significantly, as serum $1,25(OH)_2D$ concentrations vary from normal to high among adults fed diets providing normal amounts of PO_4. Even in the presence of very low serum $1,25(OH)_2D$ levels, patients with chronic renal failure exhibit significant concentration-dependent jejunal PO_4 absorption. Thus, the availability of PO_4 in the diet appears to be the major determinant of net PO_4 input to the body from the intestine.

Continuing absorption of dietary PO_4 is a major factor in the pathogenesis of secondary hyperparathyroidism occurring in patients with progressive kidney disease and as shown in Fig. 8, net intestinal PO_4 absorption among patients with chronic kidney disease in relation to dietary

PO_4 intake over the range of 10–50 mmol/day (310–1,550 mg P/day) is nearly identical to the relationship in normal subjects. Intestinal PO_4 absorption is also not apparently significantly reduced among patients with disorders associated with chronic hyperphosphatemia such as hypoparathyroidism and tumoral calcinosis.

Because of the ability of Al^{3+} and of Ca^{2+} to form insoluble PO_4 salts and thus limit intestinal PO_4 absorption, aluminum hydroxide gel, aluminum carbonate and, more recently in an attempt to prevent the potential toxicity of aluminum, calcium carbonate, and calcium acetate are routinely used in the care of patients with advanced renal failure. Chronic abuse of aluminum-containing antacids, by inhibiting absorption of dietary PO_4 and reabsorption of PO_4 entering the lumen of the gut in intestinal secretions, can rarely result in PO_4 depletion. PO_4 malabsorption can also occur with diffuse disease of the small intestine.

SELECTED REFERENCES

1. Alpers DH: Absorption of vitamins and divalent minerals. In: Sleisenger MH, Fortran JS (eds) *Gastrointestinal Disease. 4th Ed.* WB Saunders Company, Philadelphia, 1989
2. Nordin BEC (ed): *Calcium, Phosphate and Magnesium Metabolism* Churchill Livingstone, Edinburgh, 1976
3. Gallagher JC, Riggs BL, Eisman J, Hamstra A: Intestinal calcium absorption and serum vitamin D metabolites in normal subjects and osteoporotic patients. *J Clin Invest* 64:729–736, 1979
4. Kaplan RA, Haussler MR, Deftos LJ, Bone H, Pak CYC: The role of 1α-25-dihydroxyvitamin D in the mediation of intestinal hyperabsorption of calcium in primary hyperparathyroidism and absorptive hypercalciuria. *J Clin Invest* 59:756, 1977
5. Sheikh MS, Ramirez A, Emmett M, et al.: Role of vitamin D-dependent and vitamin D-independent mechanisms in absorption of food calcium. *J Clin Invest* 81:126, 1988
6. Wilz DR, Gray RW, Dominguez JH, Lemann J Jr: Plasma 1,25-$(OH)_2$-vitamin D concentrations and net intestinal calcium, phosphate and magnesium absorption in humans. *Am J Clin Nutr* 32: 2052–2060, 1979

9. Urinary Excretion of Calcium, Magnesium, and Phosphorus

Jacob Lemann, Jr., M.D.

Nephrology Division, Medical College of Wisconsin, Milwaukee, Wisconsin

As elemental substances, neither calcium (Ca), magnesium (Mg), nor phosphorus (P) [phosphate (PO_4)] are metabolized to other substances in the body. Thus, the quantities of Ca, Mg, and PO_4 excreted in the urine must ultimately be derived either from the diet (as determined by the dietary content and the efficiency of intestinal absorption of these minerals or from body stores (as determined by net rates of mineral deposition in tissues during growth or losses from tissues during senescence or disease) or from both of these sources.

Measurements of urinary mineral excretion can be viewed in several different ways that may be useful in the evaluation of patients with disorders of mineral metabolism, including metabolic bone disease or nephrolithiasis:

Absolute mineral excretion rates per unit time, as in the 24-hr urine collections, are useful in detecting lower or higher than normal excretion rates—e.g., the detection of hypercalciuria. These measurements require accurately timed and complete urine collections with measurement of urinary mineral concentration and urinary volume in order to calculate daily mineral excretion, as well as measurement of urinary creatinine concentration with calculation of daily creatinine excretion rate to verify that the urine collection is complete in relation to the weight, sex, and age of the patient (men: 20–27 mg creatinine/kg/day or 0.17–0.24 mmol creatinine/kg/day; women: 15–22 mg creatinine/kg/day or 0.13–0.19 mmol creatinine/kg/day; less in both sexes with absolute loss of muscle mass or low muscle mass in relation to total body weight as with obesity). Urinary mineral concentration may also be factored by creatinine concentration to take into account possible collection errors.

Urinary mineral excretion rates factored by glomerular filtration, the latter usually estimated from serum and urinary creatinine concentrations, may be evaluated in relation to serum mineral concentrations to assess the role of the kidney in determining abnormally low or high serum mineral concentrations. For example, the normal rates of urinary PO_4 excretion/glomerular filtration rate (GFR) despite hypophosphatemia among patients with X-linked hypophosphatemic rickets indicate renal PO_4 wasting, and the low rates of urinary Ca excretion/GFR despite hypercalcemia among patients with familial hypocalciuric hypercalcemia indicate abnormal renal Ca retention. These measurements require only a random and untimed ("spot") urine collection, preferably obtained while the patient is fasting, together with a simultaneously obtained blood sample. The urinary excretion of a substance, such as Ca, per unit GFR is formally described by the expression:

$U_{Ca}V/GFR$, mmol/L

$$= \frac{(UCa, \text{mmol/L}) (\text{Urine Flow Rate, V, L/day})}{\dfrac{(U_{creatinine} \text{ mmol/L} (\text{Urine Flow Rate, V, L/day})}{(S_{creatinine}, \text{mmol/L})}} \quad [1]$$

However, it is evident that the urine flow rate, V, appears in both the numerator and the denominator of this expression. Thus it is not necessary to obtain a timed urine collection. The expression therefore becomes:

$U_{Ca}V/GFR$, mmol/L

$$= \frac{(U_{Ca}, \text{mmol/L}) (S_{creatinine}, \text{mmol/L})}{(U_{creatinine}, \text{mmol/L})} \quad [2]$$

Mass concentration units, mg/dl (mg/100 ml), are also often used in these calculations. It is thus important to be sure that the concentration units are the same for creatinine and the mineral being evaluated.

Estimation of the quantity of a mineral excreted in the urine as a fraction or as a percentage of the quantity of that mineral that is filtered by the glomeruli may also be estimated using the measurements in a random urine and a simultaneous blood sample:

% Excreted/Filtered PO_4 (%E/FPO_4)

$$= \frac{(U_{PO_4}, \text{mmol/L}) (\text{Serum}_{creatinine}, \text{mmol/L}) (100)}{(\text{Serum } PO_4, \text{mmol/L}) (U_{creatinine}, \text{mmol/L})} \quad [3]$$

The percentage of the filtered PO_4 that is reabsorbed by the kidney tubules can then be estimated as (100) − %E/FPO_4.

The urinary concentration of a mineral in a 24-hr or a random urine may also be usefully evaluated. For example, the urinary Ca concentration in relation to other urinary constituents (oxalate, citrate, monohydrogen phosphate, dihydrogen phosphate, and sulfate) in the assessment of the relative saturation of the urine with respect to the potentially insoluble salts calcium oxalate and apatite that are the most common constituents of urinary stones.

CALCIUM

Among healthy adults in the steady-state who are eating diets providing 20 mmol Ca/day (800 mg Ca/day), net intestinal Ca absorption averages ~4 mmol/day (160 mg/day) or 20% of dietary Ca intake. Although bone is continuously remodeled, there is no net bone resorption or net bone formation. Thus, in order to sustain the steady state where intake is matched by output and balance is zero, the kidneys must excrete 4 mmol Ca/day (160 mg/day). Serum total [Ca] averages 2.4 mmol/L (9.6 mg/dL) but only 60% is ultrafilterable across the glomeruli, the remainder being bound to serum proteins, chiefly albumin. Serum ionized $[Ca^{2+}]$ averages 50% of total [Ca]. In a healthy adult with a GFR of 175 L/day (122 mL/min) and a serum ultrafilterable [Ca] ($[UF_{Ca}]$) of 1.44 mmol/L (5.8 mg/dL), 252 mmol of Ca/day are filtered (7 mg/min or about 10,100 mg/day). Because urinary Ca excretion is only 4 mmol/day, >98% of filtered Ca is reabsorbed by the tubules and <2% of filtered Ca is excreted into the urine.

Figure 1 summarizes the major factors influencing urinary Ca excretion. The maximum range of daily urinary Ca excretion in healthy adults is from ~1 mmol/day (40 mg/day) to 7.5 mmol/day (300 mg/day), whereas in disease urinary Ca excretion may be <1 mmol/day and can range upward to as much as 20 mmol/day (800 mg/day). Urinary Ca excretion declines to low levels among patients with kidney disease as a consequence of both the fall in GFR and the early onset of secondary hyperparathyroidism

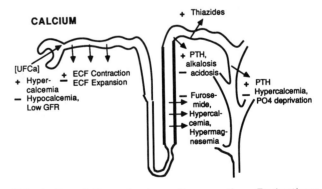

FIG. 1. Regulation of urinary Ca excretion. Reductions (−) in GFR of Ca reduce urinary Ca excretion, whereas inhibition (−) of renal tubular Ca reabsorption increase urinary Ca excretion.

that stimulates renal tubular reabsorption of filtered Ca. Hypocalcemic disorders, typified by hypoparathyroidism, are generally accompanied by very low rates of urinary Ca excretion as a consequence of the decline in glomerular filtration of Ca, although rare patients with tubulointerstitial kidney disease may exhibit hypercalciuria despite hypocalcemia—evidence for a renal Ca "leak." Hypercalcemic disorders, with the exception of familial hypocalciuric hypercalcemia (FHH), are generally associated with hypercalciuria and, as shown in Fig. 2, evaluation of $U_{Ca}V/GFR$ in relation to serum [Ca] may provide useful preliminary diagnostic information in the evaluation of patients that are found to exhibit hypercalcemia. Among healthy adults with normal serum total [Ca] concentrations ranging from 2.2 to 2.6 mmol/L (8.8–10.4 mg/dL), $U_{Ca}V/GFR$ does not exceed 0.035 mmol/L GFR (0.14 mg/100 mL GFR). Among patients with FHH, $U_{Ca}V/GFR$ is normal despite hypercalcemia emphasizing the role of augmented renal tubular Ca reabsorption in causing the hypercalcemia. Among patients with primary hyperparathyroidism, $U_{Ca}V/GFR$ ranges from normal to values generally not exceeding 0.1 mmol/L GFR (0.4 mg/100 mL GFR), because the stimulation by parathyroid hormone (PTH) of renal tubular reabsorption of filtered Ca tends to offset the increase in glomerular filtration of Ca and the inhibition of renal tubular Ca reabsorption by hypercalcemia (Fig. 1). Patients with hypercalcemia in relation to cancer or to a granuloma such as sarcoid generally exhibit $U_{Ca}V/GFR$ exceeding 0.1 mmol/L GFR (0.4 mg/100 mL GFR), because PTH secretion is inhibited by hypercalcemia, 1,25-dihydroxyvitamin D or both, and thus the effect of PTH to stimulate tubular reabsorption of filtered Ca is minimized.

Among healthy adults eating diets providing 15–30 mmol Ca/day (600–1,200 mg/day), urinary Ca excretion averages 4 mmol/day (160 mg/day), but ranges from 1 to 7.5 mmol/day (40–300 mg/day). The wide range is accounted for by the integrated effects of individual variations in the efficiency of intestinal Ca absorption, net bone

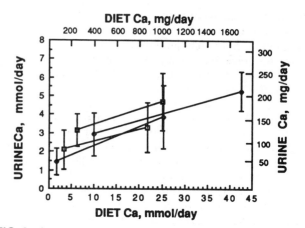

FIG. 3. Average variation in daily urinary Ca excretion ± SD as dietary intake is varied in healthy adults.

resorption, GFR, serum [UF_{Ca}], and other dietary and hormonal factors that modulate renal tubular Ca reabsorption. Among normal subjects, as shown in Fig. 3, daily urinary Ca excretion increases on the average by ~8% or 0.08 mmol/day per mmol/day increment in dietary Ca (8 mg/day/100 mg increment in dietary Ca), as dietary Ca intake varies from low intakes of 2–10 mmol/day (80–400 mg/day) to intakes of 20–40 mmol/day (800–1,600 mg/day). Urinary Ca excretion falls within 2–4 days when subjects are fed diets providing 5 mmol Ca/day (200 mg/day) or less. Even after subjects are adapted to such diets for long periods individual minimum urinary Ca excretion rates vary widely from ~0.5 to 5 mmol/day (20–200 mg/day), presumably because of individual differences in net bone resorption and the regulation of renal tubular Ca reabsorption.

Urinary Ca excretion increases as dietary NaCl intake increases, the increments being in the range of 0.6–1.2 mmol/100 mmol increment in daily urinary NaCl excretion (25–50 mg/100 mmol NaCl) as dietary NaCl intake varies over the usual extremes in health from 10 to 350 mmol/day. This effect appears to be mainly related to inhibition of proximal tubular Ca reabsorption accompanying salt-induced extracellular fluid (ECF)-volume expansion, but inhibition of Ca reabsorption in the distal nephron may also contribute.

Metabolic acidosis is accompanied by increased urinary Ca excretion as a result of inhibition of distal renal tubular Ca reabsorption. The effect of acidosis is independent of PTH. As serum [HCO_3] falls to the range of 16–20 mmol/L and GFR remains normal, urinary Ca excretion can reach rates of 15–20 mmol/day. Increasing dietary protein intake is accompanied by increased urinary Ca excretion related to the increased production of fixed acid as amino acid-sulfur is oxidized to sulfate, apparently an effect of both mild acidosis and the ability of sulfate to complex Ca within renal tubular fluid, thus limiting Ca reabsorption. Conversely, metabolic alkalosis or the administration $NaHCO_3$ or K-citrate reduces urinary Ca excretion due to enhanced distal tubular Ca reabsorption. Potassium may have an additional effect to enhance tubular Ca reabsorption, because $KHCO_3$ or K-citrate reduce urinary Ca to

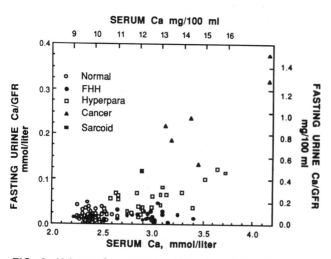

FIG. 2. Urinary Ca excretion/GFR in relation to serum total [Ca] in health and hypercalcemic disorders. *FHH*, familial hypocalciuric hypercalcemia; *Hyperpara*, primary hyperparathyroidism.

a greater degree than equivalent amounts of $NaHCO_3$ or Na-citrate. Ingestion of rapidly metabolizable nutrients such as glucose, sucrose, and ethanol is accompanied by increased urinary Ca excretion, also as a consequence of inhibition of tubular Ca reabsorption. Extreme degrees of dietary PO_4 restriction (<10 mmol/day or <300 mg/day) are associated with increased urinary Ca excretion that is the result of inhibition of PTH secretion and thus the effect of PTH to enhance renal tubular Ca reabsorption, as well as a direct effect of PO_4 deprivation to inhibit tubular Ca reabsorption.

The administration of furosemide, bumetanide, or other diuretics acting on the thick ascending loop of Henle is accompanied by inhibition of tubular Ca reabsorption at this site and increased urinary Ca excretion. By contrast, administration of thiazide diuretics is accompanied by increased tubular Ca reabsorption in the distal renal tubule and a fall in urinary Ca excretion. The administration of chlorthalidone, amiloride, or indapamide also reduce urinary Ca excretion.

Hypercalciuria (urinary Ca excretion >7.5 mmol/day; >300 mg/day or >0.1 mmol/kg/day; >4 mg/kg/day), in the absence of hypercalcemia, occurs among ~50% of patients having kidney stones composed of calcium oxalate and/or apatite and is one of the risk factors for the crystallization of these insoluble salts. Rates of glomerular filtration of Ca in the upper normal range and subtle suppression of PTH are believed to be the mechanisms involved. Increased intestinal Ca absorption is the major source of the extra Ca appearing in the urine of these patients due either to activation of 1,25dihydroxyvitamin D production or a vitamin D-independent mechanism. Nevertheless, fasting $U_{Ca}V$/GFR may be higher than normal (>0.05 mmol/L GFR or >0.14 mg/100 ml GFR), despite a normal serum [Ca], suggesting that either accelerated bone turnover or a renal Ca leak may be contributing to the hypercalciuria among some of these patients.

Abnormally rapid rates of bone resorption as seen among suddenly immobilized patients also can result in both daily and fasting hypercalciuria.

MAGNESIUM

Among normal adults eating diets providing 15 mmol Mg/day (360 mg Mg/day), net intestinal Mg absorption averages about 6 mmol/day (144 mg/day) or ~40% of dietary Mg intake. Thus in order to preserve the steady-state where intake is matched by output and balance is near zero, the kidneys must excrete 6 mmol Mg/day (144 mg/day). Serum total [Mg] averages 0.9 mmol/L (2.2 mg/dL), but only 70% is ultrafilterable across the glomeruli, the remainder being bound to serum proteins. In a healthy adult with a GFR of 175 L/day and a serum $[UF_{Mg}]$ of 0.63 mmol/L (1.5 mg/dL), 110 mmol Mg/day are filtered (1.8 mg/min or ~2,650 mg/day). Because urinary Mg excretion is only 6 mmol/day (144 mg/day), ~95% of filtered Mg is reabsorbed by the tubules and only ~5% is excreted in the urine.

MAGNESIUM

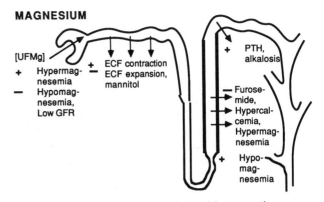

FIG. 4. Regulation of urinary Mg excretion.

Figure 4 summarizes the major factors influencing urinary Mg excretion. In health, urinary Mg excretion declines as serum [Mg] falls. The fractional excretion of Mg rises as GFR falls among patients with progressive kidney disease, thus preventing a rise in serum Mg concentration until renal failure is severe. As shown in Fig. 5, urinary Mg excretion among healthy adults is directly related to dietary Mg as intake varies from 0.5 mmol/day (12 mg/day) or less to 33 mmol/day (800 mg/day). Urinary Mg excretion falls to sustained low levels of <0.5 mmol/day (<12 mg/day) within 3–6 days when dietary Mg is reduced to 0.5 mmol/day (12 mg/day) or less.

Urinary Mg excretion increases with inhibition of proximal tubular reabsorption by ECF-volume expansion or osmotic diuretics such as mannitol. Hypermagnesemia and hypercalcemia inhibit tubular Mg reabsorption in the thick ascending loop of Henle, as does furosemide and bumetanide that act at this site. Some other drugs, notably cis-platinum, also inhibit Mg reabsorption in Henle's loop. Hypomagnesemia enhances Mg reabsorption. PTH and metabolic alkalosis enhance Mg reabsorption in the distal tubule.

PHOSPHATE

Among healthy adults who are eating diets providing 40 mmol PO_4/day (1,240 mg P/day), net intestinal PO_4 ab-

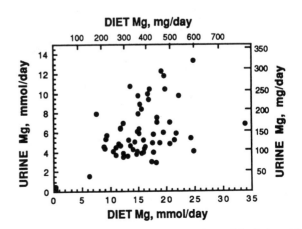

FIG. 5. Variation in urinary Mg excretion with dietary Mg intake in healthy adults.

sorption averages ~25 mmol/day (775 mg P/day) or ~60% of dietary PO_4 intake. Although bone is continuously remodeled and PO_4 in muscle and all other tissues is cycled to and from the ECF in the course of metabolism, there is no net gain or loss of PO_4 from these processes. Thus, in order to maintain the steady-state where intake is matched by output and balance is near zero, the kidneys must excrete 25 mmol PO_4/day (775 mg P/day). Serum total $[PO_4]$ concentration averages 1.2 mmol/L (3.7 mg P/dL) and is generally considered to be completely ultrafilterable across the glomeruli. However, a small fraction, 10% or less, may be bound to protein or otherwise complexed and not filterable. In a healthy adult with a GFR of 175 L/day (12 mL/min), ~210 mmol PO_4/day are filtered (4.5 mg P/min or ~6500 mg P/day). Because urinary PO_4 excretion is only 25 mmol/day, ~88% of filtered PO_4 is reabsorbed by the tubules and ~12% is excreted into the urine.

Figure 6 summarizes the major factors influencing urinary PO_4 excretion. Urinary PO_4 excretion appears to increase as serum $[PO_4]$ increases both as a result of increased filtration of PO_4, as well as inhibition of renal tubular PO_4 reabsorption. As GFR falls progressively among patients with kidney disease, the early development of secondary hyperparathyroidism inhibits renal tubular PO_4 reabsorption and, despite the fall in glomerular filtration of PO_4, preserves normal rates of urinary PO_4 excretion, thereby preventing hyperphosphatemia until GFR falls to ~25% of normal.

As shown in Fig. 7, urinary PO_4 excretion among healthy adults is directly related to dietary PO_4, as intakes vary from 2 to 80 mmol/day (62–2,480 mg P/day). Urinary PO_4 excretion falls to <0.5 mmol/day (<15 mg P/day) within 3–5 days when dietary PO_4 is reduced to only 2–4 mmol/day (62–124 mg P/day). Such avid renal PO_4 conservation can occur either without a detectable change in serum $[PO_4]$ or with only minor reductions to levels that are within the normal range for serum $[PO_4]$ of 0.9–1.5 mmol/L (2.8–4.6 mg P/dL). Measurement of $U_{PO_4}V$/GFR in a fasting or a spot urine in relation to serum $[PO_4]$ may

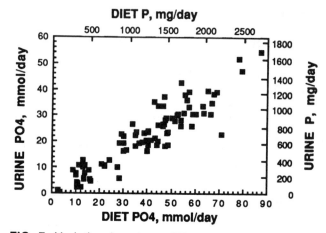

FIG. 7. Variation in urinary PO_4 excretion with dietary PO_4 intake in healthy adults.

be useful in the initial assessment of patients that exhibit hypophosphatemia. Patients who are hypophosphatemic as a consequence of dietary PO_4 deprivation or diarrheal PO_4 losses would be expected to exhibit maximum renal PO_4 conservation and thus a $U_{PO_4}V$/GFR of <0.01–0.02 mmol/L GFR or <0.03–0.06 mg/100 mL GFR. By contrast patients who are hypophosphatemic as a consequence of inhibition of renal tubular PO_4 reabsorption exhibit normal or near-normal rates of urinary PO_4 excretion in the steady-state and $U_{PO_4}V$/GFR is in the normal range of 0.06–0.25 mmol/L GFR or 0.18–0.78 mg/100 mL GFR. Such patients include those with primary hyperparathyroidism, with hereditary hypophosphatemic disorders (X-linked hypophosphatemic rickets, familial hypophosphatemic rickets with hypercalciuria) or acquired hypophosphatemia as in oncogenic hypophosphatemia, Cushing's syndrome, and with chronic glucocorticoid therapy.

Urinary PO_4 excretion is normal in childhood and among patients with acromegaly, despite higher than normal serum $[PO_4]$ concentrations. The effect of growth hormone or, perhaps a somatomedin, is to augment tubular PO_4 reabsorption (Fig. 6). Normal rates of urinary PO_4 excretion despite hyperphosphatemia are also observed in patients with tumoral calcinosis.

SELECTED REFERENCES

1. Suki WN, Rouze R: Renal transport of calcium, magnesium and phosphorus. In: Brenner BM, Rector FC Jr (eds) *The Kidney, Chap 10,* 4th ed. WB Saunders Company, Philadelphia 1991
2. Contanzo LS, Windhager EE: Renal tubular transport of calcium. In: Windhager EE (ed) *Handbook of Physiology,* Chap 36. Section 8: Renal Physiology. Oxford University Press, New York, 1992
3. Dennis V: Phosphate homeostasis. In: Windhager EE (ed) *Handbook of Physiology,* Chap 37. Section 8: Renal Physiology. Oxford University Press, New York, 1992
4. Coe FL, Favus MJ (eds): *Disorders of Bone and Mineral Metabolism.* Raven Press, New York, 1992

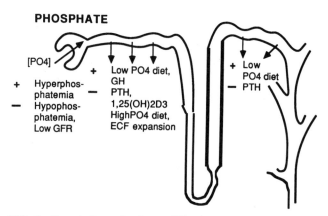

FIG. 6. Regulation of urinary PO_4 excretion.

10. Secretion, Metabolism, and Circulating Heterogeneity of Parathyroid Hormone

Gino V. Segre, M.D.

Department of Medicine, Massachusetts General Hospital, and Harvard Medical School, Boston, Massachusetts

It is important to distinguish parathyroid hormone (PTH) gene regulation and control of PTH *synthesis* from control of PTH *secretion* by parathyroid cells. The following discussion, which concerns factors that influence the plasma concentration of PTH, would be remiss without a brief consideration of the regulation of the PTH gene and PTH secretion. The PTH gene appears to be nearly maximally active under normal physiological conditions; mRNA levels for prepro-PTH fall after dispersed parathyroid cells are cultured in hypercalcemic medium for a few days (1), and with exposure to 1,25-dihydroxyvitamin D (2), whereas mRNA levels do not appear to rise with exposure of parathyroid cells to hypocalcemia. Levels of prepro-PTH mRNA also fall *in vivo*, when rats are treated with active vitamin D metabolites (3).

SECRETION

The extracellular fluid-ionized calcium concentration is the major determinant of PTH secretion. Catecholamines and other biogenic amines (4), ions [such as magnesium (5,6) and aluminum (7)], hormones [including active vitamin D metabolites (8,9), glucagon (10), secretin (10), cortisol (11)], calcitonin (12), histamine (13,14), and other agents (15) have been shown to influence PTH secretion, but their relevance to normal physiology is uncertain. Several of these agents, however, influence PTH secretion in pathophysiological states. For example, both chronic magnesium depletion (16,17) and severe hypermagnesemia (18) inhibit PTH secretion. Aluminum, which inhibits PTH secretion *in vitro* (7), may influence hormone secretion in patients with severe renal impairment, who are treated with aluminum-containing phosphate binders for control of hyperphosphatemia.

PTH secretory dynamics have been studied *in vitro* in calves (19) and humans (20) during infusion of calcium and of calcium chelators, such as EDTA. These dose-response curves describe inverse sigmoidal relationships between blood PTH and ionized calcium concentrations. In humans, perturbation of the blood-ionized calcium level by as little as 0.4 mM promptly changes PTH secretion. PTH secretion dramatically increases when ionized calcium levels are decreased to ~1 mM; further lowering of the calcium level, however, does not elicit additional increase in PTH levels. Upon raising the blood-ionized calcium, PTH secretion falls; however, it is not completely suppressed, even when blood calcium levels are strikingly elevated. PTH secretion under normal, steady-state physiological circumstances is only slightly higher than the maximally suppressed levels; this allows the gland to respond to a hypocalcemic challenge with a marked increase in PTH secretory rate.

PTH secretory dynamics in most patients with hyperparathyroidism show that the level of calcium at which PTH secretion is one-half of maximal is higher than in normal subjects (21,22). Factors responsible for this "set-point" error are under intense study, but may relate to defective calcium-sensing mechanisms in diseased cells. Additionally, PTH secretory response to a change in ambient calcium concentration is relatively insensitive *in vitro*, when there is concomitant exposure of parathyroid cells to high lithium concentrations (21) or when the cells are incubated under conditions favorable to cell division, rather than to cell growth (22). Very recent data also indicate that estrogen treatment of postmenopausal women lowers the setpoint, perhaps contributing to estrogen-induced calcium-balance changes (23).

METABOLISM OF CIRCULATING PARATHYROID HORMONE

Intact PTH is cleared very rapidly from the circulation with a half-life of less than 4 min (24). Clearance by high-capacity hepatic and renal sites removes virtually all intact hormone from the circulation (25–27); some hormone is cleared, however, through low-capacity, saturable sites that presumably involve receptor-mediated processes in bone and kidney, and perhaps in liver (28). Hepatic clearance exceeds renal clearance, and is a complex process involving at least three different mechanisms: 1) hepatic macrophages, Kupffer cells, take up most of the hormone and appear to degrade it to free amino acids or very small fragments (29); 2) Kupffer cells, also, cleave the hormone into discrete fragments and release some of them into the circulation (30); and 3) hepatocytes take up a small amount of the hormone, perhaps through receptor-mediated mechanisms (28). Kupffer cell clearance is high capacity, and may not discriminate between active and inactive hormone, whereas uptake by hepatocytes is of low capacity, but specifically removes active hormone. The carboxy-terminal fragments (C-terminal fragments) generated and released by Kupffer cells *in vitro* reflect cleavage of the hormone mostly between residues 33–34 and 36–37 of the intact molecule (29). These are the same fragments that appear *in vivo* in the circulation of animals injected with intact hormone (30,31). C-terminal fragments persist in the circulation for 5–10 times longer than intact hormone, principally because they are cleared nearly exclusively by glomerular filtration; these fragments are minimally taken up by the liver, if at all (32,33).

The fate of amino-terminal fragments that presumably result from cleavage by endopeptidase(s) is uncertain, but the weight of evidence suggests that they are not released back into the circulation, or alternatively, they are released at rates too low to be detected by the methods thus far used (34). Although the biological consequences of these events remain obscure, the release by Kupffer cells of C-terminal fragments accounts for at least a substantial part of the heterogeneity of circulating PTH.

Renal clearance mechanisms also are complex. A small amount of biologically active hormone is removed through mechanisms that are located on the basal-lateral surface of tubule cells and may be receptor-mediated, whereas the bulk of both intact hormone and C-terminal fragments are removed by glomerular filtration (35). Most studies show that neither intact hormone nor fragments are excreted in the urine (31,34). Parathyroid hormone is metabolized extensively by the kidneys, but discrete hormonal fragments, probably, are not released back into blood (34).

A great deal of interest has focused on details of PTH metabolism, principally because these events potentially could generate amino-terminal, biologically active fragments. Indeed, studies with isolated dog limbs have suggested that synthetic bovine PTH-(1–34) may have unique biological properties in bone (35). However, recent data, strongly argue against release of such fragments into the circulation, although they may be transiently present in certain organs (34,36).

HETEROGENEITY OF CIRCULATING PARATHYROID HORMONE

In normal humans, intact PTH comprises only 5–30% of the circulating immunoreactive hormone; inactive fragments that mostly consist of the C-terminal two-thirds of the intact hormone molecule account for the remaining 70–95%. Although circulating N-terminal PTH fragments have been described under certain pathological conditions (37–40), it is agreed that if they circulate at all, they comprise a very small percentage of the total plasma immunoreactive PTH. Moreover, the sequence analysis of C-terminal fragments shows that they have amino acid 34 or 37 of the intact molecule at their amino-terminus; thus, there is no evidence that PTH 1–34 is a naturally occurring fragment. Fragments comprising the middle portion of the hormone also have been reported (38,41). Because glomerular filtration is the major clearance mechanism for these fragments, their relative plasma concentration increases strikingly, as compared with that of intact hormone, when renal function is impaired (26,32).

Peripheral metabolism of intact hormone and release of PTH fragments by the glands both appear to contribute to plasma hormone heterogeneity. As previously described, a fraction of intact hormone is metabolized to C-terminal fragments, which constitute a substantial portion of the total immunoreactive hormone in circulation because they are cleared slowly. However, hormonal fragments have been detected in extracts of parathyroid glands (42,43), are released by parathyroid tissue *in vitro*

(44,45), are present in the venous effluent of normal glands, particularly when the animals are made hypercalcemic (19), and can be detected in parathyroid effluent samples collected from hypercalcemic patients with hyperparathyroidism (45). The relative concentration of intact hormone and C-terminal fragments has been shown to change during calcium chloride and EDTA infusions in man, as well as in canine and bovine species. The most striking changes were found during hypocalcemia; intact hormone became the dominant circulating form of the hormone, as compared with its relative concentration under basal conditions, when it constituted no more than 25% of total plasma immunoreactive PTH (46). Very recent studies of the calcium–PTH relationship during dynamic testing, in which levels of immunoreactive hormones were determined by assays with specificity only for intact hormone, and for epitopes in mid- and C-terminal regions of PTH showed that C-terminal fragments predominate during both hypercalcemia and hypocalcemia, but that their relative concentration is lower during hypocalcemia, as compared with intact hormone (47). The relative contribution of glandular secretion and postsecretory metabolism to the heterogeneity of PTH in circulation has not been clearly established.

REFERENCES

1. Russell J, Lettieri D, Sherwood LM: Direct regulation by calcium of cytoplasmic messenger RNA coding for pre-pro-parathyroid hormone in isolated bovine parathyroid cells. *J Clin Invest* 72:1851–1855, 1983
2. Silver J, Russell J, Sherwood LM: Regulation by vitamin D metabolites of messenger RNA for preproparathyroid hormone in isolated bovine parathyroid cells. *Proc Natl Acad Sci USA* 82:4279–4273, 1985
3. Silver J, Naveh-Many T, Mayer H, et al.: Regulation by vitamin D metabolites of parathyroid hormone gene transcription in vivo in the rat. *J Clin Invest* 78:1296–1301, 1986
4. Heath H III: Biogenic amines and the secretion of parathyroid hormone and calcitonin. *Endocrinol Rev* 1:319–338, 1980
5. Habener JF, Potts JT Jr: Relative effectiveness of magnesium and calcium on the secretion and biosynthesis of parathyroid hormone in vitro. *Endocrinology* 98:197–202, 1976
6. Brown EM, Thatcher JG, Watson EJ, Leombruno R: Extracellular calcium potentiates the inhibitory effects of magnesium on parathyroid function in dispersed bovine parathyroid cells. *Metabolism* 33:171–176, 1984
7. Morrissey J, Slatopolsky E: Effect of aluminum on parathyroid hormone secretion. *Kidney Int* 29(suppl):S41–44, 1986
8. Dietel M, Dorn G, Montz R, Altenahr E: Influence of vitamin D₃, 1,25-dihydroxyvitamin D₃, and 24,25-dihydroxyvitamin D₃ on parathyroid hormone secretion, adenosine 3',5'-monophosphate release, and ultrastructure of parathyroid glands in organ culture. *Endocrinology* 105:237–245, 1979
9. Chertow BS, Baker GR, Henry HL, Norman AW: Effects of vitamin D metabolites on bovine parathyroid hormone release in vitro. *Am J Physiol* 238:E384–E387, 1980
10. Windeck R, Brown EM, Gardner GD, Aurbach GE: Effect of gastrointestinal hormones on isolated bovine parathyroid cells. *Endocrinology* 103:2020–2025, 1978
11. Au WYW: Cortisol stimulation of parathyroid hormone secretion by rat parathyroid glands in organ culture. *Science* 193:1015–1017, 1976
12. Fischer JA, Oldham SB, Sizemore GW, Arnaud CD: Calcitonin stimulation of parathyroid hormone secretion in vitro. *Horm Metab Res* 3:223–224, 1971
13. Brown EM: Histamine receptors on dispersed parathyroid cells

from pathological human parathyroid tissue. *J Clin Endocrinol Metab* 51:1325–1329, 1980

14. William GA, Longley RS, Bowser EN, et al.: Parathyroid hormone secretion in normal man and in primary hyperparathyroidism: Role of histamine H₂ receptors. *J Clin Endocrinol Metab* 52:122–127, 1981

15. Brown EM: PTH secretion in vivo and in vitro. *Miner Electrolyte Metab* 8:130–150, 1982

16. Anast CS, Mohs JM, Kaplan SL, Burns TW: Evidence of parathyroid failure in magnesium deficiency. *Science* 177:606–608, 1972

17. Anast CS, Winnacker JL, Forte LF, Burns TW: Impaired release of parathyroid hormone in magnesium deficiency. *J Clin Endocrinol Metab* 42:707–717, 1976

18. Cholst IN, Steinberg SF, Tropper PJ, et al.: The influence of hypermagnesemia on serum calcium and parathyroid hormone levels. *N Engl J Med* 301:1221–1225, 1984

19. Mayer GP, Hurst JG: Sigmoidal relationship between parathyroid hormone secretion rate and plasma calcium concentration in calves. *Endocrinology* 102:1036–1042, 1978

20. Ramirez JA, Goodman WG, Gornbein JG, Menezes C, Moulton L, Segre GV, Salusky IB: Direct in vivo comparison of calcium-regulated parathyroid hormone secretion in normal volunteers and patients with secondary hyperparathyroidism. *J Clin Endocrinol Metab* 1993 (in press)

21. Brown EM, Wilson RE, Thatcher JC, Marynich SP: Abnormal calcium-regulated PTH release in normal parathyroid gland from patient with an adenoma. *Am J Med* 71:565–570, 1981

22. LeBoff MS, Rennke HG, Brown EM: Abnormal regulation of parathyroid cell secretion and proliferation in primary cultures of bovine parathyroid cells. *Endocrinology* 113:277–284, 1983

23. Boucher A, D'Amour P, Hamel L, Fugere P, Gascon-Barre M, Lepage R, Ste-Marie JG: Estrogen replacement decreases the set point of parathyroid hormone stimulation by calcium in normal postmenopausal women. *J Clin Endocrinol Metab* 68:831–836, 1989

24. Segre GV, Niall HD, Habener JF, et al.: Metabolism of parathyroid hormone: Physiological and clinical significance. *Am J Med* 56:774, 1974

25. Martin KJ, Hruska KA, Greenwalt A, et al.: Selective uptake of intact parathyroid hormone by the liver: Differences between hepatic and renal uptake. J Clin Invest 58:781–788, 1976

26. Hruska KA, Korkor A, Martin K, Slatopolsky E: Peripheral metabolism of intact parathyroid hormone: Role of liver and kidney and the effect of chronic renal failure. *J Clin Invest* 67:885, 1981

27. D'Amour P, Huet P, Segre GV, Rosenblatt M: Characteristics of bovine parathyroid hormone extraction by dog liver in vitro. *Am J Physiol* 241:E208, 1981

28. Rouleau MF, Warshawsky H, Goltzman D: Parathyroid hormone binding in vivo to renal hepatic and skeletal tissues of the rat using a radioautographic approach. *Endocrinology* 118:919, 1986

29. Segre GV, Perkins AS, Witters LA, Potts JT Jr: Metabolism of parathyroid hormone by isolated rat Kupffer cells and hepatocytes. *J Clin Invest* 67:449–457, 1981

30. Segre GV, D'Amour P, Potts JT Jr: Metabolism of radioiodinated bovine parathyroid hormone in the rat. *Endocrinology* 99:1645–1652, 1976

31. Segre GV, Niall HD, Sauer RT, et al.: Edman degradation of radioiodinated parathyroid hormone: Application to sequence analysis and hormone metabolism in vivo. *Biochemistry* 16:2417, 1977

32. Segre GV, D'Amour P, Hultman A, Potts JT Jr: Effects of hepatectomy, nephrectomy and nephrectomy/uremia on the metabolism of parathyroid hormone in the rat. *J Clin Invest* 67:439–448, 1981

33. Hruska KA, Kopelman R, Rutherford WE, et al.: Metabolism of immunoreactive parathyroid hormone in the dog: the role of the kidney and the effects of chronic renal disease. *J Clin Invest* 56:39–48, 1975

34. Bringhurst FR, Stern AM, Yotts M, et al.: Peripheral metabolism of parathyroid hormone: Fate of the biologically active amino-terminus in vivo. *Am J Physiol* 255:E866–893, 1988

35. Martin KJ, Hruska KA, Freitage JJ, et al.: The peripheral metabolism of parathyroid hormone. *N Engl J Med* 301:1092–1098, 1979

36. Martin KJ, Hruska KA, Greenwalt A, et al.: Selective uptake of intact parathyroid hormone by the liver: Differences between hepatic and renal uptake. *J Clin Invest* 50:808, 1977

37. Canterbury JM, Levey GS, Reiss E: Activation of renal cortical adenylate cyclase by circulating immunoreactive parathyroid hormone fragments. *J Clin Invest* 52:524–527, 1973

38. Silverman R, Yalow RS: Heterogeneity of parathyroid hormone. Clinical and physiological implications. *J Clin Invest* 52:1958–1971, 1973

39. Goltzman D, Henderson B, Loveridge M: Cytochemical bioassay of parathyroid hormone. Characteristics of the assay and analysis of circulating hormonal forms. *J Clin Invest* 65:1309–1317, 1980

40. Grunbaum D, Wexler M, Antos M, Gasoon-Barré M, Goltzman D: Bioactive parathyroid hormone in canine progressive renal insufficiency. *Am J Physiol* 247:E442–E448, 1984

41. Segre GV, Habener JF, Powell D, et al.: Parathyroid hormone in human plasma: Immunochemical characterization and biological implications. *J Clin Invest* 51:3163–3172, 1972

42. DiBella FP, Gilkinson JB, Flueck J, Arnaud CD: Carboxyl-terminal fragments of human parathyroid tumors: Unique new source of immunogens for the production of antisera potentially useful in the radioimmunoassay of parathyroid hormone in human serum. *J Clin Endocrinol Metab* 46:604–612, 1978

43. MacGregor RR, Hamilton JW, Kent GN, et al.: The degradation of proparathormone and parathormone by parathyroid and liver cathepsin B. *J Biol Chem* 254:4428–4433, 1979

44. Hanley DA, Takatsuki K, Sultan JM, et al.: Direct release of parathyroid hormone fragments from functioning bovine parathyroid glands in vitro. *J Clin Invest* 62:1247–1254, 1978

45. Flueck JA, Dibella FB, Edis AJ, et al.: Immunoheterogeneity of parathyroid hormone in venous effluent serum from hyperfunctioning parathyroid glands. *J Clin Invest* 60:1367–1375, 1977

46. D'Amour P, Labelle F, Lecavalier L, Plourde V, Harvey D: Influence of serum calcium concentration on circulating forms of PTH in three species. *Am J Physiol* 251(6 pt 1):E680–687, 1986

47. D'Amour P, Palardy J, Bahsali G, Mallette LE, DeLean A, Lepage R: The modulation of circulating parathyroid hormone immunoheterogeneity in man by ionized calcium concentration. *J Clin Endocrinol Metab* 74:525–532, 1992

11. Parathyroid Hormone: Mechanism of Action

Henry M. Kronenberg, M.D.

Endocrine Unit, Massachusetts General Hospital,
Boston, Massachusetts, and Harvard Medical School,
Boston, Massachusetts

Parathyroid hormone (PTH) regulates the levels of calcium and phosphate in blood by modulating the activity of specific cells in bone and kidney. These actions serve to: 1) stimulate release of calcium and phosphate from bone; 2) stimulate reabsorption of calcium and inhibit reabsorption of phosphate from glomerular filtrate; and 3) stimulate the renal synthesis of 1,25 dihydroxyvitamin D [$1,25(OH)_2D$], thereby increasing intestinal absorption of calcium and phosphate. The net result of these actions is to raise the level of blood calcium and lower the level of blood phosphate. Blood calcium, in turn, is the major regulator of PTH secretion; a rise in blood calcium decreases PTH secretion. The mutual regulatory interactions of PTH and calcium serve to keep the blood level of calcium constant, despite moderate fluctuations in diet, bone metabolism, and renal function. In this chapter, we shall first detail the physiologic actions of PTH and then examine the cellular and subcellular mechanisms responsible for those actions.

Parathyroid hormone has complex and still poorly understood actions on bone. Parathyroid hormone administration leads to release of calcium from a rapidly turning over pool of calcium near the surface of bone; after several hours calcium is also released from an additional pool that turns over more slowly (1). Chronic administration of PTH (or increased secretion of PTH associated with primary hyperparathyroidism) leads to an increase in osteoclast cell number and activity (2). The release of calcium is accompanied by the release of phosphate and matrix components, such as collagen. Paradoxically, at low intermittent doses, PTH administration leads to the deposition of increased amounts of trabecular bone (3). The physiologic role of this anabolic action of PTH is uncertain.

Even though PTH causes a release of phosphate from bone, PTH administration leads to a fall in the blood level of phosphate, because of the phosphaturia caused by PTH. This phosphaturia reinforces the effect of PTH on bone, because low levels of blood phosphate independently lead to resorption of bone (4). The normal dominance of the renal phosphaturic effect of PTH is well illustrated by the effect of PTH on blood phosphate in severe renal failure. In that setting, where PTH can effect little change in renal phosphate handling, the effects of PTH on bone dominate, and parathyroidectomy leads to a *fall* in blood phosphate (5,6).

Phosphate is normally reabsorbed from glomerular filtrate both in the proximal and distal tubules. Reabsorption at both these sites is inhibited by PTH (7). Parathyroid hormone administration leads to a decrease in calcium reabsorption in the proximal tubule as well, but the net effect of PTH on the kidney is to increase calcium reabsorption, due to the effects of PTH on distal tubular sites (7). This increased reabsorption of calcium synergizes with PTH-induced bone resorption to increase the blood level of calcium.

Even though the PTH-stimulated kidney more efficiently reabsorbs calcium, the absolute amount of calcium in the urine usually increases when PTH blood levels are high. This increase in urine calcium is caused by the substantial increase in filtered load of calcium resulting from increased bone resorption and increased intestinal absorption of calcium (see below).

Parathyroid hormone and vitamin D interact in a number of complex ways. In the kidney, PTH activates 25-hydroxyvitamin D 1-hydroxylase (8). This enzyme in the proximal tubule catalyzes the synthesis of the most active metabolite of vitamin D, $1,25(OH)_2D_3$, which, in turn, is a potent inducer of intestinal calcium absorption. Calcium absorption can increase from 10% to 70% in response to $1,25(OH)_2D_3$; this effect synergizes with the effect of PTH on bone and kidney to raise blood calcium. In the absence of vitamin D metabolites, bone is poorly mineralized. PTH cannot mobilize calcium efficiently from this poorly mineralized bone. At high levels, in contrast, $1,25(OH)_2D_3$ causes bone resorption directly, without requiring PTH.

The important role of $1,25(OH)_2D_3$ in partially mediating the effect of PTH on blood calcium has led to its widespread use, along with oral calcium, to treat hypoparathyroidism. Because $1,25(OH)_2D_3$ cannot mimic the *renal* effects of PTH, however, urine calcium rises quickly when hypoparathyroid patients are treated with $1,25(OH)_2D_3$. The blood calcium is best kept in the low normal range in such patients, in order to avoid the consequences of hypercalciuria.

CELLULAR ACTIONS OF PTH

Although the most obvious histologic consequence of PTH action on bone is an increase in osteoclast number and activity, osteoclasts paradoxically contain no PTH receptors, and PTH has no direct effects on isolated osteoclasts (9). Instead, PTH receptors are found on bone-forming osteoblasts. When isolated osteoblasts are treated with PTH, they secrete factor(s) that, in turn, stimulate osteoclasts to resorb bone. This functional linkage of osteoblasts and osteoclasts may partly explain the increase in osteoblast activity that accompanies the increased osteoclast activity in hyperparathyroidism. The increase in osteoclast cell number caused by PTH has been studied in a tissue culture system designed to analyze the development of differentiated osteoclasts from mononuclear progenitor cells that originate in the bone marrow (2). In this *in vitro* system, PTH stimulates the final steps in the differentiation of cells committed to the osteoclast pathway. Whether this effect of PTH is mediated indirectly by osteoblasts, or instead is a direct effect of PTH on preosteoclasts, has not been established.

The kidney responds to PTH without the dramatic changes in cellular composition found in bone. Instead, the activities of specific individual tubular cells are simulated. In the best-studied proximal tubule cell, phosphate is transported into the cell against an electrochemical gradient. The ATP used to accomplish this task does so indirectly: ATP fuels the sodium pump, which drives sodium from the cell. Sodium then travels back into the cell in response to the concentration gradient established by the sodium pump. Phosphate transport is coupled to the entry of sodium back into the cell (10). Parathyroid hormone blocks this sodium-dependent phosphate cotransport. In the distal tubule, presumably PTH has a similar effect on phosphate transport. Also in the distal tubule, PTH stimulates calcium absorption against an electrochemical gradient. After PTH is administered *in vivo*, the V_{max} of the sodium-calcium exchanger in subsequently isolated basolateral membrane vesicles is increased (11). The 1-hydroxylase responsible for hydroxylating 25-hydroxyvitamin D is located in mitochondria in proximal tubular cells and is activated both by PTH and low blood levels of phosphate.

INITIAL ACTIONS OF PTH

Intact PTH does not act directly in the cytoplasm of its target cells in kidney and bone. Instead, PTH binds to specific receptors on the surface of target cells; this binding triggers the release of cytoplasmic "second messengers" that then mediate the multiple distal effects of PTH. Binding of PTH to its receptors requires only the first 34 residues of the PTH molecule, which contains 84 amino acids. The function of the carboxyl portion of the molecule is unknown. The recently discovered factor made by certain tumors that causes humorally mediated hypercalcemia (PTHrP) resembles PTH in its first 13 residues (12). Peptide fragments of this protein bind to PTH receptors in bone and kidney (13); this action probably explains many of the activities of the protein and the similarities between hyperparathyroidism and the humoral hypercalcemia of malignancy (see Chapter 12).

The number of PTH receptors on cells is regulated; this regulation probably modulates the effects of PTH on target cells. Prolonged exposure of cultured cells to PTH leads to a dramatic decrease in the number of receptors on the surface of such cells. This action may partly explain the decreased sensitivity to PTH of experimental animals after prolonged exposure to PTH (14).

The best-characterized mediator of PTH's action is cAMP. Exposure of bone or kidney cells to PTH results in a rapid intracellular accumulation of cAMP and an outpouring of cAMP into the urine (15). The rise in urinary cAMP occurs only in response to PTH and to the PTH-like factor associated with the humoral hypercalcemia of malignancy. Although an elevation in urinary cAMP cannot be used to distinguish hyperparathyroidism from malignant hypercalcemia, the measurement of renal cAMP generation has provided a useful bioassay of PTH action in clinical investigation.

Administration of analogs of cAMP can mimic many of the effects of PTH. The rapid elevation of cAMP in response to PTH and the actions of cAMP strongly suggest that cAMP mediates the effects of PTH. Binding of PTH to its receptor on the external surface of the cell triggers the release of GDP from an intracellular protein called G_s and permits the binding of intracellular GTP to G_s. GTP-G_s then stimulates membrane-bound adenylate cyclase. The cAMP produced by adenylate cyclase then binds to the regulatory subunit of cAMP-dependent protein kinase A. This binding causes the regulatory subunit to dissociate from the catalytic subunit of protein kinase. The free catalytic subunit then phosphorylates specific serines and threonines in target proteins. The relevant target proteins and their precise modes of action remain uncharacterized, although proteins that activate genes responsive to cAMP and ion channel proteins are strong candidates.

The human disease pseudohypoparathyroidism (Chapter 46) provides evidence for the physiologic relevance of the mechanism of PTH action outlined previously, and also raises intriguing problems. Patients with pseudohypoparathyroidism are unresponsive to PTH. PTH levels in their blood are high, and yet they are hypocalcemic and hyperphosphatemic. Urinary cAMP does not rise in response to administration of exogenous PTH, a key diagnostic finding. Most of these patients have only 50% of the expected amount of G_s in membranes from a variety of accessible cells (16). This loss of G_s may well cause the unresponsiveness to PTH. Why loss of half of the normal amount of G_s leads to complete unresponsiveness to PTH is not understood. Further, the similar loss of half the normal amount of G_s in patients with pseudohypoparathyroidism, who exhibit *normal* responsiveness to PTH, remains unexplained (17). Although the explanation of pseudohypoparathyroidism thus remains incomplete, what we already know strongly supports the role of cAMP in mediating PTH's effects. Further, bone cells engineered to contain a protein kinase unresponsive to cAMP have blunted responses to PTH (18). Thus, multiple types of evidence support the model that PTH action is mediated at least in part by cAMP.

Reality may be more complicated than this straightforward model, however. PTH stimulates phosphotidylinositol turnover in cultured cell lines (19), causes a rapid rise in levels of free cytosolic calcium (20), and causes a shift of protein kinase C to the cell membrane (21). These effects are different from the actions of cAMP analogs and suggest that multiple second messengers may mediate some actions of PTH. The physiologic importance of metabolites of phosphotidylinositol and intracellular calcium as PTH-induced second messengers has not yet been established.

This brief summary illustrates the recently delineated complexities associated with PTH action. Parathyroid hormone acts on several different tissues, sometimes with apparently paradoxical actions. For example, when administered continuously to animals, PTH causes net bone resorption; yet when it is administered by once daily injection, PTH can cause net bone formation. Further, PTH acts through more than one second messenger system. Most intriguingly, both PTH and PTHrP, the mediator of the humoral hypercalcemia of malignancy, seem to bind to the same receptor. How can the same receptor mediate the carefully regulated calcium homeostatic functions of PTH and, at the same time, mediate actions of PTHrP, a peptide that has no obvious involvement in feedback-regulated, normal calcium homeostasis?

The recent cloning of DNA encoding rat, opposum, and human PTH/PTHrP receptors has begun to clarify the mechanisms involved in the PTH signaling system (22,23). The DNA sequence encoding the receptor predicts that the receptor is a member of the large family of receptors that span the plasma membrane seven times and work by activating G proteins on the inner surface of the membrane. The PTH/PTHrP receptor belongs to a newly appreciated subfamily of that large family. Members of this new sub-family, which includes receptors for calcitonin and secretin, closely resemble each other in their primary sequences and in several functional properties, but only bear a distant relationship to other members of the family. Precisely the same receptor is found in bone and kidney, both in rats and in humans. When the cloned receptor is expressed in cultured cells that do not normally bear PTH receptors, PTH binding stimulates both adenylate cyclase and phospholipase C. Thus, this one receptor is capable of stimulating both of the known second messenger pathways used by PTH. The receptor binds and responds to PTH and to amino-terminal fragments of PTHrP equally well. Further, messenger RNA for the receptor is found not only in traditional PTH target tissues, but also in putative PTHrP target tissues, such as early embryonic cells. This one receptor is, therefore, apparently quite versatile: it mediates actions of both PTH and PTHrP in multiple tissues and signals through more than one second message pathway. Data discussed in the next chapter suggest that PTHrP may well work through more than one receptor; the number of receptors for PTH is less certain. Further analysis of the properties of the cloned PTH/PTHrP receptor and the continuing search for more receptors should lead to a greater understanding of the biochemical underpinnings of this complicated physiologic signaling network.

REFERENCES

1. Talmage RV, Elliott JR: Removal of calcium from bone as influenced by the parathyroids. *Endocrinology* 62:717–722, 1958
2. Mundy GR, Roodman GD: Osteoclast ontogeny and function. In: Peck WA (ed) *Bone and Mineral Research*, vol 5. Elsevier, Amsterdam, pp 209–280, 1987
3. Slovik DM, Rosenthal DI, Doppelt SH: Restoration of spinal bone in osteoporotic men by treatment with human parathyroid hormone (1–34) and 1,25 dihydroxyvitamin D. *J Bone Min Res* 1:377–381, 1986
4. Raisz LG, Niemann I: Effect of phosphate, calcium and magnesium on bone resorption and humoral responses in tissue culture. *Endocrinology* 85:446–452, 1969
5. Gill G, Pallotta J, Kashgarian M, Kessner D, Epstein FH: Physiological studies in renal osteodystrophy treated by subtotal parathyroidectomy. *Am J Med* 46:930–940, 1969
6. Neer RM: Calcium and inorganic phosphate homeostasis. In: DeGroot LJ (ed) *Endocrinology*, vol II. New York: Grune and Stratton, pp 927–954, 1989
7. Bringhurst FR: Calcium and phosphate distribution, turnover, and metabolic actions. In: DeGroot LJ (ed) *Endocrinology*, vol II. New York: Grune and Stratton, pp 805–843, 1989
8. Garabedian M, Holick MF, DeLuca HF, et al.: Control of 25-dihydroxycalciferol metabolism by the parathyroid glands. *Proc Natl Acad Sci USA* 69:1673–1676, 1972
9. McSheehy PMJ, Chambers TJ: Osteoblastic cells mediate osteoclastic responsiveness to parathyroid hormone. *Endocrinology* 118:824–828, 1986
10. Cheng L, Sacktor B: Sodium gradient-dependent phosphate transport in renal brush border vesicles. *J Biol Chem* 256:1556–1564, 1981
11. Jayakumar A, Cheung L, Liang CT, Sacktor B: Sodium-gradient-dependent calcium uptake in renal basolateral membrane vesicles. *J Biol Chem* 259:10827–10833, 1984
12. Suva LJ, Winslow GA, Wettenhall REH: A parathyroid hormone-related protein implicated in malignant hypercalcemia: Cloning and expression. *Science* 237:893–896, 1987
13. Jüppner H, Abou-Samra AB, Uneno S, Gu WX, Potts JT Jr, Segre GV: The PTH-like peptide associated with humoral hypercalcemia of malignancy and PTH bind to the same receptor on the plasma membrane of ROS 17/2.8 cells. *J Biol Chem* 263:8557–8560, 1988
14. Mahoney CA, Nissenson RA: Canine renal receptors for parathyroid hormone—Down regulation *in vivo* by exogenous parathyroid hormone. *J Clin Invest* 72:411–421, 1983
15. Chase LR, Aurbach GD: Parathyroid function and the renal excretion of 3′,5′-adenylic acid. *Proc Natl Sci USA* 58:518–525, 1967
16. Farfel Z, Brickman AS, Kaslow HR, Brothers VM, Bourne HR: Defect in receptor-cyclase coupling protein in pseudohypoparathyroidism. *N Engl J Med* 303:237–242, 1980
17. Levine MA, Downs RW, Moses AM, et al.: Resistance to multiple hormone in patients with pseudohypoparathyroidism. *Am J Med* 74:545–556, 1983
18. Bringhurst FR, Zajac JD, Daggett AS, Skurat RN, Kronenberg HM: Inhibition of parathyroid hormone responsiveness in clonal osteoblastic cells expressing a mutant form of 3′,5′-cyclic adenosine monophosphate-dependent protein kinase. *Mol Endocrinol* 3:60–67, 1989
19. Meltzer V, Weinreb S, Bellorin-Font E, Hruska KA: Parathyroid hormone stimulation of renal phosphoinositide metabolism is a cyclic nucleotide-independent effect. *Biochem Biophys Acta* 712:258–267, 1982
20. Yamaguchi DT, Hahn TJ, Iida-Klein A, Kleeman CR, Muallem S: Parathyroid hormone-activated calcium channels in an osteoblast-like clonal osteosarcoma cell line. *J Biol Chem* 262:7711–7718, 1987
21. Abou-Samra AB, Jüppner H, Westerberg D, Potts JT Jr, Segre GV: Parathyroid hormone causes translocation of protein kinase-C activity from cytosol to membranes in rat osteosarcoma cells. *Endocrinology* 124:1107–1113, 1989
22. Jüppner H, Abou-Samra AB, Freeman M, Kong XF, Schipani E, Richards J, Kolakowski LF, Kronenberg HM, Segre GV: A G protein-linked receptor for parathyroid hormone and parathyroid hormone-related peptide. *Science* 254:1024–1026, 1991
23. Abou-Samra AB, Jüppner H, Force T, Freeman MW, Kong XF, Schipani E, Urena P, Richards J, Bonventre JV, Potts JT Jr, Kronenberg HM, Segre GV: Expression cloning of a common receptor for parathyroid hormone and parathyroid hormone-related peptide from rat osteoblast-like cells: A single receptor stimulates intracellular accumulation of both cAMP and inositol triphosphates and increases intracellular free calcium. *Proc Natl Acad Sci USA* 89:2732–3736, 1992

12. Parathyroid Hormone-Related Protein

Gordon J. Strewler, M.D. and Robert A. Nissenson, Ph.D.

Departments of Medicine and Physiology, Veterans Administration Medical Center and University of California, San Francisco, California

A second member of the parathyroid hormone (PTH) family, the PTH-related protein (PTHrP) has recently been discovered. Over the past 5 years the elucidation of the structure of PTHrP and our nascent understanding of its unique biological role has changed our view of hypercalcemia and expanded our concept of the role of the PTH/PTHrP family beyond the horizons of calcium homeostasis to include developmental and regulatory functions in a variety of tissues (1).

Parathyroid hormone-related protein was first identified as the cause of hypercalcemia in malignancy. The characteristics of the clinical syndrome of humoral hypercalcemia are discussed in Chapter 33. As in primary hyperparathyroidism, hypercalcemia in malignancy is characterized by a decreased renal threshold for phosphate, leading to hypophosphatemia, and by increased urinary excretion of cAMP (2). Yet PTH is suppressed in malignancy-associated hypercalcemia. The finding that PTH was suppressed in a syndrome that so resembled primary hyperparathyroidism biochemically suggested that a distinct molecule secreted by tumors could mimic PTH, and led to the development of bioassay techniques to search for a PTH-like factor in tumors that produced hypercalcemia. These assays guided the isolation and ultimate identification of what proved to be a PTHrP (also called PTH-like protein). As predicted, the tumor-derived protein proved to be an able mimic of PTH, for reasons that became clear when its structure could be determined.

As disclosed by molecular cloning, the amino acid sequence of PTHrP is homologous with the sequence of PTH only at the amino-terminus, where 8 of the first 13 amino acids in PTH and PTHrP are identical (Fig. 1). This homologous domain, limited as it is, involves a crucial region of the molecule that is known to be required for activation of the PTH receptor. Beyond this region the sequences of PTH and PTHrP have little in common. Even in the primary receptor binding domain (amino acids 18–34), PTH and PTHrP do not have recognizable primary sequence similarities (however, the binding domain has a common α-helical secondary structure in both peptides). Compared with the 84 amino acid peptide PTH, PTHrP is considerably longer, apparently existing in three isoforms of 139, 141, and 173 amino acids, whose sequence is identical through amino acid 139. These isoforms arise from alternative RNA splicing. Their relative secretory rates and their relative importance in normal physiology or in the pathophysiology of humoral hypercalcemia are unknown.

Human PTHrP is encoded by a single-copy gene located on chromosome 12. The human *PTHrP* gene, with three promoters, eight exons, and complex patterns of alternative exon splicing, is much more complicated than the PTH gene. Yet it is clear from the protein structure and from similarities in gene organization that both arose from a common ancestral gene.

Parathyroid hormone-related protein and PTH bind with equivalent affinity to a common receptor (3), and consequently have a very similar range of biological activities. Both produce hypercalcemia, hypophosphatemia as a consequence of reduced renal reabsorption of phosphate, and accelerated production of 1,25-dihydroxyvitamin D [1,25(OH)$_2$D] by the kidney (1,3). Despite the latter action, patients with PTHrP-induced hypercalcemia have considerably lower serum levels of 1,25(OH)$_2$D than are seen in primary hyperparathyroidism (2) (see Chapter 33).

There is little doubt that PTHrP is the major cause of hypercalcemia in malignancy. Infusion of PTHrP can reproduce most aspects of the clinical syndrome of hypercalcemia, serum levels of PTHrP are increased in hypercalcemia (4,5) (see Chapter 33), and neutralizing antibodies to PTHrP can reverse hypercalcemia induced in animals by human tumor cells (6). This indicates that secretion of PTHrP is not merely associated with hypercalcemia but necessary for hypercalcemia.

The specific tumors that characteristically produce hormonal hypercalcemia by secreting PTHrP include squamous, renal, and breast carcinoma. Parathyroid hormone-related protein also plays a causative role in the hypercalcemia that is occasionally associated with islet cell tumors and pheochromocytoma and is frequently seen in the adult T-cell leukemia syndrome, where PTHrP is produced by malignant T lymphocytes infected with the etiologic agent of this disorder, the human T-cell lymphotrophic virus.

The normal circulating level of PTHrP is considerably lower than the level of PTH, and it is doubtful that PTHrP has a major role in the day-to-day maintenance of calcium homeostasis. It is clear, however, that PTHrP has vital functions in normal physiology, primarily local ones at the cell or tissue level. Parathyroid hormone-related protein is widely present in fetal tissues, including cartilage, heart, distal renal tubules, hair follicles, and many epithelial surfaces (7). It has recently been possible to disrupt both copies of the PTHrP gene in the mouse by targeted mutations introduced by the technique of homologous recombination. Although mice heterozygous for the loss of PTHrP are phenotypically normal, in the homozygous state loss of the *PTHrP* gene is an embryonic lethal mutation. Homozygotes survive until near the time of parturition and have multiple anomalies in the development of cartilage and bone. From these results it is apparent that PTHrP is crucial for normal development of the skeleton; further studies of this model may well disclose other developmental effects of PTHrP as well.

The *PTHrP* gene is widely expressed in normal tissues of the embryo and the adult, and has been postulated to have a number of other physiological functions. The gene

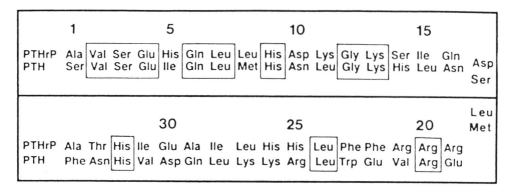

FIG. 1. Amino-terminal amino acid sequence of PTHrP is compared with that of PTH.

is expressed in a variety of endocrine tissues, in the central nervous system (8), uterus (9), placenta, and vascular smooth muscle and other smooth muscle beds (10), where it acts to relax smooth muscle. Parathyroid hormone-related protein is present in the fetal parathyroid glands, and it has been suggested that PTHrP is an important regulator of placental calcium transport (11). The hormone is also present in lactating mammary tissue under the control of prolactin and is secreted into milk at concentrations 10,000-fold higher than its serum concentration. It is not clear whether these findings reflect a role in lactation itself, in the neonate who ingests large quantities of PTHrP in milk, or both. Expressed in epidermal keratinocytes (the parental cells for squamous carcinomas that characteristically secrete PTHrP as the cause of hypercalcemia), PTHrP may be involved in differentiation of the epidermis (12). Although none of these putative functions is fully understood, the list is already impressively long (Table 1).

The foregoing illustrates how the discovery of PTHrP has widened our perspectives on the role of "calciotropic" hormones in development and differentiation. Reports on the heterogeneity of secreted PTHrP have also broadened our view of the relationships between structure and function of this peptide family. A midregion fragment of PTHrP beginning with amino acid 38 is secreted (13), and a carboxyl-terminal fragment recognized by PTHrP (109–138) antibodies is also detectable in the circulation (it could arise from peripheral, rather than cellular processing of PTHrP). It has been suggested that the actions of PTHrP on placental calcium transport (11) and renal bicarbonate transport may be functions not of the PTH-like amino-terminus but of the midregion of the molecule. It is thus conceivable that, like the neuropeptide proopiomelanocortin—the precursor of not only of ACTH, but also of opiate peptides and melanocyte-stimulating hormones—PTHrP may be a multifunctional molecule. To date, studies of PTHrP binding in its target tissues have identified only a PTH/PTHrP receptor coupled to adenylyl cyclase with kinetic characteristics of the renal/bone PTH/PTHrP receptor. However, it is attractive to speculate that some of the actions of PTHrP in "nonclassical" target tissues are initiated by binding to specific PTHrP receptors, some of which may recognize determinants in the midregion or carboxyl-terminus of PTHrP. Our understanding of PTHrP and its distinct biological actions is in its infancy.

TABLE 1. *Sites of expression and proposed actions of parathyroid hormone-related protein*

Sites of expression	Proposed actions
Fetal tissues	
Parathyroid	Stimulate placental calcium transport
Cartilage and perichondrium	Regulate chondrogenesis and mineralization
Heart, kidney, epithelia, hair follicles	Unknown
Endocrine tissues	Unknown
Pituitary	
Pancreatic islets	
Parathyroid adenomas	
Smooth muscle	
Vascular smooth muscle	Vasodilator
Urinary bladder	Relaxor
Myometrium	Regulation of parturition
Lactating mammary gland	Regulation of lactation
	Regulation of neonatal metabolism
Epidermis	Regulation of differentiation
Central nervous system	Unknown

REFERENCES

1. Halloran BP, Nissenson RA (eds): *Parathyroid Hormone-Related Protein: Normal Physiology and Its Role in Cancer.* CRC Press, Boca Raton, 1992
2. Stewart AF, Horst R, Deftos LJ, Cadman EC, Lang R, Broadus AE: Biochemical evaluation of patients with cancer-associated hypercalcemia. *N Engl J Med* 303:1377, 1980
3. Orloff JJ, Wu TL, Stewart AF: Parathyroid hormone-like proteins: Biochemical responses and receptor interactions. *Endocr Rev* 10:476, 1989
4. Budayr AA, Nissenson RA, Klein RF, Pun KK, Clark OH, Diep D, Arnaud CD, Strewler GJ: Increased serum levels of a parathyroid hormone-like protein in malignancy-associated hypercalcemia. *Ann Intern Med* 111:807, 1989
5. Burtis WJ, Brady TG, Orloff JJ, Ersback JB, Warrell RP Jr, Olson BR, Wu TL, Mitnick ME, et al.: Immunochemical characterization of circulatilng parathyroid hormone-related protein in

patients with humoral hypercalcemia of cancer. *N Engl J Med* 322:1106, 1990

6. Kukreja SC, Shevrin DH, Wimbiscus SA, Ebeling PR, Danks JA, Rodda CP, Wood WI, Martin TJ: Antibodies to parathyroid hormone-related protein lower serum calcium in athymic mouse models. *J Clin Invest* 82:1798, 1988
7. Moseley JM, Hayman JA, Danks JA, Alcorn D, Grill V, Southby J, Horton MA: Immunochemical detection of parathyroid hormone-related protein in human fetal epithelia. *J Clin Endocrinol Metab* 73:478, 1991
8. Weir EC, Brines ML, Ikeda K, Burtis WJ, Broadus AE, Robbins RJ: Parathyroid hormone-related peptide gene is expressed in the mammalian central nervous system. *Proc Natl Acad Sci USA* 87:108, 1990
9. Thiede MA, Daifotis AG, Weir EC, Brines ML, Burtis WJ, Ikeda K, Dreyer BE, Garfield RE, Broadus AE: Intrauterine occupancy controls expression of the parathyroid hormone-related peptide gene in preterm rat myometrium. *Proc Natl Acad Sci USA* 87:6969, 1990

10. Hongo T, Kupfer J, Enomoto H, Sharifi B, Giannella-Neto D, Forrester JS, Singer FR, Goltzman D, Hendy GN, Pirola C, Fagin JA, Clemens TL: Abundant expression of parathyroid hormone-related protein in primary rat aortic smooth muscle cells accompanies serum-induced proliferation. *J Clin Invest* 88:1841, 1991
11. Abbas SK, Pickard DW, Rodda CP, Heath JA, Hammonds RG, Wood WI, Caple IW, Martin TJ, Care AD: Stimulation of ovine placental calcium transport by purified natural and recombinant parathyroid hormone related protein (PTHrP) preparations. *Q J Exp Physiol* 74:549, 1989
12. Kremer R, Karaplis AC, Henderson J, Gulliver W, Banville D, Hendy G, Goltzman D: Regulation of parathyroid hormone-like peptide in cultured normal human keratinocytes. *J Clin Invest* 87:884, 1991
13. Soifer NE, Dee KE, Insogna KL, Burtis WJ, Matovcik LM, Wu TL, Milstone LM, Broadus AE, Philbrick WM, Stewart AF: Parathyroid hormone-related protein. Evidence for secretion of a novel mid-region fragment by three different cell types. *J Biol Chem* 267:18236, 1992

13. Vitamin D: Metabolism and Mechanism of Action

Anthony W. Norman, Ph.D., and Helen L. Henry, Ph.D.

Department of Biochemistry, Division of Biomedical Sciences, University of California–Riverside, Riverside, California

In the last two decades, a new concept concerning the mode-of-action of the fat-soluble vitamin D has emerged. The cornerstone of this concept is that in terms of its availability, metabolism, and mechanism of action it is more accurate to consider vitamin D a steroid hormone than a vitamin in the classical sense. Synthesis in the skin on exposure to ultraviolet light obviates the dietary necessity for vitamin D, a classical part of the definition of a vitamin. The chemical transformations through which the various derivatives of vitamin D are produced are of the same kind as those that characterize the metabolism of other steroid hormones, such as the glucocorticoid and sex steroids. The close regulation of the renal production of 1,25-dihydroxyvitamin D_3 [$1,25(OH)_2D_3$], the most potent of the naturally occurring derivatives of vitamin D, is very suggestive of its hormonal nature. The most compelling argument for the considerations of vitamin D as a steroid (pro-) hormone is the presence in classical target tissues, such as intestine, kidney, and bone of a specific, high-affinity nuclear receptor for its active metabolite, $1,25(OH)_2D_3$.

The most thoroughly studied target tissue for $1,25(OH)_2D_3$ is the intestine that depends on the hormone for adequate absorption of dietary calcium (1,2). In the intestinal mucosa, the steroid-receptor complex induces the synthesis of a specific calcium binding protein (MS = 28,000), the precise role of which in calcium absorption has yet to be elucidated (3,4). This receptor and the induction of the vitamin D-dependent 28K calcium binding protein have been identified in tissues not previously recognized as targets for vitamin D, such as the pancreas, pituitary, and brain (5,6). The biological response of these tissues to $1,25(OH)_2D_3$ and the role that the hormone plays in their differentiated functions is currently an area of active investigation.

In addition to the endocrine actions of $1,25(OH)_2D_3$ in the classical target tissues of vitamin D, in which the actions of the hormone contribute to the body's maintenance of calcium homeostasis, and the more recently recognized target tissues, such as those mentioned above, evidence suggests interaction of $1,25(OH)_2D_3$ with the hemopoietic (7) and immune systems (8). Many different cell types representing these systems respond to $1,25(OH)_2D_3$, presumably through the specific receptors that have been identified in these cells, with changes in their patterns of growth and differentiation. These interactions may be of a more paracrine or autocrine nature as indicated, e.g., by the ability of activated macrophages to convert $25OHD_3$ to $1,25(OH)_2D_3$.

The actions of $1,25(OH)_2D_3$ alluded to above appear to involve changes in gene expression in the target cells (9–11). In the intestine (12) and bone osteoblast cells (13), components of calcium transport have been identified that respond very rapidly to $1\alpha,25(OH)_2D_3$ and are thought to be mediated by nongenomic mechanisms. Investigations in this area may well provide a backdrop for nongenomic actions of other steroid hormones.

REGULATION OF VITAMIN D METABOLISM

The primary source of circulating dihydroxylated metabolites of vitamin D is the kidney. In the kidney mito-

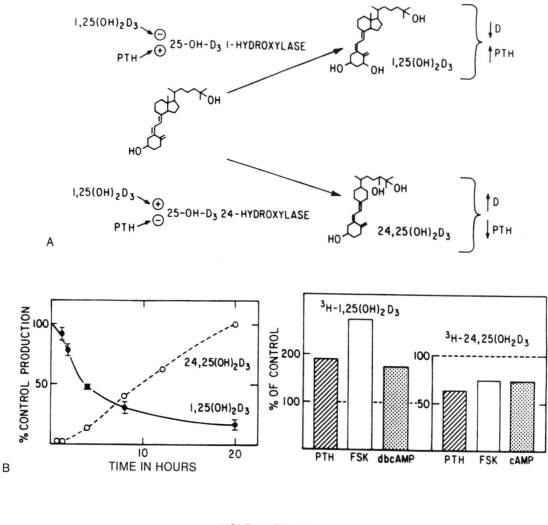

FIG. 1. Regulation of vitamin D metabolism. **A:** Conversion of 25OHD₃ to 1,25(OH)₂D₃ is downregulated by 1,25(OH)₂D₃ and upregulated by PTH. The two hormones have the opposite effects on 24,25(OH)₂D₃ production. **B:** Time course of the effect of 1,25(OH)₂D₃ on its own production *(solid symbols* and *solid line)* and on that of 24,25(OH)₂D₃ *(open symbols* and *dashed line)* in cultured chick kidney cells is shown on the *left*. On the *right* is summarized the data supporting the involvement of the cAMP intracellular signaling cascade in the regulation of 1,25(OH)₂D₃ and 24,25(OH)₂D₃ production *(FSK,* forskolin; *dbcAMP,* dibutyryl cAMP.) **C:** Transport of electrons from NADPH to ferredoxin reductase (a flavoprotein, *FP*) to ferredoxin *(FD)* and to cychrome P-450 to support the reduction of molecular oxygen to water and to the hydroxyl group to incorporate into the steroid by mitochondrial mixed-function oxidases. For further details see refs. 14 and 19.

chondrion, 25OHD₃, the major circulating form of vitamin D, is converted to either 1,25(OH)₂D₃ or 24,25(OH)₂D₃ (Fig. 1A). The predominant dihydroxylated product formed will depend on the vitamin D and parathyroid hormone (PTH) status of the individual.

In the vitamin D-deficient state, 1-hydroxylase is high and 24-hydroxylase is low. This is because, as has been shown in cell culture (Figure 1B), 1,25(OH)₂D₃ represses 1-hydroxylase and induces 24-hydroxylase activity, prob-

ably through effects on the synthesis of specific proteins. Parathyroid hormone, elevated by the hypocalcemia resulting from vitamin D deficiency, increases 1-hydroxylase activity and decreases 24-hydroxylase activity. As has been shown in cell culture, cAMP mediates this effect of PTH, but protein kinase C may also be involved in 25OHD₃ metabolisms, because 12-0-tetradecanoylphorbol-13 acetate (TPA) exerts effects opposite to those of PTH (Figure 1B). Thus, the absence of 1,25(OH)₂D₃ and the presence of PTH combine to keep $24,25(OH)_2D_3$ production low. In the vitamin D replete state, the opposite set of effects occur, resulting in lowered $1,25(OH)_2D_3$ and elevated $24,25(OH)_2D_3$ production.

Both the 1- and 24-hydroxylases are classical mitochondrial mixed-function oxidases involving the transfer of electrons from NADPH through a flavoprotein (renal ferredoxin reductase) and an iron sulfur protein (renal ferredoxin) to cytochrome P-450. All three components are located in or adjacent to the inner mitochondrial membrane. Exactly how, on a molecular level $1,25(OH)_2D_3$ and PTH exert their effects on these enzyme systems is currently under study (14).

MOLECULAR MECHANISM OF ACTION OF $1,25(OH)_2D_3$

As previously mentioned, there is emerging evidence that the spectrum of biological responses generated by $1\alpha,25(OH)_2D_3$ may be mediated by more than one fundamental mechanism; Fig. 2 summarizes this point. Historically over the past two decades much research has documented the extensive involvement of $1\alpha,25(OH)_2D_3$ in generating biological responses via genomic pathways, involving the nuclear receptor (9). In the past 5–7 years, evidence has emerged that $1\alpha,25(OH)_2D_3$ may also have the capability to generate biological responses via activation of voltage-dependent Ca^{2+} channels that are "coupled" via appropriate signal transduction pathways to the generation of biological responses (6,13,15). Examples of biologic responses supporting both genomic and nongenomic pathways is provided.

Figure 3 presents a model of the proposed regulation by $1,25(OH)_2D_3$ (designated S) and its receptor (designated R) of gene expression in a generic target cell. Target organs and cells for $1,25(OH)_2D_3$ by definition contain receptors for the secosteroid that confers on them the ability to modulate genomic events according to the prevailing concentration of $1,25(OH)_2D_3$. The interaction of $1,25(OH)_2D_3$ and its receptor with genomic material is thought to be analogous to the mode of action of other steroid hormones.

A target cell must have three key components in order for its genes to be regulated by a steroid hormone. These include 1) a protein receptor for the steroid hormone that contains both a unique binding domain for the steroid in question and also a DNA binding domain that allows the occupied receptor to locate the genes in the nucleus of the cell it will regulate; 2) hormone-responsive elements that consist of specific sequences of DNA nucleotides that facilitate/promote an interaction between the occupied receptor and the genes to be regulated (either upward or downward) in that particular cell; and 3) access to the steroid hormone in question (normally the steroid hormone is delivered through the blood compartment on a specific transport protein).

The $1,25(OH)_2D_3$ receptor is a protein of 51,000 Da, with exquisite specificity and high affinity ($K_D = 1 \times 10^{-10}$) for its ligand. The primary amino acid structure of a major portion of the chicken intestinal $1,25(OH)_2D_3$ receptor has been deduced from a complementary DNA clone. Strong homologies occur in the putative DNA binding region of the receptor with the DNA-binding domains of all the other steroid hormone receptors and also the v-erb-A oncogene. This suggests that the $1,25(OH)_2D_3$ receptor belongs to the same supergene family as that of all the other classic steroid hormone receptors (9,11). The $1,25(OH)_2D_3$ receptor protein is expressed in almost every tissue that has been examined thus far (see lower right-hand corner of Fig. 5). In target cells this receptor is partitioned between the nucleus and the cytoplasm. When $1,25(OH)_2D_3$ is delivered to the target cell, it is believed that it diffuses through the cell membrane, enters the cytoplasmic compartment, and then encounters an unoccupied receptor either in the cytoplasm or in the nucleus. The steroid-receptor complex then interacts through its

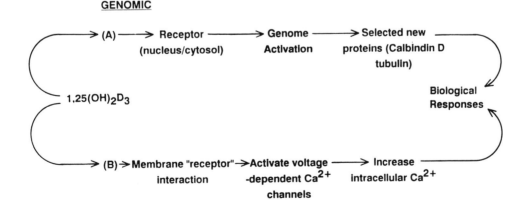

FIG. 2. Pathways of signal transduction utilized by vitamin D for generation of biological responses (see text for explanation). The spectrum of biological responses produced by the seco–steroid $1,25(OH)_2D_3$ may be mediated by two different mechanisms. **A:** GENOMIC **B:** NONGENOMIC. See ref. 20 for a further explanation.

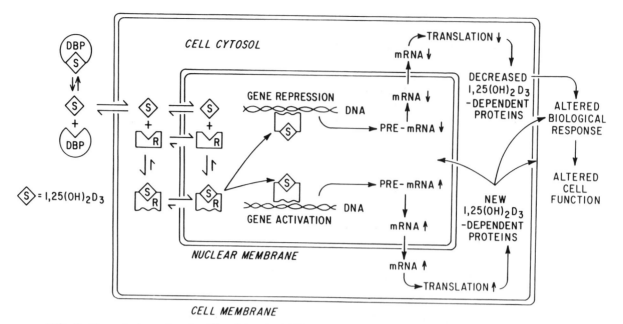

FIG. 3. Generic target cell utilized by $1\alpha,25(OH)_2D_3$ for generation of biologic responses via regulation of gene activation and/or gene repression. $1\alpha,25(OH)_2D_3$, S; DBP, plasma vitamin D binding protein; R, nuclear receptor for $1\alpha,25(OH)_2D_3$. See refs. 9–11 for further elaboration.

DNA-binding domain with the hormone-responsive elements in the genome of the cell. This process aligns the steroid-receptor complex with the promoter region of the genes that it may regulate, allowing selective up- and downregulation of the gene in question; thus either the production of mRNA is turned "on" or "off." This will result either in the increased or decreased production of the protein for which messenger RNA codes so that there will ultimately be an alteration in the cell function related to the presence of the steroid hormone.

DIVERSITY OF THE BIOLOGICAL ACTIONS OF $1,25(OH)_2D_3$

Figure 4 summarizes the actions of $1,25(OH)_2D_3$ in three widely differing systems in which this secosteroid has been shown to be capable of producing specific biological responses: the classical genomic actions calcium-metabolizing tissues as exemplified by the intestine; the more recently recognized and probably genomic actions in cell growth and differentiation; and nongenomic actions in the intestine.

The classical target organs for vitamin D and its hormonal daughter metabolite, $1,25(OH)_2D_3$, are the intestine, bone, and kidney. It is in this setting that the vitamin D endocrine systems affects mineral homeostasis, particularly with respect to inorganic phosphate and calcium. Illustrated in Fig. 4A are the biological actions of intestinal Ca^{2+} absorption and bone Ca^{2+}-mobilizing activity that have been known for decades to be stimulated *in vivo* by dietary vitamin D_3, and more recently appreciated to occur as a consequence of the metabolism of vitamin D_3 into $1\alpha,25(OH)_2D_3$, which is the immediate agonist of both of these responses.

Figure 4B describes the interaction of $1\alpha,25(OH)_2D_3$ with cells of the bone marrow. In the hematopoietic cells, $1,25(OH)_2D_3$ has been shown to promote the differentiation of promonocytes into monocytes, then macrophages, and finally into osteoclasts (16). Osteoclasts are cells that promote bone resorption, but which are devoid of receptors for $1,25(OH)_2D_3$. Thus $1,25(OH)_2D_3$, a known mediator of bone resorption (see the bone calcium mobilizing response in Fig. 4A), achieves this response not by interacting directly with the osteoclast, but by generating through its cell differentiating actions, an increased number of osteoclasts. Very recently it has been shown that γ-interferon, which is produced by activated T-lymphocytes, mediates the production in activated macrophages of a $25(OH)D_3$-1-hydroxylase, thus conferring on these cells the ability to produce limited quantities of $1,25(OH)_2D_3$ (see lower left-hand box of Fig. 5). This biological response is reflective of a wide involvement of the vitamin D endocrine system and $1\alpha,25(OH)_2D_3$ in cell differentiation processes present in bone marrow (7), the immune system (8), and the epidermis (17).

Although the majority of biological responses generated by $1,25(OH)_2D_3$ are believed to occur as a consequence of occupied nuclear receptor interaction with selected genes, it is, as emphasized in Fig. 2, unlikely that absolutely all $1,25(OH)_2D_3$-mediated biological responses occur are achieved through this mechanism. Figure 4C illustrates how rapidly $1\alpha,25(OH)_2D_3$ may stimulate the process of intestinal Ca^{2+} absorption in the perfused chick duodenum. The transport of $^{45}Ca^{2+}$ from the lumen of the intestine, across the intestinal epithelial cell, and its appearance in the blood compartment occur within minutes of application of the agonist $1\alpha,25(OH)_2D_3$ to the basal lateral side of the epithelial cell (18). The transcal-

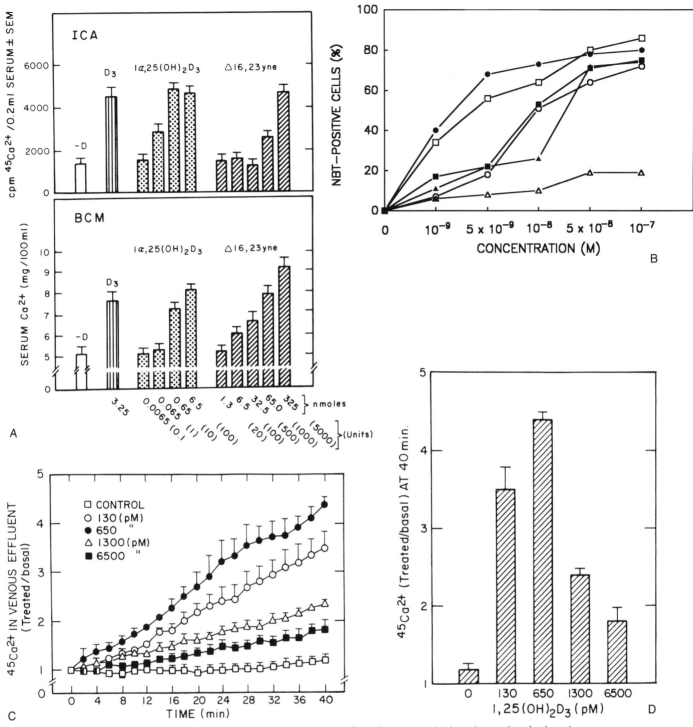

FIG. 4. Diversity of the biological actions of $1\alpha,25(OH)_2D_3$ in classical and nonclassical systems. **A:** Mineral metabolism: stimulation of intestinal Ca^{2+} absorption *(ICA)* and bone Ca^{2+}-mobilizing activity *(BCM)* in the vitamin D-deficient chick $(-D)$ by increasing doses of $1\alpha,25(OH)_2D_3$ or an analog $1\alpha,25(OH)_2$-16-ene-23-yne-D3. The vitamin D compounds were given intramuscularly to vitamin D-deficient chicks 12 hr before assay. The control vitamin D_3 (D_3) was given 48 hr before assay. A detailed description of the methods is given in refs. 21 and 22. **B:** Cell differentiation: dose-response of $1\alpha,25(OH)_2D_3$ (0–0) and five structurally related vitamin D analogs on differentiation of HL-60 cells. The results are expressed as a percentage of untreated HL-60 cells for reduction of nitroblue tetrazolium *(NBT),* which is a measure of differentiation of the HL-60 cell into a macrophage-like cell. Experimental details are provided in ref. 22. **C and D:** Nongenomic effect of $1\alpha,25(OH)_2D_3$ on the appearance of $^{45}Ca^{2+}$ in the venous effluent of perfused duodena from vitamin D-replete chicks by the process of transcaltachia (the rapid hormonal stimulation of intestinal Ca^{2+} transport). **C:** Very rapid onset of increased appearance of $^{45}Ca^{2+}$ (within 2–6 min) after introduction of varying doses of $1\alpha,25(OH)_2D_3$. **D:** Replotting of the data obtained after 40 min and illustration of the biphasic nature of the transcaltachic response. In this assay each duodena is filled with $^{45}Ca^{2+}$, and the agonist $1\alpha,25(OH)_2D_3$ is perfused through the celiac artery. The transcaltachic assay quantitates the transfer of $^{45}Ca^{2+}$ from the lumen of the intestine to the blood compartment. Experimental details are provided in ref. 17.

tachic process is not blocked by actinomycin D, an inhibitor of DNA-directed RNA synthesis (12), but is inhibited by drugs such as nifedipine, which are known blockers of voltage-gated Ca^{2+} channels (15). It is to be anticipated that there will be further description of the involvement of $1\alpha,25(OH)_2D_3$ in nongenomic biologic responses in the immediate future.

OVERVIEW OF THE VITAMIN D ENDOCRINE SYSTEM

Figure 5 summarizes the biologic events that 1) support the production of vitamin D (upper left); 2) are involved with its metabolism to its hormonally active form, namely $1,25(OH)_2D_3$, in the kidney (upper center), including the regulatory involvement of a number of other classical hormones (upper right); 3) describe the interaction of $1,25(OH)_2D_3$ in its classical target organs of intestine,

bone, and kidney (lower center); 4) describe the interaction of $1,25(OH)_2D_3$ in a lengthy list of "new" target organs/cells, some of which produce calbindin-D (lower right); and 5) describe the existence of a paracrine system for the production and interaction of $1,25(OH)_2D_3$ in cells of hematopoiesis.

$24,25(OH)_2D_3$ is a second dihydroxylated metabolite of vitamin D_3 that is produced by the kidney (Fig. 5). There is emerging evidence that $24R,24(OH)_2D_3$ has the capability to generate selected physiological responses different from $1,25(OH)_2D_3$ (5). A discussion of this topic is beyond the scope of this review.

Thus, although the arena of action of $1,25(OH)_2D_3$ is vast, there have emerged some unifying principles with respect to its actions as a steroid hormone. It is now definitely an accepted fact that $1,25(OH)_2D_3$ belongs in the family of steroid hormones. This is justified not only on chemical grounds, but on the grounds of fundamental similarities in their metabolism and modes of action.

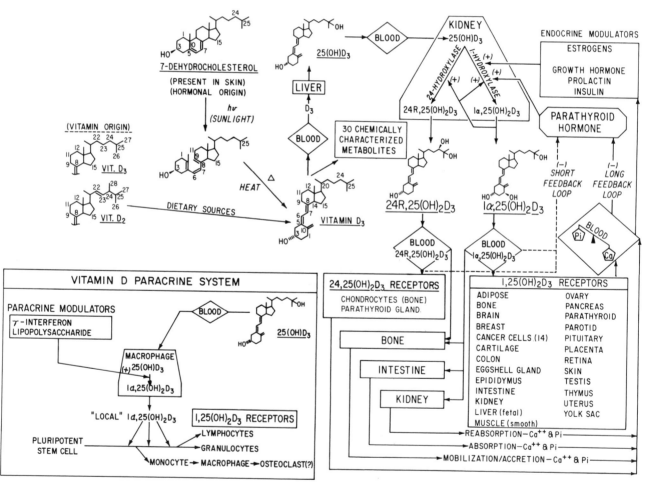

A. W. NORMAN

FIG. 5. Overview of the vitamin D endocrine system. *CaBP*, calcium binding protein, or calbindin-D_{28k}, which is induced by $1\alpha,25(OH)_2D_3$; *hv*, ultraviolet irradiation; *Pi*, inorganic phosphate; *Ca²⁺*, inorganic calcium ions. The *inset* in the *lower right-hand corner* lists cells and or organs that contain receptors for $1\alpha,25(OH)_2D_3$ and some of which contain calbindin-D_{28k}. The *inset* in the *lower left-hand corner* diagrams schematically a vitamin D paracrine system postulated to be operative in the bone marrow. See refs. 11 and 23 for more details.

CLINICAL CORRELATES

Conceptually, human clinical disorders related to vitamin D can be considered as those arising because of 1) altered availability of the parent vitamin D; 2) altered conversion of vitamin D to its principal daughter metabolites $1,25(OH)_2D_3$ and $24R,25(OH)_2D_3$; 3) conditions that may be due to variations in organ responsiveness to these dihydroxylated metabolites; and 4) perturbations in the integrated interactions of these metabolites with PTH and calcitonin. Figure 6 presents a schematic diagram of the relationship between human diseases states related to vitamin D and the vitamin D endocrine system.

It is possible to identify diseases that are present in the intestine (e.g., malabsorption and tropical sprue; see

Chapter 65) or diseases of the parathyroid gland (hyper- and hypoparathyroidism; see Chapters 29 and 45), of the bone (e.g., osteomalacia, renal osteodystrophy, or osteoporosis), or the kidney, such as chronic renal failure (Chapter 73). All of these in their own way reflect a disturbance in or a malfunctioning of the body's normal endocrine processing of vitamin D and its interaction with the other calcemic hormones. It is to be anticipated that new insights into the pathogenesis of disease related to the vitamin D endocrine system will arise as a consequence of our greatly increased knowledge concerning the scope and diversity of tissues in which both $1,25(OH)_2D_3$ and $24,25(OH)_2D_3$ interact to produce biological responses. Other chapters describe in more detail some of these disease states (e.g., osteoporosis and hypercalcemia of malignancy).

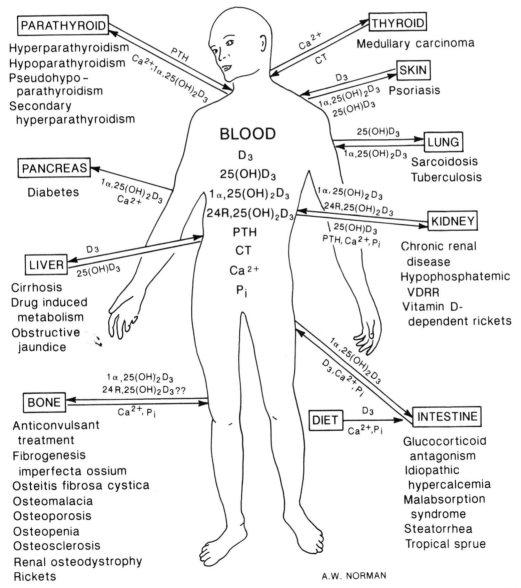

FIG. 6. Human disease states related to vitamin D and the vitamin D endocrine system. *PTH,* parathyroid hormone; *CT,* calcitonin; *Pi,* inorganic phosphate; *Ca²⁺,* calcium. See ref. 23 for more details.

ACKNOWLEDGMENT

This work was supported by U.S. Public Health Service Grant DK-09012-029.

REFERENCES

1. Nemere I, Norman AW: Transport of calcium. In: Field M, Frizzel RA (eds) *Handbook of Physiology.* Bethesda, American Physiological Society, pp 337–360, 1991
2. Theofan G, Nguyen AP, Norman AW: Regulation of calbindin-D28K gene expression by 1,25-dihydroxyvitamin D_3 is correlated to receptor occupancy. *J Biol Chem* 261:16943–16947, 1986
3. Minghetti PP, Cancela L, Fujisawa Y, Theofan G, Norman AW: Molecular structure of the chicken vitamin D-induced calbindin-D28K gene reveals eleven exons, six Ca^{2+}-binding domains, and numerous promoter regulatory elements. *Mol Endocrinol* 2: 355–367, 1988
4. Leathers VL, Linse S, Forsen S, Norman AW: Calbindin-D28K, a 1α,25-dihydroxyvitamin D_3-induced calcium-binding protein, binds five or six Ca^{2+} ions with high affinity. *J Biol Chem* 265: 9838–9841, 1990
5. Norman AW, Roth J, Orci L: The vitamin D endocrine system: Steroid metabolism, hormone receptors and biological response (calcium binding proteins). *Endocr Rev* 3:331–366, 1982
6. Walters MR: Newly identified actions of the vitamin D endocrine system. *Endocr Rev* 13:719–764, 1992
7. Reichel H, Koeffler HP, Norman AW: Production of 1α,25-dihydroxyvitamin D_3 by hematopoietic cells. *Prog Clin Biol Res* 332: 81–97, 1990
8. Manolagas SC, Hustmyer FG, Yu XP: 1,25-Dihydroxyvitamin D-3 and the immune system (42915). *Exp Biol Med* 52:238–245, 1989
9. Pike JW: Vitamin D_3 receptors: Structure and function in transcription. *Annu Rev Nutr* 11:189–216, 1991
10. Minghetti PP, Norman AW: 1,25(OH)2-Vitamin D_3 receptors: Gene regulation and genetic circuitry. *FASEB J* 2:3043–3053, 1988
11. Lowe KE, Maiyar AC, Norman AW: Vitamin D-mediated gene expression. *Crit Rev Eukar Gene Exp* 2:65–109, 1992
12. Nemere I, Yoshimoto Y, Norman AW: Studies on the mode of action of calciferol. LIV. Calcium transport in perfused duodena from normal chicks: Enhancement with 14 minutes of exposure to 1,25-dihydroxyvitamin D_3. *Endocrinology* 115:1476–1483, 1984
13. Caffrey JM, Farach-Carson MC: Vitamin D_3 metabolites modulate dihydropyridine-sensitive calcium currents in clonal rat osteosarcoma cells. *J Biol Chem* 264:20265–20274, 1989
14. Henry HL: Vitamin D hydroxylases. *J Cell Biochem* 49:4–9, 1992
15. Deboland AR, Nemere I, Norman AW: Ca^{2+}-channel agonist bay K8644 mimics 1,25(OH)2-vitamin D_3 enhancement of Ca^{2+} transport in chick perfused duodenum. *Biochem Biophys Res Commun* 166:217–222, 1990
16. Suda T, Shinki T, Takahashi N: The role of vitamin D in bone and intestinal cell differentiation. *Ann Rev Nutr* 10:195–211, 1990
17. Holick MF: Skin: Site of the synthesis of vitamin D and a target tissue for the active form, 1,25-dihydroxyvitamin D_3. *Ann NY Acad Sci* 548:14–26, 1988
18. Zhou L-X, Norman AW: 1,25(OH)2-Vitamin D_3 analog structure-function assessment of the rapid stimulation of intestinal calcium absorption (transcaltachia). *J Bone Min Res* 7:457–463, 1992
19. Henry HL, Norman AW: Vitamin D: Metabolism and biological action. *Ann Rev Nutr* 4:493–520, 1984
20. Norman AW, Nemere I, Zhou L-X, et al.: 1,25(OH)2-Vitamin D_3, a steroid hormone that produces biologic effects via both genomic and nongenomic pathways. *J Steroid Biochem Mol Biol* 41:231–240, 1992
21. Hibberd KA, Norman AW: Comparative biological effects of vitamins D_2 and D_3 and dihydrotachysterol 2 and dihydrotachysterol 3 in the chick. *Biochem Pharmacol* 18:2347–2355, 1969
22. Norman AW, Zhou J-Y, Henry HL, Uskokovic MR, Koeffler HP: Structure-function studies on analogues of 1a,25-dihydroxyvitamin D_3: Differential effects on leukemic cell growth, differentiation, and intestinal calcium absorption. *Cancer Res* 50: 6857–6864, 1990
23. Reichel H, Koeffler HP, Norman AW: The role of the vitamin D endocrine system in health and disease. *N Engl J Med* 320: 980–991, 1989

14. Calcitonin

Leonard J. Deftos, M.D.

Department of Medicine, University of California–San Diego, and San Diego Veterans Affairs Medical Center, La Jolla, California

Calcitonin (CT) is a 32-amino-acid peptide that is secreted primarily by thyroidal C-cells. Its main biological effect is to inhibit osteoclastic bone resorption. This property has led to CT's use for disorders characterized by increased bone resorption. Calcitonin is currently approved by the Food and Drug Administration for the treatment of Paget's disease, osteoporosis, and for the hypercalcemia of malignancy. The secretion of CT is regulated acutely by blood calcium and chronically by gender and perhaps age. Calcitonin is metabolized by the kidney and the liver. Calcitonin is also a tumor marker for medullary thyroid carcinoma, the signal tumor of Multiple Endocrine Neoplasia (MEN) type II (1–3).

BIOCHEMISTRY

The structure has been determined for 12 species of CT, including human (3) (Fig. 1). Common features include a 1–7 amino terminal disulfide bridge, a glycine at residue 28, and a carboxy-terminal proline amide residue. Five of the nine amino-terminal residues are identical in all CT species. The greatest divergence resides in the interior 27 amino acids. Basic amino acid substitutions enhance potency. Thus, the nonmammalian CTs have the most potency, even in mammalian systems. Unlike parathyroid hormone (PTH), a biologically active fragment of CT has

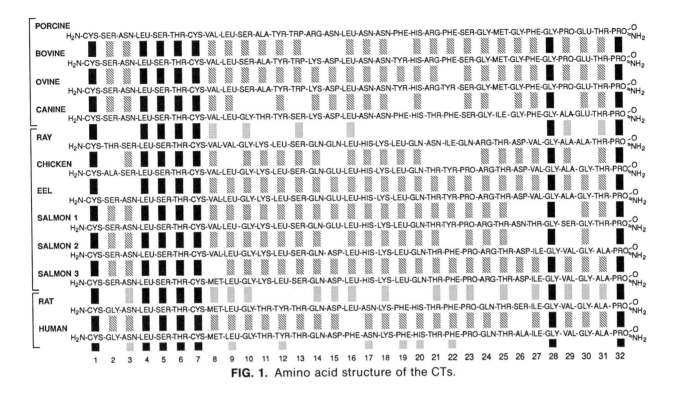

FIG. 1. Amino acid structure of the CTs.

not been discovered. However, an amphipathic backbone seems to enhance potency.

MOLECULAR BIOLOGY

The CT gene consists of 6 exons separated by introns (3) (Fig. 2). Two distinct, mature mRNAs are generated from differential splicing of the exon regions in the initial gene transcript. One translates as a 141-residue CT precursor, the other a 128-residue precursor for calcitonin gene-related peptide (CGRP). Calcitonin is the major posttranslationally processed peptide in C-cells, whereas CGRP, a 37-amino-acid peptide, is the major processed peptide in neurons. The main biological effect of CGRP is vasodilation, but it also functions as a neurotransmitter and does react with the CT receptor. The relevance of CGRP to skeletal metabolism is unknown, but it may be produced locally in skeletal tissue. Another alternate splicing pathway for the CT gene has been recently described. It produces a carboxy-terminal C-pro CT with 8 different terminal amino acids (7). The CT gene predicts the presence of other processed peptides, and there is more than one copy of this gene (4–7).

BIOSYNTHESIS

Thyroidal C-cells are the primary source of CT in mammals and the ultimobranchial gland is in submammals (1–5). C-cells are neural crest derivatives and also produce CGRP, the second CT gene product. Other tissue sources of CT have been described, notably the pituitary cells and widely distributed neuroendocrine cells (5,8,9). Although CT may have paracrine effects at these sites, the nonthyroidal sources of CT are not likely to contribute to its peripheral concentration. However, malignant transformation can occur in both eutopic and ectopic cells that produce CT, and the peptide then becomes a tumor marker. The best example of the former is medullary thyroid carcinoma of the latter small cell lung cancer. Many of the tumors associated with ectopic CT production probably derive this potential from their common neural crest origin with thyroidal C-cells (1).

BIOLOGICAL EFFECTS

The main biological effect of CT is to inhibit osteoclastic bone resorption (10). Within minutes of its administration, CT causes the osteoclast to shrink in size and to decrease its bone-resorbing activity (10,11). This dramatic and complex event is accompanied by the production of cAMP and by increased cytosolic calcium in the osteoclast (1–3,11). In a situation where bone turnover is sufficiently high, CT will produce hypocalcemia and hypophosphatemia. Calcitonin has also been reported to inhibit osteocytes and stimulate osteoblasts, but these effects are controversial (10). Analgesia is a commonly reported effect of CT treatment (4). Calciuria, phosphaturia, and gastrointestinal effects on calcium flux have been reported for CT, but they occur at concentrations of the hormone that are supraphysiologic (1). It should be noted however,

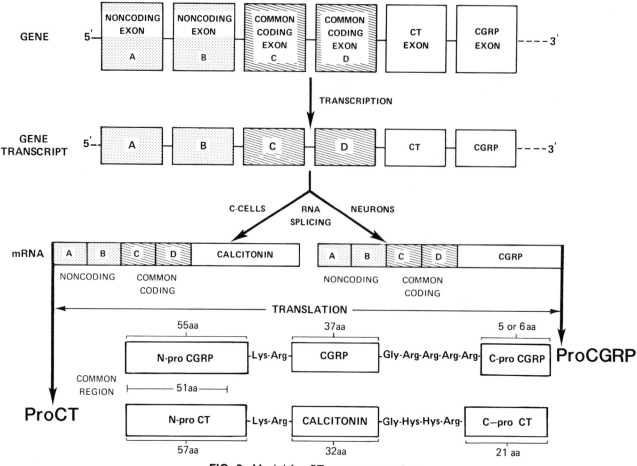

FIG. 2. Model for CT gene expression.

that the concentration of the peptide at its several sites of biosynthesis may be sufficiently high to explain some extraskeletal effects of CT by a paracrine mechanism (12). Thus, CT may exert physiological effects on the pituitary and central nervous system (5,8). Furthermore, the demonstration of CT and CT receptors at intracranial sites may qualify CT as a neurotransmitter (13). Other effects of CT have been reported. It has been observed to act as an antiinflammatory agent, to promote fracture and wound healing, to be uricosuric, to be antihypertensive, and to impair glucose tolerance. Calcitonin may regulate and be regulated by other calcitropic hormones, and there is some evidence to suggest that CT exerts an autoregulatory effect (12). The importance of these effects is yet to be determined (1–3).

CT as a Drug

The main biological action of CT—its inhibition of osteoclastic bone resorption—has resulted in its successful use in disease states characterized by increased bone resorption and the consequent hypercalcemia. Calcitonin is widely used in Paget's disease where osteoclastic bone resorption is dramatically increased. Calcitonin is also used in osteoporosis where increased bone resorption may be more subtle and in the treatment of hypercalcemia of malignancy (14). Newer pharmacological preparations of CT may have improved therapeutic effects (17). Nasal preparation of CT is receiving increasing clinical application (18).

SECRETION

Calcium

Ambient calcium concentration is the most important regulator of CT secretion (1). When blood calcium rises acutely, there is a proportional increase in CT secretion, and an acute decrease in blood calcium produces a corresponding decrease in plasma CT. However, the effects of chronic hypercalcemia and chronic hypocalcemia are not fully defined and conflicting results have been reported (19,20). It seems likely that the C-cells can respond to sustained hypercalcemia by increasing CT secretion; but, if the hypercalcemia is severe and/or prolonged, the C-cells probably exhaust their secretory reserve (1). The inhibitory effect on CT secretion by hypocalcemia is difficult to demonstrate. Chronic hypocalcemia seems to decrease the secretory challenge to C-cells and they increase their stores of CT; these stores can be released on appropriate stimulation (21).

Metabolism

The metabolism of CT is a complex process that involves many organ systems. Evidence has been reported for degradation of the hormone by kidney, liver, bone, and even the thyroid gland (3). Like many other peptide hormones, CT disappears from plasma in a multiexponential manner that includes an early half-life measured in minutes. In most studies, the kidney seems to be the most important organ of clearance for CT. Inactivation of the hormone seems more important than renal excretion, because relatively little CT can be detected in urine (1–4).

Gastrointestinal Factors

Gastrointestinal peptides, especially those of the gastrin-cholecystokinin family, are potent CT secretagogues when administered parenterally in supraphysiological concentrations (1,2). This observation has led to the postulate that there is an entero-C-cell regulatory pathway for CT secretion. However, only meals that contain sufficient calcium to raise the blood calcium have been demonstrated to increase CT secretion in humans (19). Thus, the secretory relationship between the gastrointestinal tract and C-cells in human needs further exploration to determine its physiological significance.

Other Factors

Although a variety of neuroendocrine and ionic factors have been demonstrated to regulate CT secretion under experimental conditions (1), it is unlikely that these agents participate in the physiological regulation of CT secretion (1–5).

Provocative Testing for CT-Producing Tumors

The stimulatory effect of calcium and gastrin-related peptides, especially pentagastrin, on CT secretion has led to the use of these agents as provocative tests for the secretion of CT (2). These procedures are widely used in patients suspected of having medullary thyroid carcinoma (MTC), especially when the basal concentration of the hormone is not diagnostically elevated. Medullary thyroid carcinoma is a neoplastic disorder of thyroidal C-cells that can occur in a familial pattern as part of MEN type II. Most tumors respond with increased CT secretion to the administration of either calcium or pentagastrin or their

combination, but either agent can sometimes give misleading results. Therefore, in clinically compelling situations both agents should be considered for diagnostic testing. Calcitonin measurements can also be used to evaluate the effectiveness of therapy in patients with CT-producing tumors.

Gender and Age

Most investigators find that females have lower CT levels than males (22,23). The mechanism of this difference is unclear, but may be accounted for in part by a stimulating effect of gonadal steroids on CT secretion (24,25). The effect of age on CT secretion is more controversial (22,23,26); newborns seem to have a higher serum level of the hormone and a progressive decline in adults with age has been reported by several laboratories (1,22,26). However, stable adult levels have also been observed (23). It is likely that the different assay procedures used in different studies account for the conflicting results (Fig. 3). Thus, the serum concentration of some forms of CT may decline with age whereas others do not (22,23). The physiological significance of the various circulating forms of CT measured by different assay procedures has not been defined. Nonmonomeric, as well as monomeric, forms of circulating CT species are biologically active (1,27), and some procedures may not accurately reflect biologically active CT in blood.

CLINICAL ABNORMALITIES OF CT SECRETION

Medullary Thyroid Carcinoma

Medullary thyroid carcinoma is a tumor of the CT-producing C-cells of the thyroid gland (2). Although a rare tumor, it can occur in a familial pattern as part of MEN type II (Table 1). Medullary thyroid carcinoma is generally regarded as intermediate between the aggressive behavior of anaplastic thyroid carcinoma and the more indolent behavior of papillary and follicular thyroid carcinoma. The most common presentation is a thyroid nodule and the most common symptom is diarrhea. These tumors usually produce diagnostically elevated serum concentrations of CT. Therefore, the radioimmunoassay for CT in serum can be used to diagnose the presence of MTC with an exceptional degree of accuracy and specificity. In a small but increasing percentage of patients, however, basal hormone levels are indistinguishable from normal. Many of these subjects represent the early stages of C-cell neoplasia or hyperplasia most amenable to surgical cure. To identify these patients with early disease, provocative tests for CT secretion, previously discussed, have been developed that can identify MTC in a patient whose diagnosis could have been missed if only basal CT determinations had been performed (see Appendix).

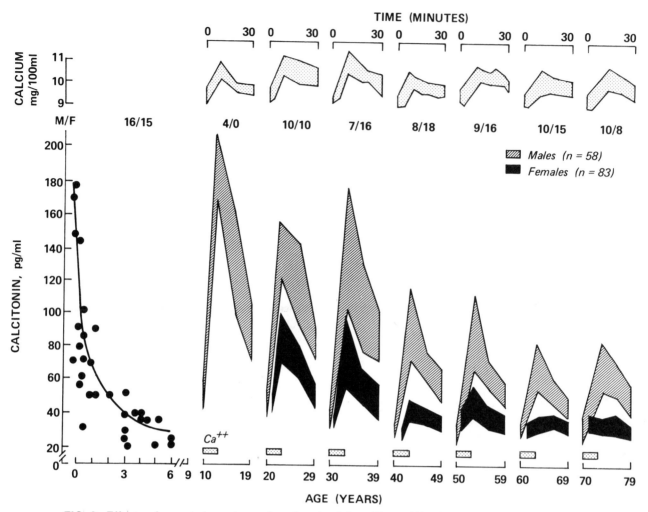

FIG. 3. Effects of age and gender on basal and calcium (3 mgs/10 min)-stimulated CT secretion in humans. (Data from refs. 22 and 26.)

Other CT-Producing Neoplasms

Neoplastic disorders of other neuroendocrine cells can also produce abnormally elevated amounts of CT. The

TABLE 1. *Components of Multiple Endocrine Neoplasia MEN type II and their frequency*

Component	MEN type IIA (%)	MEN type IIB (%)
Medullary thyroid carcinoma	97	90
Pheochromocytoma	30	45
Hyperparathyroidism	50	Rare
Mucosal neuroma syndrome	—	100

best known example is small cell lung cancer. However, other tumors, such as carcinoids and islet cell tumors of the pancreas, can do the same (1,2).

Renal Disease

There are increases in immunoassayable CT with both acute and chronic renal failure, but considerable disagreement exists regarding the mechanism and significance of these increases (1–3). Because the secretion and/or metabolism of CT is abnormal in renal disease and because renal osteodystrophy is characterized by increased bone resorption, CT, which acts to inhibit bone resorption, has been implicated in the pathogenesis of uremic osteodystrophy (3).

Hypercalciuria

Elevated levels of CT have been demonstrated in patients with hypercalciuria (28). The physiologic significance of enhanced CT secretion is unknown but may represent a compensatory response to intestinal hyperabsorption of calcium. Although CT in high concentrations has both phosphaturic and calciuric actions in man, it is not likely that a primary alteration in CT secretion contributes to the development of hypercalciuria (1).

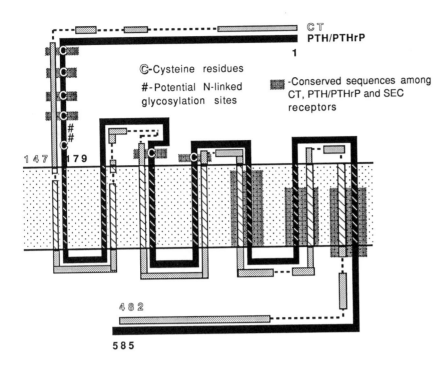

FIG. 4. Comparison of the deduced amino acid sequences of the receptors for CT, PTH/PTH-related protein, and secretin *(SEC).* Breaks in the sequences have been inserted to align the conserved amino acids. *Shaded areas* represent the regions of greatest identity and similarity. (From Lin HY, et al.: Expression cloning of an adenylate cyclase-coupled calcitonin receptor. *Science* 254:1022–1024, 1991.)

Bone Disease

No skeletal disease has been conclusively attributed to CT abnormalities (3,27). Although females have lower CT levels than males, there is conflicting evidence as to whether endogenous secretion of the hormone contributes to the pathogenesis of osteoporosis (25,29,30). That it does so is additionally supported by studies in which CT has been of therapeutic benefit in osteoporosis (17). Reduced CT reserve in females may contribute to the greater severity of osteitis fibrosa cystica in women with primary hyperparathyroidism (20).

Hypercalcemia and Hypocalcemia

Calcium challenge is a well-documented stimulus for CT secretion. Although increased CT secretion has only inconsistently been associated with chronic hypercalcemia (19,20), an exaggerated response of CT to secretagogues has been convincingly observed in several hypocalcemic states (21).

Calcitonin Receptor

The CT receptor has been recently cloned (31). It has seven putative transmembrane domains, but it shows no homology to other classical receptor families. Rather it is structurally related to the secretin receptor and the PTH/PTH-related protein receptor (Fig. 4). The CT receptor subserves a dual signal transduction function in that it can activate effector pathways mediated by both cAMP and by the phosphoinositol/Ca^{2+} pathway (32). The availability of CT receptor-specific probes will allow better elucidation of the function of CT than has been possible by imprecise binding studies.

Role of Calcitonin in Mineral Metabolism

The role of CT in calcium homeostasis and skeletal metabolism has not been established in humans, and many questions remain unanswered about the significance of this hormone in humans. Does CT secretion decline with age? Do gonadal steroids regulate the secretion of CT? Do the lower levels of serum CT in females contribute to the pathogenesis of age-related loss of bone mass and osteoporosis? Do extrathyroidal sources of CT participate in the regulation of skeletal metabolism? Are there primary and secondary abnormalities of CT secretion in diseases of skeletal and calcium homeostasis? The conclusive answer to these questions awaits clinical studies with an assay procedure that directly measures the biological activity of CT in blood. Furthermore, accurate local measurements of CT and its effects may be necessary to elucidate the emerging role of CT as a paracrine and autocrine agent.

ACKNOWLEDGMENTS

This work was supported by the National Institutes of Health, the National Cancer Institute, and the Department of Veterans Affairs.

REFERENCES

1. Deftos LJ: Calcitonin and medullary thyroid carcinoma. In: Wyngaarden, Smith, Bennett (eds) *Cecil Textbook of Medicine, 19th* ed. WB Saunders, Philadelphia, pp 1420–1423, 1991

2. Deftos LJ: Calcitonin secretion in humans. In: Cooper CW (ed) *Current Research on Calcium Regulating Hormones*. Univ. of Texas Press, Austin, pp 79–100, 1987

3. Deftos LJ: *Medullary Thyroid Carcinoma*. S Karger Publishing Co. New York, pp 1–114, 1983

4. Deftos LJ, Roos B: Medullary thyroid carcinoma and calcitonin gene expression. In: Peck WA (ed) *Bone and Mineral Research*. Excerpta Medica, Amsterdam pp 267–316, 1989

5. Fischer JA, Born W: Calcitonin gene products: evolution, expression and biological targets. *Bone and Mineral* 2:347–353, 1987

6. Cote GJ, Gould JA, Huang SC, Gagel RF: Studies of short-term secretion of peptides produced by alternative RNA processing. *Mol Cell Endocrinol* 53:211–219, 1987

7. Minvielle S, et al.: A novel calcitonin carboxyl-terminal peptide produced in medullary thyroid carcinoma by alternative RNA processing of the calcitonin/calcitonin gene-related peptide gene. *J Biol Chem* 266:24627–24631, 1991

8. Deftos LJ: Pituitary cells secrete calcitonin in the reverse hemolytic plaque assay. *Biophys Research Commun* 146:1350–1356, 1987

9. Becker KL, Monaghan KG, Silva OL: Immunocytochemical localization of calcitonin in Kulchitsky cells of human lung. *Arch Pathol Lab Med* 104:196–198, 1980

10. Deftos LJ, Glowacki J: Mechanisms of bone metabolism. In: Kem DC, Frohlich E (eds) *Pathophysiology*. JB Lippincott Co., Philadelphia, pp 445–468, 1984

11. Moonga BS, et al.: Regulation of cystosolic free calcium in isolated osteoclasts by calcitonin. *J Endocrinol* 132:241–249, 1992

12. Deftos LJ, Burton DW, Brown TF, Fieck A, Brandt DW: Calcitonin responsive elements are present in the calcitonin and PTH-like protein genes. *J Bone Min Res* 7:5235, 1992

13. Goltzman D, Tannenbaum GS: Induction of hypocalcemia by intracerebroventricular injection of calcitonin: evidence for control of blood calcium by the nervous system. *Brain Res* 416:1–6, 1987

14. Avioli LV: Calcitonin therapy for bone disease and hypercalcemia. *Arch Intern Med* 142:2076–2080, 1982

15. Singer FR, Schiller AL, Pyle EB, Krane SM: Paget's disease of bone. In: Avioli LV, Krane SM (eds). Academic Press, New York, pp 490–567, 1978

16. Gruber H, Ivey JL, Baylink DJ, Matthews M, Nelp WB, Sisom K, Chestnut CH III: Long-term calcitonin therapy in postmenopausal osteoporosis. *Metabolism* 33:295–298, 1984

17. Buclin T, Randin JP, Jacquet AF, Azria M, Attinger M, Gomez F, Burckhardt P: The effect of rectal and nasal administration of salmon calcitonin in normal subjects. *Calcif Tiss Int* 41:252–254, 1987

18. Carslens JH, Feinblatt JD. Future horizons for calcitonin. *J Bone Min Res* 49:2–6, 1991

19. Austin LA, Heath H III: Calcitonin—Physiology and pathophysiology. *N Engl J Med* 304:269–278, 1981

20. Parthemore JG, Deftos LJ: Secretion of calcitonin in primary hyperparathyroidism. *J Clin Endocrinol Metab* 49:223–226, 1979

21. Deftos LJ, Powell D, Parthemore JG, Potts JT Jr: Secretion of calcitonin in hypocalcemic states in man. *J Clin Invest* 52:3109–3114, 1973

22. Deftos LJ, Weisman MH, Williams GH, Karpf DB, Frumar AM, Davidson BH, Parthemore JG, Judd HL: Influence of age and sex on plasma calcitonin in human beings. *N Engl J Med* 302:1351–1353, 1980

23. Tiegs RD, Body JJ, Barta JM, Health H III: Secretion and metabolism of monomeric human calcitonin: Effects of age, sex, and thyroid damage. *J Bone Min Res* 1:339–343, 1986

24. Foresta C, Scanelli G, Zanatta GP, Busnardo B, Scandellari: Reduced calcitonin reserve in young hypogonadic osteoporotic men. *Hormone Metab Res* 19:275–278, 1987

25. Stevenson JC, White MC, Joplin GF, MacIntyre I: Osteoporosis and calcitonin deficiency. *Br Med J* 285:1010–1011, 1982

26. Klein GL, Wadlington EL, Collins ED, Catherwood BD, Deftos LJ: Calcitonin levels in sera of infants and children: Relations to age and periods of bone growth. *Calcif Tiss Int* 36:635–638, 1984

27. Tashjian AH Jr: Calcitonin 1976: A review of some recent advances. In: James VHT (ed) *Excerpta Medica International Congress Series Proceedings of the V International Congress of Endocrinology*. Amsterdam, New York, pp 256–261, 1976

28. Ivey JJ, Roos BA, Shen FH, Baylink DJ: Increased immunoreactive calcitonin in idiopathic hypercalciuria. *Metab Bone Dis Rel Res* 3:29–32, 1981

29. Taggart HM, Ivey JJ, Sisom K, Chestnut CH III, Baylink DJ, Huber MB: Deficient calcitonin response to calcium stimulation in postmenopausal osteoporosis. *Lancet* 1:475–478, 1982

30. Tiegs RD, Body JJ, Wahner HW, Barta J, Riggs BL, Heath H III: Calcitonin secretion in postmenopausal osteoporosis. *N Engl J Med* 312:1097–2000, 1985

31. Lin HY, et al.: Expression cloning of an adenylate cyclase-coupled calcitonin receptor. *Science* 254:1022–1024, 1991

32. Chabre O, et al.: A recombinant calcitonin receptor independently stimulates $3'5'$-cAMP and Ca^{2+}/inositol phosphate signalling pathways. *Mol Endocrinol* 6:551–556, 1992

15. Regulation of Bone Mineral Homeostasis: An Integrated View

Daniel D. Bikle, M.D., Ph.D.

Department of Medicine, University of California, San Francisco, and Veterans Administration Medical Center, San Francisco, California

Regulation of bone mineral homeostasis simply stated refers to controlling the intra- and extracellular levels of three ions [calcium (Ca), magnesium (Mg), and phosphate (Pi)] with three hormones {parathyroid hormone (PTH), calcitonin (CT), and 1,25-dihydroxyvitamin D [$1,25(OH)_2D$]} acting on three target tissues (bone, intestine, and kidney). This simple conceptual framework of bone mineral homeostasis only partially reflects the true situation. Other ions are involved; levels of pH, sodium, potassium, chloride, bicarbonate, and sulfate all alter the cellular handling of Ca, Pi, and Mg. Likewise other hormones, including prolactin, glucocorticoid hormones, growth hormone, insulin, insulin-like growth factors, and a large number of cytokines, contribute in important ways to the regulation of bone mineral homeostasis. Finally, we now recognize that a large number of tissues other than bone, intestine, and kidney serve as target tissues for the calciotropic hormones in ways that contribute to bone mineral homeostasis. However, in this chapter we will focus on the interactions among PTH, CT, and $1,25(OH)_2D$ as they regulate Ca, Mg, and Pi levels in serum through actions on bone, intestine, and kidney. Clinical examples will be provided to illustrate how this integration takes place in the patient. Details for individual tissues, hormones, and ions are to be found in the preceding chapters.

INTEGRATION OF HORMONE ACTION AT THE TISSUE LEVEL

Figure 1 illustrates the interactions between PTH and $1,25(OH)_2D$ in their regulation of serum Ca and Pi levels through their actions on bone, kidney, and intestine. Calcitonin is not included in this figure principally because its physiologic role in regulating bone mineral homeostasis is modest relative to that of PTH and $1,25(OH)_2D$. Magnesium is also not included in this figure, because its regula-

	Ca, Pi	Ca, Pi	Ca, Pi	Ca, Pi
PTH	↑,↑	—	↑,↓	↑,↓
CT	↓,↓	—	↓,↓	↓,↓
1,25D	↑,↑	↑,↑	—	↑,↑
	Bone	Gut	Kidney	Net

FIG. 2. Effect of calciotropic hormones on the blood level of Ca and Pi via their actions on their target tissues. *Arrows* indicate the effect the hormones have on Ca or Pi levels when acting on their target tissues on the x-axis.

tion by these hormones is either nonexistent or inadequately defined. However, as will be described, both CT and Mg play important roles in the etiology and treatment of certain disorders of bone mineral homeostasis. Figure 2 summarizes these actions of the calciotropic hormones with respect to their ability to regulate blood Ca and Pi levels at the different target tissues. Figure 3 illustrates the feedback and feed forward mechanisms by which Ca and Pi as well as the calciotropic hormones themselves regulate calciotropic hormone production and secretion.

As shown in Fig. 1, Ca and Pi enter the blood from the intestine, leave it through the kidney, and are stored in the body principally in bone. In order to maintain homeostasis, the net absorption of Ca and Pi in the intestine must be precisely balanced by net excretion of these ions by the kidney. Absorption of these ions by the gut is not a continuous process, but depends on dietary intake. The efficiency at which absorption occurs for a given dietary load is the regulated variable. Glomerular filtration of these ions by the kidney is relatively constant, so the kidney must be able to adjust its ability to reabsorb Ca and Pi as a function of body needs. It is the efficiency of reabsorption of these ions that is regulated. Bone provides the major buffer for maintaining relatively constant blood levels of these ions. This is achieved by balancing bone formation (which deposits these ions in bone) with bone resorption (which releases these ions to the blood stream). Different hormones act on the different tissues by different mechanisms. Yet, their effects are well coordinated to ensure increased supply of bone minerals during periods of growth, steady-state levels during middle life, but gradual loss during aging.

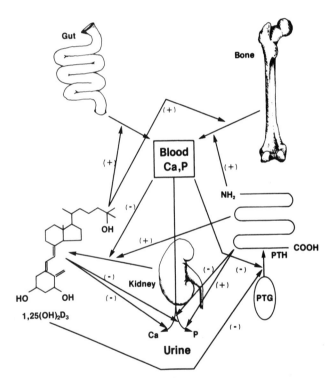

FIG. 1. Integrated view of bone mineral homeostasis. Interactions of the two principal calciotropic hormones [PTH and $1,25(OH)_2D$] acting on the three principal organs (bone, gut, and kidney) governing Ca and Pi homeostasis are shown. 1,25-Dihydroxyvitamin D is produced in the kidney under the regulation of Ca, Pi, and PTH. It stimulates intestinal Ca and Pi absorption, and with PTH regulates bone turnover and renal excretion of Ca and Pi. Parathyroid hormone is produced by the parathyroid gland *(PTG)* under the regulation of Ca and $1,25(OH)_2D$. It stimulates bone turnover, renal Pi excretion, and renal Ca reabsorption. The net effect of $1,25(OH)_2D$ is to raise serum Ca and Pi while decreasing PTH. The net effect of PTH is to raise serum Ca and $1,25(OH)_2D$ while decreasing serum Pi.

Intestinal Absorption of Calcium and Phosphate

1,25-Dihydroxyvitamin D stimulates intestinal Ca and Pi absorption. Hypocalcemia and hypophosphatemia

	Ca	Pi	PTH	1,25
PTH	↓	—	—	↓
CT	↑	?	?	?
1,25	↓	↓	↑	↓
	Ca	Pi	PTH	1,25

FIG. 3. Regulation of calciotropic hormone production and secretion. *Arrows* indicate the effect the agents on the x-axis have on the production and secretion of the hormones on the y-axis.

characterize the patient with vitamin D deficiency or vitamin D resistance principally because intestinal Ca and Pi absorption are impaired. As described in Chapter 13, 1,25(OH)$_2$D acts through both genomic and nongenomic mechanisms to regulate intestinal Ca and Pi absorption. Of interest is that the site of the intestine most sensitive to 1,25(OH)$_2$D-stimulated Ca transport (duodenum) differs from the site most sensitive to 1,25(OH)$_2$D-stimulated Pi transport (jejunum). Likewise, the mechanisms underlying Ca and Pi transport appear to be different, although little is known at the molecular level regarding 1,25(OH)$_2$D-stimulated Pi transport in the intestine. Intestinal Ca transport is quite dependent on adequate levels of 1,25(OH)$_2$D; Pi transport is less dependent on 1,25(OH)$_2$D but is clearly stimulated by 1,25(OH)$_2$D; Mg absorption is little affected by 1,25(OH)$_2$D. Parathyroid hormone does not directly regulate intestinal Ca and Pi transport, but by increasing the renal production of 1,25(OH)$_2$D provides more 1,25(OH)$_2$D to the intestine and, so, indirectly increases the absorption of these minerals.

Autoregulation of Calcium and Phosphate Absorption

Ca and Pi also alter their own and each other's absorption from the intestine. Calcium and Pi each have direct actions to limit the absorption of the other ion. Thus, calcium salts (calcium carbonate or citrate) can be used therapeutically to reduce Pi absorption in patients with renal failure who have the tendency to develop hyperphosphatemia because they are unable to excrete it from their diseased kidneys. Likewise, phosphate salts (potassium or sodium phosphate) have been used to reduce Ca absorption in patients with idiopathic hypercalciuria resulting from increased intestinal Ca absorption. Calcium and Pi also act indirectly to regulate their own intestinal absorption by controlling the circulating levels of 1,25(OH)$_2$D (Fig. 3). Low levels of Ca and/or Pi in the blood stimulate the renal production of 1,25(OH)$_2$D either by direct action on the renal 25OHD 1α-hydroxylase [the enzyme responsible for producing 1,25(OH)$_2$D from its substrate 25OHD] or through another hormone that controls 1,25(OH)$_2$D production. For Ca this other hormone is PTH. Low levels of Ca stimulate PTH secretion which then stimulates 1,25(OH)$_2$D production. Magnesium acts like Ca in controlling PTH secretion in that it stimulates PTH secretion at low levels and inhibits it at high levels. However, at very low levels of Mg, PTH secretion is inhibited. This is an important consideration to remember when facing a subject with combined hypomagnesemia and hypocalcemia as can occur in patients with malabsorption or following binge drinking. Under these circumstances treatment with Mg is far more efficacious in raising serum Ca than is Ca alone. Low levels of Pi do not act through PTH but appear to stimulate the secretion of a pituitary factor which in turn stimulates the 1α-hydroxylase. The identity of this Pi-sensitive pituitary factor is not completely established, but appears to be growth hormone that directly or indirectly through its ability to stimulate insulin-like growth factor 1 can also increase 1,25(OH)$_2$D production. Conceivably, patients with pituitary tumors or following pituitary resection could have difficulties regulating 1,25(OH)$_2$D production through this Pi-dependent mechanism, but this has not been described.

PTH-Regulated Renal Reabsorption of Calcium and Phosphate

Just as 1,25(OH)$_2$D is the principal regulator of intestinal Ca and Pi absorption, PTH is the principal regulator of the renal reabsorption of Ca and Pi. Parathyroid hormone inhibits the renal reabsorption of Pi in both the proximal and distal tubule, while enhancing the reabsorption of Ca in the distal tubule. The renal effect of PTH to inhibit Pi reabsorption dominates its countervailing actions to raise serum Pi by increasing bone resorption (releasing both Ca and Pi to the blood stream) or by increasing intestinal Pi absorption [through 1,25(OH)$_2$D] (Fig. 2). In contrast, the renal effect of PTH to stimulate Ca reabsorption combines with its actions to increase bone resorption and intestinal Ca absorption all leading to hypercalcemia (Fig. 2). Thus, primary hyperparathyroidism is characterized by hypophosphatemia and hypercalcemia. This reduction in serum Pi may contribute to the ability of PTH to stimulate 1,25(OH)$_2$D production, because as mentioned previously, hypophosphatemia stimulates the renal 1α-hydroxylase.

Autoregulation of Renal Calcium Excretion

Although PTH increases the renal reabsorption of Ca, hypercalciuria is often found in patients with primary hyperparathyroidism. The reason for this is twofold. With the development of hypercalcemia, the filtered load of Ca is increased. Furthermore, Ca reabsorption in the ascending loop of Henle and collecting duct is impaired by hypercalcemia. The ability of PTH to stimulate Ca reabsorption in the distal tubule cannot compensate for these opposing actions of hypercalcemia on Ca excretion.

In addition to its inhibition of renal Ca reabsorption, hypercalcemia inhibits PTH secretion, resulting in decreased renal production of 1,25(OH)$_2$D and decreased intestinal Ca absorption. Clinically this situation is well illustrated by patients with cancers secreting a PTH-like peptide that has all the known actions of PTH. Patients with these malignancies become quite hypercalcemic but have low PTH and lower levels of 1,25(OH)$_2$D than are seen in patients with primary hyperparathyroidism. On the other hand primary hyperparathyroidism tends to be accompanied by elevated 1,25(OH)$_2$D levels presumably because the degree of hypercalcemia in these patients is modest and not high enough to counter the stimulation by PTH and low Pi of the renal 1α-hydroxylase.

Renal Actions of 1,25-Dihydroxyvitamin D and Calcitonin

Although studies demonstrating a role for 1,25(OH)$_2$D and other vitamin D metabolites in stimulating Ca and Pi reabsorption by the kidney have been published, these actions appear not to be of major physiologic importance. In contrast, CT has been shown to be calciuric and phosphaturic, although these actions may be more important for the pharmacologic than the physiologic effects of this hormone. Regardless, such actions of CT would antagonize the effects of PTH on Ca excretion but potentiate the effects of PTH on Pi excretion, leading to a reduction in both serum Ca and Pi (Fig. 2).

Both CT and 1,25(OH)$_2$D have been shown to regulate the renal production of 1,25(OH)$_2$D. 1,25-Dihydroxyvitamin D not only inhibits its own production but stimulates the enzymes (such as the 24-hydroxylase) responsible for its catabolism. By this means, 1,25(OH)$_2$D self-regulates its own levels and limits the deleterious effects accompanying vitamin D intoxication. Calcitonin has been shown to stimulate 1,25(OH)$_2$D production *in vitro*, but its ability to do so *in vivo* in physiologic concentrations has not been demonstrated. Such an action of CT would be counter to its overall ability to reduce serum calcium through its inhibition of renal Ca reabsorption and bone resorption.

Regulation of Bone Remodeling

The regulation by PTH, CT, and 1,25(OH)$_2$D of bone formation and resorption is complex and not yet fully understood (see Chapter 6). Two major cell types are involved in bone remodeling: the osteoblasts that are responsible for bone formation (see Chapter 3) and the osteoclasts that are responsible for bone resorption (see Chapter 5). The osteoblasts contain receptors for both PTH and 1,25(OH)$_2$D. The osteoclasts do not possess receptors for either PTH or 1,25(OH)$_2$D, although they do have receptors for CT. Parathyroid hormone exerts its effects on the osteoblast in part through cAMP; CT also increases cAMP but in the osteoclast. The means by which 1,25(OH)$_2$D acts on osteoblasts is less clear but appears to involve transcriptional regulation of specific genes.

Bone Resorption

In vitro, both PTH and 1,25(OH)$_2$D stimulate bone resorption, whereas CT inhibits bone resorption. Neither PTH nor 1,25(OH)$_2$D can stimulate bone resorption in a culture of pure osteoclasts; osteoblasts are needed to convey the signal. In contrast CT can act directly on the osteoclast to inhibit its activity. These actions of PTH and 1,25(OH)$_2$D on bone resorption include both relatively acute changes in osteoclast activity, as well as longer term changes in osteoclast cell number. Both PTH and 1,25(OH)$_2$D stimulate the differentiation of osteoclasts from hematogenous precursors in the presence of osteoblasts. Through these mechanisms both PTH and 1,25(OH)$_2$D raise blood levels of Ca and Pi, actions that are antagonized by CT (Fig. 2).

Bone Formation

Although the effects of PTH and 1,25(OH)$_2$D on bone resorption are readily demonstrated *in vitro*, both agents can lead to a net increase in bone formation *in vivo*. Presumably, the ability of these hormones to regulate both bone formation and resorption reflects differing actions of these hormones on the osteoblast—one set of actions leads to osteoclast activation and another set of actions leads to bone formation. 1,25-Dihydroxyvitamin D and PTH may promote osteoblast differentiation as they do osteoclast differentiation. Because the osteoblast passes through different stages in which it progresses from a proliferating cell to a cell laying down a matrix and finally to a cell mineralizing that matrix, PTH and 1,25(OH)$_2$D could alter the function of the osteoblast differently at different stages of that progression. Thus, depending on the timing and dose administered, PTH and 1,25(OH)$_2$D could produce net formation or net resorption. Furthermore, the formation process requires adequate amounts of Ca and Pi. 1,25-Dihydroxyvitamin D may stimulate bone formation *in vivo* principally by providing adequate amounts of these minerals to the bone-forming surface. Patients with a hereditary form of vitamin D-resistant rickets who lack a functional vitamin D receptor can be cured by infusions of Ca and Pi. Conceivably PTH may be less effective in promoting bone formation if it circulates at sufficiently high concentrations to reduce blood Pi levels (by stimulating renal Pi excretion) to a point at which bone mineralization is impaired.

It is likely that the blood levels of Ca and Pi alter the response of bone to these hormones, although this has not been adequately explored. However, rickets (in children) and osteomalacia (in adults), the bone disease associated with vitamin D deficiency, can be seen in hypophosphatemic states despite adequate levels of 1,25(OH)$_2$D indicating that Pi is essential for normal mineralization. Calcium deficiency has also been reported as a cause of rickets, but this is less well established. Vitamin D deficiency is accompanied by increased levels of PTH because of the reduced blood levels of Ca and because 1,25(OH)$_2$D has a direct suppressive effect on PTH synthesis that would be lost in vitamin D deficiency. The increase in PTH would further aggravate the hypophosphatemia associated with vitamin D deficiency, potentially contributing to the development of osteomalacia.

CONCLUSIONS

The calciotropic hormones interact not only among themselves but with the minerals they are regulating in their role as regulators of bone mineral homeostasis. Although numerous target tissues are involved, as are numerous ions and hormones, the most important are PTH, CT, and 1,25(OH)$_2$D acting on bone, kidney, and intestine to regulate blood levels of Ca and Pi. Regulation entails control of how much comes into the body from the diet, how much leaves the body through the kidney, and how much is stored and released from the bone. Both feed forward and feedback mechanisms are involved. The mechanisms regulating Ca and Pi flux in one tissue differ from those in other tissues. Different hormones act on different tissues. Nevertheless, it is quite apparent that the different hormones, ions, and tissues involved communicate with each other, sending and receiving clear messages to ensure the precise regulation of these important minerals.

SELECTED REFERENCES

1. Bikle DD: Regulation of intestinal calcium transport by vitamin D (1,25(OH)$_2$D). In: Aloia RC, Curtain LM, Gordon LM (eds) *Membrane Transport and Information Storage.* Wiley-Liss, New York, pp 191–219, 1990
2. Bushinsky DA, Riera GS, Favus MJ, Coe FL: Evidence that blood ionized calcium can regulate serum 1,25(OH)$_2$D independently of parathyroid hormone and phosphorus in the rat. *J Clin Invest* 76:1599–1604, 1985
3. Cole JA, Forte LR, Eber S, Thorne PK, Poelling RE: Regulation of sodium-dependent phosphate transport by parathyroid hormone in opossum kidney cells: adnosine 3′,5′-monophosphate-dependent and independent mechanisms. *Endocrinology* 122:2981–2989, 1988
4. Fraser DR: Regulation of the metabolism of vitamin D. *Physiol Rev* 60:551–613, 1980
5. Gesek FA, Friedman PA: On the mechanism of parathyroid hormone stimulation of calcium uptake by mouse distal convoluted tubule cells. *J Clin Invest* 90:749–758, 1992
6. Gray RW, Garthwaite TL: Activation of renal 1,25-dihydroxyvitamin D synthesis by phosphate deprivation: Evidence for a role for growth hormone. *Endocrinology* 116:189–193, 1985
7. Owen TA, Aronow MS, Barone LM, Bettencourt B, Stein GS, Lian JB: Pleiotropic effects of vitamin D on osteoblast gene expression are related to the proliferative and differentiated state of the bone cell phenotype: Dependency upon basal levels of gene expression, duration of exposure, and bone matrix competency in normal rat osteoblast cultures. *Endocrinology* 128:1496–1504, 1991
8. Pocotte SL, Ehrenstein G, Fitzpatrick LA: Regulation of parathyroid hormone secretion. *Endocr Rev* 12:291–301, 1991
9. Suda T, Takahashi N, Martin TJ: Modulation of osteoclast differentiation. *Endocr Rev* 13:66–80, 1992

Clinical Evaluation of Bone and Mineral Disorders

16. History and Physical Examination

Michael P. Whyte, M.D.

*Metabolic Research Unit, Shriners Hospital for Crippled Children, and
Division of Bone and Mineral Diseases, Washington University School of
Medicine, St. Louis, Missouri*

"The more resources we have, and the more complex they are, the greater are the demands upon our clinical skill. These resources are calls upon judgment and not substitutes for it. Do not, therefore, scorn clinical examination; learn it sufficiently to get from it all it holds, and gain in it the confidence it merits."
  Sir F.M.R. Walshe [1888–1973] Canadian Medical Association Journal 67:395, 1952.

A complete medical history and thorough physical examination are the foundation for accurate diagnosis, effective patient management, and sound clinical investigation. Unfortunately, there is increasing risk that the important and accelerating technological progress in medicine will obscure this axiom for some physicians. When the clinician encounters an individual with a metabolic bone disease or deranged mineral homeostasis, the medical history and physical examination are of paramount importance. Some of the reasons are emphasized briefly below.

MEDICAL HISTORY

The patient with metabolic bone disease or abnormal mineral homeostasis will often be challenging to the physician because a great variety of nutritional, environmental, genetic, toxic, pharmacologic, and age-dependent factors can affect the skeleton and alter calcium or phosphate metabolism. Perusal of this primer will illustrate how diverse these influences can be. In children, their impact may be especially complex, because bone growth and modeling are occurring in addition to skeletal remodeling. The clinician may need some of the skills of the endocrinologist, nutritionist, nephrologist, geneticist, and perhaps the pediatrician or gerontologist to assess these factors and thereby effectively diagnose and treat his/her patient. Familiarity with skeletal radiology and pathology may also be necessary, as well as with orthopedics, rheumatology, and rehabilitation medicine if there is significant deformity. Accordingly, an accurate and detailed medical history will be essential to disclose the appropriate clinical considerations and put them into proper perspective. This will be necessary not only to achieve a correct diagnosis, but also to ensure safe and effective medical therapy.

The chief complaint may readily lead to the diagnosis, as with hip fracture from osteoporosis or bowing deformity of the legs from rickets. Often, however, the patient's principal concern will reflect a more subtle presentation. For example, the above conditions may present with gradual loss of height with kyphosis, or short stature with knock-knee deformity, respectively. In either extreme, the clinician must not lose sight of the chief complaint of the patient as the complexities of diagnosis and therapy are pursued.

Because most metabolic bone diseases are chronic conditions, the history of the present illness should provide an important understanding of the evolution of the disorder. Has the osteopenia been life-long, or has there been substantial recent loss of skeletal mass that should prompt different diagnostic considerations and interventions? Only by talking with the patient will the physician learn that previous medical records or radiographs are available to help answer many such important clinical questions. Nutritional influences should be considered at this time, because mineral and vitamin D status are both influenced by diet. Environmental factors such as sunlight exposure and exercise or work history may all be important. Indeed, until more effective regimens become available to prevent bone loss or to restore diminished skeletal mass, much of what the clinician can do to benefit a child or adult with osteopenia may come from caution against potentially traumatic activities at play or work (1). The drug history must be assessed because a great variety of pharmacologics can adversely affect the skeleton or disturb mineral homeostasis (e.g., glucocorticoids and anticonvulsants). The same is true for some "over-the-counter" preparations (e.g., vitamin A, calcium supplements, and antacids). What the patient means by "medications" should be explored, because many will not consider vitamins, mineral supplements, and antacids as such. Furthermore, use of some drugs may confound interpretation of biochemical studies, because they affect mineral homeostasis (e.g., diuretics that increase or decrease urine calcium levels and increase serum alkaline phosphatase activity). Assessment of a patient's likely compliance for therapy may be necessary to formulate not only an effective, but also a safe treatment plan as well. This is especially so when dealing with the pediatric or aged patient population. The literature is replete with cases of renal failure from vitamin D intoxication where patient education and follow-up were inadequate.

A thorough family history is important, because many of the metabolic bone diseases are heritable, and a correct diagnosis may depend on investigation of the kindred [e.g., familial benign (hypocalciuric) hypercalcemia]. Furthermore, great benefit may come from screening families or kindreds at risk for these disorders and then treating and/or educating other affected individuals (e.g., medullary carcinoma of the thyroid) or providing appropriate genetic counseling (e.g., osteogenesis imperfecta).

PHYSICAL EXAMINATION

A great variety of clinical signs as well as important skeletal deformities can accompany the metabolic bone diseases (2). Many of these disorders have phenotypic expression that includes diagnostic physical clues. Occasionally, the correct diagnosis relies importantly on the identification of such a finding; e.g., blue or gray sclerae (osteogenesis imperfecta), café-au-lait spots (McCune–Albright disease), tumor (oncogenic rickets/osteomalacia), or premature loss of deciduous teeth (hypophosphatasia). Unless these physical signs are correctly identified, a diagnosis may be missed. In some types of metabolic bone disease, the *constellation* of physical findings helps importantly in diagnosis, but it should also focus attention to significant goals of treatment (e.g., deformity) and may be the concern for critical aspects of patient education. For example in rickets the clinician may expect short stature, dentition changes, a painful skeleton, myopathy, flared wrists from metaphyseal widening, lower extremity deformity, a Harrison's groove (rib cage ridging from diaphragmatic pull), a rachitic "rosary" (enlargement of the costochondral junctions), and craniotabes (flattened posterior skull). Paget bone disease can cause an enlarging calvarium with bulging temporal arteries, asymmetrical bowing of the limbs, as well as localized areas of bone pain and warmth. In osteoporosis, one examines for loss of vertebral height that can manifest with kyphosis or a gibbus (Dowager's hump), a protuberant abdomen (that the patient may confuse with obesity), and ribs within the pelvic rim that may be bruised, as well as paravertebral muscle spasm and thin skin (McConkey's sign).

The skeletal deformity that accompanies metabolic bone disease can be the cause of much of its morbidity. Without a detailed physical examination, important clinical problems may be ignored. Insertion of something as inexpensive as a shoe lift can be of considerable benefit to the patient, but must come from accurate evaluation of leg-length inequality if further complications are to be avoided. Clinical quantitation, photographic documentation, and even videotaping of disturbances may be helpful to assess progression or response of deformity to therapy.

CONCLUSIONS

The complex interaction of the many endogenous and exogenous factors that impact on mineral homeostasis and skeletal physiology discussed throughout this primer account for why patients with metabolic bone disease are especially challenging. These individuals require and typically benefit greatly from time and effort on their behalf when they first present to a physician. Demonstration of concern for and commitment to the patient by a complete medical history and thorough physical examination helps to win his/her confidence and trust. This rapport will likely be essential for effective management of their condition. It should be self-evident that the information gathered by the medical history and physical examination will be the guide to the great myriad of biochemical, radiologic, and other technologies that are important for subsequent diagnosis and treatment. Finally, as reviewed throughout this primer, effective therapies are available for most of the metabolic bone diseases. Once the proper clinical foundation based on the medical history and physical examination is in place, the physician can then be rewarded by a patient that he/she has helped.

REFERENCES

1. Whyte MP: *Osteoporosis.* In Rakel RE (ed) *Conn's Current Therapy 1992.* WB Saunders, New York, pp 523–527, 1992
2. Parsons V: *Color Atlas of Bone Disease.* Year Book Medical Publishers, Inc., Chicago, 1980

17. Collection, Preservation, and Analysis of Urine in the Evaluation of Mineral Metabolism, Bone Disease, and Nephrolithiasis

Jacob Lemann, Jr., M.D.

Nephrology Division, Medical College of Wisconsin, Milwaukee, Wisconsin

Random or "spot" urine specimens can be collected at any time but are preferably obtained when patients have not eaten for 8 hr or more and are not receiving either intravenous fluids or drugs. Twenty-four-hour urine specimens must be accurately timed and completely collected. Patients are instructed to begin the collection by voiding into the toilet so that the collection is begun with their bladder empty and noting the time. They then collect all urine passed at each voiding during the ensuing day, completing the collection by voiding and saving the urine passed exactly 24 hr after the collection began. They should be reminded to urinate before defecating, because of the potential for inadvertent loss of urine during defecation.

Containers for the collection of urine specimens must be clean. Appropriate containers are preferably provided

TABLE 1. *Some commonly measured urinary constituents*

Substance	Units	Preservative required	Methods of measurement	Analytical interference	Range of daily excretion rate in health
Volume	mL/day or L/day	No	1. Direct using graduated cylinder. 2. Indirect by weighing and subtracting weight of container. Because urine specific gravity ranges from 1.001 to 1.032, urine volume is negligibly overestimated by <3%.	None	400 mL/day when solute excretion and fluid intake are low to >5,000 mL/day.
Creatinine Formula wt. = 113	mg/day or mmol/day	No	1. Colorimetric 2. Enzymatic	Acetone and acetoacetate increase measurement with most colorimetric techniques.	20–26 mg/kg/day (0.18–0.23 mmol/kg/day) in men and 15–21 mg/kg/day (0.13 to 0.19 mmol/kg/day) in women. 10–15 mg/kg/day in preadolescent children
Calcium Formula wt. = 40 Equivalent wt. = 20	mg/day or mmol/day or mEq/day	HCl or thymol + phenyl mercuric nitrate	1. Colorimetric 2. Atomic absorption spectrometry	Therapeutic administration of EDTA reduces and highly pigmented urines increase the measurement with colorimetric techniques.	40–300 mg/day (to 250 mg/day in women) or 1.0–7.5 mmol/day (to 6.25 mmol/day in women); <4 mg/kg/day or <0.1 mmol/kg/day.
Phosphorus Formula wt. = 31 (inorganic phosphate, PO_4, is actually measured and expressed as P)	mg/day or mmol/day	No	1. Colorimetric	None	300–1,800 mg/day (10–60 mmol/day) reflecting diet. Falls to <0.5 mmol/day when diet P reduced to ~3 mmol/day.
Magnesium Formula wt. = 24 Equivalent wt. = 12	mg/day or mmol/day or mEq/day	No	1. Colorimetric 2. Atomic absorption spectrometry	None	50–350 mg/day (2–15 mmol/day) reflecting diet. Falls to <0.5 mmol/day when diet reduced to 0.5 mmol/day or less.
Hydroxyproline Formula wt. = 131	mg/day or mmol/day	Toluene or thymol + phenylmercuric nitrate	1. Colorimetric 2. High-pressure liquid chromatography	None	15–45 mg/day (0.11–0.34 mmol/day).
cAMP	µmol/day or nmol/100 ml GFR	No	1. Radioimmunoassay 2. High-pressure liquid chromatography	None	2.5–8.0 µmol/day or 1.3–3.7 nmol/100 ml GFR.
Sodium Formula wt. = 23	mmol/day	No	1. Ion-selective electrode 2. Emission spectrometry 3. Atomic absorption spectrometry	None Electrode response may not be linear at Na concentrations <30 mmol/L.	0–350 mmol/day or more. Reflects dietary intake.
Potassium Formula wt. = 39	mmol/day	No	1. Ion-selective electrode 2. Emission spectrometry 3. Atomic absorption spectrometry	None	30–100 mmol/day. Reflects dietary intake.
Chloride Formula wt. = 35.5	mmol/day	No	1. Ion-selective electrode 2. Coulometric titration	None	0–350 mmol/day or more. Reflects dietary intake.

TABLE 1. *Continued.*

Substance	Units	Preservative required	Methods of measurement	Analytical interference	Range of daily excretion rate in health
Urea (as urea-N; formula wt. = 28)	g/day	HCl or toluene or thymol + phenylmercuric nitrate	1. Enzymatic	None	5–25 g/day. Reflects dietary protein intake.
pH		Toluene or thymol + phenylmercuric nitrate	1. Ion-selective electrode	None	4.5–7.5
Oxalate (as oxalic acid; formula wt. = 90)	mg/day or mmol/day	HCl	1. Enzymatic 2. Ion chromatography	*In vitro* nonenzymatic conversion of ascorbic acid to oxalate in alkaline urines.	9–41 mg/day (0.10–0.46 mmol/day)
Citrate (as citric acid; formula wt. = 210)	mg/day or mmol/day	Toluene or thymol + phenylmercuric nitrate	1. Enzymatic	None	Men: 210–1,200 mg/day (1–5.8 mmol/day. Women: 400–1,400 mg/day (2–6.5 mmol/day). Falls with acidosis.
Uric acid Formula wt. = 168	mg/day or mmol/day	Toluene or thymol + phenylmercuric nitrate	1. Enzymatic	None	Men: <800 mg/day (<4.8 mmol/day). Women: <750 mg/day (<4.5 mmol/day).

by the physician or laboratory and must be so provided if preservatives are used in the containers. If patients use their own containers, such as an empty 1 gallon plastic milk bottle, the container must be thoroughly washed with hot soapy water and then thoroughly rinsed until the rinse water no longer foams (at least five rinses).

Whether preservatives should be used in containers for urine collections depends on how quickly the specimen can be delivered to the laboratory for analysis, the type of analysis that is to be made, and knowledge regarding the possible interfering effects of the preservative on the analytical measurement. Preservatives should not be used unless required to prevent degradation of the urinary constituent that is to be measured during the urine collection and transport of the specimen to the laboratory. The advent of new techniques and new instruments for analysis makes it essential that physicians recognize the potential of preservatives to interfere with analytical measurements and ask their laboratory for specific advice regarding the use of preservatives.

Approximately 20 ml of 6 N HCl may be used to preserve 24-hr urines during collections. Acetic acid or boric acid are also sometimes used. Alternatively, two or three small crystals of thymol, together with a few grains of phenylmercuric nitrate dispensed with a small narrow spatula, effectively prevent bacterial growth in containers used for 24-hr urine collections. Containers are not initially sterile and, in any event, may become colonized by bacteria shed from the glans and prepuce or vulva during micturition. If urine pH is to be measured accurately, the loss of dissolved CO_2 must be prevented or minimized. A small aliquot of a random urine can be drawn into a syringe immediately after voiding, any remaining air rapidly expelled, and the syringe capped. To prevent CO_2 loss during 24-hr urine collections, a layer of mineral oil

or toluene is placed in the container. Twenty-four-hour urines may also be refrigerated during collection, but refrigeration is generally inconvenient when patients collect urines outside of the hospital.

The currently preferred techniques for preservation of urine collections for the measurement of some urinary constituents, the methods of analyses, and some interferences are summarized in Table 1. The table also presents the normal ranges for daily urinary composition in healthy adults.

The creatinine concentration of 24-hr urines must be measured, multiplied by the urine volume to estimate daily urinary creatinine content (= creatinine excretion rate), and the latter value assessed in relation to the patient's age, sex, and body weight to determine the accuracy of the urine collection. Creatinine production and thus daily urinary excretion of creatinine in the steady-state reflects muscle mass. Men excrete 20–26 mg creatinine/kg body weight/day (0.18–0.23 mmol/kg/day), whereas women, whose muscle mass is a relatively smaller proportion of their total body weight, excrete 15–21 mg creatinine/kg body weight/day (0.13–0.19 mmol/kg/day). Alternatively, as muscle mass declines with age, urinary creatinine excretion (mg/kg/day) can be approximated among adults by (1):

Men: $U_{creatinine}V$, mg/kg/day $= 28 - 0.2 \times$ age, years

Women: $U_{creatinine}V$, mg/kg/day $= 23.8 - 0.17 \times$ age, years

To convert mg creatinine to mmol, divide by 113, the formula weight of creatinine.

Patients who are malnourished and exhibit muscle wasting or who are markedly obese will, of course, excrete relatively less creatinine in relation to their total weight so that urinary creatinine must be assessed in relation to the clinical evaluation of individual patients. It must be emphasized that the total urine volume, which reflects intake of water and other fluids relative to extrarenal water losses, is never a reliable estimate of the accuracy of a 24-hr urine collection.

The urinary creatinine concentration must also always be measured in random or spot specimens together with the measurement of the creatinine concentration in a simultaneously collected blood (serum or plasma) specimen to permit estimation of renal excretion of other substances per unit of glomerular filtrate (see section on urinary excretion of calcium, phosphate, and magnesium).

SELECTED REFERENCES

1. Mitch WE, Walser M: Chapter 41. In: Brenner BM, Rector FC Jr (eds) *Nutritional Therapy of the Uremic Patient*. The Kidney, 3rd ed. WB Saunders Co., Philadelphia, p 1762, 1986
2. NCCLS: *Collection and Preservation of Timed Urine Specimens*: National Committee for Clinical Laboratory Standards (NCCLS). NCCLS Document GP-13-P. vol 7. no 8, 1987

18. Blood Calcium, Phosphorus, and Magnesium

Anthony A. Portale, M.D.

Departments of Pediatrics and Medicine, University of California at San Francisco, San Francisco, California

SERUM CALCIUM CONCENTRATION

Calcium in serum exists in three separately definable fractions: protein-bound calcium (40%), which is not ultrafilterable by the kidney, and ionized (48%) and complexed (12%) calcium, which are ultrafilterable (1). Complexed calcium is that bound to various cations, such as phosphate, citrate, and bicarbonate. For clinical purposes, the total concentration of calcium in serum is the most commonly evaluated index of calcium status.

Total Calcium Concentration

Albumin accounts for 90% of the protein-binding of calcium in serum; globulins account for the remainder. Calcium binds to anionic carboxylate groups on the albumin molecule, and in normal serum, the binding sites are largely unoccupied. Conditions that change the concentration of albumin in serum, such as nephrotic syndrome or hepatic cirrhosis, will affect the measurement of total calcium concentrations. A decrease in serum albumin concentration of 1 g/dL results in a decrease in protein-bound and hence total calcium concentration of ~0.8 mg/dL. For routine clinical interpretation of serum calcium levels, the total serum calcium concentration can be "corrected" for changes in albumin concentration as follows:

Corrected total calcium concentration (mg/dL)

= measured total calcium concentration (mg/dL)

+ 0.8 × [4 − albumin concentration (g/dL)].

Several algorithms or nomograms, such as that of McLean and Hastings, have been developed to "correct" the calcium concentration for abnormal values of total protein, albumin, and phosphorus, or to estimate the "free" calcium concentration. Given that the measurement of blood ionized calcium concentration is now widely available in clinical laboratories, the use of such "corrected" values should be abandoned.

Calcium binding to albumin is strongly pH-dependent, between pH 7 and 8; an acute increase or decrease in pH of 0.1 pH units will increase or decrease, respectively, protein-bound calcium by ~0.12 mg/dL. In hypocalcemic patients with metabolic acidosis, rapid correction of acidemia with sodium bicarbonate can precipitate tetany, due to increased binding of calcium to albumin and thus to a decrease in ionized calcium concentration.

The total calcium concentration in serum exhibits a circadian rhythm characterized by a single nadir and peak, with amplitude (nadir to peak) of ~0.5 mg/dL (Table 1) (2,3). This rhythm is thought to reflect hemodynamic changes in serum albumin concentration that result from changes in body posture (4). Prolonged upright posture or venostasis can cause hemoconcentration and thus potentially misleading increases of 0.4–0.6 mg/dL in serum calcium concentration. There is negligible difference between values taken in fasting and nonfasting states.

Normal values for serum total calcium concentration vary somewhat among clinical laboratories, and in general range from ~9.0–10.6 mg/dL. The concentration decreases with advancing age in men, from a mean of ~9.6 mg/dL at age 20 to ~9.2 mg/dL at age 80 years, and the decrease can be accounted for by decrease in serum albumin concentration (5). In women, no change is observed with age. In children, the serum calcium concentration is higher than in adult subjects, being highest at 6–24 months of age, mean ~10.2 mg/dL, decreasing to a plateau of ~9.8 mg/dL at 6–8 years, and decreasing further to adult values at 16–20 years (6) (Table 2).

For routine determination of total serum calcium concentration, most clinical laboratories use automated spectrophotometric techniques, such as the *o*-cresolphthalein complexone method; the reference method is atomic ab-

TABLE 1. *Characteristics of the circadian rhythms in blood mineral concentration in humans*

	Concentration (mg/dL)		Amplitude (mg/dL)	Phase (hr)	
	Fasting	24-hr mean	(Nadir to peak)	Nadir	Peak
Total serum calcium	9.6	9.4	0.5	0300	1300
Blood ionized calcium	4.67	4.52	0.3	1900	1000
Serum phosphorus	3.6	4.0	1.2	1100	0200

Data are from refs. 2 and 13.

sorption spectrophotometry (7). Calcium concentrations expressed in mg/dL can be converted to mmol/L or mM by dividing by 4, and to mEq/L by dividing by 2. The atomic weight of calcium is 40.08 and its valence is 2.

Ionized Calcium

Ionized calcium is the fraction of plasma calcium that is important for physiologic processes, such as muscle contraction, blood coagulation, nerve conduction, hormone secretion (parathyroid hormone and 1,25-dihydroxyvitamin D) and action, ion transport, bone mineralization, and integrity of plasma membranes. In the past, measurement of blood-ionized calcium concentration has been technically difficult and not widely available in clinical settings. With the advent of newer, semiautomated instruments using ion-selective electrodes, the concentration of ionized calcium can now be readily and accurately measured (8). This measurement is most useful in critically ill patients, particularly those in whom serum protein levels are decreased, acid-base disturbances are present, or to whom large amounts of citrated blood products are given, such as with cardiac surgery or liver transplantation.

The range of values of ionized calcium for normal individuals must be established for each laboratory, and will vary depending on which technique is used, and whether the measurement is made in serum, plasma, or heparin-

ized whole blood. Measured with currently available, ion-selective electrodes, normal serum ionized calcium concentrations in adult men and women range from ~4.6–5.3 mg/dL, without significant sex differences (7,8). In healthy infants, ionized calcium levels decrease from ~5.8 mg/dL at birth to a nadir of 4.9 mg/dL at 24 hr of life (9), and increase slightly during the first week of life (10). Values in young children are slightly higher (~0.2 mg/dL) than those in adults until after puberty.

Blood ionized calcium concentrations exhibit a circadian rhythm characterized by a peak at 1000 and a nadir at 1800-2000, with amplitude (nadir to peak) of 0.3 mg/dL (2). Thus, specimens for analysis drawn after the morning give slightly lower values. Specimens must be obtained anaerobically to avoid spurious results due to *ex vivo* changes in pH. Measurements made in heparinized whole blood tend to be slightly lower than those in serum, due to binding of calcium by heparin. Calcium binding to heparin can be minimized by using calcium-titrated heparin (Radiometer Corporation, Copenhagen, Denmark) at a concentration of 50 IU/mL or less, or sodium or lithium heparin at a concentration of 15 U/mL or less (11); under these circumstances, values from serum, plasma, or whole blood are similar. For hospitalized patients, it is recommended that specimens be obtained in the morning fasting state to avoid possible effects of posture, diurnal variation, and food ingestion.

TABLE 2. *Representative normal values for serum concentrations of total calcium, phosphorus, and magnesium*

	Age (yr)	Total calcium (mg/dL)	Phosphorus (mg/dL)	Magnesium (mg/dL)
Infants	0–0.25	8.8–11.3	4.8–7.4	1.6–2.5
	1–5	9.4–10.8	4.5–6.2	
Children	6–12	9.4–10.3	3.6–5.8	1.7–2.3
Males	20	9.1–10.2	2.5–4.5	1.7–2.6
	50	8.9–10.0	2.3–4.1	1.7–2.6
	70	8.8–9.9	2.2–4.0	1.7–2.6
Females	20	8.8–10.0	2.5–4.5	1.7–2.6
	50	8.8–10.0	2.7–4.4	1.7–2.6
	70	8.8–10.0	2.9–4.8	1.7–2.6

Values are approximate and normal ranges must be determined for each laboratory. Data are from refs. 5, 6, 8–10, and 16–18.

SERUM PHOSPHORUS CONCENTRATION

Phosphorus exists in plasma in two forms: an organic form principally consisting of phospholipids and an inorganic form (12). Of the total phosphorus in plasma of ~14 mg/dL, ~8 mg/dL is in the organic form and ~4 mg/dL in the inorganic form. In clinical settings, only the inorganic orthophosphate form is routinely measured. About 15% of total inorganic phosphorus in plasma is protein-bound. The remaining 85%, which is ultrafilterable, exits principally either as the undissociated or "free" ions, $HPO_4^=$ and $H_2PO_4^-$, which are present in serum in a ratio of 4:1 at pH 7.4, or as phosphate complexed with sodium, calcium, or magnesium.

The terms "phosphorus concentration" and "phosphate concentration" are often used interchangeably, and for clinical purposes the choice matters little. It is phosphorus in the form of the phosphate ion, which circulates in blood, is filtered by the glomerulus, and is transported across plasma membranes. However, the content of "phosphate" in plasma, urine, tissue, or foodstuffs is measured and expressed in terms of the amount of elemental phosphorus contained in the specimen, hence use of the term "phosphorus concentration."

In healthy subjects ingesting typical diets, the serum phosphorus concentration exhibits a circadian rhythm, characterized by a decrease to a nadir just before noon, an increase to a plateau in late afternoon, and a small further increase to a peak shortly after midnight (Table 1) (2,13). The amplitude (nadir to peak) is ~1.2 mg/dL, or 30% of the 24-hr mean level. Increases or decreases in dietary intake of phosphorus induces substantial increases or decreases in serum phosphorus levels during late morning, afternoon, and evening, but less or no change in morning-fasting phosphorus levels (13). To minimize the effect of dietary phosphorus on the serum phosphorus concentration, specimens for analysis should be obtained in the morning fasting state. Specimens obtained in the afternoon are more affected by diet, and may be more useful in monitoring the effect of changes in dietary phosphorus on serum levels of phosphorus, as in patients with renal insufficiency receiving phosphorus binders to suppress secondary hyperparathyroidism. With administration of aluminum hydroxide, a phosphorus binding agent, a decrease in morning-fasting phosphorus levels can underestimate the severity of hypophosphatemia that obtains throughout much of the day (13,14).

Factors other than time of day and diet can affect the serum phosphorus concentration. Presumably by inducing movement of phosphorus into the cell, a decrease in phosphorus concentration can be acutely induced by intravenous infusion of glucose or insulin, ingestion of carbohydrate-rich meals, acute respiratory alkalosis, and infusion or endogenous release of epinephrine. The decrease in phosphorus level induced by acute respiratory alkalosis can be as great as 2.0 mg/dL (15). An increase in serum phosphorus concentration can be acutely induced by metabolic acidosis and by intravenous infusion of calcium.

There are substantial effects of age on the fasting serum concentration of phosphorus. Phosphorus levels are very high in infants, ranging from 4.8 to 7.4 mg/dL (mean 6.2) in the first 3 months of life and decreasing to 4.5–5.8 mg/dL (mean 5.0) at age 1–2 years (16). In mid-childhood, values range from 3.5 to 5.5 mg/dL (mean 4.4) and decrease to adult values by late adolescence (6,17). In adult males, serum phosphorus levels decrease with age from ~3.5 mg/dL at age 20 years to 3.0 mg/dL at age 70 (5,17). In women, the values are similar to those of men until after the menopause, when they increase slightly from ~3.4 mg/dL at age 50 to 3.7 mg/dL at age 70.

The normal range for serum phosphorus concentration is laboratory-specific. The most commonly used methods for determination of phosphorus concentration use automated spectrophotometric techniques based on the reaction of phosphate ions with molybdate (7). In males, representative normal ranges are ~2.5–4.5 mg/dL at age 20, 2.3–4.1 mg/dL at age 50, and 2.2–4.0 mg/dL at age 70. In women, representative normal ranges are ~2.7–4.4 mg/dL at age 50 and 2.9–4.8 mg/dL at age 70 (Table 2).

Phosphorus concentrations should be determined in serum or plasma that has been separated promptly from red blood cells. Prolonged standing or hemolysis of the specimen can lead to a spurious increase in phosphorus concentration. Concentrations of phosphorus expressed as mg/dL can be converted to mmol/L by dividing by 3.1. The atomic weight of phosphorus is 30.98. Because plasma phosphate is a mixture of monovalent and divalent ions, the composite valence of phosphorus in serum (or intravenous solutions) at pH 7.4 is 1.8. At this pH, 1 mmol phosphorus is equal to 1.8 mEq.

SERUM MAGNESIUM CONCENTRATION

As with calcium, magnesium exists in serum in three distinct forms, protein-bound magnesium (30%), which is not ultrafilterable, and ionized (55%) and complexed (15%) magnesium, which are ultrafilterable (11). Magnesium is bound principally to albumin in a pH-dependent manner similar to that of calcium. Ionized magnesium is the fraction that is important for physiologic processes, including neuromuscular transmission and cardiovascular tone. Measurement of ionized magnesium concentration is rarely available, and for most clinical purposes, the total concentration of magnesium in serum is determined. Most laboratories use automated spectrophotometric techniques; the reference method is atomic absorption spectrophotometry (7).

The serum concentration of magnesium is closely maintained within the narrow range of ~1.7–2.6 mg/dL. There are no significant differences in magnesium concentration between men and women, nor with respect to age, the values in children being similar to those in adults (Table 2). The circadian variation in magnesium concentration is of low amplitude and not clinically significant.

Prolonged standing or hemolysis of the specimen can lead to a spurious increases in serum magnesium concentration. Concentrations expressed as mg/dL can be converted to mmol/L by dividing by 2.4, and to mEq/L by dividing by 1.2. The atomic weight of magnesium is 24.31.

REFERENCES

1. Moore EW: Ionized calcium in normal serum, ultrafiltrates, and whole blood determined by ion-exchange electrodes. *J Clin Invest* 49:318–334, 1970
2. Markowitz M, Rotkin L, Rosen JF: Circadian rhythms of blood minerals in humans. *Science* 213:672–674, 1981
3. Halloran BP, Portale AA, Castro M, Morris RC Jr, Goldsmith RS: Serum concentration of 1,25-dihydroxyvitamin D in the human: Diurnal variation. *J Clin Endocrinol Metab* 60:1104–1110, 1985
4. Jubiz W, Canterbury JM, Reiss E, Tyler FH; Circadian rhythm in serum parathyroid hormone concentration in human subjects: Correlation with serum calcium, phosphate, albumin, and growth hormone levels. *J Clin Invest* 51:2040–2046, 1972
5. Keating FR Jr, Jones JD, Elveback LR, Randall RV: The relation of age and sex to distribution of values in healthy adults of serum, calcium inorganic phosphorus, magnesium, alkaline phosphatase, total proteins, albumin, and blood urea. *J Lab Clin Med* 73:825–834, 1969
6. Arnaud SB, Goldsmith RS, Stickler GB, McCall JT, Arnaud

CD: Serum parathyroid hormone and blood minerals: interrelationships in normal children. *Pediatr Res* 7:485–493, 1973

7. Pesce AJ, Kaplan LA (eds): *Methods in Clinical Chemistry*, CV Mosby Company, St. Louis, 1987

8. Bowers GN, Brassard C, Sena S: Meaurement of ionized calcium in serum with ion-selective electrodes: A mature technology that can meet the daily service needs. *Clin Chem* 32:1437–1447, 1986

9. Loughead JL, Mimouni F, Tsang RC: Serum ionized calcium concentrations in normal neonates. *Am J Dis Child* 142:516–518, 1988

10. David L, Anast CS: Calcium metabolism in newborn infants: The interrelationship of parathyroid function and calcium, magnesium, and phosphorus metabolism in normal, "sick," and hypocalcemic newborns. *J Clin Invest* 54:287–296, 1974

11. Boink ABTJ, Buckley BM, Christiansen TF, Covington AK, Maas AHJ, Muller-Plathe O, Sachs C, Siggaard-Andersen O: IFCC recommendation: Recommendation on sampling, transport and storage for the determination of the concentration of ionized calcium in whole blood, plasma and serum. *Clin Chim Acta* 202:S13–S22, 1991

12. Marshall RW: Plasma fractions. In: Nordin BEC (ed) *Calcium, Phosphate and Magnesium Metabolism*. Churchill Livingston, London, pp 162–185, 1976

13. Portale AA, Halloran BP, Morris RC Jr: Dietary intake of phosphorus modulates the circadian rhythm in serum concentration of phosphorus: Implications for the renal production of 1,25-dihydroxyvitamin D. *J Clin Invest* 80:1147–1154, 1987

14. Cam JM, Luck VA, Eastwood JB, de Wardener HE: The effect of aluminum hydroxide orally on calcium, phosphorus and aluminum metabolism in normal subjects. *Clin Sci Mol Med* 51:407–414, 1976

15. Mostellar ME, Tuttle EP: Effects of alkalosis on plasma concentration and urinary excretion of inorganic phosphate in man. *J Clin Invest* 43:138–149, 1964

16. Brodehl J, Gellissen K, Weber HP: Postnatal development of tubular phosphate reabsorption. *Clin Nephrol* 17:163–171, 1982

17. Greenberg BG, Winters RW, Graham JB: The normal range of serum inorganic phosphorus and its utility as discriminant in the diagnosis of congenital hypophosphatemia. *J Clin Endocrinol Metab* 20:364–379, 1960

18. Meites S (ed): *Pediatric Clinical Chemistry*. The American Association for Clinical Chemistry, Washington, 1981

19. Parathyroid Hormone and Calcitonin

*Lawrence E. Mallette, M.D., Ph.D., and †Robert F. Gagel, M.D.

*Division of Endocrinology and Metabolism, Baylor College of Medicine,
Veterans Administration Medical Center, Houston, Texas, and †Division of
Endocrinology, M. D. Anderson Cancer Center, Houston, Texas

PARATHYROID HORMONE

The ability to measure circulating parathyroid hormone (PTH) accurately has simplified the evaluation of disorders of calcium metabolism. Although excess parathyroid function can be surmised indirectly, for example from elevated serum chloride values or radiographic subperiosteal bone resorption, these changes either are nonspecific or occur too rarely to be reliable. Measurement of PTH in serum is a more useful method of assessing parathyroid function. Because of the improved utility of the newer PTH assays, diagnostic practice has changed. Twenty years ago it was considered appropriate to arrive at a diagnosis of presumptive primary hyperparathyroidism only after excluding occult malignancy with extensive radiographic examination. Today, when the serum PTH value is elevated in a well-validated assay, screening for malignancy can usually be limited to those simple steps that would be appropriate for the general examination of any patient of similar age. This improved diagnostic accuracy comes mainly from increased assay sensitivity, which may also have presented us with a dilemma, because it is now possible to document mild cases of primary hyperparathyroidism for which the proper management is uncertain.

This section will outline the methods currently available for PTH measurement, review a few clinical situations in which PTH measurement may be useful, and make suggestions for timing of sampling to enhance diagnostic discrimination.

Background: Hormone Secretion and Catabolism

The chief biologically active secretory form of PTH is an 84-amino-acid straight-chain polypeptide (1). Several quirks of nature complicated the task of developing an adequate immunological assay for PTH (Table 1). The first problem was that the hormone circulates at low concentrations, the normal range for the intact PTH molecule being ~10–55 ng/L (1–5 pmol/L) (2,3). The intact, biologically active hormone has a short half-life (2–4 min), which may account in part for its extremely low level in serum (2). It is cleared by the kidney, via peritubular uptake (4) and by the liver (5).

The second problem was that PTH undergoes extensive catabolism, both in the parathyroid cell and in the liver. The catabolic products are missing most of the amino-terminal 27 amino acids (5–7) and thus are devoid of hypercalcemic, hypocalciuric, and phosphaturic activity (8). Because these fragments have a long half-life, they accumulate in serum to a level in normal subjects that is perhaps 5- to 20-fold greater than that of intact hormone. Their presence complicates the immunologic measurement of the biologically active hormone (9).

In a simplified view, two types of PTH fragments are present in serum, those of hepatic origin and those of parathyroid gland origin (Fig. 1). The first type is formed when enzymes on the surface of the hepatic Kupffer cells cleave the hormone in its 34–43 region (5). These fragments are formed at a rate determined largely by the concentration of intact PTH. The amino-terminal fragment is either de-

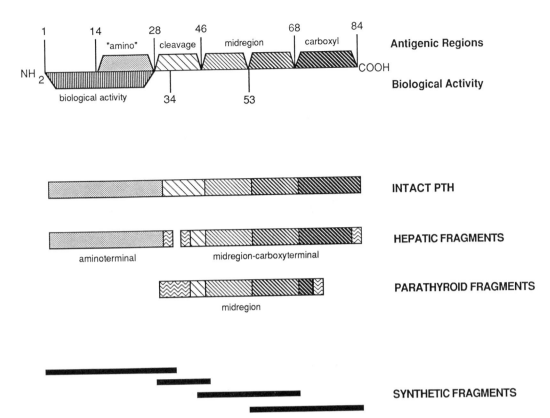

FIG. 1. Stylized diagram of antigenic and functional regions in the PTH molecule, circulating peptide fragments of the hormone, and available synthetic peptide fragments of PTH. Five antigenic regions may be differentiated *(top panel)*. Assays specific for each region have been developed. Biological activity requires a major portion of the 1–28 region, but antibodies recognizing this region usually react with the more antigenic 14–28 portion. Four types of PTH peptides are present in serum *(middle panels)*, but the concentration of amino-terminal fragment in serum is very low. *Wavy segments* in the fragments indicate regions of uncertain or variable length. Four synthetic peptide fragments *(straight lines* in *bottom panel)* are widely available for establishing specificity or for use as radioligands.

graded within the liver or cleared rapidly from the circulation, so is present only at very low concentrations in normal serum (10). The second type of PTH fragments, those arising from the parathyroid cell itself, are abbreviated at each end of the molecule—they do not react in assays specific for either the 1–34 or 65–84 region (11). Again, the amino-terminal fragment is not thought to be secreted by the parathyroid cell in significant amounts. At high calcium concentrations the parathyroid cell suppresses the secretion of intact PTH to near zero, but fragments continue to be released (12,13). These fragments are detectable in the serum of patients with nonparathyroid forms of hypercalcemia (14). Both the hepatic and the parathyroid fragments of PTH are cleared by the kidney and will accumulate in subjects with renal insufficiency.

TABLE 1. *Facts about parathyroid hormone that made assay difficult*

Short circulating half-life with low circulating levels
Extensive catabolism with long-lived products
Multiple antigenic epitopes in the molecule

The third quirk of nature that complicated measurement of PTH was the fact that the intact PTH molecule is large enough to possess at least five different antigenic epitopes (9). Thus, antisera generated against the intact PTH molecule will contain several species of antibodies, each recognizing a different region of the PTH molecule (Fig. 1). This fact, together with the presence in serum of several forms of PTH, made it advantageous to develop assays specific for a single region within the PTH molecule in order to simplify interpretation of assay results.

Measurement Methods

Two techniques for the measurement of PTH are currently widely available, the traditional radioimmunoassay (RIA) and the two-site immunoradiometric assay (IRMA). The RIA technique uses an antibody against the target molecule and a radiolabeled version of the target molecule, called the radioligand or tracer (Fig. 2). Antibody and tracer are present at the same concentration in every tube in the assay run, whereas the concentration of the unlabeled target molecule (added in the experimental sam-

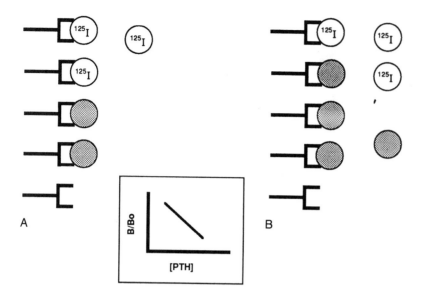

FIG. 2. Radioimmunoassay for PTH. Antibody *(stick figures)* and ^{125}I-labeled PTH fragment *(light circles)* are present at a constant concentration in each assay tube. Variable concentrations of unlabeled PTH *(dark circles)* compete with labeled PTH for binding to the available antibody sites. Moving from a lower concentration of unlabeled PTH **(A)** to a higher concentration **(B)** diminishes the number of counts bound to antibody *(inset)*. B/Bo, counts bound to antibody in presence of the unknown or standard amount of unlabeled PTH divided by antibody bound counts without added unlabeled PTH.

ple) varies. Tracer and unlabeled target molecule compete for binding to the antibody: higher concentrations of unlabeled target molecule cause less radioligand to be bound. Measurement of the fraction of tracer bound to antibody thus provides an estimate of the amount of unlabeled target molecule.

Early RIAs for human PTH were often not sensitive enough to detect normal levels of the hormone. Insufficient sensitivity made it impossible to discriminate low from normal PTH values and blurred the discrimination between normal and modestly elevated values. New reagents for RIA were developed to provide sufficient sensitivity. Antibodies of higher affinity were generated using human PTH as antigen, rather than heterologous PTHs (bovine or porcine) that had been used earlier (15–17). Fragments of PTH were synthesized for establishing regional assay specificity and for use as tracers (Fig. 1) (8). These fragments have more favorable chemical properties for use as radioligands than the native PTH-(1–84) molecule originally used (18).

Use of the hormone fragment as tracer is the easiest way to narrow the specificity of the assay to a single region of the PTH molecule, because an assay can detect only antigenic sites that are present in its tracer molecule. Region-specific PTH RIAs of three types have been the most widely used: the midregion, carboxy-terminal, and amino-terminal assays. We will not discuss amino-terminal assays, because they have mostly been supplanted by the IRMA for intact PTH (see below).

Midregion-specific assays use a form of PTH-(44–68) as radioligand. They may recognize the 44–53 region, the 53–68 region, or both (Fig. 1), but the distinction is clinically unimportant, because measurements with 44–53 specific and 53–68 specific assays correlate well on direct comparison (19). Midregion assays often have the advantage of extreme sensitivity, being able to distinguish even among varying degrees of hypoparathyroidism (20). Assay sensitivity is not a function of specificity, however, but rather a function of antibody-ligand affinity and tracer specific activity. Some midregion assays may use a lower

affinity antibody and thus not possess this ability to discriminate low levels of PTH. Another advantage of midregion assays is that they detect all three important circulating PTH fragments, including those of parathyroid origin. Some parathyroid adenomas release large amounts of PTH fragments (11), and, for detection of these, the midregion assay may be the most useful type assay.

Carboxy-terminal specific assays, measuring the 69–84 region, perform differently from midregion-specific assays. They do not detect the PTH fragments of parathyroid origin. Thus they give lower values for total immunoreactivity and are not as useful for diagnosis of the parathyroid adenoma or for venous sampling studies for parathyroid tumor localization.

The terms midregion-specific and carboxy-terminal–specific have sometimes been loosely applied. Midregion assays have sometimes been called "midmolecule–carboxy-terminal," a term that technically should imply recognition of the entire 44–84 region. The recommended terminology defines PTH assays according to what specific region is being recognized, as established using the easily available synthetic PTH fragments (Fig. 1).

Readers of the older literature should be aware that RIAs originally were termed carboxy-terminal–specific if they did not detect the 1–34 synthetic peptide, which at the time was the only peptide fragment available for testing. Some of the more useful of these assays were later found in fact to be midregion-specific (21,22). The term carboxy-terminal–specific should now be reserved for assays that read the 69–84 region.

A newer development in the field of PTH measurement is the IRMA for intact PTH (3,23). This type of assay uses two different antibodies against the PTH molecule, each recognizing a separate region (Fig. 3). One antibody is bound to a solid phase and is present in great excess so that it can extract all the intact PTH from the serum sample, even in the presence of large amounts of PTH fragments, which will also be extracted. The second antibody, directed against the other end of the molecule, is radiola-

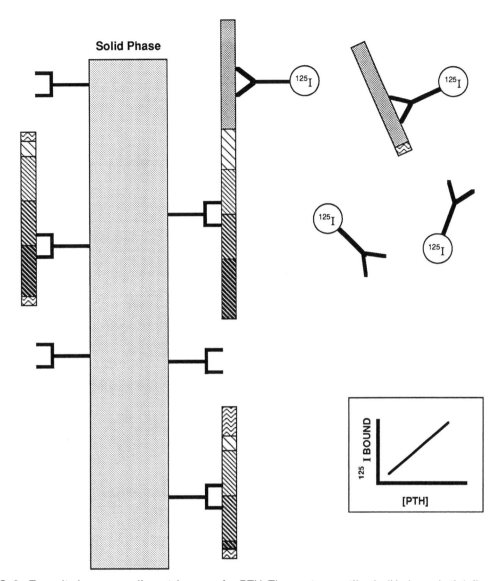

FIG. 3. Two-site immunoradiometric assay for PTH. The capture antibody *(U-shaped stick figures)* is bound to a solid phase (plastic bead or test-tube wall) and is used to extract PTH from the serum sample. In this example the capture antibody is midregion-specific and captures the three types of PTH peptides. Intact PTH is completely captured but an excess of unoccupied capture antibody remains. The bound intact PTH is the only captured species that will bind the ^{125}I-labeled "signal antibody" (amino-terminal–specific in this example; *Y-shaped stick figures*). Any amino-terminal PTH fragments that are present will also bind the ^{125}I-labeled antibody, but will be washed away when the solid phase is rinsed before counting. The number of counts bound to the solid phase after washing increases in direct proportion to the amount of intact PTH in the sample *(insert)*. Parathyroid hormone regions are coded here as in Fig. 1.

beled and is used as a "probe" to detect bound molecules that bear both epitopes. Each molecule of the probe antibody can (unlike the tracer PTH used for RIA) be radiolabeled at several sites. This "hotter" tracer enhances the sensitivity of the IRMA. By proper choice of the two antibodies, an assay that will detect essentially only the intact PTH molecule can be developed (Fig. 3). Caution should be exercised, however, in equating PTH values from the IRMA with biological activity, because minor structural changes in the PTH molecule, such as cleavage of even one or two amino acids from its amino-terminal end or

oxidation of its methionine might reduce its biological activity but not its recognition by the IRMA. At present there is no knowledge about whether these modifications actually occur *in vivo*.

Other methods have been described for measurement of PTH in serum or plasma. Bioassays have been an invaluable research tool, but are not likely to be used routinely for clinical diagnosis (2,24). Bioassay methods that are sensitive enough to detect normal circulating levels use tissue slices and quantitative histochemical techniques, so that only small numbers of samples can be measured in each run and the expense is great. Enzyme-linked immunosorbent assays (ELISAs), of either the colorometric or fluorescence variety, are potentially useful tools that will probably see more widespread usage in the future (10).

Criteria for an Adequate PTH Assay

Regardless of assay type, several criteria define an adequate PTH assay. An adequately sensitive assay should discriminate almost completely between normal subjects and patients with total hypoparathyroidism (14). This ability is the most reliable clinical criterion of diagnostic sensitivity. More research is needed into how total hypoparathyroidism is to be defined, but a temporary working definition might be the requirement for at least 50,000 U/day of vitamin D or the equivalent for adequate treatment.

The binding value representing zero PTH should be established in each assay run by reference to a panel of sera from totally hypoparathyroid individuals, rather than to assay buffer (25). If buffer is used for the zero reference, nonspecific effects of serum proteins on tracer binding will be interpreted as representing PTH immunoreactivity, thereby giving too high a normal range.

Between-assay and within-assay coefficients of variance should be below 10%, and samples should be run at least in duplicate. In the PTH RIA, samples should also be assayed at two or more different dilutions, to help in detecting false positives, which usually will not "dilute out" in parallel with the standard curve. Such false-positives may occur in up to 2% of samples (26).

The laboratory performing the assay should routinely provide the following information with their reports: the precise regional specificity of the assay, the expected ranges for totally hypoparathyroid patients and normal subjects, assay precision, and number of replicates/dilutions performed. Failure to follow these guidelines and to provide normative information in the past has led to false-positive or false-negative diagnoses.

Units

PTH results need not be expressed in SI units. PTH RIAs, even those with well-defined regional specificity, detect a mixture of peptides of varying molecular weight in serum. Thus, expression of results in pmol/L is not appropriate, and PTH RIA results may validly be expressed in arbitrary units (µL-Eq or ng-Eq of an in-house standard, for example), as long as the normal range is well established. Comparison of results between laboratories may be facilitated if the in-house standard is calibrated against the World Health Organization International Research Standard for Human Parathyroid Hormone for Immunoassay (27), with assay results expressed in units of ng-Eq/L. For biterminal assays for intact PTH, expression of results in pmol/L is more appropriate, although there is still uncertainty about whether all species of PTH being measured have equimolar biologic and immunologic potencies with intact PTH.

Influence of Renal Function on PTH Assay Results

Fragments of PTH are cleared largely by glomerular filtration. Midregion and carboxy-terminal assays are therefore sensitive to renal function. The glomerular filtration rate must be considered in interpreting the results of these assays. Glomerular filtration rates below 40 mL/min will cause an increase in midregion PTH values, even before significant parathyroid hyperplasia is thought to have occurred. Midregion PTH values also increase with aging, largely a result of the declining glomerular filtration rate, although a slight increase in parathyroid function may accompany aging (28).

Intact PTH is cleared by the liver as well as the kidney. In the kidney, intact PTH is cleared by peritubular uptake rather than glomerular filtration (4), and this process is less influenced by declining renal function. Intact PTH values obtained by the IRMA are therefore less sensitive to declining glomerular filtration rates than are midregion and carboxy-terminal RIA values. Renal failure may, however, prolong the half-life of bioactive PTH by a factor of roughly two (2). Thus, in the first 20 min after parathyroidectomy, intact PTH values may fall less rapidly in those with renal insufficiency (29).

Specific Uses of PTH Assays

Differential Diagnosis of Hypercalcemia

PTH assays are important for the differentiation of *primary hyperparathyroidism* from other (nonparathyroid-mediated) forms of hypercalcemia, such as malignancy, sarcoidosis, and thyrotoxicosis. Approximately 95% of patients with primary hyperparathyroidism will have elevated values with an adequate midregion-specific assay (14,21). The percentage with elevations in the IRMA for intact PTH may be slightly less (30), perhaps because fragments are not being detected and perhaps because the upper limit of normal for the IRMA may be harder to define because of pulsatile hormone secretion (see below). Either assay may be used for initial diagnosis, with the other performed selectively to confirm equivocal or unexpected results or resolve diagnostic problems.

Midregion PTH values are depressed by 20–40% in patients with *nonparathyroid hypercalcemia,* but significant immunoreactivity is still detectable in serum of ~50–70% of the subjects (relative to hypoparathyroid subjects) (14,21). This immunoreactivity is thought to be derived from the parathyroid cell itself, which continues to release PTH fragments even at high ambient calcium concentrations (12,13). In nonparathyroid hypercalcemia patients with significant degrees of renal failure (creatinine clearance below 40 mL/min), these PTH fragments will accumulate, giving an apparent false elevation of the midregion PTH value (14). When serum creatinine values are above ~2.0 mg/dL, use of an assay for intact PTH is probably preferred.

Intact PTH values by IRMA are suppressed below the normal range in many patients with nonparathyroid hypercalcemia, and at least into the lower half of the normal range in the remainder. In a group of 52 patients with malignancy hypercalcemia, all PTH values were below 25 pg/mL in an assay with an upper limit of normal of 55 pg/mL (31). Decreased renal function in nonparathyroid hypercalcemia patients still has an influence on the intact PTH value. In our hypercalcemic cancer patients, intact PTH values between 18–25 pg/mL were often associated with significant renal insufficiency (31).

Differential Diagnosis of Hypocalcemia

Parathyroid hormone measurement with either RIA or IRMA may help in evaluating hypocalcemia. Parathyroid hormone values should be undetectable in hypocalcemia due to total hypoparathyroidism, but may lie within the normal range in hypocalcemia due to partial loss or inhibition of parathyroid function (partial hypoparathyroidism or magnesium deficiency for example). Parathyroid hormone values can differentiate *hypoparathyroidism* from *pseudohypoparathyroidism,* but the discrimination of type I from type II pseudohypoparathyroidism requires study of the phosphaturic and cAMP excretory responses to infusion of synthetic PTH-(1–34)(32) (see Appendix vii). When *deficiency of vitamin D action* (low vitamin D supply or resistance to its action) causes hypocalcemia, the condition is often chronic, with markedly increased PTH values (33). With hypocalcemia of shorter duration, PTH will be less elevated. Measurement of PTH can detect mild degrees of secondary hyperparathyroidism and is useful in situations where *milder vitamin D deficiency* might be expected (less severe degrees of intestinal malabsorption or dietary-environmental vitamin deficiency). Serum 25-hydroxyvitamin D measurements may be of value in this setting (see Chapter 21), but may be a less sensitive means of detecting mild deficiency (28). Parathyroid hormone values may also be used to monitor the adequacy of treatment of secondary hyperparathyroidism. Adequate treatment should eventually restore normal PTH values, although in long-standing hypocalcemia this may require many weeks of normocalcemia (33).

Evaluation of Renal Osteodystrophy

One of the goals of managing *renal failure* patients is to minimize the rate of parathyroid growth. The midregion PTH RIA may be used to assess the degree of parathyroid hyperfunction in renal failure if it has been validated in a set of patients well characterized as to severity of hyperparathyroid bone disease. One such assay was shown to give values from 4- to 40-fold elevated in advanced renal failure patients without clinical evidence of bone disease who were just beginning hemodialysis, whereas hemodialysis patients with radiographic and clinical evidence of significant hyperparathyroid bone disease showed values from 60- to 600-fold above normal (14). Hemodialysis patients with hypercalcemia unrelated to the parathyroid glands showed midregion PTH values 4- to 20-fold elevated. In contrast, hemodialysis patients with true auton-

omous (tertiary) hyperparathyroidism showed values more than 40-fold elevated.

The IRMA for intact PTH can provide similar information, but with greater day-to-day or minute-to-minute variability. Intact PTH values change rapidly with a change in serum calcium, and serum calcium in patients with renal disease shows marked day-to-day variation in response to fluctuations in dietary phosphate absorption and episodes of dialysis. Intact PTH values in fact have been shown to change rapidly as serum calcium changes during hemodialysis (34).

Use in Other Metabolic Bone Diseases

Measurement of PTH is indicated in other metabolic bone diseases. Patients with *Paget's disease* who develop primary or secondary hyperparathyroidism have an accelerated course of their bone disease, presumably because the Pagetoid bone cells remain responsive to PTH. Furthermore, the incidence of hyperparathyroidism is increased to as high as 12–18% in Paget's disease (35). It thus may be wise to screen patients with symptomatic Paget's disease for occult hyperparathyroidism by measurement of PTH.

Parathyroid hormone measurement may be useful in the assessment of normocalcemic hypophosphatemia. Serum PTH values in the *hereditary form of hypophosphatemic rickets/osteomalacia* are usually normal unless treatment with neutral phosphate has been instituted. Other forms of hypophosphatemia, however, may show parathyroid hyperfunction. Patients with mild degrees of *vitamin D deficiency* may present with hypophosphatemia and a low-normal serum calcium value, but with a significant increase in PTH. Patients with the syndrome of *hypophosphatemia related to prostatic carcinoma* or other malignancies show low serum 1,25-dihydroxyvitamin D values and may show increased PTH values if their dietary calcium intake is deficient. In the rare syndrome of *masked primary hyperparathyroidism*, a parathyroid adenoma is present but is unable to cause hypercalcemia because of concomitant vitamin D deficiency. These patients usually present with normal serum calcium, hypophosphatemia, elevated serum alkaline phosphatase, and markedly elevated PTH values.

Timing of the Sample: Influence of Ultradian Variation, Episodic Secretion, and Other Factors on PTH Assay Results

Secretion of PTH occurs episodically in normal subjects, with secretory spikes in the intact hormone occurring several times a day and lasting several minutes. Because a normal range is presumably defined by a set of samples randomly obtained, episodic secretion makes the upper limit of normal for the intact PTH assay difficult to define. Unexpectedly high values should therefore be verified by assay of a second sample or measurement of PTH in a midregion assay. The midregion assay, because of the longer half-life of the peptides it detects, tends to integrate these secretory bursts over time and shows less minute-to-minute variation than does an assay for intact PTH. The device of pooling three samples obtained at intervals of several minutes has been used for other hormones that are episodically secreted, but seems too cumbersome for routine application.

When possible, midregion PTH values for diagnosis should be obtained before 11 AM. In some normal subjects midregion PTH values increase in the afternoon. When a rise occurs it usually begins between 1130 and 1300 hr (36). Thus, a wider normal range must be used for afternoon samples, with the upper limit increased by ~33%. An even greater increase in midregion PTH values may occur at night (21), and nocturnal samples are not recommended for diagnosis. Changes in the normal range for intact PTH values as a function of time of day have not been reported, and fasting morning samples are therefore preferred.

Like normal parathyroid glands, most parathyroid adenomas vary their secretion of PTH as an inverse function of the ambient serum calcium value. This fact can be used to enhance the diagnostic discrimination of PTH assays. Parathyroid hormone values in those with primary hyperparathyroidism will be more elevated if the sample is obtained after serum calcium has been lowered a bit by the initial treatment (e.g., by dietary calcium restriction or hydration). These maneuvers will not increase PTH values above normal in those with nonparathyroid forms of hypercalcemia unless hypocalcemia occurs.

In hypocalcemic conditions, the differentiation of secondary hyperparathyroidism (vitamin D deficiency and pseudohypoparathyroidism) from hypoparathyroidism is enhanced if the PTH value is measured before treatment is instituted (33). Treatment of secondary hyperparathyroidism will lower the PTH value, thus lessening the diagnostic separation between groups.

For monitoring of renal failure patients, the optimal timing of intact PTH samples in relationship to hemodialysis has not been determined. Values obtained before dialysis might reflect the maximum stress on the parathyroid glands, whereas values taken after dialysis when serum calcium has increased might give an estimate of parathyroid suppressibility. More study of this question is needed.

In summary, PTH can now be measured reliably by a number of methods, and these measurements are clinically useful in many situations.

CALCITONIN MEASUREMENT

Measurement Methods

Measurement of serum calcitonin is useful in several clinical situations. It is the primary diagnostic tool for diagnosis of medullary thyroid carcinoma (37) and may be useful for diagnosis of other tumors in which ectopic production of calcitonin is observed (38). Serum calcitonin measurement has not proven diagnostically useful for any bone disease, although abnormalities of calcitonin secretion have been reported in Williams' syndrome. It is

now possible to measure normal circulating concentrations of calcitonin by utilizing one of several methods.

The *first method* is a standard radioimmunoassay utilizing polyclonal antisera raised by injection of synthetic human calcitonin into rabbits (39–42) or goats (17). The sensitivity of these assays varies considerably, with the more sensitive assays capable of detecting normal circulating concentrations of calcitonin (2–10 pg/mL). Commercial kits are available that rival the sensitivity of the best research assays.

A *second method* utilizes a concentration technique. Calcitonin and other small peptides are adsorbed by passage of 10–50 mL of serum through a silica cartridge. The peptides are then eluted from the column. The eluate is dried and diluted in a small volume of assay buffer, to be assayed in a sensitive standard radioimmunoassay (43–46). The advantages of this technique include sensitivity (detection limit of 0.5 pg/mL) and elimination of other substances present in serum that may cause a false-positive elevation of the serum calcitonin (44). Disadvantages include the requirement for concentration of each sample and the exclusion of high molecular weight forms of calcitonin (procalcitonin) produced by lung carcinomas and other tumors (44,45,47,48).

A *third method* for calcitonin measurement is the two-site IRMA, which uses affinity-purified polyclonal antibodies directed against two epitopes within the calcitonin monomer (49,50) to provide a specific and sensitive (10 pg/mL) assay for calcitonin monomer (Fig. 4). A similar technique has been applied to the development of a colorimetric ELISA for calcitonin using monoclonal antibodies (51). A two-site IRMA with specificity only for procalcitonin has also been developed (52). Its antisera are directed against an epitope in the sequence for calcitonin monomer and a second in the flanking region of calcitonin (katacalcin or carboxy-terminal adjacent peptide) (Fig. 4). From the available reports, the sensitivity of the IRMA and ELISA techniques for calcitonin is less than for the RIA or the concentration RIA, but not direct comparative studies have been performed.

Specific Uses of Calcitonin Assays

Measurement of serum calcitonin is most frequently used for the diagnosis and management of medullary thyroid carcinoma. The best diagnostic accuracy is provided by use of a provocative stimulation technique such as the pentagastrin test (37,46,53) (Fig. 5), the combined calcium-pentagastrin test (54), or the short calcium infusion (see Appendix) (39). Interpretation of calcitonin values from these tests is usually straightforward. There are, however, diagnostic pitfalls. In 1–5% of tests, measurement of calcitonin with a standard RIA will give an elevated basal serum calcitonin with no additional increase after the provocative stimulation (Fig. 5) (37,44). This type of result is consistent with one of three possibilities. First, the elevated serum calcitonin may represent a nonspecific RIA result. Such false-positive test results are usually assay-specific, and reassay of the samples with a RIA using a different antiserum or by the concentration

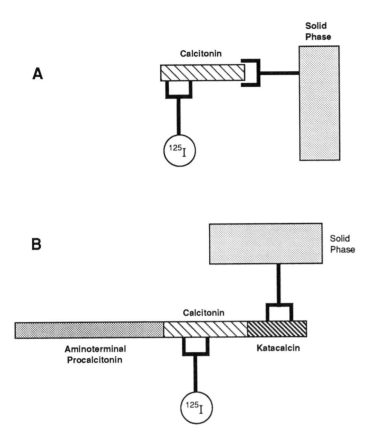

FIG. 4. Two-site immunoradiometric assay for calcitonin **(A)** or procalcitonin **(B)**. Calcitonin is extracted by antibody bound to a solid phase. This antibody recognizes an antigenic site that is present only after cleavage of the carboxyl flanking peptide of the procalcitonin molecule (katacalcin), so procalcitonin is not extracted. The bound calcitonin is then quantitated with a second antibody labeled with ^{125}I. The assay for procalcitonin utilizes an extracting antibody against katacalcin and a labeled antibody against calcitonin.

technique will usually yield a normal result. A second possibility is that the elevated value represents a higher molecular weight form of calcitonin, ectopically produced by a tumor other than a medullary thyroid carcinoma; release of calcitonin from such tumors may not be increased by calcium or pentagastrin (38). A third rare possibility is calcitonin production by a medullary thyroid carcinoma that responds poorly to a provocative stimulus.

In summary, measurement of circulating concentrations of calcitonin is easily performed by one of several techniques. Sensitive standard RIA kits and measurement of calcitonin by the concentration technique are commercially available. Measurement of calcitonin and procalcitonin by two-site IRMA is currently limited to the research laboratory.

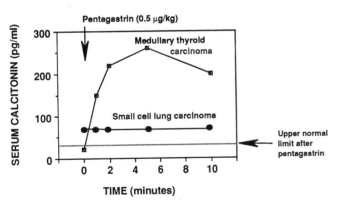

FIG. 5. Pentagastrin test for diagnosis of medullary carcinoma of the thyroid. Pentagastrin was injected intravenously, and serum calcitonin was measured by a standard calcitonin RIA at the indicated time points (see Appendix vii). The upper limit of normal after pentagastrin stimulation is indicated. The result with higher calcitonin values is consistent with C-cell hyperplasia or microscopic medullary thyroid carcinoma, whereas the elevated basal value with a flat response is consistent either with the ectopic production of calcitonin by a malignancy such as small cell carcinoma of the lung or with an assay artifact.

REFERENCES

1. Keutmann HT, Sauer MM, Hendy GN, O'Riordan JLH, Potts JT Jr: Complete amino acid sequence of human parathyroid hormone. *Biochemistry* 17:5723–5729, 1978
2. Goltzman D, Gomolin H, DeLean A, Wexler M, Meakins JL: Discordant disappearance of bioactive and immunoreactive parathyroid hormone after parathyroidectomy. *J Clin Endocrinol Metab* 58:70–75, 1984
3. Nussbaum SR, Zahradnik RJ, Lavigne JR, et al.: Highly sensitive two-site immunoradiometric assay of parathyrin, and its clinical utility in evaluating patients with hypercalcemia. *Clin Chem* 33:1364–1367, 1988
4. Martin KJ, Hruska KA, Lewis J, Anderson C, Slatopolsky E: The renal handling of parathyroid hormone. Role of peritubular uptake and glomerular filtration. *J Clin Invest* 60:808–814, 1977
5. Segre GV, Perkins AS, Witters LA, Potts JT Jr: Metabolism of parathyroid hormone by isolated rat Kupffer cells and hepatocytes. *J Clin Invest* 67:449–457, 1981
6. Segre GV, Nial HD, Sauer RT, Potts JT Jr: Edman degradation of radioiodinated parathyroid hormone: Application to sequence

analysis and hormone metabolism in vivo. *Biochemistry* 16: 2417–2427, 1977

7. MacGregor RR, McGregor DH, Lee SH, Hamilton JW: Structural analysis of parathormone fragments elaborated by cells cultured from a hyperplastic human parathyroid gland. *Bone and Mineral* 1:41–50, 1986

8. Rosenblatt M: Parathyroid hormone: Chemistry and structure-activity relations. In: Ioachim HL (ed) *Pathobiology Annual*. Raven Press, New York, pp 53–86, 1981

9. Segre GV, Habener JF, Powell D, Tregear GW, Potts JT Jr: Parathyroid hormone in human plasma: Immunochemical characterization and biological implications. *J Clin Invest* 51: 3163–3172, 1972

10. Klee GG, Preissner CM, Schryver PG, Taylor RL, Kao PC: Multisite immunochemiluminometric assay for simultaneously measuring whole-molecule and amino-terminal fragments of human parathyrin. *Clin Chem* 38:628–635, 1992

11. Marx SJ, Sharp ME, Krudy A, Rosenblatt M, Mallette LE: Radioimmunoassay for the middle region of human parathyroid hormone: Studies with a radioiodinated synthetic peptide. *J Clin Endocrinol Metab* 53:76–84, 1981

12. Hanley DA, Takatsuki K, Sultan JM, Schneider AB: Direct release of parathyroid hormone fragments from functioning bovine parathyroid glands in vitro. *J Clin Invest* 62:1247–1254, 1978

13. Mayer GP, Deaton JA, Hurst JG, Habener JF: Effects of plasma calcium concentration on the relative proportion of hormone and carboxyl fragments in parathyroid venous blood. *Endocrinology* 104:1778–1784, 1979

14. Mallette LE, Tuma SN, Berger RE, Kirkland J: Radioimmunoassay for the middle region of human parathyroid hormone using an homologous antiserum with a carboxy-terminal fragment of bovine PTH as radioligand. *J Clin Endocrinol Metab* 54: 1017–1024, 1982

15. Fischer JA, Binswanger U, Dietrich FM: Human parathyroid hormone. Immunological characterization of antibodies against a glandular extract and the synthetic amino-terminal fragments 1–12 and 1–34 and their use in the determination of immunoreactive hormone in human sera. *J Clin Invest* 85:1382–1394, 1974

16. Manning RM, Hendy GN, Papapoulos SE, O'Riordan JLH: Development of homologous immunological assays for human parathyroid hormone. *J Endocrinol* 85:161–170, 1980

17. Mallette LE: General techniques for raising antisera against parathyroid hormone and calcitonin. In Bickle DD (ed) *Assay of Calcium Regulating Hormones*. Springer-Verlag, New York, pp 169–189, 1983

18. Sharp M, Marx SJ: Radioimmunoassay for the middle region of human parathyroid hormone: Comparison of two radioiodinated synthetic peptides. *Clin Chim Acta* 145:59–68, 1985

19. Mallette LE: Radioimmunoassays for the midregion of parathyrin. Characterization of 44–53 versus 53–68 specific assays (abstract). *Clin Chem* 30:1041, 1984

20. Mallette LE, Cooper J, Kirkland JL: Transient congenital hypoparathyroidism. Possible association with lesions of the pulmonary valve. *J Pediatr* 101:928–931, 1982

21. Arnaud CD, Tsao HS, Littledike T: Radioimmunoassay of human parathyroid hormone in serum. *J Clin Invest* 50:21–34, 1971

22. Gallagher JC, Riggs BL, Jerpbak CM, Arnaud CD: The effect of age on serum immunoreactive parathyroid hormone in normal and osteoporotic women. *J Lab Clin Med* 95:373–385, 1980

23. Blind E, Schmidt-Gayk H, Scharla S, et al.: Two-site assay of intact parathyroid hormone in the investigation of primary hyperparathyroidism and other disorders of calcium metabolism compared with a midregion assay. *J Clin Endocrinol Metab* 67: 353–360, 1988

24. Chambers DJ, Dunham J, Zanelli JM, et al.: A sensitive bioassay of parathyroid hormone in plasma. *Clin Endocrinol* 9:375–379, 1978

25. Habener JF, Potts JT Jr: Radioimmunoassay of parathyroid hormone. In Antoniades HN (ed) *Hormones in Human Blood*. Harvard University Press, Cambridge, pp 551–558, 1976

26. Mallette LE, Nammour H: False elevation of the midregion PTH value. Inhibition of tracer binding by heterophilic antibody in patient serum (abstract). *J Bone Mineral Res 2* (suppl 1):102, 1987

27. Zanelli JM, Gaines Das RE: International collaborative study of N.I.B.S.C. Research Standard for human parathyroid hormone for immunoassay. *J Endocrinol* 86:291–304, 1980

28. Marcus R, Madvig P, Young G: Age-related changes in parathyroid hormone and parathyroid hormone action in normal humans. *J Clin Endocr Metab* 58:223–230, 1983

29. Ryan MF, Jones SR, Barnes AD: Clinical evaluation of a rapid parathyroid hormone assay. *Ann Clin Biochem* Jan 29(pt 1): 48–51, 1992

30. Endres DB, Villanueva R, Sharp CF Jr, Singer FR: Measurement of parathyroid hormone. *Endocrinol Metab Clin North Am* 18:611–630, 1989

31. Mallette LE, Beck P, VandePol C: Malignancy hypercalcemia: Evaluation of parathyroid function and response to treatment. *Am J Med Sci* 302:205–210, 1991

32. Mallette LE, Kirkland JL, Gagel RF, Law WM Jr, Heath H III: Synthetic human parathyroid hormone-(1–34) for the study of pseudohypoparathyroidism. *J Clin Endocrinol Metab* 67: 964–972, 1988

33. Mallette LE, Wilson DP, Kirkland JL: Evaluation of hypocalcemia with a highly sensitive homologous radioimmunoassay for the midregion of parathyroid hormone. *Pediatrics* 71:64–69, 1983

34. Felsenfeld AJ, Ross D, Rodriguez M: Hysteresis of the parathyroid hormone response to hypocalcemia in hemodialysis patients with low turnover aluminum bone disease. *J Am Soc Nephrol* 2:1136–1143, 1991

35. Siris ES, Clemens TP, McMahon D, et al.: Parathyroid function in Paget's disease of bone. *J Bone Miner Res* 4:75–80, 1989

36. Mallette LE, Kirkland JL: Fine regulation of serum calcium. Acute midday decreases in calcium ion concentration trigger a parathyroid response. In Cohn DV, Fujita T, Potts J Jr (ed) *Endocrine Control of Bone and Calcium Metabolism*. Elsevier, New York, pp 268–271, 1984

37. Gagel RF, Tashjian AH Jr, Cummings T, et al.: The clinical outcome of prospective screening for multiple endocrine neoplasia type 2a. An 18-year experience. *N Engl J Med* 318:478–844, 1988

38. Samaan NA, Castillo S, Schultz PN, Khalil KG, Johnston DA: Serum calcitonin after pentagastrin stimulation in patients with bronchogenic and breast cancer compared to that in patients with medullary thyroid carcinoma. *J Clin Endocrinol Metab* 51: 237–241, 1980

39. Parthemore JG, Bronzert D, Roberts G, Deftos LJ: A short calcium infusion in the diagnosis of medullary thyroid carcinoma. *J Clin Endocrinol Metab* 39:108–111, 1974

40. Parthemore JG, Deftos LJ: Calcitonin secretion in normal human subjects. *J Clin Endocrinol Metab* 47:184–188, 1978

41. Gagel RF, O'Briain DS, Voelkel EF, et al.: Pituitary immunoreactive calcitonin-like material: Lack of evidence for cross-reactivity with pro-opiomelanocortin. *Metabolism* 32:686–696, 1983

42. Heath H III, Sizemore GW: Plasma calcitonin in normal man: differences between men and women. *J Clin Invest* 60: 1135–1140, 1977

43. Body JJ, Heath H III: Estimates of circulating monomeric calcitonin: Physiological studies in normal and thyroidectomized man. *J Clin Endocrinol Metab* 57:897–903, 1983

44. Body JJ, Heath H III: "Nonspecific" increases in plasma immunoreactive calcitonin in healthy individuals: Discrimination from medullary thyroid carcinoma by a new extraction technique. *Clin Chem* 30:511–514, 1984

45. Heath H III, Body JJ, Fox J: Radioimmunoassay of calcitonin in normal human plasma: Problems, perspectivs and prospects. *Biomed Pharmacother* 38:241–245, 1984

46. Gharib H, Kao PC, Heath H III: Determination of silica-purified plasma calcitonin for the detection and management of medullary thyroid carcinoma: Comparison of two provocative tests. *Mayo Clin Proc* 62:373–378, 1987

47. Deftos LJ, Roos BA, Bronzert D, Parthemore JG: Immunochemical heterogeneity of calcitonin in plasma. *J Clin Endocrinol Metab* 40:409–412, 1975

48. Lee JC, Parthemore JG, Deftos LJ: Immunochemical heterogeneity of calcitonin in renal failure. *J Clin Endocrinol Metab* 45: 528–533, 1977

49. Motte P, Ait-Abdellah M, Vauzelle P, et al.: A two-site immuno-radiometric assay for serum calcitonin using monoclonal anti-peptide antibodies. *Henry Ford Hospital Medical J* 35:129–132, 1987

50. Motte P, Vauzelle P, Alberici G, et al.: Utilization of synthetic peptides for the study of calcitonin and biosynthetic precursors for calcitonin. *Int J Rad Appl Instrum* 14:289–294, 1987

51. Seth R, Motte P, Kehely A, et al.: A sensitive and specific two-site enzyme-immunoassay for human calcitonin using monoclonal antibodies. *J Endocrinol* 119:351–357, 1988

52. Ghillani P, Motte P, Bohuon C, Bellet D: Monoclonal antipeptide antibodies as tools to dissect closely related gene products. A model using peptides encoded by the calcitonin gene. *J Immunol* 141:3156–3163, 1988

53. Wells SA Jr, Ontjes DA, Cooper CW, et al.: The early diagnosis of medullary carcinoma of the thyroid gland in patients with multiple endocrine neoplasia type II. *Ann Surg* 182:362–370, 1975

54. Wells SA Jr, Baylin SB, Linehan WM, et al.: Provocative agents and the diagnosis of medullary carcinoma of the thyroid gland. *Ann Surg* 188:139–141, 1978

20. Parathyroid Hormone-Related Protein Assays

William J. Burtis, M.D., Ph.D.

Department of Medicine, West Haven Veterans Affairs Medical Center,
West Haven, Connecticut, and Yale University School of Medicine,
New Haven, Connecticut

Parathyroid hormone-related protein (PTHRP) is a complex protein, recently purified from tumors of patients with humoral hypercalcemia of malignancy (HHM), which has amino acid sequence homology with parathyroid hormone (PTH) in the aminoterminal region (see Chapters 12 and 33) (1–5). The gene encoding PTHRP, unlike the gene for PTH itself, is expressed in many different tissues of the body (skin and other epithelia, the CNS, many endocrine glands, islet cells, breast, uterus, urinary bladder, and others). Even the non-PTH-like portion of the amino acid sequence of PTHRP is highly conserved across avian and mammalian species, suggesting that PTHRP probably plays important, although incompletely understood, roles in normal physiology.

There is emerging evidence that the cDNA-encoded protein undergoes complex posttranslational processing and is proteolytically cleaved into several smaller, biologically active fragments (6). For example, a midregion fragment, PTHRP(67–86)amide, has been shown to stimulate a placental calcium pump, whereas a carboxyterminal region, PTHRP(107–111), may inhibit osteoclastic bone resorption (7,8). Only the aminoterminal region [e.g., PTHRP(1–36)], has homology with PTH and is able to stimulate PTH receptors. In addition to classical PTH-like effects on bone and kidney, aminoterminal PTHRP also causes smooth muscle relaxation, vasodilatation, and complex tissue-specific effects on growth and differentiation (9–11). It is not clear whether all of these effects of aminoterminal PTHRP are mediated through the recently cloned PTH receptor, or if there is a unique PTHRP receptor (12,13). In normal physiology, these biologically active peptides are probably usually acting at the local tissue level (paracrine, autocrine, or possibly even intracellular or "intracrine" effects). When PTHRP is produced in an unregulated fashion by tumors, however, plasma levels of PTHRP rise and the protein may begin to act systemically, in an endocrine manner. Thus, tumors expressing PTHRP cause hypercalcemia by secreting large amounts of the aminoterminal PTH-like region, which binds to and stimulates classical PTH receptors throughout the body.

Whether there are more subtle endocrinological effects of PTHRP in normal physiology (e.g., effects on calcium metabolism during lactation or pregnancy) is currently under investigation.

BIOASSAYS

Using a sensitive cytochemical bioassay, it was demonstrated over 10 years ago that circulating levels of PTH-like bioactivity are on average ~10-fold elevated in patients with HHM compared with normal volunteers, despite normal levels of PTH itself (14). Because of the labor-intensive nature of this cytochemical bioassay, it is rarely performed today and is not clinically available.

Nephrogenous cyclic AMP (NcAMP) excretion represents a sort of *in vivo* bioassay for PTH-like activity. In fact, the existence of PTHRP was originally postulated largely because of the observation of increased NcAMP excretion in the urine of patients with HHM, despite normal serum levels of PTH (15). The assay requires both plasma and (acidified) spot urine samples. A radioimmunoassay (RIA) is used to measure the urine cAMP (UcAMP) and plasma cAMP (PcAMP) concentrations. The cAMP produced in the kidney itself, NcAMP, is then calculated by subtracting the cAMP in the glomerular filtrate from the total UcAMP excretion:

$$NcAMP = UcAMP \times (S_{Cr}/U_{Cr}) - PcAMP$$

where the units are nmol/100 mL of glomerular filtrate (16). Nephrogenous cAMP accounts for roughly half of the total UcAMP. Nephrogenous cAMP excretion results almost entirely from PTH-like stimulation of the proximal renal tubule (other hormones, e.g., vasopressin, whose action on the nephron is also mediated by intracellular cAMP, contribute relatively little NcAMP excretion).

Nephrogenous cAMP excretion is elevated in patients with hypercalcemia resulting either from hyperparathyroidism or from HHM. However, the NcAMP assay alone cannot be used to differentiate between these, the two most common causes of hypercalcemia, because both PTH and PTHRP are equipotent in stimulating renal adenylate cyclase in the proximal tubule and raising NcAMP. One approach is to measure both NcAMP and serum PTH, and if PTH is normal assume that an elevated NcAMP is due to PTHRP. A more direct approach is to measure plasma PTHRP itself, using immunoassays that have recently become commercially available.

IMMUNOASSAYS

Within the past several years, a number of immunoassays have been developed that are capable of measuring circulating levels of PTHRP (17–24). These assays utilize antibodies directed at various regions of the protein. Because the proteolytic processing and metabolism of PTHRP is still incompletely worked out, the exact forms of PTHRP peptides existing in the circulation are unknown. There is no a priori reason to expect that all of these peptides circulate at the same molar concentrations, or that their levels distinguish equally well between normal physiology and HHM, so each PTHRP assay must be validated against appropriate clinical controls. Furthermore, because the peptides are subject to proteolytic degradation following sample collection, specimens should in general be obtained in tubes containing protease inhibitors, kept on ice, and the plasma separated and frozen promptly before being sent for assay (24).

The two most common types of immunoassays today are RIAs and immunoradiometric assays (IRMAs). There are several fundamental differences between the RIA and IRMA techniques (25). Radioimmunoassays utilize *polyclonal* antiserum raised against the peptide of interest. A given antiserum must be used at a specific, *limited* concentration such that it binds ~30% of "trace" amounts of ^{125}I-labeled peptide added to the assay tube. The RIA technique involves *competition* of cold and radiolabeled peptide for the limited number of antibody binding sites. Sensitivity is determined by the minimum concentration of cold peptide that will "displace" a significant amount of labeled peptide from these binding sites. In contrast, IRMAs utilize two *affinity-purified* or *monoclonal* antibodies. These antibodies are used at high concentrations, as *excess* reagents in the chemical reaction. There is no radiolabeled "trace" peptide, and *no competition* for limited binding sites. Cold peptide binds to the "capture antibody" (attached to a plastic surface) and also binds ^{125}I-labeled "signal antibody" (in solution, generally directed toward a second "site" on the peptide) (Fig. 1). Sensitivity is determined by the minimum concentration of cold peptide that will cause a statistically significant increase in counts of bound ^{125}I-labeled antibody above background. Often, IRMAs can be made more sensitive than RIAs because they are able to utilize much higher concentrations of antibody.

The author's laboratory has developed RIAs for N-terminal PTHRP(1–36), midregion PTHRP(37–74), C-terminal PTHRP(109–138), "tail-region" PTHRP(141–173), and a two-site IRMA for N-terminal PTHRP(1–74)

(18,26,27). Of these assays, only the PTHRP(1–74) IRMA and the C-terminal PTHRP(109–138) RIA are clinically useful at the present time. Other laboratories have also developed IRMAs and/or RIAs directed at various regions of PTHRP (19–24,28).

Our N-terminal PTHRP(1–74) IRMA utilizes affinity-purified anti-PTHRP(37–74) as the capture antibody and ^{125}I-labeled, affinity-purified anti-PTHRP(1–36) as the signal antibody (18). Only peptides containing epitopes recognized by *both* of these antibodies are measured. Thus the assay is specific for fairly large forms of amino-terminal PTHRP; there is no cross-reactivity with PTH itself. Using this assay on plasma collected in tubes containing protease inhibitors, we found PTHRP(1–74) levels to average ~21 pmol/L in patients with HHM, whereas most normal subjects had low (<5) or undetectable (<1 pmol/L) levels (Fig. 2). In contrast to patients with HHM, cancer patients with hypercalcemia caused by direct bone involvement [local osteolytic hypercalcemia (LOH)] and with low UcAMP excretion had low or undetectable PTHRP(1–74) levels, as did patients with primary hyperparathyroidism or miscellaneous causes of hypercalcemia. Patients with cancer and normal serum calcium levels occasionally had slightly elevated PTHRP(1–74)

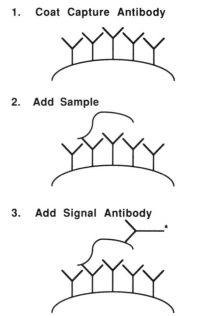

1. Coat Capture Antibody

2. Add Sample

3. Add Signal Antibody

FIG. 1. Immunoradiometric assay methodology. *1*, Capture antibody, directed at one end of the protein of interest, is coated in excess on a solid plastic surface (e.g., bead). *2*, Sample containing the protein of interest (assay standard or unknown) is added, incubated, and any unbound sample is then washed away. *3*, Signal antibody, directed at a second site on the protein and prelabeled with radioiodine (*asterisk*), is added in excess, incubated, and then any unbound labeled antibody is washed away. The remaining bound signal antibody, measured in a gamma counter, is proportional to the amount of protein in the sample. For the PTHRP(1–74) IRMA (18), the capture antibody is affinity-purified anti-PTHRP(37–74), and the signal antibody is radiolabeled anti-PTHRP(1–36).

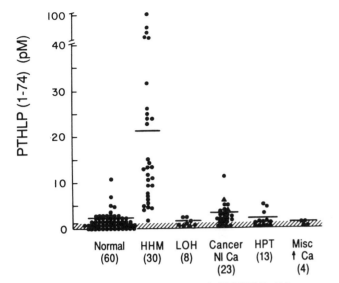

FIG. 2. Plasma concentrations of PTHRP(1–74) measured by IRMA. Normal volunteers (*n* = 60) usually had undetectable (<1 pmol/L) or low concentrations. Patients with malignancy-associated hypercalcemia (*n* = 38) were divided into two groups: those with elevated UcAMP excretion (HHM, *n* = 30) were found to have elevated PTHRP concentrations (mean 21 pmol/L), whereas those with normal UcAMP excretion (LOH, *n* = 8) were found to have low or undetectable PTHRP concentrations. Patients with cancer and normal serum calcium (*n* = 23), hyperparathyroidism (*n* = 13), or miscellaneous causes of hypercalcemia (*n* = 4) also had low or undetectable PTHRP(1–74) concentrations. (From Burtis WJ, Brady TG, Orloff JJ et al.: Immunochemical characterization of circulating parathyroid hormone-related protein in patients with humoral hypercalcemia of cancer. *N Engl J Med* 322:1106–1112, 1990.)

levels; some of these patients subsequently became hypercalcemic several months later. In this series of 38 unselected patients with malignancy-associated hypercalcemia, ~80% had HHM, whereas 20% had LOH, confirming earlier observations suggesting that PTHRP-induced HHM is the most common cause of hypercalcemia in patients with cancer (15,29).

Our C-terminal PTHRP(109–138) RIA utilizes a rabbit polyclonal antiserum raised against Tyr[109]-PTHRP(109–138) (18). This assay is quite specific for short species of C-terminal PTHRP; PTHRP(107–138) and Tyr[109]-PTHRP(109–138) are recognized about equally well, but PTHRP(1–141) is <10% as potent. Using this assay on plasma collected in tubes containing protease inhibitors, we found PTHRP(109–138) levels to average ~24 pmol/L is patients with HHM, similar to the molar concentrations of PTHRP(1–74) in these patients. The measured N- and C-terminal peptides circulate in HHM as separate, unconnected species, however, because an anti-PTHRP(1–36) antibody column removed PTHRP(1–74) immunoactivity, but failed to remove PTHRP(109–138) immunoactivity from plasma. We found levels of C-terminal PTHRP to be undetectable (<2 pmol/L) in most normal subjects and in patients with hypercal-

cemia caused by hyperparathyroidism, vitamin D intoxication, or granulomatous diseases. However, in patients with renal insufficiency C-terminal PTHRP levels are elevated. As creatinine clearance falls below ~20 mL/min, PTHRP(109–138) levels begin to rise, reaching on average 30 pmol/L in patients on dialysis. This finding suggests that a C-terminal PTHRP species is released into the circulation in patients without cancer, is renally cleared, and becomes measurable when it accumulates in renal failure.

The experience with our midregion PTHRP(37–74) and tail region PTHRP(141–173) RIAs is more limited, but suggests that the species measured using these assays circulate at higher levels in normal subjects, but that the levels are not significantly elevated above normal in patients with HHM (26,27). Ratcliffe et al. reported a similar finding using their midregion PTHRP(37–67) RIA; molar concentrations were relatively high, but there was a large overlap between normal levels and levels in patients with HHM (22). These investigators also reported unexpectedly disparate results in two N-terminal RIAs they developed; their direct RIA measured levels of 190 pmol/L, but failed to differentiate patients with HHM from normal subjects, whereas their extraction RIA measured levels of only 11 pmol/L in patients with HHM, but these low levels were clearly higher than those of normal subjects (22). One possible explanation is that the extraction RIA measures a large, "intact N-terminal," biologically active PTH-like species similar to that measured by IRMA, whereas the direct RIA measures a species inactivated by proteolytic cleavage at the Arg[19–21] residues (5). Whatever the explanation, the important point is that not all PTHRP assays measure peptides whose levels correlate closely with the HHM syndrome, so the tract record of each assay in terms of its ability to diagnose HHM must be carefully scrutinized.

Normal circulating levels of aminoterminal PTHRP are still poorly defined, because they are below or just slightly above the detection limits of assays developed to date. The most sensitive IRMAs now have reported detection limits ~0.1 pmol/L, yet most normal individuals still have undetectable levels in these assays. Midregion PTHRP RIAs, on the other hand, are much less sensitive, but may be capable of detecting circulating species in normal subjects. It might be hoped that the ability to measure changes of PTHRP within the normal range would elucidate normal physiologic functions of the protein, but to the extent that these actions are autocrine or paracrine in nature, circulating concentrations may poorly reflect events at the tissue or cellular level.

Elevated circulating levels, in contrast, are readily detectable with most current PTHRP assays in patients with HHM. In using the current PTHRP assays clinically for the differential diagnosis of hypercalcemia, several important points must be kept in mind (30,31). First, as previously discussed, different assays will provide different degrees of discrimination between patients with HHM and those without; IRMAs measuring large N-terminal regions seem to be best in this regard. Second, not all patients with hypercalcemia caused by malignancy will have elevated levels of PTHRP in even the best assay; ~20% will have LOH rather than HHM, so that PTHRP levels will be low. Third, not all patients with elevated PTHRP levels will have a malignant tumor. C-terminal levels are elevated in patients with renal insufficiency, and N-terminal levels may be elevated in patients with nonmalignant pheochromocytomas. In addition, rare patients with hypercalcemia due to mammary hypertrophy or lymphedema may be elevated PTHRP levels (32,33).

The use of PTHRP as a "tumor marker" must still be considered investigational, although the expected variations in PTHRP levels have been seen following therapeutic intervention in a small number of patients with PTHRP-producing tumors (18–20). It is not yet clear how commonly elevations in PTHRP antedate the development of hypercalcemia. Clearly, the assays with the most potential in this regard would be those providing the largest difference between normal levels and levels in HHM. Open questions at the present time are whether tumors produce unique, abnormally processed forms of PTHRP, or indeed which tissues contribute to the normal circulating levels of the various PTHRP peptides.

ACKNOWLEDGMENTS

This work was supported by a Merit Review grant from the Department of Veterans Affairs. The author would like to gratefully acknowledge the expert secretarial assistance of Charleen Stewart.

REFERENCES

1. Stewart AF, Broadus AE: Clinical review 16: Parathyroid hormone-related proteins: coming of age in the 1990s. *J Clin Endocrinol Metab* 71:1410–1414, 1990
2. Strewler GJ, Nissenson RA: Hypercalcemia in malignancy. *West J Med* 153:635–640, 1990
3. Bilezikian JP: Parathyroid hormone-related peptide in sickness and in health. *N Engl J Med* 322:1990, 1990
4. Mallette LE: The parathyroid polyhormones: New concepts in the spectrum of peptide hormone action. *Endocr Rev* 12: 110–117, 1991
5. Burtis WJ: Parathyroid hormone-related protein: Structure, function, and measurement. *Clin Chem* 38:2171–2183, 1992
6. Soifer NE, Dee KE, Insogna KL, et al.: Parathyroid hormone-related protein: Secretion of a novel mid-region fragment by three different cell lines in culture. *J Biol Chem* 267: 18236–18243, 1992
7. Care AD, Abbas SK, Pickard DW, et al.: Stimulation of ovine placental transport of calcium and magnesium by mid-molecule fragments of human parathyroid hormone-related protein. *J Exp Physiol* 75:605–608, 1990
8. Fenton AJ, Kemp BE, Hammonds RG, et al.: A potent inhibitor of osteoclastic bone resorption within a highly conserved pentapeptide region of parathyroid hormone-related protein; PTHrP(107–111). *Endocrinology* 129:3424–3426, 1991
9. Orloff JJ, Wu TL, Stewart AF: Parathyroid hormone-like proteins: Biochemical responses and receptor interactions. *Endocr Rev* 10:476–495, 1989
10. Yamamoto M, Harm SC, Grasser WA, Thiede MA: Parathyroid hormone-related protein in the rat urinary bladder: A smooth muscle relaxant produced locally in response to mechanical stretch. *Proc Natl Acad Sci USA* 89:5326–5330, 1992
11. Kaiser S, Laneuville P, Bernier SM, Rhim JS, Kremer R, Goltzman D: Enhanced growth of a human keratinocyte cell line induced by antisense RNA for parathyroid hormone-related peptide. *J Biol Chem* 267:13623–13628, 1992
12. Jueppner H, Abou-Samra A, Freeman M, et al.: A G protein-linked-receptor for parathyroid hormone and parathyroid hormone-related peptide. *Science* 254:1024–1026, 1991
13. Orloff JJ, Ganz MB, Ribaudo AE, et al.: Analysis of parathyroid hormone-related protein binding and signal transduction mechanisms in benign and malignant squamous cells. *Am J Physiol* 262 (Endocrinol Metab 25) E599–E607, 1992
14. Goltzman D, Stewart AF, Broadus AE: Malignancy-associated hypercalcemia: Evaluation with a cytochemical bioassay for parathyroid hormone. *J Clin Endocrinol Metab* 53:899–904, 1981
15. Stewart AF, Horst R, Deftos LJ, Cadman EC, Lang R, Broadus AE: Biochemical evaluation of patients with cancer-associated hypercalcemia: Evidence for humoral and nonhumoral groups. *N Engl J Med* 303:1377–1383, 1980
16. Broadus AE: Nephrogenous cyclic AMP. *Recent Prog Horm Res* 37:667–701, 1981
17. Budayr AA, Nissenson RA, Klein RF, et al.: Increased serum levels of a parathyroid hormone-like protein in malignancy-associated hypercalcemia. *Ann Intern Med* 111:807–812, 1989
18. Burtis WJ, Brady TG, Orloff JJ, et al.: Immunochemical characterization of circulating parathyroid hormone-related protein in patients with humoral hypercalcemia of cancer. *N Engl J Med* 322:1106–1112, 1990
19. Henderson JE, Shustik C, Kremer R, Rabbani SA, Hendy G, Goltzman D: Circulating concentrations of parathyroid hormone-like peptide in malignancy and in hyperparathyroidism. *J Bone Miner Res* 5:105–112, 1990
20. Kao PC, Klee GG, Taylor RI, Heath H: Parathyroid hormone-related peptide in plasma of patients with hypercalcemia and malignant lesions. *Mayo Clin Proc* 65:1399–1407, 1990
21. Ratcliffe WA, Norbury S, Heath DA, Ratcliffe JG: Development and validation of an immunoradiometric assay of parathyrin-related protein in unextracted plasma. *Clin Chem* 37:678–685, 1991
22. Ratcliffe WA, Norbury S, Stott RA, Heath DA, Ratcliffe JG: Immunoreactivity of plasma parathyrin-related peptide: Three region-specific radioimmunoassays and a two-site immunoaradiometric assay compared. *Clin Chem* 37:1781–1787, 1991
23. Grill V, Ho P, Body JJ, et al.: Parathyroid hormone-related protein: Elevated levels in both humoral hypercalcemia of malignancy and hypercalcemia complicating metastatic breast cancer. *J Clin Endocrinol Metab* 73:1309–1315, 1991
24. Pandian MR, Morgan CH, Carlton E, Segre GV: Modified immunoradiometric assay of parathyroid hormone-related protein: Clinical application in the differential diagnosis of hypercalcemia. *Clin Chem* 38:282–288, 1991
25. Ekins R: More sensitive immunoassays. *Nature* 284:14–15, 1980
26. Burtis WJ, Gaich G: Measurement of mid-region PTH-related protein in plasma using a novel PTHRP(37–74) RIA. *J Bone Miner Res* 6(suppl 1):S229, 1991
27. Burtis WJ, Debeyssy M, Philbrick WM, et al.: Evidence for the presence of an extreme carboxyterminal parathyroid hormone-related peptide in biological specimens. *J Bone Min Res* 7(Suppl 1):S225, 1992
28. Budayr AA, Halloran BP, King JC, Diep D, Nissenson RA, Strewler GJ: High levels of parathyroid hormone-like protein in milk. *Proc Natl Acad Sci USA* 86:7183–7185, 1989
29. Godsall JW, Burtis WJ, Insogna KL, Broadus AE, Stewart AF: Nephrogenous cyclic AMP, adenylate cyclase-stimulating activity, and the humoral hypercalcemia of malignancy. *Recent Prog Horm Res* 42:705–750, 1986
30. Gaich GA, Burtis WJ: The diagnosis and treatment of malignancy-associated hypercalcemia. *The Endocrinologist* 1:371–379, 1991
31. Bilezikian JP: Clinical utility of assays for parathyroid hormone-related protein. *Clin Chem* 38:179–181, 1992
32. Khosla S, VanHeerden JA, Gharib H, et al.: Parathyroid hormone-related protein and hypercalcemia secondary to massive mammary hyperplasia. *N Engl J Med* 322:1157, 1990
33. Braude S, Graham A, Mitchell D: Lymphoedema/hypercalcemia syndrome mediated by parathyroid hormone-related protein. *Lancet* 337:140–141, 1991

21. Vitamin D and Metabolites

Thomas L. Clemens, Ph.D., and John S. Adams, M.D.

Division of Endocrinology and Metabolism, Cedars-Sinai Medical Center,
University of California–Los Angeles School of Medicine,
Los Angeles, California

The ability to measure with precision vitamin D metabolites in human serum or plasma has improved dramatically in the last 10–15 years. Before 1971 when the first competitive protein binding assays for 25-hydroxyvitamin D (25OHD) were described (1,2), an estimate of the circulating concentration of active vitamin D metabolites was obtained solely by bioassay (3,4). In the ensuing years three significant advances have permitted the detection and accurate quantitation of the less plentiful metabolites of 25OHD: 1) the realization that many if not all of the biological actions of vitamin D on human mineral ion homeostasis are initiated by binding of 1,25-dihydroxyvitamin D [$1,25(OH)_2D$] to a specific intracellular binding protein (the vitamin D receptor); 2) introduction of sophisticated techniques for chromatographic purification of lipid extracts of serum; and 3) the synthesis of radioligands of high specific activity. Despite rapid progress in terms of the number of vitamin D metabolites isolated and structurally identified in mammalian species, only measurement of serum concentrations of 25OHD and $1,25(OH)_2D$ have proven clinical utility. For this reason particular attention will be paid to a description of the methods and clinical significance of assaying these two metabolites in human serum.

ANALYTICAL METHODS

Sample Preparation for Measurement of 25-Hydroxyvitamin D and 1,25-Dihydroxyvitamin D

Prior to quantitation of vitamin D metabolites by competitive protein binding assay (CPBA) or high-pressure liquid chromatography (HPLC) with UV absorption, serum samples must be deproteinized or extracted and partially purified. Extraction or deproteinization frees the metabolites that are almost completely associated with vitamin D binding protein (DBP) and albumin (5). Ethanol, methanol, and acetonitrile effectively free 25OHD and $1,25(OH)_2D$ by deproteinization. Two-phase liquid-liquid partition with a variety of solvents—including chloroform-methanol, methylene chloride-methanol, ethylacetate-cyclohexane, hexane-isopropanol, and diethyl ether—provides a less contaminated extract (6). Of these, more selective solvents such as diethyl ether produce the cleanest extracts (7). Backwashing nonpolar organic extracts with weakly basic solutions removes acidic lipids. Extracts are purified by preparative column chromatography to separate vitamin D metabolites and eliminate lipid and other interfering substances extracted from serum. In particular, silicic acid or silica minicolumns

have been recognized for their convenience and ability to separate D, 25OHD, and dihydroxylated metabolites (8,9). More recently, methods based on solid-phase extraction and preparative chromatography on a single octadecyl (C-18) silica reverse phase cartridge have been reported for 25OHD and $1,25(OH)_2D$ (10–13). Before the introduction of the method illustrated in Fig. 1, competitive radioreceptor assays for $1,25(OH)_2D$ required HPLC to eliminate interfering compounds. This new method (Fig. 1) has significantly reduced the technical, instrumental, and specimen volume requirements for the measurement of $1,25(OH)_2D$ by competitive radioreceptor assay.

Methods requiring extraction and chromatography must be monitored for recovery of the analyte of interest and include solvent or column blanks. Losses are monitored and the final result corrected by equilibrating serum with a small but known amount of purified tritiated $25OHD_3$ or $1,25(OH)_2D_3$ of high specific activity before initiating the extraction and chromatography. If total 25OHD or $1,25(OH)_2D$ is to be measured by CPBA, care must be taken to ensure D_2 and D_3 metabolites are not separated and are recovered equally. Solvents, chromatographic media, and cartridges may contain substances that interfere with CPBA, especially with DBP resulting in the inaccurate measurement of 25OHD. Undetectable levels of the vitamin D metabolites should be found when water blanks are treated identically to specimens.

MEASUREMENT OF 25-HYDROXYVITAMIN D

Serum 25OHD is most often measured by CPBA and occasionally by direct quantitation by UV absorption on HPLC. Of these, CPBA has been most widely utilized because of the availability of reagents, modest specimen requirements, and ease of performance. Rat serum diluted ~1:50,000 (V/V), which contains a high-affinity DBP, is commonly used as the specific binder with tritiated $25OHD_3$ of high-specific activity (>100 Ci/mmol) as tracer. Because rat DBP does not significantly discriminate between $25OHD_2$ and $25OHD_3$ (14), these assays measure the total 25OHD concentration. Methods utilizing direct quantitation by UV absorption after separation by HPLC can quantitate $25OHD_2$ and $25OHD_3$ independently (15). Individual measurements of $25OHD_2$ and $25OHD_3$ do not generally provide any advantage over total 25OHD in assessing vitamin D status in clinical practice, particularly in the United States where foods are supplemented with either D_2 or D_3.

Competitive protein binding assay with DBP requires extraction and chromatographic purification as described previously. Inasmuch as DBP has the highest affinity for

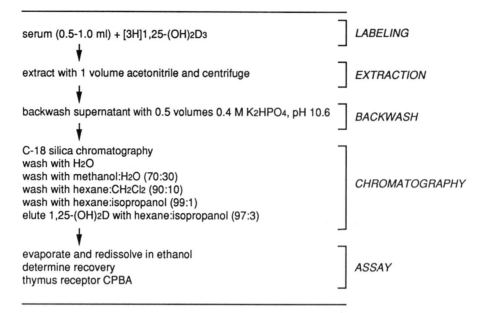

FIG. 1. Purification and quantitation of 1,25-(OH)$_2$D: the single silica cartridge system.

25OHD$_3$-26,23-lactone; equal affinity for 25OHD$_2$, 25OHD$_3$, 24,25(OH)$_2$D$_3$, and 25,26(OH)$_2$D$_3$; somewhat less affinity for 24,25(OH)$_2$D$_2$ and 25,26(OH)$_2$D$_2$; and less affinity for 1,25(OH)$_2$D and vitamin D (14,16), methods that do not chromatographically separate 25OHD from these cross-reacting steroids will overestimate its concentration. Perhaps of more importance are the other nonspecific substances extracted from serum even with selective solvents that cross-react in nonchromatographic assays increasing the apparent concentration of 25OHD (17,18). The practice of preparing standards in vitamin D free serum to "blank out" nonspecific effects should be discouraged, because these effects undoubtedly vary between individuals in health and disease. Although few assays have difficulty recognizing supranormal levels of 25OHD, separation of normal and subnormal levels is more difficult, requiring well-validated chromatographic assays free of solvent, cartridge, and serum interference (19).

Radioimmunoassays (18) have been reported for 25OHD, however they require chromatographic purification to eliminate nonspecific serum interferences and do not measure 25OHD$_2$. Recently, an antiserum has been produced that recognizes 25OHD$_2$ and 25OHD$_3$ equally (20). However, vitamin D and other metabolites of D$_2$ and D$_3$ cross-react in this nonchromatographic assay. A recent advance has been the development of a radioimmunoassay using an antibody raised against the 23,24,25, 26,27-pentanor-C-22 carboxylic acid of vitamin D with iodinated 25OHD as radioligand (21). Because of the ease and speed of performance, this assay should achieve widespread use in the near future.

HPLC coupled with direct UV quantitation can provide the best estimate of true 25OHD [25OHD$_2$ and 25OHD$_3$] (15,18,19). Unfortunately, the need for extraction and preparative chromatography of a relatively large sample volume (1–5 mL) and the expensive instrumental requirements have prevented the widespread use of this method by the clinical laboratory.

Because serum levels of 25OHD are influenced by sunlight, normal valves are dependent on season and latitude as indicated in Table 1.

Measurement of 1,25-Dihydroxyvitamin D

Introduction of a simplified method for assay of 1,25(OH)$_2$D in 1984 (12,13) that does not require HPLC has substantially increased the availability of this analysis. This unique method combined solid-phase extraction with

TABLE 1. Serum 25-hydroxyvitamin D and 1,25-dihydroxyvitamin D in healthy individuals and normal relative variations

	25OHD	1,25(OH)$_2$D
Normal adults	10–50 ng/mL[a,b]	15–60 pg/mL[a,b]
Elderly	↓, →	↓, →, ↑
Children	→	→
Pregnancy	→	↑
Summer/fall	↑	→
Winter/spring	↓	→
Increasing latitude	↓	→

[a] SI units can be calculated as indicated below. The conversion factors are for 25OHD and 1,25(OH)$_2$D standards and assume D$_2$ and D$_3$ forms are measured on an equimolar basis. 25OHD ng/mL × 2.50 = nmol/L; 1,25(OH)$_2$D pg/mL × 2.40 = pmol/L.

[b] Both 25OHD and 1,25(OH)$_2$D are relatively stable in serum, however, samples should be frozen until assayed. Although serum and plasma yield similar results, serum is preferred because of its greater ease in handling. Interassay precision expressed as the coefficient of variation is typically 10–15% in the normal range.

a competitive radioreceptor assay utilizing vitamin D receptor from bovine thymus with a nonequilibrium delayed addition of tracer (Fig. 1). Utilization of bovine thymus vitamin D receptor provides a number of advantages over the previously used chick intestinal receptor. The thymus receptor recognizes $1,25(OH)_2D_2$ and $1,25(OH)_2D_3$ equivalently, unlike the chick intestinal receptor (12,14) that underestimates $1,25(OH)_2D_2$. Bovine thymus provides a relatively unlimited and reproducible source of stable receptor. Thymus receptor appears to be less sensitive to lipid interference and other nonspecific interferences extracted from serum, eliminating the need for extensive purification including HPLC. When 1 mL of serum is extracted, a sensitivity of 2–5 pg/mL is achieved with the thymus receptor and delayed addition of tracer. Dihydrotachysterol (DHT)-treated patients have falsely elevated levels of $1,25(OH)_2D_3$ in the chick intestinal but not thymus receptor assay (22). Several radioimmunoassays (23) have been reported for the measurement of $1,25(OH)_2D$ in serum. Because these antisera cross-react with other metabolites to a much greater extent than the vitamin D receptor, more extensive sample preparation including HPLC is required. Perhaps more importantly, most antisera discriminate against $1,25(OH)_2D_2$ and do not provide an overall measurement of $1,25(OH)_2D$. Until these deficiencies are resolved, it is likely that radioimmunoassays will increase not decrease interlaboratory variation in $1,25(OH)_2D$ measurements (24).

Serum levels of $1,25(OH)_2D$ vary with age and increase during pregnancy as indicated in Table 1. There is still no consensus whether $1,25(OH)_2D$ levels go down (25), up (26), or do not change in aging normal adults. The serum $1,25(OH)_2D$ concentration is generally not affected by fluctuation in the circulating level of its natural substrate 25OHD. An exception is some patients with granuloma-forming diseases or those with very low serum 25OHD levels who experience a rapid influx of vitamin D into the circulation (i.e., after sunlight exposure) (27).

Measurement of Vitamin D

Quantitation of vitamin D in serum is difficult because of its limited solubility, low concentration, and comigration with contaminating lipid. Existing methods require extraction, preparative chromatography, and one or more HPLC steps. Levels are measured with HPLC and UV absorption (15,28) or CPBA with DBP (16,29). Vitamin D binding protein from most species discriminates against D_2 underestimating its concentration (29). Vitamin D levels do not provide a good indication of vitamin D status, because its low concentration compared with 25OHD, dependence on sunlight exposure, and rapid disappearance from serum (27). Holick and colleagues have described a vitamin D (fat-soluble vitamin) "absorption test" that measures serum levels of vitamin D after oral administration of a standard vitamin D_2 dose (30).

Vitamin D assays have also been used to monitor the vitamin D content of foods and fortified dairy products. A noteworthy application was a recent study that found striking discrepancies in the reported and measured vita-

min D content of randomly selected milk and infant formulae (31).

Measurement of 24,25-Dihydroxyvitamin D

Next to 25OHD, $24,25(OH)_2D$ is the most abundant vitamin D metabolite in serum. This steroid has been measured with CPBA following extraction, preparative chromatography, and HPLC (16). As with vitamin D, DBP does not recognize $24,25(OH)_2D_2$ and $24,25(OH)_2D_3$ equally, resulting in underestimation of total $24,25(OH)_2D$ (14,16). Normal phase HPLC on cyano-bonded silica or silica with methylene chloride-isopropanol separates $25OHD_2$-23,26-lactone, a metabolite not adequately resolved from $24,25(OH)_2D$ with previous systems (16,32). Routine clinical determination of $24,25(OH)_2D$ is not indicated at this time until the controversy regarding its role, if any, in mineral metabolism in man is resolved.

Free 25-Hydroxyvitamin D and
1,25-Dihydroxyvitamin D

Circulating vitamin D and its metabolites are almost completely bound by serum proteins, primarily DBP and secondarily albumin. In normal individuals ~0.4% of the $1,25(OH)_2D$ and 0.03% of the 25OHD are free (33,34). Because of alterations in the concentration of DBP and albumin, total levels of vitamin D metabolites do not provide an accurate estimate of free levels in various physiologic or pathophysiologic conditions. Although methods have been reported for the determination of free vitamin D metabolites (32,33), their availability is currently limited.

CLINICAL UTILITY OF THE VITAMIN D
METABOLITE ASSAYS

There are in general four circumstances that prompt the clinician to investigate a patient's vitamin D status: 1) an abnormal serum calcium concentration; 2) renal stone disease and hypercalciuria; 3) metabolic bone disease; and 4) monitoring a patient's response to vitamin D therapy. The most frequently encountered clinical states that result in disordered calcium and bone metabolism that may present with an abnormal serum concentration of 25OHD or $1,25(OH)_2D$ are presented in Table 2.

The Hypocalcemic Patient

When confronted with a hypocalcemic patient, it is useful to consider whether the reduction in the serum ionized calcium concentration is due to a deficiency in one or both of the classical calcemic hormones: $1,25(OH)_2D$ and parathyroid hormone (PTH). In the case of the former hormone, measurement of the serum 25OHD concentration provides the most valuable information. Due to its high affinity for binding to the circulating vitamin D binding protein and its long serum half-life (15–60 days), mea-

TABLE 2. *Vitamin D metabolite concentrations in patients with disordered calcium homeostasis*

	25OHD	1,25(OH)$_2$D
Hypocalcemia		
Vitamin D deficiency	D	D,I,N
Severe hepatocellular disease	D	D,N
Nephrotic syndrome	D	D,N
Renal failure	N	D
Hyperphosphatemia	N	D
Hypoparathyroidism	N	D,N
Pseudohypoparathyroidism	N	D,N
Hypomagnesemia	N	D,N
Vitamin D-dependent rickets, type I	N,I	D
Vitamin D-dependent rickets, type II	N,I	I
Hypercalcemia/hypercalciuria:		
Vitamin D, 25OHD intoxication	I	N,D
1,25(OH)$_2$D intoxication	N	I
Granuloma-forming diseases	N	I
Lymphoma	N	D,I
Hyperparathyroidism	N	D,I
Williams syndrome	N	I
Idiopathic hypercalciuria	N	I
Idiopathic osteoporosis	N	N,I
PTHrP-associated	N	D

D, decreased; I, increased; N, normal.

surement of the 25OHD concentration provides an excellent index of the amount of vitamin D that is metabolized in the liver to 25OHD. In the hypocalcemic patient, a frankly low 25OHD level almost always indicates deficient cutaneous synthesis and dietary intake of vitamin D. Patients with severe hepatocellular disease or nephrotic syndrome may have a low total serum calcium and 25OHD concentration owing to either a decrease in hepatic synthesis or urinary loss of proteins that bind calcium (albumin and prealbumin) and 25OHD (DBP, albumin) in the circulation. In such cases a low serum ionized calcium concentration and a compensatory elevation in the circulating PTH concentration may aid in establishing the presence of true 25OHD deficiency. Hypocalcemia with a normal or elevated 25OHD concentration points either to deficiency or decrease in bioeffectiveness of PTH, an acquired abnormality in metabolism of 25OHD to 1,25(OH)$_2$D (i.e., renal failure, hyperphosphatemia), an inherited defect in 1,25(OH)$_2$D synthesis, or a defect in the action of 1,25(OH)$_2$D at its target tissue. The latter two situations, both rare, can usually be distinguished on biochemical grounds by the circulating 1,25(OH)$_2$D concentration. It will be low or non-detectable in patients with vitamin D-dependent rickets type I, and often dramatically increased in patients with vitamin D-dependent rickets type II (Chapter 66). In patients with hypocalcemia and diminished synthesis, release, or end-organ effectiveness of PTH (i.e., patients with hypoparathyroidism, pseudohyperparathyroidism, or magnesium deficiency), the 1,25(OH)$_2$D concentration will be inappropriately low. However, because of overlap of the serum 1,25(OH)$_2$D concentration into the normal range in such patients, measurement of this metabolite is not always helpful in establishing the diagnosis of hypoparathyroidism.

The Hypercalcemic/Hypercalciuric Patient

The utility of the 25OHD assay in the evaluation of a hypercalcemic patient is limited. Only if 25OHD is present in high concentrations in the circulation and it (or its metabolites) binds to high-affinity receptor for 1,25(OH)$_2$D is it capable of producing hypercalcemia. 25-Hydroxyvitamin D intoxication may arise after ingestion of large amounts of vitamin D or 25OHD$_3$. In 25OHD intoxication the serum 1,25(OH)$_2$D concentration may be normal or even reduced unless there is some additional abnormality in regulation of the 1-hydroxylation of 25OHD. Normal individuals do not become vitamin D-intoxicated from endogenously synthesized vitamin D; the endogenous photosynthesis of vitamin D is regulated by the conversion of previtamin D to nonbiologically active photoisomers in the skin (35).

The usefulness of the 1,25(OH)$_2$D assay in evaluating a patient with hypercalcemia and/or hypercalciuria is, for the most part, restricted to patients with suppressed PTH secretion; an elevation in the serum 1,25(OH)$_2$D concentration may be an accompaniment of primary hyperparathyroidism (unless renal failure is present), and there is little need for this metabolite to be measured when that diagnosis is certain or highly likely. Therefore, an inappropriate elevation in the serum 1,25(OH)$_2$D concentration and a suppressed PTH concentration in a patient with hypercalciuria and/or hypercalcemia is highly suggestive of: 1) exogenous intoxication with 1(OH)D$_3$, DHT, or 1,25(OH)$_2$D; 2) endogenous intoxication with 1,25(OH)$_2$D as may occur in sarcoidosis, other granulomatous diseases, and lymphoma; 3) idiopathic absorptive hypercalciuria (36); or 4) idiopathic osteoporosis, a condition of premature bone loss observed principally, but not exclusively, in men (37). Determination of the serum 1,25(OH)$_2$D concentration may also be helpful in discerning the presence of primary hyperparathyroidism in patients who are suspected to harbor the disease, but in whom confirmatory laboratory data are lacking; measurement of the serum 1,25(OH)$_2$D concentration like measurement of the urinary cAMP concentration is an index of the bioactivity of circulating PTH. Hypercalcemia in patients with the syndrome of humoral hypercalcemia of malignancy (HHM) is caused by tumor-derived parathyroid hormone-related protein (PTHrP) that activates the PTH receptor (38). Surprisingly, however, patients with HHM have reduced (not elevated) circulating 1,25(OH)$_2$D levels. It is possible that these tumors release additional factors that suppress 25OHD-1-hydroxylase activity. Alternatively, other disease-related processes, such as severe hypercalcemia, might override any stimulatory effect of PTHrP.

REFERENCES

1. Belsey RE, Deluca HF, Potts JT Jr: Competitive protein binding assay for vitamin D and 25-OH vitamin D. *J Clin Endocrinol Metab* 33:554–557, 1971

2. Haddad JG, Chyu KJ: Competitive protein binding radioassay for 25-hydroxy-cholecalciferol. *J Clin Endocrinol Metab* 33: 992–995, 1971

3. McCollum FG, Simmonds N, Shipley PG, Park EA: Studies on experimental rickets. XVI. A delicate biological test for calcium-depositing substances. *J Biol Chem* 54:41–50, 1922

4. Schacter D, Rosen SM: Active transport of Ca^{45} by the small intestine and its dependence on vitamin D. *Am J Physiol* 196: 357–365, 1959

5. Haddad JG Jr: Transport of vitamin D metabolites. *Clin Orthop Res* 142:249–261, 1979

6. Jones G, Seamark DA, Trafford DJH, Makin HLJ: Vitamin D: Cholecalciferol, ergocalciferol and hydroxylated metabolites. *Chromatogr Sci* 30:73–128, 1985

7. Taylor GA, Peacock M, Pelc B, Brown W, Holmes A: Purification of plasma vitamin D metabolites for radioimmunoassay. *Clin Chim Acta* 108:239–246, 1980

8. Koshy KT: Chromatography of vitamin D_3 and metabolites. *Adv Chromatogr* 20:83–138, 1982

9. Adams JS, Clemens TL, Holick MF: Silica Sep-Pak preparative chromatography for vitamin D and its metabolites. *J Chromatogr* 226:198–201, 1981

10. Rhodes CJ, Claridge PA, Trafford DJH, Makin HLJ: An evaluation of the use of Sep-Pak C-18 cartridges for the extraction of vitamin D_3 and some of its metabolites from plasma and urine. *J Steroid Biochem* 19:1339–1354, 1983

11. Hollis BW, Frank NE: Solid phase extraction system for vitamin D and its major metabolites in human plasma. *J Chromatogr* 343:43–49, 1985

12. Reinhardt TA, Horst RL, Orf JW, Hollis BW: A microassay for 1,25-dihydroxyvitamin D not requiring high performance liquid chromatography: Application to clinical studies. *J Clin Endocrinol Metab* 58:91–98, 1984

13. Hollis BW: Assay of circulating 1,25-dihydroxyvitamin D involving a novel single-cartridge extraction and purification procedure. *Clin Chem* 32:2060–2063, 1986

14. Jones G, Byrnes B, Palma F, Segev D, Mazur Y: Displacement potency of vitamin D_2 analogs in competitive protein-binding assays for 25-hydroxyvitamin D_3, 24,25-dihydroxyvitamin D_3 and 1,25-dihydroxyvitamin D_3. *J Clin Endocrinol Metab* 50: 773–775, 1980

15. Jones G: Assay of vitamins D_2 and D_3 and 25-hydroxyvitamins D_2 and D_3 in human plasma by high-performance liquid chromatography. *Clin Chem* 24:287–298, 1978

16. Horst RL, Littledike ET, Riley JL, Napoli JL: Quantitation of vitamin D and its metabolites and their plasma concentrations in five species of animals. *Anal Biochem* 116:189–203, 1981

17. Dorantes LM, Arnaud SB, Arnaud CD: Importance of the isolation of 25-hydroxyvitamin D before assay. *J Lab Clin Med* 91: 791–796, 1978

18. Bouillon R, Van Herck E, Jans I, Tan BK, Van Baelen H, De Moor P: Two direct (nonchromatographic) assays for 25-hydroxyvitamin D. *Clin Chem* 30:1731–1736, 1984

19. Mayer E, Schmidt-Gayk H: Interlaboratory comparison of 25-hydroxyvitamin D determination. *Clin Chem* 30:1199–1204, 1984

20. Hollis BW, Napoli JL: Improved radioimmunoassay for vitamin D and its use in assessing vitamin D status. *Clin Chem* 31: 1815–1819, 1985

21. Hollis BW, Kamerad JQ, Selvaag SR, Lorenz JD, Napoli JL: Determination of vitamin D status by radioimmunoassay using an [I^{125}]-labeled tracer. *Clin Chem* 39:529–533, 1992

22. Taylor A, Norman ME: 1,25(OH)₂D levels in dihydrotachysterol-treated patients: Influence on 1,25(OH)₂D assays. *J Bone Miner Res* 2:567–570, 1987

23. Bouillon R, De Moor P, Baggiolini EG, Uskokovic MR: A radioimmunoassay for 1,25-dihydroxycholecalciferol. *Clin Chem* 26: 562–567, 1980

24. Jongen MJM, Van Ginkel FC, van der Vijgh WJF, Kuiper S, Netelenbos JC, Lips P: An international comparison of vitamin D metabolite measurements. *Clin Chem* 30:399–403, 1984

25. Quesada JM, Coopmans W, Ruiz B, Aljama P, Jans I, Bouillon R: Influence of vitamin D on parathyroid function in the elderly. *J Clin Endocrinol Metab* 75:494–501, 1992

26. Ebeling PR, Sandgren ME, DiMagno EP, Lane AW, DeLuca HF, Riggs BL: Evidence of an age-related decrease in intestinal responsiveness to vitamin D: Relationship between serum 1,25-dihydroxyvitamin D_3 and intestinal vitamin D receptor concentrations in normal women. *J Clin Endocrinol Metab* 75:176–82, 1992

27. Adams JS, Clemens TL, Parrish JA, Holick MF: Vitamin D synthesis and metabolism after ultraviolet radiation of normal and vitamin D deficient subjects. *N Engl J Med* 306:722–725, 1982

28. Clemens TL, Adams JS, Nolan JM, Holick MF: Measurement of circulating vitamin D in man. *Clin Chim Acta* 121:301–308, 1982

29. Hollis BW, Roos BA, Lambert PW: Vitamin D in plasma: Quantitation by a nonequilibrium ligand binding assay. *Steroids* 37: 609–619, 1981

30. Lo CW, Paris PW, Clemens TL, Nolan J, Holick MF: Vitamin D absorption in healthy subjects and in patients with intestinal malabsorption syndromes. *Am J Clin Nutr* 42:644–649, 1985

31. Holick MF, Shao Q, Liu WW, Chen TC: The vitamin D content of fortified milk and infant formula. *N Engl J Med* 326: 1178–1181, 1991

32. Jones G: Chromatographic separation of 24(R), 25-dihydroxyvitamin D_3 and 25-hydroxyvitamin D_3-26,23-lactone using a cyano-bonded phase packing. *J Chromatogr* 276:69–74, 1983

33. Bikle DD, Gee E, Halloran B, Kowalski MA, Ryzen E, Haddad JG: Assessment of the free fraction of 25-hydroxyvitamin D in serum and its regulation by albumin and the vitamin D-binding protein. *J Clin Endocrinol Metab* 63:954–959, 1986

34. Bikle DD, Siiteri PK, Ryzen E, Haddad JG: Serum protein binding of 1,25-dihydroxyvitamin D: A re-evaluation by direct measurement of free metabolite levels. *J Clin Endocrinol Metab* 61: 969–975, 1985

35. Holick MF, MacLaughlin JA, Doppelt SH: Factors that influence the cutaneous photosynthesis of previtamin D_3. *Science* 211:590–593, 1981

36. Broadus AE, Insogna KL, Lang R, Mallette LE, Oren DA, Gertner JM, Kligor AS, Ellison AF: A consideration of the hormonal basis and phosphate leak hypothesis of absorptive hypercalciuria. *J Clin Endocrinol Metab* 58:161–169, 1984

37. Zerwekh JE, Sakhaee K, Breslau NA, Gottschalk F, Pak CYC: Impaired bone formation in male idiopathic osteoporosis: Further reduction in the presence of concomitant hypercalciuria. *Osteoporosis Int* 2:128–34, 1992

38. Martin TJ, Mosley JM, Gillespie MT: Parathyroid hormone-related protein: Biochemistry and molecular biology. *Crit Rev Biochem Mol Biol* 26:377–95, 1991

22. Markers of Bone Formation and Resorption

Pierre D. Delmas, M.D., Ph.D.

*Department of Rheumatology and Metabolic Bone Diseases, INSERM
Research Unit 234, Hôpital E. Herriot, and University Claude Bernard,
Lyon, France*

The rate of formation and degradation of bone matrix can be assessed either by measuring a prominent enzymatic activity of the bone forming or resorbing cells, such as alkaline and acid phosphatase activity, or by measuring bone matrix components released into the circulation during formation or resorption (Table 1). These markers are of unequal specificity and sensitivity, and some of them have not been yet fully investigated. None of these markers is disease-specific, but a given marker may be more sensitive to assess bone turnover in one metabolic bone disease than in another one. For example, serum osteocalcin is more sensitive than serum alkaline phosphatase to measure the subtle changes of bone formation in osteoporosis, but the opposite is true in Paget's disease of bone. Measurement of the urinary excretion of the pyridinoline cross-links of collagen has emerged recently as a sensitive marker of bone resorption that appear to be useful in the clinical investigation of patients with metabolic bone disease.

BIOCHEMICAL MARKERS OF BONE FORMATION

Serum Alkaline Phosphatase

Serum alkaline phosphatase activity is the most commonly used marker of bone formation and it is the best index to monitor the activity of Paget's disease of bone. Because only half of the circulating levels are normally derived from bone in adults, serum alkaline phosphatase lacks sensitivity in conditions with a mild increase in bone turnover such as osteoporosis. In addition, a moderate increase of serum alkaline phosphatase is ambiguous, because it may reflect a mineralization defect, or the effect of one of the numerous medications that have been shown to increase the hepatic isoenzyme of alkaline phosphatase. In an attempt to improve the specificity and sensitivity of serum alkaline phosphatase measurement, techniques have been developed to differentiate the bone and the liver isoenzymes that only differ by posttranslational modifications as they are coded by a single gene. These techniques rely on the use of differentially effective activators and inhibitors (heat, phenylalanine, and urea), separation by electrophoresis, lectin precipitation, and the use of antibodies (1–3). In general, these assays have slightly enhanced the sensitivity of this marker, but most of them are indirect and/or technically cumbersome. A real improvement should be obtained by using a monoclonal antibody recognizing the bone isoenzyme with a much higher affinity than the liver isoenzyme, a reagent that has been recently available (4).

Serum Osteocalcin

Osteocalcin, also called bone Gla-protein, is a small noncollagenous protein that is specific for bone tissue and dentin, although its precise function remains unknown (5). Osteocalcin is predominantly synthesized by the osteoblasts and incorporated into the extracellular matrix of bone, but a fraction of newly synthesized osteocalcin is released into the circulation where it can be measured by radioimmunoassay (6,7). Serum osteocalcin correlates with skeletal growth at the time of puberty and is increased in a variety of conditions characterized by increased bone turnover such as primary and secondary hyperparathyroidism, hyperthyroidism, Paget's disease, and acromegaly. Conversely, it is decreased in hypothyroidism, hypoparathyroidism, and in glucocorticoid-treated patients. Because antibodies directed against bovine osteocalcin cross-react with human osteocalcin, most systems have been developed with bovine osteocalcin as a tracer, standard, and immunogen. Depending on the epitopes recognized by the antibody, some polyclonal antisera (but also monoclonal antibodies) may see, in addition to the intact molecule, fragments of osteocalcin, the significance of which is still unclear (8,9). In most cases, however, serum osteocalcin is a valid marker of bone turnover when resorption and formation are coupled, and is a specific marker of bone formation whenever formation and resorption are uncoupled (10–13). Sandwich assay using monoclonal antibodies recognizing different epitopes of human osteocalcin have been recently available that are likely to improve the sensitivity of the assay (14).

Procollagen I Extension Peptides

During the extracellular processing of collagen I, there is a cleavage of the aminoterminal (p-coll-I-N) and carboxyterminal (p-coll-I-C) extension peptides before fibril formation. These peptides circulate in blood where they might represent useful markers of bone formation, because collagen is by far the most abundant organic component of bone matrix. It has been shown that a single dose of 30 mg of prednisone suppresses serum p-coll-I-C measured by radioimmunoassay without decreasing urinary hydroxyproline (15); suggesting that, indeed, circulating p-coll-I-C reflects bone formation. Serum p-coll-I-C is weakly correlated with histological bone formation, with *r* values ranging from 0.36 to 0.50, in patients with vertebral osteoporosis (16). The menopause induces a significant but marginal (+20%) increase in serum p-coll-I-C that is not correlated with the subsequent rate of bone loss

TABLE 1. *Biochemical markers of bone turnover*

Formation	Resorption
Serum	Plasma
Serum osteocalcin (bone Gla protein)	Tartrate-resistant acid phosphatase
Total and bone alkaline phosphatase	Pyridinoline and pyridinoline-containing peptides (?)
Serum procollagen I extension peptide (carboxyterminal)	Urine
	Urinary pyridinoline and deoxypyridinoline (collagen cross-links) and corresponding peptides
	Fasting urinary calcium and hydroxyproline
	Urinary hydroxylysine glycosides

measured by densitometry (17). The reasons for this lack of sensitivity are not clear. Despite its potential value, this marker does not stand currently as a valid alternative to the previously described markers of bone formation.

BIOCHEMICAL MARKERS OF BONE RESORPTION

Urinary Calcium and Hydroxyproline

Fasting urinary calcium measured on a morning sample and corrected by creatinine excretion is certainly the cheapest assay of bone resorption. It is useful to detect a marked increase of bone resorption but lacks sensitivity. Most of the endogenous hydroxyproline present in biologic fluids is derived from the degradation of various forms of collagen. As half of human collagen resides in bone, where its turnover is probably faster than in soft tissues, excretion of hydroxyproline in urine is regarded as a marker of bone resorption. Actually, the relationship of urinary hydroxyproline excretion to the metabolism of collagen is complex. Hydroxyproline can be derived from some fragments of the complement and undergoes an active liver metabolism so that free and peptide-bound urinary hydroxyproline represents only a fraction of total collagen catabolism (18). As a consequence of its tissue origin and metabolism pattern, urinary hydroxyproline is poorly correlated with bone resorption assessed by calcium kinetics or bone histomorphometry (19), and there is an obvious need for a more sensitive and convenient marker of bone resorption.

Urinary Pyridinoline

Pyridinoline (Pyr) and deoxypyridinoline (D-Pyr) are nonreducible cross-links that stabilize the collagen chains within the extracellular matrix (20). Pyridinoline is pres-

ent in bone and cartilage matrix and in minute amounts in some other connective tissues. Significant amounts of D-Pyr are only found in bone collagen, at a concentration of 0.07 mol/mol of collagen. The relative proportion of Pyr and D-Pyr in bone matrix is variable according to the species. In human bone, the ratio Pyr/D-Pyr is 2:3. Pyridinoline and D-Pyr are likely to be released from bone matrix during its degradation by the osteoclasts. As both cross-links result from a posttranslational modification of collagen molecules already secreted and incorporated into the extracellular matrix, they cannot be reutilized during collagen synthesis. Available data suggest that Pyr and D-Pyr are not metabolized *in vivo*. They are excreted in urine in free form (~40%) and in peptide bound form (60%), and the total amount can be measured by fluorimetry after reversed-phase HPLC of a cellulose-bound extract of hydrolized urine (21,22). Urinary Pyr and D-Pyr are markedly higher in children than in adults (23), are increased by 50–100% at the time of menopause, and go down to premenopausal levels under estrogen therapy (24). In patients with vertebral osteoporosis, the urinary cross-link levels, especially of D-Pyr are correlated with bone turnover measured by calcium kinetics (25) and bone histomorphometry (26). Pyridinoline and D-Pyr appear to be more sensitive than hydroxyproline in Paget's disease of bone and are reduced markedly by bisphosphonate therapy (27). Pyr and D-Pyr are also significantly increased in patients with primary hyperparathyroidism (27) and normalized after surgical removal of the adenoma contrasting with persistent subnormal excretion of hydroxyproline (28). In patients with malignant hypercalcemia, the urinary excretion of Pyr and D-Pyr is two- to threefold increased on the average, but the decrease under bisphosphonate therapy is less pronounced and retarded as compared with the fall of urinary calcium, suggesting a dissociation between the effect of this treatment on bone mineral and bone matrix (29). The urinary cross-link excretion is increased in osteomalacia, in patients with hyperthyroidism (30) and appears to be a sensitive index of bone metabolism in hypothyroid patients treated with L-thyroxine (31). In summary, the measurement of urinary cross-links appear to have several potential advantages over hydroxyproline: they are relatively specific for bone turnover, they do not appear to be metabolized *in vivo* before their urinary excretion, and the absence of intestinal absorption of Pyr and D-Pyr contained in gelatin allows to collect urine without any food restriction. Pyridinoline and D-Pyr excretion undergoes a circadian rhythm with a peak during the night and a nadir during the afternoon (32), a pattern similar to the rhythm of osteocalcin that probably reflects a nocturnal increase of bone turnover and resorption (33). Because urinary cross-link excretion decreases by 30% between 8:00 and 11:00 AM (32); the sampling time is important to obtain reproducible results. The contribution of connective tissues other than bone in the urinary excretion has not been investigated in humans but the fact that for a given assay the molar ratio of Pyr/D-Pyr is similar in normal individuals and in patients with various metabolic bone diseases suggests that Pyr and D-Pyr do not differ markedly in terms of sensitivity. So far, all the data have been obtained with the HPLC assay of the total Pyr and D-Pyr excretion. More convenient techniques are required for a broad clinical use of this marker. Immunoassays are currently being developed, using antibodies directed against either free Pyr or one of the two cross-linking domains of type I collagen (i.e., the N-telopeptide to helix and the C-telopeptide to helix domains). If their clinical validation show that they have adequate sensitivity and specificity, they should be very valuable for the investigation of metabolic bone diseases.

Other Markers of Bone Resorption

Hydroxylysine is another amino acid unique to collagen and proteins containing collagen-like sequences. Like hydroxyproline, hydroxylysine is not reutilized for collagen biosynthesis, and its glycosylated excretion is a potential marker of collagen degradation (34). The relative proportion and total content of galactosyl hydroxylysine and glucosyl-galactosyl hydroxylysine vary in bone and soft tissues that suggest that their urinary excretion might be a more sensitive marker of bone resorption than urinary hydroxyproline, although available data are still scanty. This marker deserves further evaluation, but its development is limited by the current high-pressure liquid chromatography technique.

Plasma tartrate-resistant acid phosphatase (TRAP) is another potential marker of bone resorption. In normal plasma, TRAP corresponds to plasma isoenzyme 5, which originates partly from bone. Osteoclasts contain a TRAP that is released into the circulation (35). Plasma TRAP is increased in a variety of metabolic bone disorders with increased bone turnover (36) and after oophorectomy (37), but it is not clear whether this marker is actually more sensitive than urinary hydroxyproline (37). Its clinical utility in osteoporosis remains to be investigated. The lack of specificity of plasma TRAP activity for the osteoclast, its unstability in frozen samples, and the presence of enzyme inhibitors in serum are potential drawbacks that will limit the development of enzymatic assays of TRAP. Conversely, the development of new immunoassay using monoclonal antibodies specifically directed against the bone isoenzyme of TRAP (38) should be valuable to assess the ability of this marker to predict osteoclast activity in osteoporosis.

USE OF MARKERS OF BONE TURNOVER IN OSTEOPOROSIS

Bone Turnover at Menopause

Menopause induces a dramatic increase of bone turnover that peaks 1–3 years after cessation of ovarian function and slows down thereafter for the next 8–10 years, a pattern that is also illustrated by cross-sectional studies after oophorectomy (37). Serum osteocalcin, urinary Pyr cross-links such as other markers of bone turnover are significantly increased after the menopause and return to premenopausal levels within a few months of hormone replacement therapy (24,39). Two independent studies have shown that, in untreated postmenopausal women followed for 2–4 years, serum osteocalcin is correlated with the spontaneous rate of bone loss assessed by repeated measurements of the bone mineral content of the radius and the lumbar spine (i.e., the higher bone turnover rate, the higher the rate of bone loss) (39,40). Recently, we have shown that the combination of a single measurement of serum osteocalcin, urinary hydroxyproline, and D-Pyr can predict the rate of bone loss over 2 years with an r value of 0.77 (24). Whether slow and fast losers of bone do so for a prolonged period of time after menopause is debated, but a recent long-term study suggests that the rate of bone loss measured over 12 years is increased in postmenopausal women classified as rapid losers from initial bone marker measurements (41). The combination of bone mass measurement and assessment of bone turnover by a battery of specific markers is likely to be helpful in the future for the screening of patients at risk for osteoporosis who should be treated. In addition, it has been shown that osteoporotic patients with a high bone turnover—assessed by the markers—have a better response (increase in bone mass) to antiresorption therapy than those with a low bone turnover (42).

Bone Turnover in the Elderly and in Patients with Hip Fracture

Despite the importance of hip fracture as a major health problem, few studies have been devoted to potential bone turnover abnormalities in those patients. Histological studies suggest an increased bone resorption as a consequence of secondary hyperparathyroidism. In a large group of patients studied immediately after hip fracture, we have found increased urinary cross-links excretion and decreased serum osteocalcin levels when comparing with age-matched healthy elderly (43), suggesting that increased bone resorption and decreased bone formation might be an important determinant of the low bone mass that characterizes patients with hip fracture. Vitamin K deficiency, a common finding in the elderly and in patients with hip fracture, could influence the degree of carboxylation of circulating osteocalcin that contains three residues of the vitamin K-dependent amino acid Gla. Serum noncarboxylated osteocalcin is increased in elderly patients (44) and reflects the subsequent risk of hip fracture in elderly institutionalized women (45). Thus, the level of the γ-carboxylation of osteocalcin appears to reflect the poor nutritional status of elderly patients with hip fracture, and its significance deserves further investigations.

In conclusion, there has been important developments in the field of bone biomarkers in recent years. Some of these new markers need to be further characterized, especially in terms of clearance and metabolism. It should be remembered that circulating and urinary markers reflect the overall level of bone turnover of the entire skeleton, and do not allow, so far, to discriminate between trabecular and cortical bone turnover, nor can they provide an analysis of cellular vs. tissular levels of activity. Different markers probably reflect different events of bone metabolism, and using a panel of markers is likely to provide more information on the complex aspects of bone formation and resorption. The use of new sensitive markers is of special interest in osteoporosis, a condition in which conventional markers are usually in the normal range.

REFERENCES

1. Moss DW: Alkaline phosphatase isoenzymes. *Clin Chem* 28:2007–2016, 1982
2. Farley JR, Chesnut CJ, Baylink DJ: Improved method for quantitative determination in serum alkaline phosphatase of skeletal origin. *Clin Chem* 27:2002–2007, 1981
3. Duda RJ, O'Brien JF, Katzmann JA: Concurrent assays of circulating bone gla-protein and bone alkaline phosphatase: Effects of sex, age, and metabolic bone disease. *J Clin Endocrinol Metab* 66:951–957, 1988
4. Hill CS, Wolfert RL: The preparation of monoclonal antibodies which react preferentially with human bone alkaline phosphatase and not liver alkaline phosphatase. *Clin Chim Acta* 186:315–320, 1989
5. Price PA: Vitamin K-dependent bone proteins. In: Cohn DV, Martin TJ, Meunier PJ (eds) *Calcium Regulation and Bone Metabolism. Basic and Clinical Aspects*, vol 9. Elsevier Science Publishers BV, New York, pp 419–426, 1987
6. Price PA, Williamson MK, Lothringer JW: Origin of vitamin K-dependent bone protein found in plasma and its clearance by kidney and bone. *J Biol Chem* 256:12760–12766, 1981
7. Price PA, Parthemore JG, Deftos LJ: New biochemical marker for bone metabolism. *J Clin Invest* 66:878–883, 1980
8. Gundberg C, Weinstein RS: Multiple immunoreactive forms in uremic serum. *J Clin Invest* 77:1762–1767, 1986
9. Tracy RP, Andrianorivo A, Riggs BL, Mann KG: Comparison of monoclonal and polyclonal antibody-based immunoassays for osteocalcin. A study of sources of variation in assay results. *J Bone Miner Res* 5:451–461, 1990
10. Brown JP, Delmas PD, Malaval L, Meunier PJ: Serum bone Gla-protein: A specific marker for bone formation in postmenopausal osteoporosis. *Lancet* 1:1091–1093, 1984
11. Delmas PD, Malaval L, Arlot M, Meunier PJ: Serum bone gla-protein compared to bone histomorphometry in endocrine diseases. *Bone* 6:329–341, 1985
12. Delmas PD, Demiaux B, Malaval L, Chapuy MC, Edouard C, Meunier PJ: Serum bone gamma carboxyglutamic acid containing protein in primary hyperparathyroidism and in malignant hypercalcemia. Comparison with bone histomorphometry. *J Clin Invest* 77:985–991, 1986
13. Bataille R, Delmas P, Sany J: Serum bone gla-protein in multiple myeloma. *Cancer* 59:329–334, 1987
14. Garnero P, Grimaux M, Demiaux P, Preaudat C, Seguin P, Delmas PD: Measurement of serum osteocalcin with a human-specific two-site immunoradiometric assay. *J Bone Miner Res* 12:1389–1398, 1992
15. Simon LS, Krane SMK: Procollagen extension peptides as markers of collagen synthesis. In: Frame B, Potts JT Jr (eds) *Clinical Disorders of Bone and Mineral Metabolism.* Excerpta Medica, Amsterdam, pp 108–111, 1983
16. Parfitt AM, Simon LS, Villanueva AR: Procollagen type I carboxyterminal extension peptide in serum as a marker of collagen biosynthesis in bone. Correlation with iliac bone formation rates and comparison with total alkaline phosphatase. *J Bone Miner Res* 2:427–436, 1987
17. Hassager C, Fabbri-Mabelli G, Christiansen C: The effect of the menopause and hormone replacement therapy on serum carboxyterminal propeptide of type I collagen. *Osteoporosis Int* 3:50–52, 1993
18. Prockop OJ, Kivirikko KI: Hydroxyproline and the metabolism of collagen. In: Gould BS (ed) *Treatise on Collagen.* New York, Academic Press, pp 215–246, 1968
19. Delmas PD: Biochemical markers of bone turnover for the clinical assessment of metabolic disease. *Endocrin Metab Clin North America* 19:1:1–18, 1990
20. Eyre DR: Collagen crosslinking amino-acids. *Meth Enzymol* 144:115–139, 1987
21. Black D, Duncan A, Robins SP: Quantitative analysis of the pyridinium crosslinks of collagen in urine using ion-paired reversed-phase high-performance liquid chromatography. *Anal Biochem* 169:197–203, 1988
22. Eyre DR, Koob TJ, Van Ness KP: Quantitation of hydroxypyridinium crosslinks in collagen by high-performance liquid chromatography. *Anal Biochem* 137:380–388, 1984
23. Beardsworth LJ, Eyer DR, Dickson IR: Changes with age in the urinary excretion of Lysyl-and hydroxylysylpyridinoline, two new markers of bone collagen turnover. *J Bone Miner Res* 5:671–676, 1990
24. Uebelhart D, Schlemmer A, Johansen J, Gineyts E, Christiansen C, Delmas PD: Effect of menopause and hormone replacement therapy on the urinary excretion of pyridinium crosslinks. *J Clin Endocrinol Metab* 72:367–373, 1991
25. Eastell R, Hampton L, Colwell A: Urinary collagen crosslinks are highly correlated with radio isotopic measurements of bone resorption. In: Christiansen C, Overgaard K (ed). Proceedings of the *Third International Symposium on Osteoporosis* Osteopress, Aalborg, Denmark pp 469–470, 1990
26. Delmas PD, Schlemmer A, Gineyts E, Riis B, Christiansen C: Urinary excretion of pyridinoline crosslinks correlates with bone turnover measured on iliac crest biopsy in patients with vertebral osteoporosis. *J Bone Miner Res* 6:639–644, 1991
27. Uebelhart D, Gineyts E, Chapuy MC, Delmas PD: Urinary excretion of pyridinium crosslinks: A new marker of bone resorption in metabolic bone disease. *Bone Miner* 8:87–96, 1990
28. Seibel MJ, Gartenberg F, Silverberg SJ, Ratcliffe A, Robins SP, Bilezikian JP: Urinary hydroxypyridinium crosslinks of collagen in primary hyperparathyroidism. *J Clin Endocrinol Metab* 74:481–486, 1992
29. Body JJ, Delmas PD: Urinary pyridinium cross-links as markers of bone resorption in tumor-associated hypercalcemia. *J Clin Endocrinol Metab* 74:471–475, 1992
30. Robins SP, Black D, Paterson CR, Reid DM, Duncan A, Seibel MJ: Evaluation of urinary hydroxypyridinium crosslink measurements as resorption markers in metabolic bone diseases. *Eur J Clin Invest* 21:310–315, 1991
31. Harvey RD, McHardy KC, Reid IW: Measurement of bone collagen degradation in hyperthyroidism and during thyroxine replacement therapy using pyridinium cross-links as specific urinary markers. *J Clin Endocrinol Metab* 72:1189–1194, 1991
32. Schlemmer A, Hassager C, Jensen SB, Christiansen C: Marked diurnal variation in urinary excretion of pyridinium cross-links in premenopausal women. *J Clin Endocrinol Metab* 74:476–480, 1992
33. Eastell R, Calvo MS, Burritt MF, Offord KP, Russell RGG, Riggs BL: Anomalities in circadian patterns of bone resorption and renal calcium conservation in type I osteoporosis. *J Clin Endocrinol Metab* 74:487–494, 1992
34. Krane SM, Kantrowitz FG, Byrne M, Pinnel SR, Singer FR: Urinary excretion of hydroxylysine and its glycosides as an index of collagen degradation. *J Clin Invest* 59:819–827, 1977
35. Minkin C: Bone acid phosphatase: Tartrate-resistant acid phosphatase as a marker of osteoclast function. *Calcif Tissue Int* 34:285–290, 1982
36. Stepan JJ, Silinkova-Malkova E, Havrenek T: Relationship of plasma tartrate-resistant acid phosphatase to the bone isoenzyme of serum alkaline phosphatase in hyperparathyroidism. *Clin Chim Acta* 133:189–200, 1983
37. Stepan JJ, Pospichal J, Presl J, Pacovsky V: Bone loss and biochemical indices of bone remodeling in surgically induced postmenopausal women. *Bone* 8:279–284, 1987
38. Kraenzlin M, Lau KHW, Liang L: Development of an immunoassay for human serum osteoclastic tartrate-resistant acid phosphatase. J Clin Endocrinol Metab 71:442–451, 1990
39. Johansen JS, Riss BJ, Delmas PD, Christiansen C: Plasma BGP: An indicator of spontaneous bone loss and effect of estrogen treatment in postmenopausal women. *Eur J Clin Invest* 18:191–195, 1988

40. Slemenda C, Hui SL, Longcope C, et al.: Sex steroids and bone mass. A study of changes about the time of menopause. *J Clin Invest* 80:1261–1269, 1987
41. Hansen MA, Kirsten O, Riss BJ, Christiansen C: Role of peak bone mass and bone loss in postmenopausal osteoporosis: 12 years study. *Br Med J* 303:961–964, 1991
42. Civitelli R, Gonnelli S, Zacchei F, et al.: Bone turnover in postmenopausal osteoporosis. Effect of calcitonin treatment. *J Clin Invest* 82:1268–1274, 1988
43. Akesson K, Vergnaud P, Gineyts E, Delmas PD, Obrant KJ: Biochemical evidence for decreased bone formation and in-creased bone resorption in women with hip fracture. In: Christiansen C, Overgaard K (eds) *Osteoporosis, vol 1.* Osteopress APS: Denmark pp 362–363, 1990
44. Plantalech L, Guillaumont M, Vergnaud P, Leclercq M, Delmas PD: Impairment of gamma carboxylation of circulating osteocalcin (bone gla-protein) in elderly women. *J Bone Miner Res* 6:1211–1216, 1991
45. Szulc P, Chapuy MC, Meunier PJ, Delmas PD: Noncarboxylation serum osteocalcin (ncOC) is a predictor of the risk of hip fracture in elderly women. *Bone Miner* 17:S80, abstract 40, 1992

23. Blood Aluminum in Renal Osteodystrophy

Dennis L. Andress, M.D.

Dialysis Unit, Veterans Administration Medical Center, and Division of Nephrology, University of Washington, Seattle, Washington

Aluminum accumulation in uremic patients is associated with bone disease, which is characterized by reduced bone formation (1). The most extensive accumulations of aluminum occur in association with either osteomalacia (excess unmineralized osteoid) or aplastic bone histology (normal or decreased osteoid), diseases that untreated result in bone pain and fractures. Assessment of bone aluminum and bone formation are best done with bone biopsies taken after tetracycline labeling. However, the inconvenience of the biopsy as well as the inevitable delays with tetracycline labeling and specimen processing make it worthwhile to consider less time-consuming noninvasive tests. One such test, serum aluminum, has been advocated as part of the evaluation of aluminum-related bone disease. This test, however, is helpful only if strict procedural guidelines for analysis are followed and there is awareness of potential false-positive results. In this section, the utility of blood aluminum measurements in uremia is reviewed, and recommendations are given for the use of this test in the evaluation of renal osteodystrophy.

ALUMINUM ASSAYS

Accurate measurements of aluminum in serum or plasma are best obtained using flameless electrothermal atomic absorption spectrometry (2). The advantages of this method include the elimination of sample pretreatment and the capability of measuring small volumes (<100 μL). Although problems with matrix interference and standardization may still occur, protein precipitation with nitric acid can significantly reduce anticipated matrix effects (3), and the use of uremic serum to calculate standard curves will improve the accuracy of the test in uremia.

Many of the items used in sample collection and analysis are potential sources of aluminum contamination (4). Blood collected in glass vacuum tubes using stainless steel needles should be transferred to plastic tubes soon after centrifugation. The use of heparinized collection tubes does not result in an artificially elevated aluminum concentration (5). Samples can be stored or shipped at room temperature without affecting aluminum levels (3). All glass and plastic ware used in the analytic procedure should be prewashed in acid (6); and final sample preparation should be performed in a laminar flow hood to prevent contamination by dust. Under these conditions serum aluminum is less than 10 μg/L (0.37 μmol/L) in healthy subjects.

ALUMINUM KINETICS IN RENAL FAILURE

Aluminum is absorbed in normal individuals only when large oral doses (1–3 g/per day) are given (7,8). Because aluminum is considerably more soluble at low pH, aluminum absorption most likely occurs in the stomach and small intestine (7). One exception is aluminum phosphate, which is relatively insoluble at acid pH and does not cause elevated plasma aluminum when ingested by normal subjects (7). Circulating aluminum is 90–95% protein-bound, principally to transferrin (9) and albumin (10). Although aluminum clearance is <10% of the glomerular titration rate (11), this is adequate to excrete all absorbed aluminum under normal conditions. The normal urinary aluminum excretion rate is ~15 μg/day.

In patients with impaired renal function, the complete elimination of an oral aluminum load becomes compromised (12). Consequently, nondialyzed uremic patients taking aluminum-containing phosphate binders have elevated serum aluminum (13,14) and some develop aluminum-related bone disease (15). In uremic patients who have not taken aluminum phosphate binders regularly, the finding of increased tissue stores of aluminum suggests that the uremic state may predispose to enhanced aluminum absorption (12). Consistent with this observation is the finding of elevated serum aluminum in uremic patients not taking aluminum medications (14).

Although chronic ingestion of aluminum is a long-term risk factor for aluminum bone disease (16), aluminum contamination of water used for dialysis poses a greater risk for acute intoxication syndromes. Serum aluminum levels >200 µg/L are common in patients with aluminum-related encephalopathy (14). The high percentage of aluminum bound to protein greatly facilitates the transfer of aluminum from contaminated dialysate to plasma when the water concentration of aluminum exceeds 15 µg/L. Water treatment by deionization usually maintains serum aluminum below 100 µg/L whereas reverse osmosis, the more effective method of purifying water, results in serum aluminum levels <50µg/L (14).

Because the majority of circulating aluminum is protein-bound only small amounts are available for removal by hemodialysis. Plasma aluminum concentrations <300 µg/L do not decrease appreciably during a typical 4-hr hemodialysis period using cuprophan membranes (17). However, the administration of deferoxamine increases the aluminum flux across the dialyzer and results in lower plasma aluminum levels. The improved aluminum clearance is similar whether acetate or bicarbonate is used in the dialysate (17). The increased clearance is attributed to the increased ultrafilterable fraction of the deferoxamine-aluminum complex (584 Da) and to the enhanced mobilization of tissue stores of aluminum.

BLOOD ALUMINUM IN ALUMINUM-RELATED OSTEODYSTROPHY

Mean random serum aluminum levels generally range from 150 to 225 µg/L in dialysis patients with aluminum-related osteomalacia and aplastic bone disease (Chapter 73) compared with mean values of 75–120 µg/L in patients with nonaluminum osteodystrophy (18–20). Although such values are often significantly different when group comparisons are made (18,20), the large variations within each group can make it difficult to use a single measurement to exclude the presence of aluminum bone disease. For example, a random plasma aluminum level >200 µg/L is specific for aluminum bone disease (93%) when osteomalacia is the predominant lesion in affected patients. However, the low sensitivity (43%) precludes its use in excluding the disease due to the high number of false-negatives (18). The sensitivity can be improved (77%) if the cutoff for a positive test is set at 100 µg/L or greater, although at the expense of a decrease in specificity (73%). This failure to predict accurately the presence of aluminum bone disease is partly due to the daily fluctuations related to aluminum ingestion. Consequently, random circulating levels often poorly reflect total tissue stores of aluminum.

The deferoxamine infusion test appears to be more useful than random aluminum levels in assessing total body aluminum and bone aluminum content, particularly in patients with the osteomalacic lesion. The administration of deferoxamine as a single intravenous infusion (40 mg/kg) during the last 2 hr of hemodialysis results in substantial elevations in plasma aluminum (bound to deferoxamine) within 6–24 hr (18). The sustained elevation in plasma aluminum 48 hr after the infusion correlates well with total bone aluminum content (r = 0.60) and bone surface aluminum staining (r = 0.50). As a result, an increment in plasma aluminum >200 µg/L above baseline results in a sensitivity of 94% and a specificity of 52% for the diagnosis of aluminum-related bone disease when the population under study is comprised predominantly of patients with osteomalacia (18,21).

More recently, in a prospective evaluation in asymptomatic patients on long-term hemodialysis (>8 years), it was discovered that the deferoxamine infusion test had a low specificity (35%) in diagnosing aluminum-related osteodystrophy (Table 1). In contrast, random plasma aluminum levels >100 µg/L had a 65% specificity for the diagnosis. Because almost all of the affected patients had the aplastic variety of aluminum osteodystrophy, rather than osteomalacia, the low specificity of plasma aluminum in diagnosing the disease may be attributed to the lower levels of bone and whole body aluminum in patients with the aplastic lesion when compared with patients with aluminum-related osteomalacia (22).

Other studies have suggested that the deferoxamine infusion test is nonspecific for aluminum-related osteodystrophy when compared with random aluminum levels (19,23). However, these results must be interpreted with caution due to differences in the methods used for administering deferoxamine and in the populations studied. For example, large single infusions of deferoxamine (6 g) may be less discriminatory in a dialysis population in which affected patients have only mild to moderate accumulations of bone surface aluminum (19). Moreover, giving deferoxamine at the beginning of dialysis and sampling serum too soon thereafter (3 hr) may prevent the emergence of discriminatory peak levels of aluminum in patients with significant bone aluminum accumulation (23).

The relatively low specificity of serum aluminum measurements in the diagnosis of aluminum osteodystrophy implies that factors other than aluminum have a role in causing impaired bone formation. One such factor, para-

TABLE 1. *Sensitivities, specificities, and positive predictive values for noninvasive tests in aluminum-related renal osteodystrophy*

Positive test	Sensitivity (%)	Specificity (%)	Pos. pred. value (%)
Random plasma aluminum >100 µg/L	100	65	62
Plasma aluminum increment >200 µg/L after deferoxamine	100	35	47
Plasma N-PTH in the normal range	70	76	63
2 and 3	80	67	70
1 and 3	80	88	80

Blood tests were performed during the prospective evaluation of 27 long-term hemodialysis patients. The positive predictive values were calculated based on a prevalence of 37% with aluminum-related osteodystrophy. N-PTH, aminoterminal parathyroid hormone.

thyroid hormone (PTH), appears to be permissive in the development of aluminum-related osteomalacia (24) and aplastic bone disease (16) when relatively low circulating levels coexist with elevated plasma aluminum. The close positive correlation between plasma PTH and bone formation rate and the finding of absent to minimal bone surface aluminum in patients with osteitis fibrosa (25) suggest that the influence of elevated PTH on osteoblast function may be "protective" in the presence of elevated circulating aluminum. Because dialysis patients with aluminum osteodystrophy often have intact or decreased PTH secretion (26), plasma intact or aminoterminal (N)PTH is a useful noninvasive test for aluminum bone disease when levels are within the normal range. As shown in Table 1, a normal plasma N-PTH has a 76% specificity for the diagnosis of aluminum bone disease in long-term dialysis patients. When a positive test for the disease includes both an elevated random plasma aluminum and a normal plasma N-PTH, the sensitivity is 80% and the specificity, 88%. Furthermore, for this combination the positive predictive value (i.e., the probability that a randomly selected patient with a positive test has the disease) is 80%. Thus, plasma aluminum and PTH together substantially improve the predictive value compared with the use of either alone.

CONCLUSIONS

In summary, serum or plasma aluminum measurements are most helpful in the diagnosis of aluminum osteodystrophy when low circulating levels are used to exclude the disease. Elevated random aluminum levels have a higher specificity for the correct diagnosis than the plasma aluminum increment after deferoxamine in asymptomatic long-term dialysis patients with aplastic aluminum-related bone disease. In this group of patients, the positive predictive value of serum aluminum in the diagnosis of aluminum osteodystrophy is enhanced by the addition of plasma PTH. With the inclusion of plasma PTH as a diagnostic test, the improved specificity underscores the importance of low levels of PTH in the pathogenesis of impaired bone function in this disorder.

REFERENCES

1. Sherrard DJ, Andress DL: Renal osteodystrophy. In: Schrier RW, Gottschalk CW (eds) *Diseases of the Kidney*. Little, Brown and Co., Boston, pp 3035–3062, 1988
2. Legendre GR, Alfrey AC: Measuring picogram amounts of aluminum in biological tissue by flameless atomic absorption analysis of a chelate. *Clin Chem* 22:53–56, 1976
3. Savory J, Wills MR: Analytical methods for aluminum measurement. *Kidney Int* 29(suppl 18):24–27, 1986
4. Guillard O, Piriou A, Mura P: Precautions necessary when assaying aluminum in serum of chronic hemodialyzed patients. *Clin Chem* 28:1714, 1982
5. Bertholf RL, Brown S, Renoe BW, Wills MR, Savory J: An improved method for determining aluminum in serum by furnace atomic absorption spectrophotometry. *Clin Chem* 29:1087–1089, 1983
6. Moody JR, Lindstrom RM: Selection and cleaning of plastic containers for storage of trace element samples. *Anal Chem* 49: 2264–2267, 1977
7. Kaehny WD, Hegg AP, Alfrey AC: Gastrointestinal absorption of aluminum from aluminum-containing antacids. *N Engl J Med* 296:1389–1390, 1977
8. Gorsky JE, Dietz AA, Spencer H, Osis D: Metabolic balance of aluminum studies in six men. *Clin Chem* 25:1739–1743, 1979
9. Trapp GA: Plasma aluminum is bound to transferrin. *Life Sci* 33:311–316, 1983
10. Trapp GA: Interactions of aluminum with cofactors, enzymes and other proteins. *Kidney Int* 29(suppl 18):12–16, 1986
11. Burnatowska-Hledin MA, Mayor GH, Lau K: Renal handling of aluminum in the rat: Clearance and micropuncture studies. *Am J Physiol* 249:F192, 1985
12. Alfrey AC, Hegg A, Craswell P: Metabolism and toxicity of aluminum in renal failure. *Am J Clin Nutr* 33:1509–1516, 1980
13. Berlyne GM, Pest D, Ben-Ari J, Weinberger J, Stern M, Gilmore GR, Levine R: Hyperaluminaemia from aluminum resins in renal failure. *Lancet* 2:494–496, 1970
14. Parkinson IS, Ward WK, Kerr DNA: Dialysis encephalopathy, bone disease and anaemia: The aluminum intoxication syndrome during regular hemodialysis. *J Clin Pathol* 34:1285–1294, 1981
15. Felsenfeld AJ, Gutman RA, Llach F, Harrelson JM: Osteomalacia in chronic renal failure: A syndrome previously reported only with maintenance dialysis. *Am J Nephrol* 2:147–154, 1982
16. Andress DL, Maloney NA, Endres DB, Sherrard DJ: Aluminum associated bone disease in chronic renal failure: High prevalence in a long-term dialysis population. *J Bone Miner Res* 1:391–398, 1986
17. Milliner DS, Hercz G, Miller JH, Shinaberger JH, Nissenson AR, Coburn JW: Clearance of aluminum by hemodialysis: effect of deferoxamine. *Kidney Int* 29(suppl 18):100–103, 1986
18. Milliner DS, Nebeker HS, Ott SM, Andress DL, Sherrard DJ, Alfrey AL, Slatopolsky EA, Coburn JW: Use of the deferoxamine infusion test in the diagnosis of aluminum-related osteodystrophy. *Ann Intern Med* 101:775–780, 1984
19. Hodsman AB, Hood SA, Brown P, Cordy PE: Do serum aluminum levels reflect underlying skeletal aluminum accumulation and bone histology before or after chelation by deferoxamine? *J Lab Clin Med* 106:674–681, 1985
20. Llach F, Felsenfeld AJ, Coleman MD, Keveney JJ, Pederson JA, Medlock TR: The nature course of dialysis osteomalacia. *Kidney Int* 29(suppl 18):74–79, 1986
21. Nebeker HG, Andress DL, Milliner DS, Ott SM, Alfrey AC, Slatopolsky E, Sherrard DJ, Coburn JW: Indirect methods for diagnosis of aluminum bone disease: Plasma aluminum, the desferrioxamine infusion test and serum iPTH. *Kidney Int* 29(suppl 18):96–99, 1986
22. Andress DL, Maloney NA, Coburn JW, Endres DB, Sherrard DJ: Osteomalacia and aplastic bone disease in aluminum-related osteodystrophy. *J Clin Endocrinol Metab* 65:11–16, 1987
23. Malluche HH, Smith AJ, Abreo K, Faugere MC: The use of deferoxamine in the management of aluminum accumulation in bone in patients with renal failure. *N Engl J Med* 311:140–144, 1984
24. Hodsman AB, Sherrard DJ, Wong EGC, Brickman AS, Lee DBN, Alfrey AC, Singer FR, Norman AW, Coburn JW: Vitamin D resistant osteomalacia in hemodialysis patients lacking secondary hyperparathyroidism. *Ann Inter Med* 94:629–637, 1981
25. Andress DL, Endres DB, Maloney NA, Kopp JB, Coburn JW, Sherrard DJ: Comparison of parathyroid hormone assays with bone histomorphometry in renal osteodystrophy. *J Clin Endocrinol Metab* 63:1163–1169, 1986
26. Andress DL, Felsenfeld AJ, Voigts A, Llach F: Parathyroid hormone response to hypocalcemia in hemodialysis patients with osteomalacia. *Kidney Int* 24:364–370, 1983

24. Radiologic Evaluation of Bone Mineral in Children

Andrew K. Poznanski, M.D.

Department of Radiology, Children's Memorial Hospital, Chicago, Illinois

Bone mineral evaluation in childhood is performed for different reasons than that in the adult, and the approaches used for its evaluation are consequently different. A major use of bone mineral evaluation in children is in the management of renal osteodystrophy and rickets. It is also useful in many other chronic conditions with bone loss such as inflammatory bowel disease and juvenile rheumatoid arthritis. Bone mass evaluation is also of value in congenital disorders such as osteogenesis imperfecta and osteopetrosis. In the premature, severe bone loss can occur, and evaluation may be needed to diagnose its causes as well as determine whether fractures in such infants were due to very poor bone loss or child abuse.

Bone mineral evaluation in childhood can be qualitative or quantitative. The qualitative methods are very important because they can be diagnostic of the type of bone loss. Rickets, osteoporosis, hyperparathyroidism, and other vitamin deficiencies or poisonings and osteogenesis imperfecta, may have typical appearances.

QUALITATIVE EVALUATION OR RADIOGRAPHS FOR BONE LOSS

Overall Density

This is a very inaccurate and inconsistent method for evaluation of bone loss (1). In the spine >50% of bone can be lost without any evidence on the radiograph. This is due to the fact that only the cortical bone is clearly seen on the plain radiograph, and much loss of cancellous bone can occur before it is visualized. Also, the apparent density is very dependent on the kilovoltage used; the higher the kilovoltage, the more "washed out" the bone appears (Fig. 1). Similarly, the lack of using a high ratio grid for radiography can make the bones look more osteoporotic.

Relationship of the Appearance of the Cortex of Bone to that of the Center of Bone

This sign is sometimes useful in evaluation of the vertebrae (2), although it too is technique-dependent. The appearance of a thin, very sharply defined cortex in an epiphysis with a very lucent central trabecular bone is helpful in the diagnosis of severe osteoporosis, as may be seen in scurvy. Sometimes focal areas of lucency may be associated with endosteal scalloping (2).

Appearance of Trabecular Pattern

The appearance of a coarse trabecular pattern may be useful in evaluating whether osteopenia is present and determining the type; however, it can also be quite inaccurate. In the spine the presence of many vertical striations is usually a sign of osteoporosis. Similarly, in the hip, the appearance of coarse trabeculations may have an indication of loss of bone. There is some difference in appearance between the coarse trabecular pattern in osteoporosis and hyperparathyroidism, but usually this is not a good differential sign.

Presence of Compression Fractures of the Spine or Fractures of Other Bones

The appearance of anterior wedging or concave endplate deformities in the spine, best seen in the lateral projections, is a good sign of bone loss (2) (Fig. 2).

In children compression fracture may be seen in diseases associated with severe bone loss such as osteogenesis imperfecta, rickets, juvenile rheumatoid arthritis, or Crohn disease. It may be secondary to steroid therapy. Sometimes it is the presenting sign of leukemia or neuroblastoma; other disorders producing wedged vertebrae include histiocytosis X, juvenile osteoporosis, Gaucher disease, and Scheuermann disease. Concave or square impression on the endplate may be seen in sickle cell disease. In these various disorders the spine compression fractures may occur without any history of trauma.

Bone loss can be associated with a variety of fractures of the long bones as well as the spine. In hyperparathyroidism fractures through the growth plates are not uncommon. Fracture healing with overabundant callous can be seen in osteogenesis imperfecta or osteoporosis associated with neuromuscular abnormalities, particularly myelodysplasia. In premature neonates on parenteral alimentation fractures most occur without history of trauma (Fig. 3).

Presence of Bowing of the Bones in Children

A number of conditions with osteopenia in children, particularly rickets (Fig. 4), osteogenesis imperfecta, and fibrous dysplasia will result in bowing of the long bones. This may be associated with small cortical breaks on the convex surface. After treatment for rickets the bones tend to straighten with growth.

Presence of Subperiosteal Resorption and Other Signs of Hyperparathyroidism

Subperiosteal resorption is a classical manifestation hyperparathyroidism and is pathognomonic of it (3,4). It is

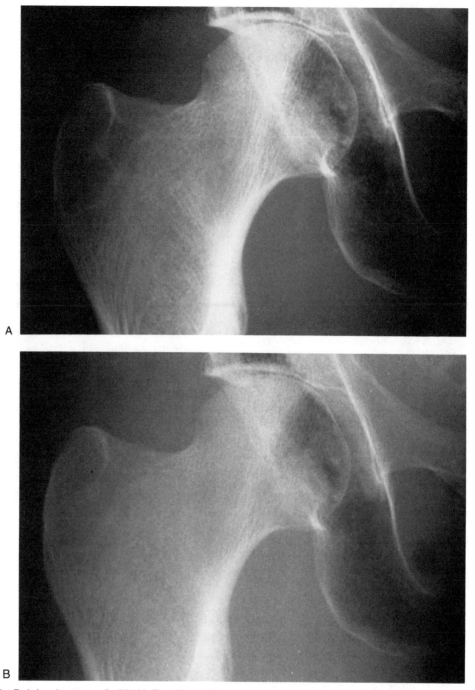

FIG. 1. Pelvic phantom. **A:** 70 kV; **B:** 120 kV. This is the same bone radiographed with two different techniques. Note how at the lower kV the bones appear dense and well mineralized, with well-defined trabeculae whereas at the higher kV they appear much more osteopenic. Other factors such as use of lower ratio grids and poor technique can also change the appearance from that of good mineralization to poor mineralization.

best seen in hand radiographs obtained with either industrial films or with mammography film screen combination, and the radiographs need to be examined with a magnifying glass. These resorptions can be easily missed if ordinary screen exposures are obtained (5). These findings are probably best seen along the radial aspect of the middle phalanges (Fig. 5A,B). The distal tufts are another good area for evaluation (Fig. 5A), but are probably not as useful as the middle phalanges, because some irregularity of the tufts can normally occur, and when these defects are subtle it is difficult to determine whether they are due to normal variation or hyperparathyroidism. Periosteal resorption may also be seen in other areas of the body. Commonly involved areas, particularly in infants and young children, include the medial side of the femoral necks and the medial aspect of the upper humerus or upper tibia (Fig. 5C) as well as near the metaphyseal areas of many other bones. The growth plate and metaphysis can have a rickets-like appearance with somewhat greater widening at the lateral and medial ends than in the center. Other changes of hyperparathyroidism include sclerosis of bone that in the spine can have a rugger jersey appear-

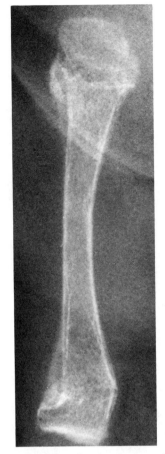

FIG. 3. Multiple fractures in the femur of a premature neonate with bronchopulmonary dysplasia. There is callous around the *upper femoral fracture*. The *lower fracture* is angulated with some callous on the lateral side. This is evidence of healing. The poorly mineralized bones in this infant fractured with no known trauma, but from normal handling in the nursery.

ance (Fig. 6) and a coarse trabecular pattern (5,6). The rugger jersey appearance may also be seen in osteopetrosis. There may be arterial calcification as well (7) (Fig. 5A). In children, slipping of various epiphyses, particularly the proximal femoral and the proximal humeral, may be seen (8) (Figs. 7 and 8). Aseptic necrosis may also be present (Fig. 8). Metaphyseal fractures can be symmetrical in various bones (Fig. 9). Well-circumscribed lucent areas from brown tumors may be seen in any part of the skeleton (Figs. 7 and 10).

Presence of Linear Striations

Linear striations (9,10) in the cortex of the second metacarpal as well as other bones can be due to hyperparathyroidism or osteomalacia or just simply increased metabolism such as in hyperthyroidism. Some striation may be seen in normal children. Abnormal striations are usually not seen in slower forms of bone loss that occurs in chronic diseases or juvenile rheumatoid arthritis. When this intracortical resorption is present on the radiographs

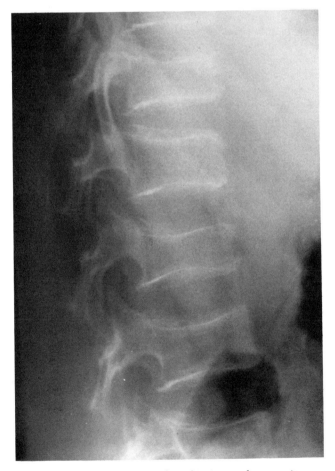

FIG. 2. Multiple compression fractures from osteoporosis in a boy with Crohn's disease. The vertebral bodies are flatter than normal with indentations on the endplates. Compared with the shape of the vertebrae in Fig. 6, their shape is more normal although in that figure the sclerotic changes are abnormal.

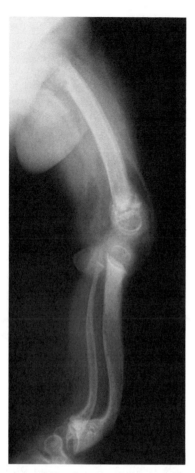

FIG. 4. Bowing of the bones of the leg of a child with treated rickets. the legs may bend in any direction, depending on the stresses involved.

of the hand, the cortical measurements are not accurate in determining bone loss, and other methods should be used.

Metaphyseal Changes in Rickets

Irregularity of the metaphysis in growing children is usually the hallmark of rickets (Fig. 11). It is associated with an increase of apparent distance between the ossified portion of the metaphysis and the epiphysis. This finding is due to the lack of ossification of osteoid that is being produced. The changes are most severe in bones with the greatest growth so that they are most pronounced in the distal femur of most ages. They are rarely seen in slow-growing bones like the tubular bones of the hand. During a growth spurt such as in adolescence, the rachitic changes may appear greater than during a period of slower growth. Widening of the anterior ribs, the rachitic rosary may also be seen radiographically (Fig. 12). Similar changes in the metaphyses may be indistinguishable from those seen in hyperparathyroidism, although in some cases of the latter, there is more erosion around the edge of the involved growth plate than is seen in rickets (6) (Fig. 13). All types of rickets have similar changes at the growth plate, and the radiologic distinction at the growth plate between the various types of rickets may be difficult and diagnosis is usually based on clinical and biochemical findings. Occasionally, radiologically differentiation is possible. For example the radiologic appearance of vitamin D-resistant rickets is somewhat different in that one never sees secondary hyperparathyroidism in untreated cases and in older children with this disease thickened bowed bones, particularly the femora, are usually present and these are not seen in other forms of rickets. Vitamin D-dependent rickets is often associated with radiologic signs of hyperparathyroidism.

During the healing of rickets the first calcification may occur at the zone of provisional calcification, leaving a lucent band between the new calcification and the irregular metaphysis. Also during healing, periosteal elevation may be present (Fig. 14).

Disorders Mimicking Rickets

There are a number of conditions that can mimic rickets (11), including copper deficiency, diaphosphonate therapy, fluorosis, hypophosphatasia, primary and secondary hyperparathyroidism, Menkes syndrome, Schwachman syndrome, and various forms of metaphyseal chondrodysplasia, particularly Jansen syndrome in the neonate, and McKusick and Schmidt forms in older children. Mucolipidosis II and osteopetrosis in infants may have manifestations similar to rickets. Among these conditions mimicking rickets, radiologic differentiation is often possible. For example, in Jansen syndrome, the epiphysis is very markedly displaced from the metaphysis much more so than in rickets (Fig. 15). Later on bizarre calcifications are seen in the cartilaginous portion that are even more characteristic. The serum calcium may be elevated in Jansen's syndrome, which also differentiates it from rickets. Hypophosphatasia usually also has different manifestations than rickets, with more punched-out appearing defects in the metaphysis rather than involving the whole growth plate evenly (Fig. 16). The rachitic-like changes of hyperparathyroidism can also sometimes be differentiated by erosion along the edge of the growth plate (Fig. 13). There are also a number of localized disorders that can mimic rickets. These include old growth plate fracture that has not been immobilized (Fig. 17), frostbite, radiation therapy, and chronic recurrent multifocal osteomyelitis.

Signs of Osteomalacia

When the growth plates are closed what is called rickets in childhood is termed osteomalacia. Radiologic differentiation from other forms of osteopenia is difficult unless Looser's zones, also called pseudofractures, are present. These are areas of cortical lucency often associated with adjacent cortical sclerosis that may not go completely through the cortex (Fig. 18). These are often seen along the medial side of the femoral neck and in the pubis or ischium. They may occur in other areas.

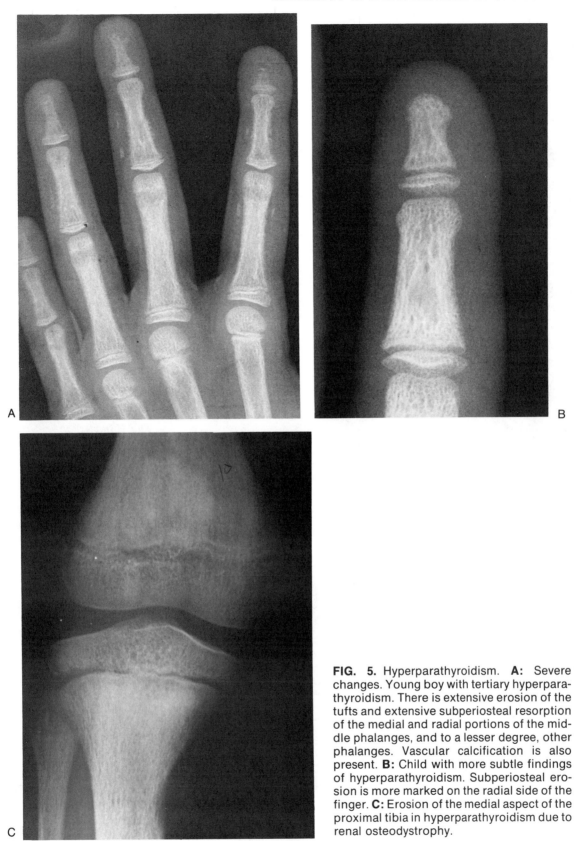

FIG. 5. Hyperparathyroidism. **A:** Severe changes. Young boy with tertiary hyperparathyroidism. There is extensive erosion of the tufts and extensive subperiosteal resorption of the medial and radial portions of the middle phalanges, and to a lesser degree, other phalanges. Vascular calcification is also present. **B:** Child with more subtle findings of hyperparathyroidism. Subperiosteal erosion is more marked on the radial side of the finger. **C:** Erosion of the medial aspect of the proximal tibia in hyperparathyroidism due to renal osteodystrophy.

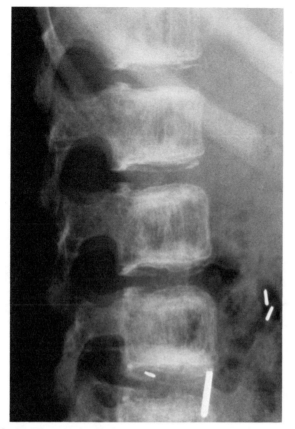

FIG. 6. "Rugger jersey" spine in a child with renal osteodystrophy. The sclerotic bands on the *upper* and *lower margins* of each vertebrae are characteristic of secondary hyperparathyroidism. Coarse trabeculae are seen in the vertebral bodies.

Increased Bone Mineral with Sclerosis

Increased bone density on radiography can be seen in a variety of bone dysplasias, the most classic of which is osteopetrosis. Although the bone appears very dense and thick, it is very brittle and prone to fracture. Bands of density may also be seen and may mimic renal osteodystrophy in the spine.

QUANTITATIVE MEASUREMENTS OF BONE LOSS IN CHILDREN

Different techniques of bone loss evaluation are used in children than adults. One of the problems of many of the newer methods is the lack of proper standards for young children. The methods that have pediatric applications are the various cortical measurements, single photon absorptiometry (SPA) and dual energy x-ray absorptiometry (DXA), the latter may be of value because it is a low radiation procedure, it can be used for various sites, and pediatric standards are becoming available.

Cortical Measurements

The Hand

Methods of Measuring

Films of the hand are obtained using a high detail film screen combination such as one used for mammography.

The most commonly used measurements (12) are of the second metacarpal, and various standards have been ob-

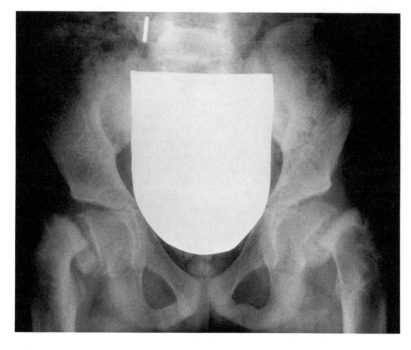

FIG. 7. Bilateral slipped capital femoral epiphyses in a child with renal osteodystrophy. Note the widened growth plate in the proximal femora and displacement of the femoral heads with respect to the neck. These are fractures through the growth plate. At the inferior margin of each growth plate, there is a small fragment of bone that probably broke from the metaphysis. The appearance is similar to that seen in congenital coxa vara. The lucency in the left femoral neck is a brown tumor, a manifestation of hyperparathyroidism.

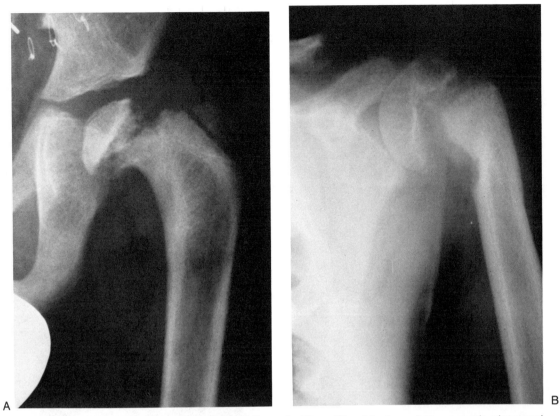

FIG. 8. Boy with tertiary hyperparathyroidism. **A:** Hip with widening of the growth plate and displacement of the capital femoral epiphysis. There is a small crescent of bone in the subcortical surface of the femoral head that is a sign of aseptic necrosis. **B:** Slipped epiphysis of the upper humerus. The growth plate is wide and irregular, and there is an erosion along the medial side of the upper femur, a manifestation of hyperparathyroidism.

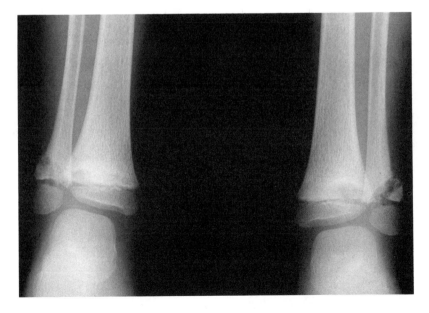

FIG. 9. Bilateral growth plate and metaphyseal fractures (Salter II) of the fibula in the same boy with renal osteodystrophy illustrated in Fig. 8. Note the rachitic changes of the tibial growth plates (partially healed).

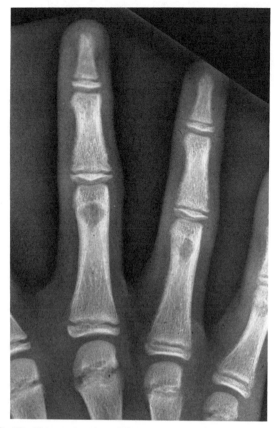

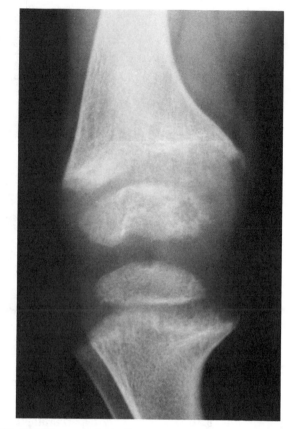

FIG. 10. Hyperparathyroidism. The lucent defects in the distal portions of the proximal phalanges are brown tumors of hyperparathyroidism. Note also the extensive subperiosteal resorption on both medial and lateral surfaces of the middle phalanges. There is also some erosion of the tufts of the distal phalanges.

FIG. 11. Characteristic findings of rickets in a child with nutritional rickets. There is widening and irregularity of the growth plate with marked fraying of the metaphyses of the distal femur and proximal tibia. The bone density is decreased, and there is some bowing.

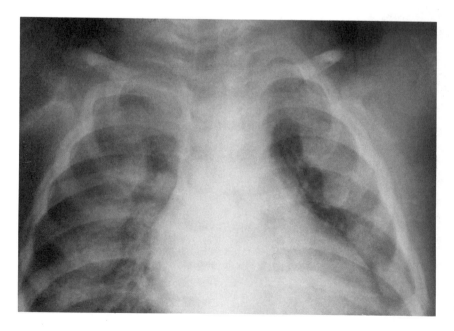

FIG. 12. Chest x-ray of the small child shown in Fig. 11. The anterior ribs are widened anteriorly. This corresponds to the rachitic rosary of rickets.

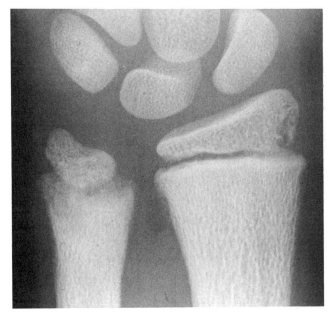

FIG. 13. Child with renal osteodystrophy with erosion of the edge of the growth plate, including a slight irregularity of the epiphysis. This has been termed the "rotten core" appearance and is typical of the growth plate of hyperparathyroidism rather than rickets.

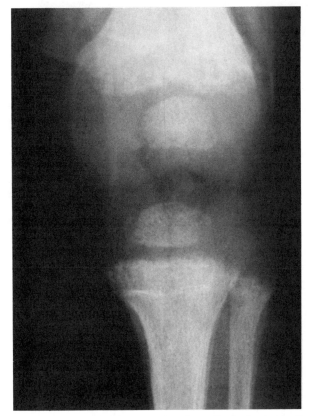

FIG. 14. Rickets with some healing. Periosteal reaction of the shafts of the tibia and fibula is a sign of some degree of healing. Also, note the distal portions of the metaphyses are more lucent than the rest. This is due to incomplete ossification of the previously unossified osteoid and is a sign of healing rickets.

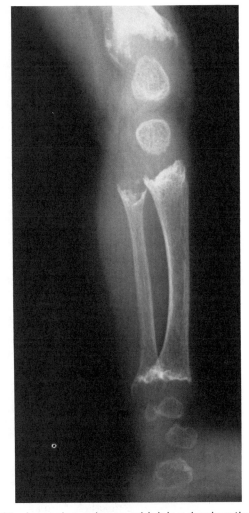

FIG. 15. Jansen's syndrome, which is a dominantly inherited metaphyseal chondrodysplasia. Note the irregular, somewhat sclerotic metaphyseal ends reminiscent of rickets. However, there is marked separation between the peculiar rounded epiphyses of the distal femur and proximal tibia and their respective metaphyses. With age this wide space fills in with irregular calcification, giving the characteristic appearance of Jansen's syndrome, which is then not confused with rickets.

tained for different population groups. The most commonly used standards in the United States have been those of Garn et al. (13). In these standards the measurements are obtained at the midpoint of the second metacarpal, the midpoint being defined as halfway between the upper margin and the notch at the bottom of the bone. The outside diameter of the bone (T) and the inside diameter of the bone (M) are measured (Fig. 19). The inside diameter is sometimes poorly defined, particularly in cases where there is rapid bone loss or permeative bone loss when the margin may appear ragged. In such cases most small projections into the medullary space are not counted. The measurements are best obtained using a comparator that is a magnifying glass with a small scale that can measure to one-tenth of a millimeter or alternately precise calipers

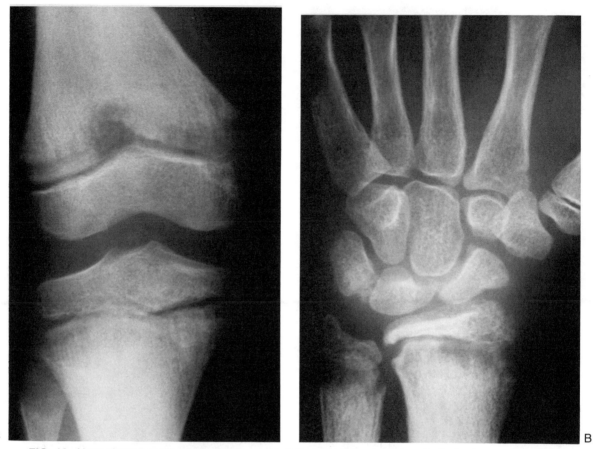

FIG. 16. Hypophosphatasia. **A:** Knee; **B:** wrist. Although there is some similarity between hypophosphatasia and rickets, the metaphyseal lucency is not the same as the fraying in rickets that extends across the whole growth plate. The metaphyseal defects appear more focal than in rickets, and parts of the growth plate appear normal. In infants, the changes of hypophosphatasia may be similar to rickets but are usually more severe and occur at birth, whereas rickets usually does not manifest itself before 3 months of age.

can be used. The cortical thickness $C = T - M$. The percentage of cortical area (PCA) can also be calculated

$$PCA = \frac{100 \ (T^2 - M^2)}{T^2}$$

Advantages of Cortical Measurements

This is the simplest, least expensive technique of measuring bone. It is particularly useful in children, because good age standards are available for both males and females of various ages and for whites, blacks, and Mexican-Americans (12). The advantage of using the cortical measurements is that it not only gives some measurements of cortical thickness, but it also gives information on what is happening at the various surfaces of the growing bone or within the cortex of the bone. For example, one can determine whether the bone loss is due to endosteal resorption or lack of subperiosteal surface apposition. In most causes of pediatric osteoporosis other than renal osteodystrophy, the usual loss is due to increased resorption along the endosteal surface resulting in a larger medullary space (14). This is true in the hand and other bones. In some growth disorders there is a lack of growth on the outside surface (13). This is particularly common in children with chronic diseases and may be seen in a variety of conditions such as osteogenesis imperfecta, abnormal nutrition states, juvenile rheumatoid arthritis, or Crohn disease (12,14). Because little or no bone can be lost from the outer surface a diminished outside diameter is indicative of lack of growth. Also, from the hand radiograph one can determine the presence or absence of subperiosteal resorption indicating hyperparathyroidism and intracortical resorption indicating rapid bone loss or hyperparathyroidism. When subperiosteal resorption or intracortical resorption is present, cortical measurements do not accurately reflect the loss of bone in the appendicular skeleton, and other methods must be used (12). Cortical measures are therefore not useful in the evaluation of renal osteodystrophy.

Another advantage of the hand radiograph in children is that bone age can be determined, and bone mineralization that is age-dependent can be considered not only relative to the chronological age, but also to skeletal matura-

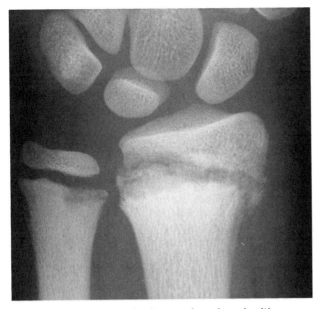

FIG. 17. Young football player who played with a sore wrist for a few weeks. The widening and irregularity of the growth plates is due to an unhealed growth plate fracture of the radius and ulna that had not been allowed to heal because of motion between the fragments. After casting healing was complete.

tion (14). The latter may be more realistic, particularly in disorders where there is marked retardation of skeletal maturation or in delayed puberty.

Disadvantages of Using the Hand Radiograph

The cortical measurement of the hand does not measure cancellous bone or intracortical resorption. The inability to measure cancellous bone mass is less of a problem in the child than in the adult because hip fractures are usually not a problem. If subperiosteal resorption or intracortical loss is seen on the hand radiograph then SPA or DXA studies can be performed for better evaluation.

Evaluation of the Humeral Cortex in Neonates

Cortical bone standards have been developed for the humerus for neonates of varying gestational ages (15). These humeral measurements are obtained at the level of the nutrient foramen of the humerus (Fig. 20). As for measurements of the second metacarpal, the outside diameter (T) and the inside diameter (M) are measured, and the difference between these is defined at the cortical thickness $C = T - M$. One can then follow a premature infant from birth to determine whether the infant is grow-

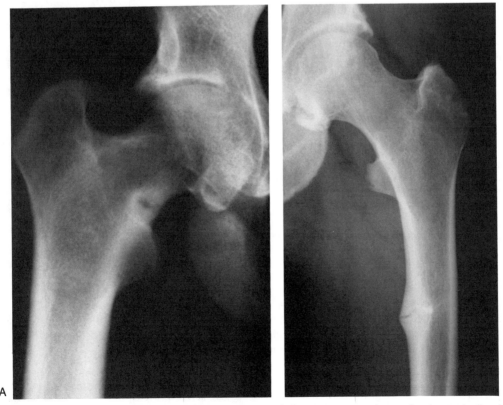

FIG. 18. Looser's zones, otherwise known as pseudofractures, are signs of osteomalacia. **A:** A female with vitamin D-resistant rickets and painful hips. The linear lucency in the medial portion of the femoral neck with sclerosis around it is typical of the pseudofractures of osteomalacia. **B:** These fractures can occur anywhere as in this child, where the pseudofracture is in the midshaft.

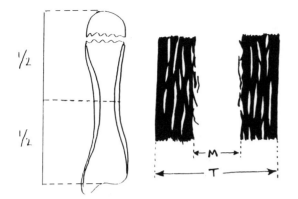

FIG. 19. Measurements taken for evaluation of cortical thickness, using the Garn method. The measurement is taken at the midpoint of the second metacarpal, the midpoint being defined as halfway between the upper margin and the notch at the bottom of the bone. The two measurements that are taken are the outside diameter (T) and the inside diameter (M). The inside diameter, M, is sometimes poorly defined, particularly in cases in which there is rapid bone loss or permeative bone loss, when the margin may appear ragged. In such cases, the inner margin is defined as a line where most of the bone is present. Small projections into the medullary space are not counted. (From Poznanski AK: The Hand in Radiologic Diagnosis with Gamuts and Pattern Profiles. W. B. Saunders, Philadelphia, 1984.)

ing along the normal curve as he/she would have done *in utero* or whether significant bone loss has occurred (Fig. 21). In severely ill premature infants, there is a rapid bone loss that occurs mainly by endosteal resorption (Fig. 22). This may predispose the infant to fractures after ordinary handling (Fig. 3).

Other Cortical Standards

Virtama and Helela (16) have developed cortical standards for a number of sites in other long bones in a Finnish population. Their values for the second metacarpal are fairly close to the Garn standards (13).

Single Photon Absorptiometry

Method

This technique (17) uses a narrow beam from a low-energy radioisotope source usually ^{125}I source and a detector, usually a sodium iodide crystal. The detector and source move together along a linear path. Any bone can be scanned but the one usually used is the shaft of the radius usually near the junction of the distal and the middle third of the forearm. The hand and forearm are held in the device with an attempt to keep them in a reproducible position if the exam is to be redone at a later date. A computer is used to obtain the change in counts at the bone edge to determine the edges of the radius and calcu-

late the bone mineral content. The values are given in g/cm, also a value in g/cm^2 is calculated by dividing the mineral content by the width of the bone. In small children the computer may have difficulty in determining the edge and this must be defined manually, which adds to the inaccuracy of the study.

Advantages

The technique will detect intracortical bone loss. It exposes the patient to a very small radiation dose and only a very narrow portion of the body is exposed. It is relatively inexpensive if a moderate number of patients are examined and the cost of the relatively short-lived isotope (half-life = 60 days) can be amortized over many patients. The isotope source needs to be replaced 3–4 times/year. It is a useful procedure in following some patients with bone loss that may occur in renal osteodystrophy.

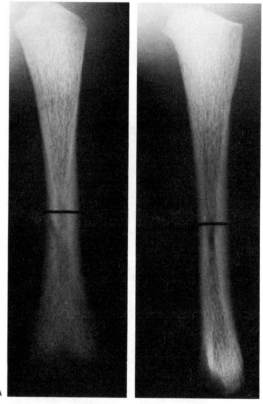

A   B

FIG. 20. Neonatal humerus in two projections. **A:** In the anteroposterior view the nutrient foramen is clearly seen. The *black line* indicates the site of measurement of the outer and inner diameters, just superior to where the nutrient canal leaves the bone. **B:** In the lateral view the more distal portion of the nutrient canal is seen as a small circle in the center of the bone. The measurement is taken 2 mm superior to this, as indicated by the *black line*. This level corresponds to the same location seen in A. (From Poznanski AK, Kuhns LR, Guire KE: New standards of cortical mass in the humerus of neonates: A means of evaluating bone loss in the premature infant. *Radiology* 134:639–644, 1980.)

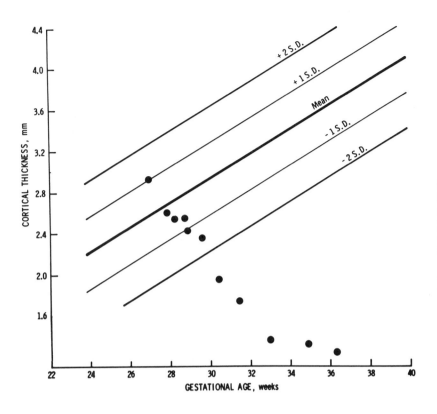

FIG. 21. Plot of cortical thickening of the humerus against gestational age. The dots are the cortical measures over time of a premature infant with severe pulmonary disease. The cortical thickness *(C)* was ±1 SD above mean at birth but decreased rapidly thereafter. At ~10 weeks after birth, equivalent to just above 36 weeks gestational age, the bone mineral was very low, much lower than even a 22-week gestational age infant. (From Poznanski AK, Kuhns LR, Guire KE: New standards of cortical mass in the humerus of neonates: A means of evaluating bone loss in the premature infant. *Radiology* 134:639–644, 1980.)

Disadvantages

The measurements when obtained at the conventional shaft site, near the distal radius, measure mostly cortical bone with only 5% trabecular bone. The more distal measurement can measure greater percentage of trabecular bone (~25%) (18); however, it is still basically a cortical bone measurement.

Another potential problem is that, if the measures are done without taking radiograph of the forearm, faulty readings may occur. If there is an old fracture, a bone island or a cortical defect at the site of the measurement, these will be measured with the bone and result in a false estimate of overall bone mass.

Single photon absorptiometry is potentially inaccurate in young children because of the lack of good standards. It is also potentially less accurate in children than in adults in follow-up studies, because the site of the measurement will not be the same each time. Since the distal end of the forearm grows faster than the proximal, the one-third measurement used for localization of the scan will not be in the same position on subsequent studies. Another problem in children is that the values are usually compared only with standards for the child's chronological age, whereas it would be more appropriate to use the bone age. Therefore if SPA is done in children, a hand and forearm radiograph should also be obtained. The technique has also been used in infants (19,20), but these data are very hard to reproduce because of the relatively small difference between the bone of the radius and the soft tissues (21). Somewhat better measurements can be obtained in the humerus or femur, but again there is a lack of standards.

MEASUREMENT OF BONE MINERAL CONTENT OF THE SPINE AND OTHER PARTS OF THE SKELETON IN CHILDREN

Three techniques are currently available. These are quantitative computed tomography (QCT), dual photon absorptiometry (DPA), and DXA (also called DEXA and DRA). Of these, DXA (which is the newest of the three) may be the most practical in children.

Quantitative computed tomography measures bone density of several computed tomography cuts of vertebra and compares these with a standard. It has the theoretical advantage over the others that it can measure only the trabecular bone and is less affected by volume than either DPA or DXA. Pediatric standards are available (22) for QCT. It, however, has several major disadvantages. It gives a high radiation dose [200–1,500 m Rem (2–15 mSv)] and also uses an expensive machine. Also QCT is difficult to do in other areas than the spine.

Dual photon absorptiometry has been used primarily in adults, and it measures the absorption of radiation from a gadolinium-153 source. It gives a lower dose than QCT (1–15 mREM) (10–150 µSv), but it has a poor spatial resolution (3–4 mm), needs expensive source replacement every 18 months, and requires relatively long exam time (20 min) that can be a problem in children. Most importantly, no good pediatric standards are available.

Dual energy x-ray absorptiometry is similar to DPA, but instead of a radioactive source it uses x-rays at two energy levels. The image produced is much sharper, with a resolution of ~1.5 mm vs. 3–4 mm for DPA. It allows faster scanning with time down to under 1 min for small parts with some units. It gives a very low dose (1–6 mR)

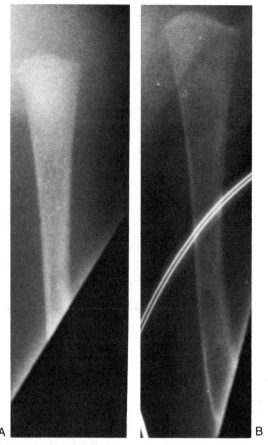

FIG. 22. Humerus of a premature infant at birth **(A)** and 6 weeks later. **(B).** Note the marked thinning of the cortex postnatally. Most of the loss has occurred by endosteal resorption. The outer diameter has shown little change, but the medullary diameter is considerably wider. This is the same infant plotted in Fig. 21. (From Poznanski AK, Kuhns LR, Guire KE: New standards of cortical mass in the humerus of neonates: A means of evaluating bone loss in the premature infant. *Radiology* 134:639–644, 1980.)

(10–20 µGy). It provides greater precision and accuracy than DPA.

Normal standards are available in children for DXA not only for age, but also for weight and Tanner stages of sexual maturity (23). This is important because major changes in bone mass occur at puberty.

Another advantage of both DXA and DPA is that measurement of other parts of the body as well as body fat and total skeletal mass can be determined with these devices.

STRATEGIES TO EVALUATE BONE LOSS IN CHILDREN

The hand radiograph obtained using mammography film screen combination is probably the method of choice as the initial method of evaluating bone loss in children. The advantages include giving qualitative and quantitative data. From the hand radiograph one can detect the pres-

ence of rickets in the distal radius and ulna. The bone age can also be determined so that proper standards for bone mineralization can be used. It also gives information of what is occurring at each bone surface whether there is or is not subperiosteal resorption and also gives a measure of the growth that has occurred at the outside surface. Good normative data for cortical measures are available not only for whites but for other races (12).

In renal osteodystrophy, if there is subperiosteal or intracortical bone loss, SPA or DXA should be used. SPA is difficult in infants but may be used in older children. If used in children, hand and forearm radiographs should also be obtained to evaluate the qualitative factors. Dual photon absorptiometry has little use in children and QCT, although a useful research tool, is not practical in clinical practice.

Radiography of the knees is the single best view to determine the presence of rickets, because this is the area where most growth is occurring; however, an anteroposterior view of the ankle or wrist may also be used. To detect the pseudofractures of osteomalacia the best views are the hips or shoulder. Radiography of painful areas should be obtained, because pseudofractures can occur in other areas.

Measurement of cortical thickness of the humerus is probably the simplest and best method for evaluation of bone loss in premature neonates. This is readily available from available chest radiographs so that additional films need not be taken. Because most of the bone loss appears to be due to endosteal resorption, this measure is an accurate means for evaluating appendicular bone loss. Single photon absorptiometry has been used in infants, but is very difficult to reproduce, particularly when using the distal radius. Dual energy x-ray absorptiometry may be potentially a useful tool in neonates, but little data are currently available.

REFERENCES

1. Epstein DM, Dalinka MK, Kaplan FS, Aronchick JM, Marinelli DL, Kundel HL: Observer variation in the detection of osteopenia. *Skeletal Radiol* 15:347–349, 1986
2. Schneider R: Radiologic methods of evaluating generalized osteopenia. *Orthop Clin North Am* 15:631–651, 1984
3. Meema HE, Oreopoulos DG: The mode of progression of subperiosteal resorption in the hyperparathyroidism of chronic renal failure. *Skeletal Radiol* 10:157–160, 1983
4. Debnam JW, Bates ML, Kopelman RC, Teitelbaum SL: Radiological pathological correlations in uremic bone disease. *Radiology* 125:653–658, 1977
5. Weiss A: Incidence of subperiosteal resorption in hyperparathyroidism studied by fine detail bone radiography. *Clin Radiol* 25:273–276, 1974
6. Parfitt AM: Clinical and radiographic manifestations of renal osteodystrophy. In: Davis DS (ed) *Calcium Metabolism in Renal Failure and Nephrolithiasis.* John Wiley & Sons, Inc., pp. 145–195, 1977
7. Meema HE, Oreopoulos DG, DeVeber GA: Arterial calcifications in severe chronic renal disease and their relationship to dialysis treatment, renal transplant, and parathyroidectomy. *Radiology* 121:315–321, 1976
8. Mehls O, Ritz E, Krempien B, Gilli G, Link K, Willich E, Scharer K: Slipped epiphyses in renal osteodystrophy. *Arch Dis Child* 50:545–554, 1975

9. Meema HE, Meema S: Comparison of microradioscopic and morphometric findings in the hand bones with densitometric findings in the proximal radius in thyrotoxicosis and in renal osteodystrophy. *Invest Radiol* 7:88–96, 1972

10. Meema HE, Oreopoulos DG, Meema S: A roentgenologic study of cortical bone resorption in chronic renal failure. *Radiology* 126:67–74, 1978

11. Frame B, Poznanski AK: Conditions that may be confused with rickets. In: DeLuca HJ (ed) *Pediatric Diseases Related to Calcium*. Elsevier, Holland/New York, pp. 269–289, 1980

12. Poznanski AK: *The Hand in Radiologic Diagnosis*. W. B. Saunders, Philadelphia, 1974

13. Garn SM, Poznanski AK, Nagy JM: Bone measurement in the differential diagnosis of osteopenia and osteoporosis. *Radiology* 100:509–518, 1971

14. Poznanski AK: Radiologic evaluation of growth. In: Davidson M (ed) *Growth Retardation Among Children and Adolescents with Inflammatory Bowel Disease: Report of Workshop Conducted in Reston, Virginia*, March 6–8, 1981. National Foundation for Ileitis and Colitis, New York; pp. 53–81, 1983

15. Poznanski AK, Kuhns LR, Guire KE: New standards of cortical mass in the humerus of neonates: A means of evaluating bone loss in the premature infant. *Radiology* 134:639–644, 1980

16. Virtama P, Helela T (eds): *Radiographic Measurements of Cortical Bone*. Turku Auraprint Oy, Stockholm, 1969

17. Sorenson JA, Cameron JR: A reliable in vivo measurement of bone-mineral content. *J Bone Joint Surg* 49-A:481–497, 1967

18. Mazess RB, Peppler WW, Chesney RW, Lange TA, Lindgren U, Smith E Jr: Does bone measurement on the radius indicate skeletal status? *J Nucl Med* 25:281–288, 1984

19. Minton SD, Steichen JJ, Tsang RC: Decreased bone mineral content in small-for-gestational-age infants compared with appropriate-for-gestational-age infants: Normal serum 25-hydroxyvitamin D and decreasing parathyroid hormone. *Pediatrics* 71:383–388, 1983

20. Vyhmeister NR, Linkhart TA, Hay S, Baylink DJ, Ghosh B: Measurement of bone mineral content in the term and preterm infant. *Am J Dis Child* 141:506–510, 1987

21. Tyson JE, Maravilla A, Lasky RE, Cope FA, Mize CE: Measurement of bone mineral content in preterm neonates. *Am J Dis Child* 137:735–737, 1983

22. Gilsanz V, Gibbens DT, Roe TF, et al.: Vertebral bone density in children: Effect of puberty. *Radiology* 166:847–850, 1988

23. Southard RN, Morris JD, Mahan JD, et al.: Bone mass in healthy children: Measurement with quantitative DXA. *Radiology* 179:735–738, 1991

25. Scintigraphy in Metabolic Bone Disease

David C. Wang, M.D., Sambasiva R. Kottamassu, M.D., and Kastytis Karvelis, M.D.

Department of Diagnostic Radiology, Division of Nuclear Medicine, Henry Ford Hospital, Detroit, Michigan

Skeletal scintigraphy in clinical practice was greatly expanded with the development of bone-seeking technetium-99m (^{99m}Tc)-Sn compounds of polyphosphate and diphosphonate that are easily prepared from readily available commercial kits. Technetium-99m is a gamma emitter with a physical half-life of 6 hr. It can be obtained from an inexpensive generator and has a gamma ray energy of 140 KeV, which is well suited for gamma camera imaging. These characteristics make it an almost ideal agent for nuclear medicine imaging [1].

Bone scanning with radionuclides has gained wide clinical acceptance for evaluation of metastatic bone disease, primary bone tumors, osteomyelitis, and aseptic necrosis. Metabolic bone disease has also been studied and detected by skeletal scintigraphy [1].

The factors that affect the rate and degree of skeletal uptake of radionuclides have not been clearly defined. Studies have shown that the initial uptake is predominately related to blood flow; however, the following factors also play a role: capillary permeability; local acid-base relationships; the quality of mineralizable bone; bone turnover; hormones; and vitamins [2].

The rapid short-term uptake of the technetium phosphate compounds, which are analogs of calcium phosphate, is believed to occur by ion exchange (a chemical rather than a metabolic process) through replacement of hydroxyl groups at vascularized bone surfaces. Thus, periosteal, endosteal, trabecular, and Haversian surfaces are the major sites of rapid ion exchange and will demonstrate increased uptake. The metaphyses of rachitic bones have been shown histologically to contain increased and dilated capillary networks, and it is likely that the increased uptake that is seen in the metaphyses is related to increased blood flow, in spite of the overall decreased rate of osteogenesis [1].

BONE SCANNING TECHNIQUE

Technetium-99m labeled methylene diphosphonate or hydroxymethylene diphosphonate is administered intravenously. Dosages range from 10 to 25 mCi. Twenty mCi is the usual adult dose, with 25 mCi sometimes given when single photon emission tomography is anticipated. Pediatric dosage is calculated based on body surface area (Table 1). Approximately 50–60% of the tracer is taken up by bone, with the remainder excreted by the kidneys [2]. Total irradiation is ~0.7 rads to the bone, and on average <0.4 rads to the ovaries or testes per 20 mCi dose of ^{99m}Tc [3].

No specific patient preparation is necessary; however, the patient should be encouraged to drink several large glasses of water (if not contraindicated) immediately after being injected to enhance renal clearance of tracer not bound to bone. This reduces the level of soft tissue activity seen on the images as well as reducing radiation to the patient.

Gamma camera imaging is performed at ~2–3 hr after injection. Scanning earlier than this may result in images that are degraded by significant blood pool activity. Ante-

TABLE 1. *Body surface area method for the calculation of radiopharmaceutical dosages for pediatric patients*

Patient wt. (kg)	Body surface area (m²)	Fraction of adult dose
2	0.15	0.09
4	0.25	0.14
6	0.33	0.19
8	0.40	0.23
10	0.46	0.27
15	0.63	0.36
20	0.83	0.48
25	0.95	0.55
30	1.08	0.62
35	1.20	0.69
40	1.30	0.75
45	1.40	0.81
50	1.51	0.87
55	1.58	0.91

From Chilton HM, Witcofski RL: Fundamentals of radiopharmaceuticals. In: Swanson DP, Chilton HM, Thrall JH (eds) *Pharmaceuticals in Medical Imaging*. Macmillan, New York, p 295, 1990.

rior and posterior images of the entire body can be obtained with either a scanning whole body camera or with multiple spot images.

Single photon emission computed tomography imaging can provide additional spatial and contrast resolution and may be helpful in localizing areas of abnormality, especially in the hips, spine, knees, and skull. Sixty-four separate images (20–30 sec each) are obtained with the camera head moving circumferentially about the patient. Computer reconstruction allows viewing of the images in the axial, sagittal, and coronal planes.

In addition to the standard delayed images, blood flow and blood pool images can be obtained. The three-phase scanning can demonstrate abnormally increased blood flow or soft tissue perfusion in a specific area. The delayed

TABLE 2. *Bone scan patterns in metabolic bone disease*

Generalized features
    Increased activity in axial skeleton
    Increased activity in long bones
    Increased activity in periarticular areas
    Prominent calvarium and mandible
    Beading of the costochondral junctions
    ''Tie'' sternum
    Faint or absent kidney images
Occasionally associated findings
    Focal tracer uptake involving one or more entire vertebrae (spinal compression fracture)
    Focal uptake in ribs or other skeletal areas (fractures, pseudofractures, stress microfractures)
    Abnormal tracer uptake in the kidneys (renal disease)
    Soft tissue tracer uptake (soft tissue calcification)

From Wahner HW: Assessment of metabolic bone disease: Review of new nuclear medicine-procedures. *Mayo Clin Proc* 60:827–835, 1985.

static bone scan is performed at 2–3 hr. A fourth phase or further delayed images can be obtained at 16–24 hr, if additional delineation between bone and soft tissue is needed.

FINDINGS ON BONE SCINTIGRAPHY

The scintigraphic diagnosis of metabolic bone disease begins with the recognition of generalized increased bone uptake. This generalized increase is often accompanied by localized uptake due to a superimposed focal pathologic process (4). Seven scintigraphic features of metabolic bone disease have been described by Fogelman et al. (Table 2). Metabolic bone disease is suggested if 3 or more of these findings are present. These findings, however, are not specific for a particular condition or group of disorders. Bone scintigraphy has low sensitivity and specificity for the diagnosis of most metabolic bone diseases compared with biochemical testing and bone biopsy (5). Attempts have been made to increase the specificity by quantification. Twenty-four hr whole-body retention of tracer can distinguish Paget's disease, osteomalacia, and primary hyperparathyroidism from normal. This tech-

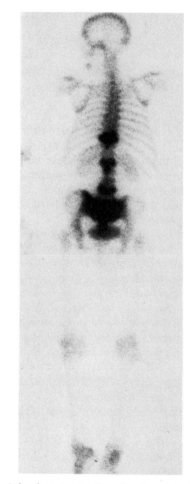

FIG. 1. Vertebral compression fractures in the thoracic and lumbar spine and sacral fracture in a patient with osteoporosis.

nique is technically demanding, and its accuracy is limited by the dependence of uptake not only on osteoblastic activity, but also on blood flow, kidney function, and other poorly understood factors (4). Although bone scanning may be of little use for early detection of metabolic bone disorders, the recognition of abnormal image patterns may be helpful in the interpretation of atypical bone scans in patients who undergo screening for a variety of disease states (5).

Primary Hyperparathyroidism

Bone scintigrams are usually unremarkable in asymptomatic patients with primary hyperparathyroidism. Quantitation of skull uptake or measurement of the 24-hr total body retention may be helpful and both are usually elevated. In more advanced cases of primary hyperparathyroidism, any or all of the common findings (Table 2)

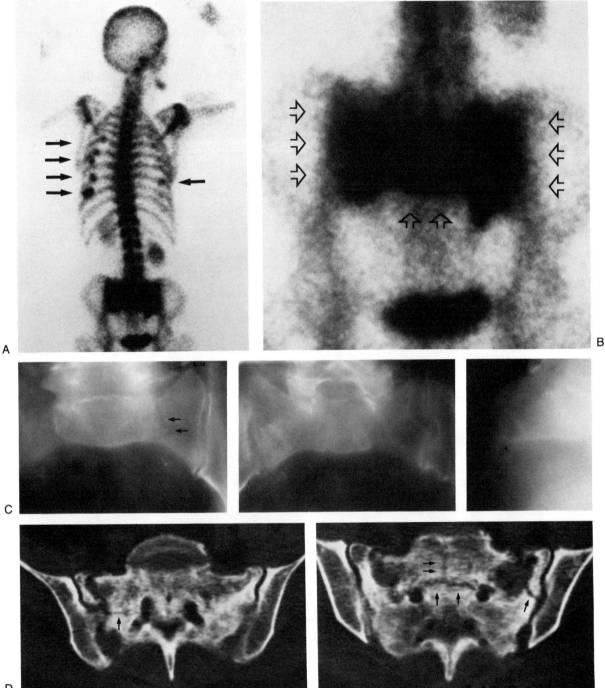

FIG. 2. Multiple insufficiency fractures with **(A)** increased uptake involving the ribs as well as **(B)** an ''H''-type fracture of the sacrum that is seen on linear tomography **(C)** and computed tomography **(D)** in this patient with osteoporosis.

may be evident. Focal abnormalities such as collapsed vertebra, cysts, or brown tumors may be seen. Cysts are generally photopenic, whereas brown tumors exhibit focal increased uptake. Increased lung or soft tissue uptake may be present in patients with renal involvement. After parathyroidectomy, the elevated lung uptake will rapidly return to normal; however, abnormal bone uptake may persist for ~1 year (5).

Skeletal Scintigraphy in Osteoporosis

Skeletal scintigraphy with ^{99m}Tc diphosphonates frequently surpasses or compliments radiographic findings in evaluating the focal complications of osteoporosis, including traumatic/insufficiency fractures, vertebral compressions, aseptic necrosis, and acute infarction. However, it is well known that routine skeletal radiographs have limited sensitivity in evaluating bone mineral content. As much as 30–40% of the bone mineral content may be lost before a decrease in bone density is radiographically evident. Most types of osteoporosis have no characteristic biochemical profile. Detection of osteoporosis is likewise imprecise when based on ^{99m}Tc diphosphonate skeletal imaging. Bone scans may demonstrate a normal or rarely a washed-out appearance with diffuse decreased skeletal uptake. Single and dual photon absorptiometry and quantitative computed tomography are sensitive techniques for measuring bone mineral content (see ref. 6 and Chapter 26).

Bone scintigraphy has a significant role in assessing the focal complications of osteoporosis. In patients with osteoporosis, back pain can occur as a result of microfractures without an obvious vertebral body collapse on radiographs. Bone scan, however, may show a localized increased uptake due to the microfractures. Total body scans are useful in assessing the location and extent of the fractures throughout the skeleton, which commonly occur in the spine (Fig. 1), femoral neck, wrist, ribs, and pubis. In vertebral fractures, the radionuclide images, while initially demonstrating markedly increased uptake, usually are negative by 18–24 months, allowing some estimate of the age of the fractures to be made (6). Pinhole or single photon emission tomography imaging, as well as magnetic resonance imaging are useful for detecting early aseptic necrosis of the femoral heads when radiographs are equivocal or negative (6).

Osteoporotic patients on sodium fluoride treatment may develop insufficiency or "stress" fractures of the calcaneus, femur or tibia due to increased number of new

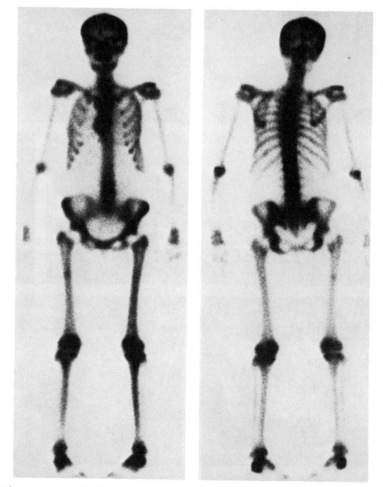

FIG. 3. *(Anterior, posterior)* Diffuse increased uptake in the axial skeleton, calvarium, sternum, and ends of long bones (bilateral hip prothesis).

resorption sites before they are subsequently filled with new bone. Within the first few weeks, radiographs may be negative, but by 4–6 weeks, there is evidence of healing fractures. Radionuclide imaging will often show these lesions before they are radiographically evident (6).

Transverse fractures of the sacrum are often not apparent on radiographs, but recognized on bone scan or computed tomography (Fig. 2B,C,D). Sacral fractures usually occur in patients with osteoporosis and other metabolic bone disease as the result of mild trauma. Clinical symptoms range from localized sacral tenderness to neurologic symptoms due to sacral nerve root irritation from cauda equina compression. The shape and anatomy of the sacrum, as well as coexistent osteopenia, makes radiographic evaluation of this osseous structure very difficult. In the case of osteoporotic sacral fractures, the bone scan is very sensitive, and the characteristic H-shaped pattern of uptake across the sacrum and sacroiliac joints suggests the correct diagnosis (7).

Skeletal Scintigraphy in Osteomalacia and Rickets

Osteomalacia is a disorder in which mineral deposition in the newly formed osteoid is impaired. In addition, in growing children, impaired calcification of maturing cartilage at the zone of provisional calcification leads to the condition known as rickets. Common causes of osteomalacia include dietary deficiency, hepatic insufficiency, malabsorption, and renal insufficiency that may be glomerular or tubular (see Section VI).

In osteomalacia, radionuclide imaging with ^{99m}Tc diphosphonates, often shows increased accumulation in the skeleton, which may involve the entire skeleton or more prominent uptake may be seen in the axial skeleton, at the ends of the long bones and in the wrists. Increased uptake in the calvarium and at the costochondral junction is also frequently noted (Fig. 3). These findings are nonspecific and may be seen in other metabolic bone diseases (8). Focal areas of increased uptake due to multiple rib fractures, or Looser's zones with or without insufficiency fractures, may be present (6).

Looser's zones are often symmetrical and are oriented at right angles to the long axis of the involved bone. The common sites of Looser's zones include the axillary aspect of the scapula, concave aspect of the long bones, pubic rami, ischium, ribs and proximal ulna. These sites are often visualized on radionuclide images prior to becoming radiographically apparent (6).

In patients with renal osteodystrophy, there is a variable degree of osteomalacia and secondary hyperparathyroidism. The bone scintigraphy often demonstrates either a nonspecific diffuse increased uptake involving the entire skeleton, or only the long bones with prominent calvarial uptake (6). Renal uptake is often faint or absent, which may reflect reduced excretion of the tracer by the kidneys due to increased skeletal uptake (8). Pulmonary uptake may be increased, usually when pulmonary calcification is severe (Fig. 4) (4). Ectopic calcification may also demonstrate focal uptake (Fig. 5).

Skeletal uptake of the radionuclide, expressed as bone-

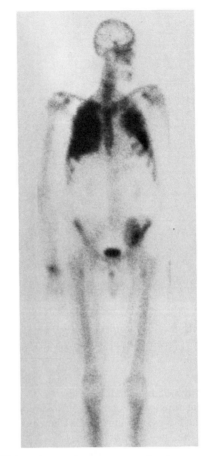

FIG. 4. Extensive pulmonary uptake in a patient with renal osteodystrophy. Note the transplanted kidney in the left pelvis.

to-soft tissue ratio, is significantly higher in osteomalacia patients than in controls. Fogelman et al. reported the mean bone-to-soft tissue uptake ratio for the osteomalacia group was 6.57 ± 1.43, whereas that in the control patients was 4.05 ± 0.69 (8).

Other Metabolic Bone Diseases

Increased growth hormone secretion in acromegaly may result in diffuse increased uptake (5). A positive relationship between uptake and basal levels of growth hormone has been shown, and changes can be seen in response to therapy. However, assessment of activity is an unreliable indicator of severity and the sensitivity and specificity of the scintigraphic changes are too low to be of practical clinical use (5).

Paget's disease is characterized by skeletal metaplasia and focal areas of intense uptake (Fig. 6). Diminished uptake can also be seen within the early lytic phase of the disease or the late sclerotic phase that no longer has active bone turnover (5). Fibrous dysplasia will also demonstrate focal areas of markedly increased uptake (5). Engelmann's disease and melorrheostosis have characteristic patterns of increased uptake corresponding to well-recog-

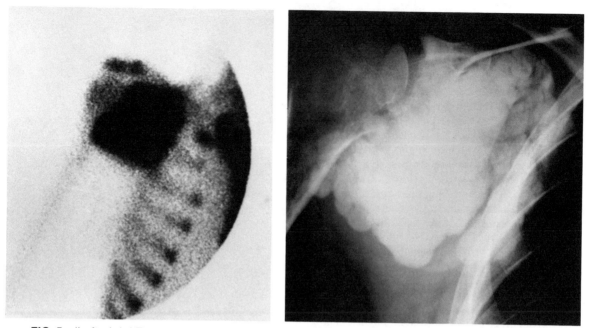

FIG. 5. *(Left, right)* Ectopic calcifications of the right shoulder on x-ray and bone scan in a patient with severe renal osteodystrophy.

nized radiographic abnormalities (see ref. 9 and Chapter 74). Hyperthyroidism will cause a diffuse increase in uptake in the long bones, and elevated 24-hr total body retention of tracer has been reported (5).

Hypertrophic osteoarthropathy exhibits a distinctive periosteal and periarticular uptake in the extremities, with early involvement of the distal third of the tibiae, fibulae, radii, and ulnae and later involvement of the femora, humeri, metacarpals, and metatarsals. The asymmetric up-take seen in ~15% of patients with hypertrophic osteoarthropathy may give the appearance of metastatic disease (5) (Fig. 7).

PARATHYROID SCANNING

Primary hyperparathyroidism is most commonly due to a solitary parathyroid adenoma (10). Because of the

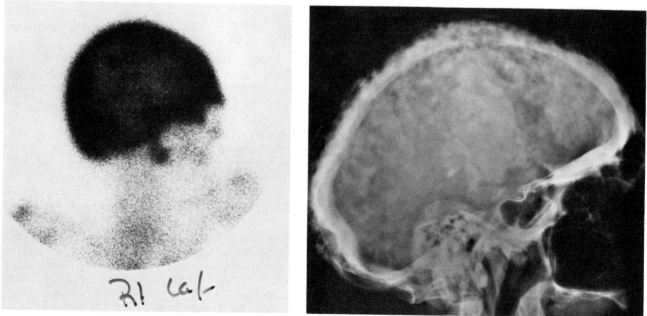

A
B

FIG. 6. Paget's disease. Intense cranial uptake **(A)** and characteristic cotton wool appearance with widening of the diploe and basilar invagination **(B)**.

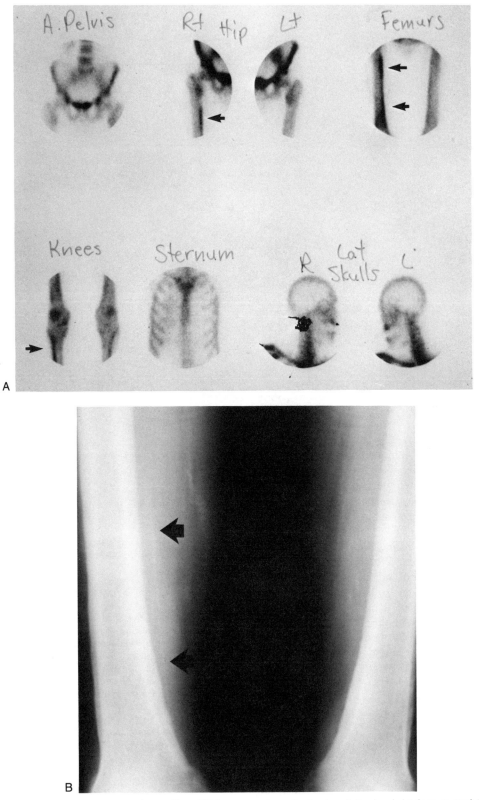

FIG. 7. Hypertrophic osteoarthropathy. **(A)** Increased periosteal uptake in right femur and tibia on bone scan *(small arrows)* and **(B)** periosteal calcification and cortical thickening on x-ray *(large arrows).*

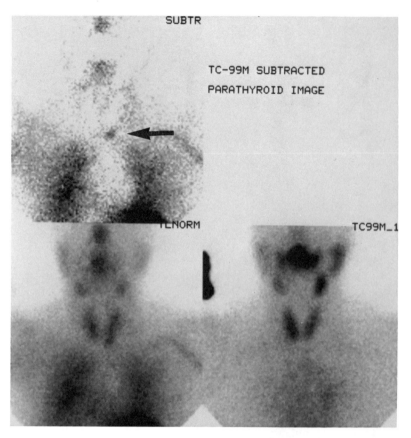

SUBTR

TC-99M SUBTRACTED
PARATHYROID IMAGE

TLNORM

TC99M_1

FIG. 8. Parathyroid subtraction scan. A small parathyroid adenoma is visible on the computer-subtracted image *(arrow)*. On their own, the ^{201}Tl scan *(bottom left)* and the ^{99m}Tc scan *(bottom right)* are relatively unremarkable.

90–95% success rate of the initial surgery, a parathyroid scan has a limited role in preoperative evaluation; however, it is most useful prior to reoperation in patients with a failed initial surgery. The scan can aid in locating an ectopic gland or an abnormal gland in a patient with surgically altered anatomy (11).

Imaging is performed utilizing both ^{99m}Tc and ^{201}Tl. Thallium is a potassium analog and distributes in relationship to blood flow and state of the Na^+, K^+-ATPase system (11). Because of their increased vascularity, both the thyroid and parathyroid glands exhibit increased uptake of thallium relative to surrounding tissue. By contrast, technetium is taken up only by the thyroid. An image of the parathyroid gland can be obtained by subtracting the ^{99m}Tc image from the ^{201}Tl image. The sensitivity of the parathyroid subtraction scan (Fig. 8) ranges from 70–90%, depending on the size of the adenoma or area of hyperplasia. Adenomas <300 mg in size are difficult to identify (10).

Palpation of the neck is necessary for correlating the scintigraphic findings. Adenomatous goiters, thyroid carcinoma, chronic thyroiditis, and lymphoma can give a false-positive appearance on a parathyroid subtraction scan (11).

REFERENCES

1. Genant HK: Bone-seeking radionuclides: An in vivo study of factors affecting skeletal uptake. *Radiology* 113:373–382, 1974
2. Mettler FA: *Essentials of Nuclear Medicine Imaging.* Grune & Stratton Inc., New York, 1985
3. MIRD: Method of calculation: "S" absorbed dose per unit cumulated activity selected radionuclides and organs, *MIRD Pamphlet* No. 11, 1975
4. Wahner HW: Assessment of metabolic bone disease. Review of new nuclear medicine procedures. *Mayo Clin Proc* 60:827–835, 1985
5. Siegel BA: *Nuclear Medicine: Self-Study Program* 1. Society of Nuclear Medicine. New York, 1988
6. McAfee JG: Radionuclide imaging in metabolic and systemic skeletal diseases. *Semin Nucl Med* 17:334–349, 1987
7. Reis T: Detection of osteoporotic sacral fractures with radionuclides. *Radiology* 146:783–785, 1983
8. Fogelman I: Role of bone scanning in osteomalacia. *J Nucl Med* 19:245–248, 1978
9. Shier CK: Ribbing's disease: Radiographic-scintigraphic correlation and comparative analysis with Engelmann's disease. *J Nucl Med* 28:244–248, 1987
10. Fine EJ: Parathyroid imaging: Its current status and future role. *Semin Nucl Med* 17:350–359, 1987
11. Winzelberg GG: Radionuclide imaging of parathyroid tumors: Historical perspectives and newer techniques. *Semin Nucl Med* 15:161–170, 1985

26. Bone Density Measurement and the Management of Osteoporosis*

*C. Conrad Johnston, Jr., M.D., and †L. Joseph Melton III, M.D.

*Department of Medicine, Indiana University School of Medicine,
Indianapolis, Indiana, and †Department of Health Sciences Research,
Mayo Clinic, Rochester, Minnesota

All agree on the importance of osteoporosis as a major public health problem (see Chapters 56–63). Any amelioration of the impact of osteoporosis depends on a reduction in its attendant fractures. Many interventions depend, in turn, on bone mass measurements, and appropriate clinical application of these technologies should be based on the following criteria: 1) bone mass can be measured accurately and safely; 2) fractures result at least in part from low bone mass; 3) bone mass measurements can estimate risk of future fracture; 4) such information cannot be obtained from other clinical evaluations; 5) clinical decisions can be based on information obtained from bone mass measurement; and 6) such decisions lead either to an intervention that would result in a reduction in future fractures or to avoidance of future diagnostic efforts and therapeutic interventions, which would reduce health care costs.

MEASUREMENT OF BONE MASS

Bone mass can be measured with good accuracy and considerable precision using currently available techniques (Table 1). All of these are far superior to standard roentgenograms and other methods available that have error rates of 30–50%. Moreover the accuracy of bone mass measurements compares favorably with that of many other accepted tests, including screening tests such as serum cholesterol.

Methods for measuring bone mass are also very safe with low radiation exposure. Single photon absorptiometry (SPA) produces a dose of <15 mRem, dual photon absorptiometry (DPA), and dual energy x-ray absorptiometry (DEXA) <5 mRem and modern quantitative computed tomography (QCT) from 100 to 1,000 mRem. These can be compared with the dose received from a chest x-ray of 20–50 mRem, full dental x-ray of 300 mRem or abdominal computed tomography of 1–6 Rem (2,3).

Relationship of Bone Mass to Fracture

There is considerable evidence that fractures result from low bone mass. Bone mineral density (BMD) is highly correlated with bone strength (4,5), accounting for 75–85% of the variance in ultimate strength of bone tissue (6). Bone mineral density diminishes with aging in the femoral neck, falling an estimated 58% in women and 39% in men between the ages of 20 and 90 years, whereas BMD of the intertrochanteric region of the proximal femur declines 53% and 35%, respectively (7).

Because bone strength is a determinant of fracture susceptibility, along with the likelihood of sustaining sufficient trauma, it follows that BMD is also correlated with fracture risk in patients (8). Indeed, there is a gradient of increasing hip fracture risk as bone mass falls. For example, cervical or intertrochanteric fractures are rare among Rochester, Minnesota, women with femoral BMD ≥ 1.0 g/cm^2, but incidence rates increase as femoral bone mass declines (Fig. 1), reaching levels of 8.3 and 16.6/1,000 person-years, respectively, among women with cervical or intertrochanteric BMD levels <0.6 gm/cm^2 (9).

Although assessment of the proximal femur by DEXA has not been available long enough for long-term prospective studies to be conducted; short-term studies indicate that such measurements can predict the risk of hip fractures (10). Theoretical models also indicate that lifetime hip fracture risk varies with femoral bone density and age. According to one model (11), for women 40 years old at the time of assessment, the estimated lifetime risk of a femur fracture is negligible among those with bone density of 1.3 g/cm^2. It is ~9.2% for a cervical femur fracture and 5.1% for an intertrochanteric fracture among those with BMD of 1.0 g/cm^2 and continues to rise as bone mass falls below that level. For bone density of 0.6 g/cm^2, the lifetime risk is estimated to be >25% for both fracture sites. For women 60 years old, the lifetime fracture risk is estimated at only 5.0% for cervical femur and 2.2% for intertrochanteric fractures among those with an initial femoral bone density of 1.0 g/cm^2, about half as much as for the 40-year-olds with the same BMD.

There are, of course, other risk factors for these fractures, especially those related to falling. For vertebral fractures, reduced bone mass [along with poor bone quality (12)] is the predominant cause of fracture; trauma plays a small role (13). On the other hand, falls are important in the etiology of hip and Colles' fractures (13). However, the risk of falls increases only from 19%/year among women age 60–64 years to 33%/year at ages 80–84 (14). Falling per se, therefore, cannot explain the exponential increase in hip fractures with aging, although a change in the type of falls may play a role (14). For example, a fall directly on the hip may be associated with a much higher risk of hip fracture than other types of falls (15). The situation is analogous to the etiology of coronary heart disease. Like heart disease, the causes of hip fractures are multi-

* Adapted from a report of the Scientific Advisory Committee of the National Osteoporosis Foundation (see ref. 1).

TABLE 1. *Comparison of bone densitometry techniques*

Technique	Site	Relative sensitivity	Precision (%)	Accuracy (%)	Duration of examination (min)	Absorbed dose (mrem)	Cost ($)
Standard techniques							
SPA	Proximal	1X	2–3	5	15	10	75
DPA	radius	2X	2–4	4–10	20–40	5	100–150
QCT	Spine, hip	3–4X	2–5	5–20	10–20	100–1,000	100–200
	Spine						
Newer developments							
SPA-R	Distal radius, calcaneus	2X	1–2	5	10–20	5–10	50[a]
DEXA	Spine, hip	2X	1–2	3–5	5	1–3	75[a]
QCT-A	Spine, hip	3–4X	1–2	5–10	10	100–300	100[a]

SPA, single photon absorptiometry; SPA-R, retilinear SPA; DPA, dual photon absorptiometry; DEXA, DPA with a dual-energy x-ray source; QCT-A, QCT with advanced software and hardware capabilities. (From Genant HK, Block JE, Steiger P, Glueer CC, Ettinger B, Harris ST: Appropriate use of bone densitometry. *Radiology* 170:817–822, 1989.)
[a] Projected cost.

factorial. Measurement of any single risk factor (bone mass, cholesterol) cannot completely explain the occurrence of the disease. Nonetheless, measurement of the factor identifies those who have the greatest risk of developing the disease and, thus, would benefit most from therapy.

Bone Mass Measurement Predicts Future Fracture

Considerable evidence now suggests that bone mass predicts the probability of future fracture. Whereas the bone mass of women with hip fractures overlaps the bone mass of women of similar age who have not had hip fractures (7,16–18), bone mass measurement is not intended to be a diagnostic test for fracture. Rather, it measures a risk factor (reduced bone mass) for future fractures and is properly used for risk stratification. This is again analo-

gous to measurement of other risk factors, like cholesterol for coronary heart disease or blood pressure for stroke.

There is ample evidence that bone mass measurements can stratify patients on the basis of fracture risk. Recently published studies have demonstrated that measuring bone mass in the radius (19–22) or os calcis (20,22,23) will predict the risk of fractures in the future. In one prospective study, women with bone mass in the lowest quintile had ~4 times the risk of subsequent fractures as women in the highest quintile; vertebral fracture incidence, for example, was inversely correlated with bone mass measured in the radius, os calcis, or lumbar vertebra (23). Another prospective study (19) has found that measurement of bone mass in the forearm predicts future fracture, even after adjusting for age (Fig. 2). This confirms the findings of earlier investigations that used densitometry of the forearm (24) but did not adjust for age. Further studies on this population have confirmed that a single measure-

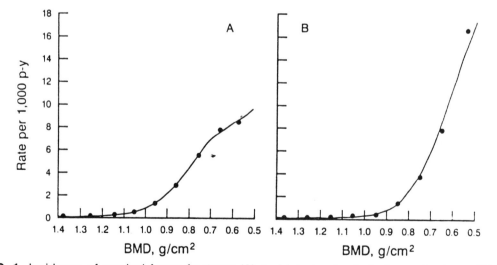

FIG. 1. Incidence of cervical femur fractures **(A)** and intertrochanteric femur fractures **(B)** by cervical and intertrochanteric BMD, respectively. (From Melton LJ, Kan SH, Wahner HW, Riggs BL: Lifetime fracture risk: An approach to hip fracture risk assessment based on bone mineral density and age. *J Clin Epidemiol* 41:985–994, 1988.)

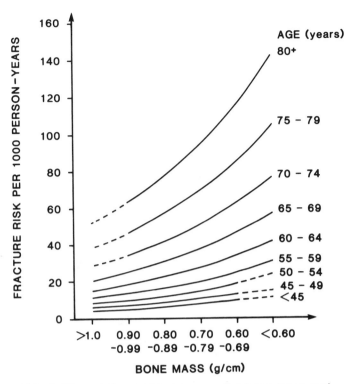

FIG. 2. The relationship between radial bone mass and subsequent fractures defined in each group *(solid lines)*. There is an increased risk of fracture with declining bone mass (plotted on the x-axis). (From Hui SL, Slemenda CW, Johnston CC Jr: Age and bone mass as predictors of fracture in a prospective study. *J Clin Invest* 81:1804–1809, 1988.)

ment of the radius predicts the risk of fracture at all sites and at the hip. For each standard deviation decline in bone mass, there was slightly more than a doubling in the fracture risk, controlling for age (25). In Fig. 3, the probability of not having a hip fracture in retirement-home

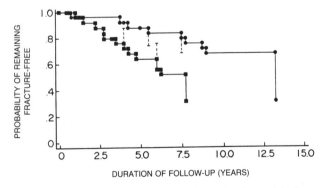

FIG. 3. A plot of the probability of not having a hip fracture over time in a retirement home for two levels of bone mass at the midshift radius; bone mass level more than 0.6 g/cm *(circles)*; <0.6 g/cm *(squares)*. Dotted vertical lines denote 95% confidence intervals at selected points. X-axis is years of follow-up. (From Hui SL, Slemenda CW, Johnston CC Jr: Baseline measurement of bone mass predicts fracture in white women. *Ann Intern Med* 111: 355–361, 1989.)

residents is plotted for two levels of bone mass. In a prospective study of 9,703 nonblack women, age 65 years and older who were followed for an average of 1.6 years, 53 hip fractures occurred (26). The risk of fracture was inversely related to bone density, with a relative risk of 1.66 for a decrease of ±1 SD in bone density at the calcaneus, 1.55 at the distal radius, and 1.41 at the proximal radius. In most of the reported studies, the relative risk of subsequent fractures was increased to between 1.5 and 2.0 for a change of ±1 SD. In fact, in this same cohort it now appears that fractures at virtually all skeletal sites are significantly associated with reduced skeletal density (27).

Although the association between bone mass and fractures had been demonstrated for measurements of bone mass at all sites, case-control studies have found that hip fracture risk is even more strongly associated with bone mass in the hip than with bone mass in the forearm (4,7), and prospective studies now bear this out (10). Similarly, vertebral fractures are more strongly associated with bone mass in the spine than with bone mass in the forearm (7,28). Consequently, the direct measurement of bone mass in the hip and spine that is now possible may have even greater predictive accuracy for hip and vertebral fractures.

Thus, it is now well established that measurement of bone mass assesses the risk of fracture. This appears to be true for all types of fractures, including vertebral and hip fractures. This relationship between bone mass and the risk of fracture is as strong or stronger than the relationship between serum cholesterol and the risk of coronary heart disease (19).

FRACTURE RISK ASSESSMENT USING CLINICAL RISK FACTORS

It is commonly believed that osteoporosis-prone individuals can be identified through common clinical observations (29,30), but this has never been demonstrated experimentally. For example, female patients who are white, short, thin, and smoke have a higher risk of osteoporosis than black, tall, obese, nonsmoking women (31–36). However, the power of these and other factors [e.g., thyroid or gastrointestinal disease (12) and heavy alcohol consumption (37,38)] for predicting fractures has not been well quantified in the few case-control studies that have considered all of them simultaneously. Moreover, these risk factors may not be independent; for example, smoking and obesity are related to each other as well as to osteoporosis (39). Other potential risk factors, such as thyrotoxicosis, malabsorption syndromes, or prolonged corticosteroid therapy, may be important but are relatively rare (40). Ideally, the ability of risk factors to predict fracture would be established by prospective studies of a population for whom therapeutic decisions are to be made—primarily perimenopausal women. Unfortunately, the limited data available suggest that a person's risk of fracture cannot be accurately estimated by assessing these risk factors (41).

There are data, however, on the association between

common risk factors and bone mass. These studies have all found that risk factors for osteoporosis based on history or physical examination are not reliable predictors of bone mass. Moreover, there is no set of risk factors that is consistently found in all studies. For example, Yano et al. (42) accounted for only 22–38% of the variability in bone mass (at the os calcis and radius) in 43- to 80-year-old females, using height, weight, age, and serum estrogen concentrations as independent variables. Others have reported r^2 values of 40% [using age, muscle area, thiazide use, hormone therapy, dietary vitamin D and vitamin D + calcium interaction as independent variables (43)], 40% [using age, with a range of 42–84 years, which is much broader than that usually seen in osteoporosis clinics (44)], 25% [using months of amenorrhea (45)], and 25–31% [using body mass index, years postmenopausal, and smoking (46)]. In a study of 49 women, ages 38–43, seven risk factors in a risk score were not significantly correlated with bone mass measured in the wrist (SPA) or spine (by QCT and DPA) (47). In a study of peri- and early postmenopausal women (i.e., a population for whom estrogen therapy would be considered), age, height, weight, calcium and caffeine intake, alcohol and tobacco use, and a urinary marker of bone turnover were used to construct a model to predict bone mass in the radius, lumbar spine, and hip. None of the models correctly identified >70% of the women with low bone mass at any site. A small subgroup (7%) with short stature, low body weight, low calcium intake, and who were heavy smokers always had low radial bone mass. Using the models, ~30% of the population could be assessed without bone mass measurement. However, predictions for spine and femur were less efficient, suggesting that direct measurements are required if decisions about therapy are to be based on bone mass at these sites (48). Together, these studies demonstrate that various risk factors, although statistically significant, account for much less than half of the variability in bone mass and, therefore, do not provide adequate precision to classify individual patients.

INDICATIONS FOR BONE MASS MEASUREMENTS

A task force of the National Osteoporosis Foundation has suggested the following clinical indications for bone mass measurements (1).

Estrogen-Deficient Women

Indication 1—In estrogen-deficient women, bone mass measurements can be used to diagnose significantly low bone mass in order to make decisions about hormone replacement therapy.

Rationale. Estrogen deficiency following menopause, oophorectomy, or prolonged amenorrhea from any cause is associated with bone loss. Bone loss, in turn, is associated with a greater risk of fractures. Bone loss and the associated risk of fractures can be prevented or slowed with estrogen replacement therapy (ERT). Not all women

will benefit equally from estrogen, however. Bone mass measurements are needed to determine which women have the lowest bone mass and will benefit the most from treatment. Thus, measurement of bone mass will allow women to make rational decisions regarding long-term ERT for protection from osteoporosis.

Background. It has been sufficiently demonstrated that there is a spectrum of bone mass in estrogen-deficient women so that those with high or low bone mass can be easily detected. As noted previously, bone mass measurements predict risk of future fractures.

Decisions for ERT to prevent bone loss can be guided by bone mass measurement. A substantial proportion of postmenopausal women receiving ERT for menopausal symptoms and other reasons that have little to do with osteoporosis are treated but treatment is typically for a limited time. It has been estimated that only 5% of postmenopausal women will get long-term ERT (10 years or more) for reasons independent of concerns about osteoporosis and, consequently, unaffected by potential bone mass measurements (1). Thus, the majority of postmenopausal women will have to weigh costs and benefits of this therapy. Because ERT has side effects and potentially serious risks and because patient acceptance may be a problem with the use of estrogen-progestin combinations that often lead to cyclical bleeding, it is important to select those at greatest risk of future fracture for long-term ERT. This determination can reliably be made only by direct measurement of bone mass.

Treatment with ERT will reduce future fractures. There is compelling evidence that long-term estrogen therapy prevents bone loss and fracture. In one clinical trial of three groups of patients followed from 6 weeks, 3 years, or 6 years after oophorectomy, estrogen (mestranol) significantly retarded bone loss for as long as estrogens were prescribed, at least 10 years (49,50). These effects of estrogen were independent of the duration of ovarian insufficiency that preceded the onset of treatment (51), and recent data show ERT to be effective in slowing bone loss up to age 70 (52). However, because the effect of treatment is to slow the rate of bone loss, greater benefits are achieved with earlier treatment because bone mass is maintained at a higher level. Similar results have been found by other investigators (53–59). There is also evidence that ERT prevents fractures as well. One randomized trial showed that 38% of oophorectomized women not on treatment experienced vertebral deformity, whereas 4% of the women on ERT had such changes (50). A retrospective study of 245 long-term estrogen users vs. 245 controls found a 50% reduction in osteoporosis-related fractures (53). This result was largely due to prevention of spine fractures. Randomized trials of ERT for hip fracture prevention are less feasible because of the long delay between menopause and the age of fracture. However, case control studies show a reduction in hip and Colles' fracture associated with long-term ERT (37,38,60–62). Most recently a retrospective cohort study was published from Framingham showing a 35% reduction in hip fracture risk among women who had ever taken postmenopausal estrogen (63). Thus, the available data consistently show that estrogen prescribed early after menopause for a minimum of 5–10 years will reduce the risk of hip fracture by ~50%.

Bone mass measurements will lead to an increase in appropriate outcomes (fewer fractures). It has been estimated that, in the absence of bone mass measurements, 15% of women over age 50 would have long-term ERT and that 10% of the entire group of perimenopausal women would experience hip fracture during a lifetime (1). In a program emphasizing bone mass measurements in the hip to identify high risk women, it was estimated that 22% of women would have long-term ERT and that only 8% of all perimenopausal women would experience a hip fracture during life. Bone mass measurements would result in treating 7% more women (from 15–22%) with ERT and might reduce the lifetime risk of hip fracture by as much as 2% (from 10 to 8%, a relative reduction of 20%).

Protocol. Women should be measured to make a diagnosis of low bone mass when ERT is being considered for the prevention of bone loss or treatment of osteoporosis. This could include women of any age who had amenorrhea of greater than 6 months' duration. The majority of these women would be perimenopausal. In addition, younger women with prolonged amenorrhea would be eligible if prevention of bone loss was of clinical concern and ERT (including oral contraceptives) was being considered.

Women who were to be placed on long-term ERT for other reasons than prevention of bone loss or treatment of osteoporosis need not be measured. Likewise, women in whom ERT is contraindicated or who refuse to consider estrogen or some other therapy to slow bone loss do not need bone mass measurements.

Bone mass can be measured in the spine by QCT or DPA or DEXA, in the hip by DPA or DEXA or in the radius or os calcis by SPA. Bone mass measurements of the hip or spine may prove to be better predictors of fractures at these sites than would measurement of the peripheral skeleton. However, this must be documented in prospective studies, because peripheral measurements have been shown to predict fractures (19–25).

Women who are amenorrheic and whose bone mass is about equal to or more than 1 SD below the mean for young (age 30–35) normals should be strongly considered for ERT. One standard deviation below the mean is close to the empirical fracture threshold of ~1.0 g/cm^2 in the proximal femur (z-score = -0.79 for cervical and -0.46 for intertrochanteric bone mineral density) and in the spine (z-score = -1.29 for lumbar spine BMD) as assessed by DPA (1). A comparable level in the distal radius (z-score = -1.0) is 0.82 g/cm by SPA. The specific method of administration of estrogen or estrogen/progestin is discussed in Chapter 56. The length of time therapy should be continued is not certain, but a minimum of 5–10 years is suggested by results of case-control studies (38).

Patients whose bone mass is greater than 1 SD above the mean for young normals are relatively protected from osteoporosis and have lower risk of fracture. They probably need no further measurement. If concern arises, measurement can be repeated in 5 or more years and ERT considered at that time. Estrogen replacement therapy is not usually indicated for patients within ±1 SD of the mean, but they may benefit from measurements after 3–5 years to see if they have developed low bone mass.

Roentgenographic Abnormalities

Indication 2—In patients with vertebral abnormalities or roentgenographic osteopenia, bone mass measurements would be used to diagnose spinal osteoporosis in order to make decisions about further diagnostic evaluation and therapy.

Rationale. Patients commonly present with roentgenographic findings consistent with spinal osteoporosis. These are either a radiologist's diagnosis of spinal osteopenia or, often, abnormalities of the thoracic or lumbar vertebrae, including anterior wedging or endplate deformities. A diagnosis of osteoporosis should prompt an evaluation to exclude treatable causes of accelerated bone loss and should stimulate aggressive therapy to prevent further bone loss or to increase spinal bone mass. The complete clinical evaluation is potentially expensive and therapy is associated with costs and health risk. Although indiscriminate treatment of such patients would lead to the maximum reduction of fracture risk, there is evidence that many individuals with vertebral abnormalities do not have significant osteoporosis. Consequently, the costs and risks associated with the clinical work-up and long-term therapy cannot be justified for them, and it becomes essential to identify among those with roentgenographic vertebral abnormalities that smaller group with reduced bone mass.

Background. There is a spectrum of bone mass in patients with vertebral abnormalities or apparent osteopenia on roentgenogram. Not all patients with roentgenographic findings suggestive of osteopenia actually have the condition. The roentgenographic appearance of osteopenia is notoriously inaccurate. In addition to insensitivity in detecting bone loss (64,65), roentgenographic osteopenia is not correlated with vertebral fractures. For example, 29% of 218 ambulatory women aged 45 or over seen as outpatients at Henry Ford Hospital had roentgenographic osteopenia, but only one-seventh of them had vertebral wedging or compression (66). Because the appearance of osteopenia can result from technical faults on the roentgenogram (67), normal individuals can be misclassified. Even vertebral fractures do not provide clear-cut evidence for osteoporosis. Some true fractures are due to episodes of severe trauma earlier in life (68), whereas others are not fractures at all but represent old juvenile epiphysitis or positioning problems on the roentgenogram (69) or normal variations in vertebral body shape (70).

Although change in vertebral shape indicate a fracture, change typically cannot be assessed due to the absence of baseline roentgenograms. Thus, fractures must often be diagnosed empirically, based on deviation from expected vertebral dimensions. The clinical setting provides little guidance, because vertebral fracture symptoms may be nonspecific (66,71,72). Inevitably, osteoporosis will be overdiagnosed in this clinical setting. Among an age-stratified random sample of Rochester, Minnesota, women,

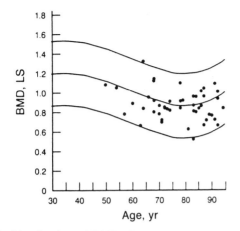

FIG. 4. Distribution of BMD of lumbar spine *(LS)*, by age, among Rochester, Minnesota women. The relation is best described by a cubic model: $\hat{\mu} = 0.517835 + 0.4922212 \times 10^{-1} \times age - 0.105822 \times 10^{-2} \times age^2 + 0.625726 \times 10^{-5} \times age^3; \hat{\sigma} = 0.158749, r^2 = 0.33$. Values for women aged 50 years and over with one or more vertebral fractures are also indicated (●). (From Melton LJ III, Kan SH, Frye MA, Wahner HW, O'Fallon WM, Riggs BL: Epidemiology of vertebral fractures in women. *Am J Epidemiol* 129: 1000–1011, 1989.)

one-fourth had vertebral abnormalities of one sort or another, but 21% of these women with apparent vertebral fractures had lumbar spine BMD values above the theoretical "fracture threshold" of 0.97 g/cm^2 (Fig. 4). As noted previously, vertebral fracture is related to bone mass and bone mass measurements predict probability of future fractures.

Bone mass measurements will lead to an increase in appropriate outcomes (reduced inappropriate evaluation and therapy for patients without osteoporosis). Practical savings to be derived from making bone mass measurements in this setting depend on the frequency with which vertebral abnormalities are encountered. It has been estimated that >2 million women between the ages 50 and 70 have vertebral fractures (73) and as many as one-fifth of these may have bone mass above the "fracture threshold." Thus, there is a potential for evaluating or treating as many as 400,000 middle-aged women when they in fact have normal bone mass.

Protocol. Any patient with a specific sign suggestive of spinal osteoporosis, including roentgenographic osteopenia or evidence suggestive of collapse, wedging, or ballooning of one or more thoracic or lumbar vertebral bodies, should have bone mass measurements, if that patient is a candidate for therapeutic intervention or extensive diagnostic evaluation. Bone mass measurements are not indicated for patients whose work-up or treatment will not be altered by bone mass measurements (e.g., patients previously evaluated for whom no specific treatment was indicated). In this setting, bone mass should be measured in the spine by DPA, DEXA, or QCT.

Patients with vertebral abnormalities and spinal BMD above the "fracture threshold" would not be considered to have fractures on the basis of osteoporosis, and consequently, would not require a work-up for metabolic bone

disease nor would they be treated for established osteoporosis, because all such therapy is aimed at preserving bone mass or increasing it. Women with vertebral abnormalities and spinal BMD below the "fracture threshold" would be considered to have osteoporotic fractures and would be further evaluated.

Glucocorticoid Therapy

Indication 3—In patients receiving long-term glucocorticoid therapy bone mass measurements would be used to diagnose low bone mass (see Chapter 61).

Steroid therapy is required for a number of diseases, such as rheumatoid arthritis, chronic active hepatitis, inflammatory bowel disease, and asthma. This therapy has a number of serious side effects, including rapid bone loss leading to vertebral and other fractures (74–77). Some, but not all, steroid-treated patients experience this excessive bone loss (Fig. 5) and not all have fractures. The importance of assessment is increased because patients are frequently on long-term therapy. Moreover, unlike involutional osteoporosis, patients may be children in whom it would need to be determined whether skeletal development was lagging behind normal adolescent development patterns. Information about bone mass may permit improved patient management through more precise adjustments of dose and duration of therapy to maximize therapeutic effects while minimizing skeletal complications.

Protocol. Patients who are to be placed on long-term (more than 1 month) glucocorticoid treatment (a dose > 7.5 mg of prednisone/day or equivalent) can

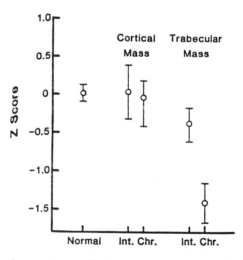

FIG. 5. Comparison of trabecular mass and cortical mass in normal controls and patients. The z-score is a function of the mean ± SD of age-adjusted and sex-adjusted values. *Int.* denotes intermittent steroid use, and *Chr.* chronic, or long-term, use. Trabecular mass in the long-term-use group was significantly smaller than in the normal ($p < 0.01$) and intermittent-use ($p < 0.03$) groups. *Bars* denote ± SEM. (From Adinoff AD, Hollister JR: Steroid-induced fractures and bone loss in patients with asthma. *N Engl J Med* 309:265–268, 1983.)

have bone mass measurements when it is possible to adjust the dose. Measurements of the spine using DPA or DEXA or QCT are advised, because trabecular bone is primarily affected (Fig. 5).

Primary Hyperparathyroidism

Indication 4—In patients with asymptomatic primary hyperparathyroidism, bone mass measurements would be used to diagnose low bone mass in order to identify those at risk of severe skeletal disease who may be candidates for surgical intervention (see Chapter 29).

The clinical spectrum at presentation of primary hyperparathyroidism has changed with the advent of routine biochemical screening (78). Previously, patients presented with symptomatic bone disease, renal stones or other complaints that alerted the physician and that lead to surgical intervention. Now, many of the patients are asymptomatic and have no obvious complications. The management of such asymptomatic individuals remains controversial (79). Primary hyperparathyroidism is associated with a decrease in bone mass in some patients, which can be detected by measurement of bone mass but not by usual radiographic evaluation (Fig. 6) (80). Such a

reduction in bone mass may be accompanied by an increased frequency of fractures of the vertebrae, distal radius, and hip (81). Thus, it can be argued that the finding of low bone mass in patients with otherwise asymptomatic hyperparathyroidism should be considered a possible indication for surgery. Following successful surgery, bone mass has generally been found to increase, although not to normal values, when measured in the radius (82–85), the spine (85) and the total body (86). Because low bone mass is related to fracture risk, an increase in bone mass should reduce the risk of subsequent fractures.

Protocol. Diagnosis of primary hyperparathyroidism should be made using acceptable clinical criteria. Those who have no symptoms that could be attributed to primary hyperparathyroidism that would lead to surgery should have measurements. Bone mass may be measured in the radius by SPA or in the spine by DPA or DEXA or QCT.

Other Potential Indications

With the improvement in technology leading to better precision and accuracy of measurement, other indications for clinical application of bone mass measurements may develop. However, at the time this information was written, insufficient data existed to meet all the criteria outlined at the outset.

Universal Screening for Osteoporosis Prophylaxis. Bone mass measurement for osteoporosis prophylaxis may meet some of the criteria for a screening test (i.e., the disease is common; screening tests are available; effective therapy is available for patients with abnormal tests; and treatment should reduce fracture incidence). However, some patients might be on effective treatment for reasons unrelated to osteoporosis, whereas others might decline therapy regardless of bone mass measurement. In addition, optimal screening regimens have not been determined. However, selective screening as outlined previously is justifiable.

Monitoring Bone Mass to Assess the Efficacy of Therapy. Some have concluded that it is difficult to assess true change in bone mass with two measurements taken closely enough together to provide relevant data for managing treatment (87,88). For example, two measurements of an individual 1 year apart, given a 2% SD of the difference between measurements and no bone loss between the measurements, would yield a 95% probability interval for the difference between the measurements extending from −5.6 to +5.6%. This results from the basic statistical fact that the variance of the difference between two measurements equals the sum of the two individual variances. Critics often note that bone loss over life is only ~1%/year in women and half that figure in men and conclude that prospects are dim for monitoring changes in bone mass reliably. However, the issue is considerably more complex than this for these three reasons: 1) recent changes in technology have improved precision of longitudinal measurement, but the extent of this improvement is not as yet clear; 2) rates of bone loss around the time of menopause may be much greater than 1%, particularly in trabecular bone; and 3) populations for whom such moni-

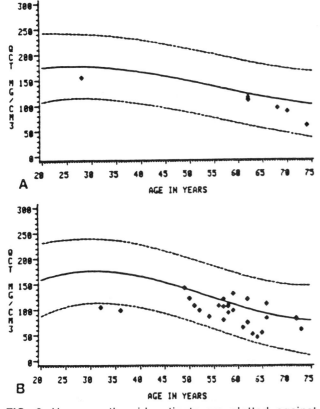

FIG. 6. Hyperparathyroid patients are plotted against normal curves as determined by QCT in males **(A)** and females **(B)**. *Solid curves* indicate the cubic regression lines and *dashed lines* indicate the 95% confidence limits for the normal subjects. (From Richardson ML, Pozzi-Mucelli RS, Kanter AS, Kolb FO, Ettinger B, Genant HK: Bone mineral changes in primary hyperparathyroidism. *Skel Radiol* 15:85–95, 1986.)

toring might be beneficial vary greatly. Considering ERT, the example given previously implies that, even with completely effective treatment (no bone loss in any subject), a small 2.5% group of individuals would have apparent bone loss exceeding 5.6%, when in fact no bone had been lost. However, such data can also be viewed in a somewhat different light. Consider, for example, a population of 100 early menopausal women receiving ERT where 15% do not respond to therapy and lose vertebral bone at a rate of 3%/year, whereas the other 85% lose no bone. (In fact, the latter group would probably experience a small gain in bone during the first years of therapy). If the 100 women were reassessed at the end of 1 year, ~2 of the 85 responders would have apparent bone loss of >5% (an arbitrary cutoff for nonresponse), whereas ~4 of the 15 nonresponders would be detected as having >5% loss/year. Therefore, about two-thirds of those designated as nonresponders would come from the true nonresponders, and 73% of the nonresponders might be missed. Although this does not provide convincing evidence for the usefulness of these methods in the estimation of changes in bone mass, slight alterations in the assumptions or in the precision of the technique greatly enhance this picture. For example, if the precision of the new methods (DEXA) is 1% (which appears to be approximately correct for spine measurements) and the same example is used (15% nonresponders) and the interval between measurements is increased to 2 years, then ~84% of the nonresponders would demonstrate bone loss exceeding 3%, whereas few or none of the responders would be misclassified.

No gain in bone has been assumed in these calculations, and as has been shown, there is a small but important increase in bone mass in patients on ERT. Including such gains in bone mass would further enhance differentiation between those responding to therapy and those not. Before deciding that measuring rates of change can be done in the clinical arena, we need evidence that good precision can be maintained over longer periods of times. Certainly, these methods are applicable to the study of patients on investigational therapy where large increases of bone mass may be seen (e.g., sodium fluoride, bisphosphonates, and low-dose parathyroid hormone). However, these would not have general clinical applicability until such therapies were Food and Drug Administration-approved.

Identifying "Fast Losers" of Bone for More Aggressive Therapy. Some have found evidence for a subgroup of postmenopausal women who lose bone at an accelerated rate (89,90). A combination of bone mass measurement and markers of bone turnover were utilized to identify those at the greatest risk of osteoporotic fractures, assuming that such rates of loss continue for long periods of time. The implication is that these women will ultimately develop clinically important fractures. It did appear that there were more vertebral fractures, but not Colles' fractures, among those losing rapidly (90). Should these data be confirmed, the most efficient way to identify those at highest fracture risk would be through a combination of markers and a bone mass measurement. Until these data

have been confirmed, the identification of rapid losers remains investigational.

REFERENCES

1. Johnston CC Jr, Melton LJ III, Lindsay R, Eddy D: Clinical indication for bone mass measurement. *J Bone Miner Res* 4(suppl 2), pp 1–28, 1989
2. Boshong S: *Radiologic Science for Technologists: Physics, Biology and Protection, 4th ed.* CV Mosby Co., St. Louis, 1988
3. Kereiakes J, Rosenstein M: *Handbook of Radiation Doses in Nuclear Medicine and Diagnostic Radiology.* CRC Press, Boca Raton, Florida, 1980
4. Mazess RB, Wahner HW: Nuclear medicine and densitometry. In: Riggs BL, Melton LJ (eds) *Osteoporosis: Etiology, Diagnosis, and Management.* Raven Press, New York, pp 251–295, 1988
5. Hayes WC, Gerhart TN: Biomechanics of bone. Applications for assessment of bone strength. Chapter 9. In: Peck WA (ed) *Bone and Mineral Research/3.* Elsevier Science Publishers V.B., Amsterdam, pp 259–294, 1985
6. Melton LJ, Chao EYS, Lane J: Biomechanical aspects of fractures. Chapter 4. In: Riggs BL, Melton LJ (eds) *Osteoporosis: Etiology, Diagnosis, and Management.* Raven Press, New York, pp 111–131, 1988
7. Riggs BL, Wahner HW, Seeman E, Offord KP, Dunn WL, Mazess RB, Johnson KA, Melton LJ: Changes in bone mineral density of the proximal femur and spine with aging: Differences between the postmenopausal and senile osteoporosis syndromes. *J Clin Invest* 70:716–723, 1982
8. Ross PD, Davis JW, Vogel JM, Wasnich RD: A critical review of bone mass and the risk of fractures in osteoporosis. *Calcif Tissue Int* 46:149–161, 1990
9. Melton LJ, Wahner HW, Richelson LS, O'Fallon WM, Riggs BL: Osteoporosis and the risk for hip fracture. *Am J Epidemiol* 124:254–261, 1986
10. Cummings SR, Black DM, Nevitt MC, Browner W, Cauley J, Ensrud K, Genant HK, Gluer CC, Hulley SB, Palermo L, Scott J, Vogt TM, and the Study of Osteoporotic Fractures Research Group: Bone density at various sites for prediction of hip fractures. *Lancet* 341(1):72–75, 1993
11. Melton LJ, Kan SH, Wahner HW, Riggs BL: Lifetime fracture risk: An approach to hip fracture risk assessment based on bone mineral density and age. *J Clin Epidemiol* 41:985–994, 1988
12. Parfitt AM, Duncan H: Metabolic bone disease affecting the spine. Chapter 13. In: Rothman RH, Simeone FA (eds) *The Spine.* W. B. Saunders, Philadelphia, pp 775–905, 1982
13. Melton LJ, Cummings SR: Heterogeneity of age-related fractures: Implications for epidemiology. *Bone Miner* 2:321–331, 1987
14. Cummings SR, Nevitt MC: Epidemiology of hip fractures and falls. In: Kleerekoper M, Krane SM (eds) *Clinical Disorders of Bone and Mineral Metabolism.* Mary Ann Liebert, Inc., New York, pp 231–236, 1989
15. Hayes WC, Piazza SJ, Zysset PK: Biomechanics of fracture risk prediction of the hip and spine by quantitative computed tomography. *Radiol Clin North Am* 29:1–18, 1991
16. Krolner B, Pors Nielsen S: Bone mineral content of the lumbar spine in normal and osteoporotic women: Cross sectional and longitudinal studies. *Clin Sci* 62:329–336, 1982
17. Cummings SR: Are patients with hip fractures more osteoporotic? Review of the evidence. *Am J Med* 78:487–494, 1985
18. Aitken JM: Relevance of osteoporosis in women with fractures of the femoral neck. *Br Med J* 288:597–601, 1984
19. Hui SL, Slemenda CW, Johnston CC Jr: Age and bone mass as predictors of fracture in a prospective study. *J Clin Invest* 81:1804–1809, 1988
20. Wasnich RD, Ross PD, Heilbrun LK, Vogel JM: Selection of the optimal site for fracture risk prediction. *Clin Orthop* 216:262–268, 1987
21. Gardsell P, Johnell O, Nilsson BE: The predictive value of bone

loss for fragility fractures in women: A longitudinal study over 15 years. *Calcif Tissue Int* 49:90–94, 1991

22. Black DM, Cummings SR, Genant HK, Nevitt MC, Palermo L, Browner W: Axial and appendicular bone density predict fractures in older women. *J Bone Miner Res* 7:633–638, 1992

23. Ross PD, Wasnich RD, Vogel JM: Detection of prefracture spinal osteoporosis using bone mineral absorptiometry. *J Bone Miner Res* 3:1–11, 1988

24. Smith DM, Khairi MRA, Johnston CC Jr: The loss of bone mineral with aging and its relationship to risk of fracture. *J Clin Invest* 56:311–318, 1975

25. Hui SL, Slemenda CW, Johnston CC Jr: Baseline measurement of bone mass predicts fracture in white women. *Ann Intern Med* 111:355–361, 1989

26. Cummings SR, Black DM, Nevitt MC, Browner WS, Cauley JA, Genant HK, Mascioli SR, Scott JC, Seeley DG, Steiger P, Vogt TM, and the Study of Osteoporotic Fractures Research Group: Appendicular bone density and age predict hip fracture in women. *JAMA* 263:665–668, 1990

27. Seeley DG, Browner WS, Nevitt MC, Genant HK, Scott JC, Cummings SR, and the Study of Osteoporotic Fractures Research Group: Which fractures are associated with low appendicular bone mass in elderly women? *Ann Intern Med* 115:837–842, 1991

28. Eastell R, Wahner HW, O'Fallon WM, Amadio PC, Melton LJ III, Riggs BL: Unequal decrease in bone density of lumbar spine and ultradistal radius in Colles' and vertebral fracture syndromes. *J Clin Invest* 83:168–174, 1989

29. Heidrich F, Thompson RS: Osteoporosis prevention: Strategies applicable for general population groups. *J Family Pract* 25:33–39, 1987

30. Davis MR: Screening for postmenopausal osteoporosis. *Am J Obstet Gynecol* 156:1–5, 1987

31. Cummings SR, Kelsey JL, Nevitt MC, O'Dowd KJ: Epidemiology of osteoporosis and osteoporotic fractures. *Epidemiol Rev* 7:178–208, 1985

32. Trotter MN, Broman GE, Peterson RR: Densities of bones of white and Negro skeletons. *J Bone Joint Surg* 42A:50–58, 1960

33. Nordin BEC, MacGregor J, Smith DA: The incidence of osteoporosis in normal women. Its relation to age and the menopause. *Quart J Med* 137:25–28, 1966

34. Alffram P: An epidemiologic study of cervical and trochanteric fractures of the femur in an urban population. *Acta Orthop Scand* (Suppl) 65:1–109, 1964

35. Smith DM, Johnston CC Jr, Yu PL: In vivo measurement of bone mass. *JAMA* 219:325–329, 1972

36. Daniels HW: Osteoporosis of the slender smoker: Vertebral compression fractures and loss of metacarpal cortex in relation to postmenopausal cigarette smoking and lack of obesity. *Arch Intern Med* 136:298–304, 1976

37. Hutchinson A, Polansky SM, Feinstein AR: Post-menopausal estrogens protect against fractures of hip and distal radius: A case-control study. *Lancet* 2:705–709, 1979

38. Paganini-Hill A, Ross RK, Gerkins JR, Henderson BE, Arthur M, Mack TM: Menopausal estrogen therapy and hip fractures. *Ann Intern Med* 95:28–31, 1981

39. Lindsay R: The influence of cigarette smoking on bone mass and bone loss (abstract). In: DeLuca HF, Frost HM, Jee WSS, Johnston CC Jr, Parfitt AM (eds) *Osteoporosis: Recent Advances in Pathogenesis and Treatment*. University Park Press, Baltimore, p 481, 1981

40. Melton LJ, Riggs BL: Clinical spectrum. In: Riggs BL, Melton LJ (eds) *Osteoporosis: Etiology, Diagnosis and Management*. Raven Press, New York, pp 155–179, 1988

41. Wasnich RD, Ross PD, Vogel JM, MacLean CJ: The relative strengths of osteoporotic risk factors in a prospective study of postmenopausal osteoporosis. *J Bone Miner Res* 2(suppl 1):343, 1987

42. Yano K, Wasnich RD, Vogel JM, Heilbrun LK: Bone mineral measurements among middle-aged and elderly Japanese residents in Hawaii. *Am J Epidemiol* 119:751–764, 1984

43. Sowers MR, Wallace RD, Lemke JH: Correlates of mid-radius bone density among postmenopausal women: A community study. *Am J Clinical Nutr* 41:1045–1053, 1985

44. Ismail F, Epstein S, Pacific R, Droke D, Thomas SB, Avioli LV: Serum bone gla protein (BGP) and other markers of bone mineral metabolism in postmenopausal osteoporosis. *Calcif Tissue Int* 39:230–233, 1986

45. Jones KP, Ravuikar VA, Tukhinsky D, Schiff: Comparison of bone density in amenorrheic women due to athletics weight loss and premature menopause. *Obstet Gynecol* 66:5–7, 1987

46. Evers SE, Orchard JW, Haddad RG: Bone density in postmenopausal North American Indians and Caucasian females. *Hum Biology* 57:719–726, 1985

47. Citron JT, Ettinger B, Genant HK: Prediction of peak premenopausal bone mass using a scale of weighted clinical variables. In: Christiansen C, Johansen JS, Riis BJ (eds) *Osteoporosis 1987*, I. Norhaven A/S, Viborg, Denmark, pp 146–149, 1987

48. Slemenda CW, Hui SL, Longcope C, Wellman H, Johnston CC Jr: Predictors of bone mass in perimenopausal women: A prospective study of clinical data using photon absorptiometry. *Ann Intern Med* 112:96–101, 1990

49. Lindsay R, Aitken JM, Anderson JB, Hart DM, McDonald EB, Clark AC: Long-term prevention of postmenopausal osteoporosis by estrogen. *Lancet* 1:1038–1041, 1976

50. Lindsay R, Hart DM, Forrest C, Baird C: Prevention of spinal osteoporosis in oophorectomized women. *Lancet* 2:1151–1154, 1980

51. Abdalla H, Hart DM, Lindsay R: Differential bone loss and effects of long-term estrogen therapy according to time of introduction of therapy after oophorectomy. In: Christiansen C, et al. (eds) *Osteoporosis 2*. Aalborg Stifsbogtrykkeri, Copenhagen, Denmark, pp 621–624, 1984

52. Quigley MET, Martin PL, Burnier AM, Brooks P: Estrogen therapy arrests bone loss in elderly women. *Am J Obstet Gynecol* 156:1516–1523, 1987

53. Ettinger B, Genant HK, Cann CE: Long-term estrogen therapy prevents bone loss and fracture. *Ann Intern Med* 102:319–324, 1985

54. Christiansen C, Christiansen MS, McNair PL, Hagen C, Stocklund KE, Transbol I: Prevention of early postmenopausal bone loss: Conducted 2-year study in 315 normal females. *Eur J Clin Invest* 10:273–279, 1980

55. Genant HK, Cann CE, Ettinger B, Gordon GS: Quantitative computed tomography of vertebral spongiosa: A sensitive method for detecting early bone loss after oophorectomy. *Ann Intern Med* 97:699–705, 1982

56. Horsman A, Gallagher JC, Simpson M, Nordin BEC: Prospective trial of estrogen and calcium in postmenopausal women. *Br Med J* 2:789–792, 1977

57. Horsman A, James M, Francis R: The effect of estrogen dose on postmenopausal bone loss. *N Engl J Med* 309:1405–1407, 1983

58. Nachtigall LE, Nachtigall RH, Nachtigall RD: Estrogen replacement therapy I: A 10-year prospective study in the relationship of osteoporosis. *Obstet Gynecol* 53:277–283, 1979

59. Recker RR, Saville PD, Heaney RP: The effect of estrogens and calcium carbonate on bone loss in postmenopausal women. *Ann Intern Med* 87:649–655, 1977

60. Weiss NS, Ure CL, Ballard JH, Williams AR, Daline G JR: Decreased risk of fractures of the hip and lower forearm with postmenopausal use of estrogens. *N Engl J Med* 303:1195–1198, 1980

61. Johnson RE, Specht EE: The risk of hip fracture in postmenopausal females with and without estrogen drug exposure. *Am J Public Health* 71:138–144, 1981

62. Kreiger N, Kelsey JL, Holford TR, O'Connor T: An epidemiological study of hip fracture in postmenopausal women. *Am J Epidemiol* 116:141–148, 1982

63. Kiel DP, Felson DT, Andereson JJ, Wilson PWF, Moskowitz MA: Hip fracture and the use of estrogens in postmenopausal women: The Framingham Study. *N Engl J Med* 317:1169–1174, 1987

64. Lachman E: Osteoporosis: The potentialities and limitations of its roentgenologic diagnosis. *Am J Roentgenol* 74:712–715, 1955

65. Lutwak L, Whedon GD: Osteoporosis. In: Dowling HF, Aldrich RA, Burnett CH, Finland M, Ingelfinger FJ, Myers JD (eds)

Disease-a-month. Bar Book Medical Publisher Inc., Chicago, pp 1–39, 1963

66. Smith RW Jr, Rizek J: Epidemiologic studies of osteoporosis in women of Puerto Rico and southeastern Michigan with special reference to age, race, national origin and to other related or associated findings. *Clin Orthop* 45:31–48, 1966
67. Genant HK, Vogler JB, Block JE: Radiology of osteoporosis. Chapter 7. In: Riggs BL, Melton LJ III (eds). *Osteoporosis: Etiology, Diagnosis and Management.* Raven Press, New York, pp 181–220, 1988
68. Riggs LB, Wahner HW: Bone densitometry and clinical decision-making in osteoporosis. *Ann Intern Med* 108:293–295, 1988
69. Doyle FH, Gutteridge DH, Joplin GF, Fraser R: An assessment of raiological criteria used in the study of spinal osteoporosis. *Br J Radiol* 40:241–250, 1967
70. Gallagher JC, Hedlund LR, Stoner S, Meeger C: Vertebral morphometry: Normative data. *Bone and Mineral* 4:189–196, 1988
71. Gerson-Cohen J, Rechtman AM, Schraer H: Asymptomatic fractures in osteoporotic spines of the aged. *JAMA* 153:625–627, 1953
72. Ettinger B, Genant HK, Cann CE: Postmenopausal bone loss is prevented by treatment with low-dosage estrogen with calcium. *Ann Intern Med* 106:40–45, 1987
73. Melton LJ III: Epidemiology of vertebral fractures: In: Christiansen C, Johansen JS, Riis BJ (eds). *Osteoporosis.* Osteopress A/S, Copenhagen, pp 33–37, 1987
74. Gennari C: Glucocorticoids and bone. In: Peck WA (ed) *Bone and Mineral Research/3.* Elsevier, Amsterdam, 1985
75. Peck W, Gennari C, Raisz L, Meunier P, Ritz E, Krane S, Nuki G, Avioli LV: Corticosteroids and bone: Round table discussion. *Calcif Tiss Int* 36:4–7, 1984
76. Baylink DJ: Glucocortocoid-induced osteoporosis. *N Engl J Med* 309:306–308, 1983
77. Richardson ML, Genant HK, Cann CE, Ettinger BE: Assessment of metabolic bone diseases by quantitative computerized tomography. *Clin Orthop* 185:224–238, 1985
78. Heath H III: Clinical spectrum of primary hyperparathyroidism: Evolution with changes in medical practice and technology. *J Bone Miner Res* 6(suppl 2):S63–S70, 1991
79. Anonymous: Consensus Development Conference Statement. *J Bone Miner Res* 6(suppl 2):S9–S13, 1991
80. Richardson ML, Pozzi-Mucelli RS, Kanter AS, Kolb FO, Ettinger B, Genant HK: Bone mineral changes in primary hyperparathyroidism. *Skel Radiol* 15:85–95, 1986
81. Peacock M, Horman A, Aaron JE, Marshall DH, Selby PL, Simpson M: The role of parathyroid hormone in bone loss. In: Christiansen C, Arnaud CD, Nordin BEC, et al. (eds) *Osteoporosis 1.* Aalborg Stifsbogtrykkeri, Copenhagen, Denmark, pp 463–467, 1984
82. Leppla DC, Snyder W, Pak CYC: Sequential changes in bone density before and after parathyroidectomy in primary hyperparathyroidism. *Invest Radiol* 17:604–606, 1982
83. Mautalen C, Reyes HR, Ghiringhelli G, Fromm G: Cortical bone mineral content in primary hyperparathyroidism: Changes after parathyroidectomy. *Acta Endocrinol* 111:494–497, 1986
84. Martin P, Bergmann P, Gillet C, Fuss M, Kinnaert P, Covilain J, Van Geertruyden J: Long-term irreversibility of bone loss after surgery for primary hyperparathyroidism. *Arch Intern Med* 150:1495–1497, 1990
85. Abugassa S, Nordenstrom J, Eriksson S, Mollerstrom G, Alveryd A: Skeletal remineralization after surgery for primary and secondary hyperparathyroidism. *Surgery* 107:128–133, 1990
86. Eastell R, Kennedy NSJ, Smith MA, Tothill P, Edwards CRW: Changes in total body calcium following surgery for primary hyperparathyroidism. *Bone* 7:269–272, 1986
87. Heaney RP: En recherche de la difference (P < 0.05)*, *Bone Miner* 1:99–114, 1986
88. Cummings SR, Black D: Should perimenopausal women be screened for osteoporosis? *Ann Intern Med* 104:817–823, 1986
89. Christiansen C, Riis BJ, Rodbro P: Prediction of rapid bone loss in postmenopausal women. *Lancet* 1:1105–1108, 1987
90. Hansen MA, Overgaard K, Riis BJ, Christiansen C: Role of peak bone mass and bone loss in postmenopausal osteoporosis: 12 year study. *Bone Miner J* 303:961–964, 1991

27. Bone Biopsy and Histomorphometry in Clinical Practice

Robert R. Recker, M.D.

Department of Medicine, Creighton University, Omaha, Nebraska

Metabolic bone disease in adult humans is fundamentally a disease of the bone remodeling system. Remodeling also occurs in children where modeling is the predominant bone system. These systems can be directly examined by performing histomorphometric analysis of microscopic sections of trabecular bone from transilial bone biopsies. Fluorochromes must be given as tissue-time markers before biopsy, and the specimens must be processed without removal of mineral.

BONE REMODELING SYSTEM

The bone remodeling system has been characterized in numerous publications in the recent past (1). A brief summary is presented herein.

Bone remodeling occurs on trabecular and Haversian bone surfaces. The first step is activation of osteoclast precursors to form osteoclasts that then begin to excavate a cavity on a surface. After removal of ~0.05 mm³ of bone tissue, the site remains quiescent for a short time, following which activation of osteoblast precursors occurs at the site and the excavation is refilled. Ideally there is no net change in the amount of bone after the work is finished. The average length of time required to complete the remodeling cycle is ~5 months (2), ~3 weeks for resorption and the rest for formation. This process serves several functions, among them the removal of aged, microdamaged bone tissue and rearrangement of the bone architecture to meet the needs of mechanical support. With normal daily use of the skeleton, bone loss, abnormal accumulation of microdamage, or errors in geometry can come about only through defects in this system. Impediments to bone cell function such as vitamin D deficiency are manifest through this system.

Frost (3) has pointed out that population dynamics can be applied to the remodeling events that occur continuously in the skeleton (3). These dynamics can be examined by the use of histomorphometry of nondecalcified sections of trabecular bone from biopsies taken after appropriate labeling with tissue-time markers.

BIOPSY PROCEDURE

The transilial approach is preferred over the vertical one by most workers, because there is less discomfort to the patient and most of the best quality normal reference data from living subjects comes from transilial biopsies (2).

Most clinicians prefer to use the biopsy site located ~2 cm posterior to the anterior superior spine immediately inferior to the crest. With the patient supine and the hip slightly elevated on a folded sheet, the biopsy site can be located by grasping the ala of the ilium with the thumb and forefinger immediately posterior to the anterior superior spine. The thumb then falls into the spot where the skin incision should be made and the trephine should be inserted. After mild sedation with intravenous benzodiazepine, the area to be prepped and the location for placement of the local anesthetic should be marked with a felt-tipped pen. The surgeon should perform a complete scrub; he should wear cap, mask, gown, and gloves; and the operative site should be prepped and draped. The core of bone should be removed through a 1.5 cm incision using blunt dissection as much as possible. The wound can be closed with two or three sutures of 5-0 monofilament. After 2 hr of quiet rest, the patient can be permitted to return to usual activities with instructions to keep the dressing dry and to avoid heavy physical activity for a few days. After 7 days, the suture can be removed.

The most important advice for the surgeon is to use very gentle pressure to advance the trephine through the ilium. This requires great patience, because the tendency is to hurry through the biopsy site pressing even harder as the trephine advances. Excessive pressure on the trephine will crush most osteopenic specimens and will create excessive artifact in others.

Complications of the procedure include mild postoperative discomfort in ~90% of the cases, moderate discomfort in ~5% of the cases, and more than moderate in ~5% of the cases. Severe complications are very rare (4). Bleeding has occurred in a few cases, usually in patients with clotting defects such as renal patients. There have been a few cases of temporary femoral nerve palsy thought to be due to hematoma formation. The procedure itself is nearly pain-free.

BIOPSY INSTRUMENT

There are several instruments that can be used (4), some that are motor-driven. It is important to use a trephine with inner diameter of 7.5–8.0 mm in order to obtain a large enough specimen for proper histomorphometric analysis. The most important feature of the instrument is that the teeth be very sharp.

Proper sharpening can be difficult to achieve. The author has solved this problem by acquiring a miniature machine tool to perform the sharpening in the bone laboratory.

TETRACYCLINE LABELING

The ideal tissue-time bone fluorochrome label for use in humans is one of the tetracycline antibiotics. Fluorochromes that are not of this class of drugs cannot be given because of safety reasons. Demeclocycline fluoresces with an orange color and all the remainder fluoresce with a light lemon color. Most observers possess enough color acuity to distinguish between these two labels. This difference in the color of fluorescence can be exploited in order to distinguish between pairs of labels given at different points in time. The author uses tetracycline hydrochloride (250 mg four times daily) or demeclocycline (150 mg four times daily). The tetracycline must be taken on an empty stomach. No dairy products or calcium supplements should be taken for one hour before and after the tetracycline.

There are practical limits for optimal timing of the labels. The minimum schedule is 2 days of label, 10 days free, 2 days of label then 5 days before biopsy (2-10-2:5). The maximum schedule is 3-14-3:5. The author routinely uses 3-14-3:5. A thorough analysis of the optimal labeling schedule has been published (5). Longer labeling schedules will result in few surfaces taking the double label because of the "label-escape" phenomenon and shorter schedules will result in labels spaced too closely together for accurate label width measurements (Fig. 1).

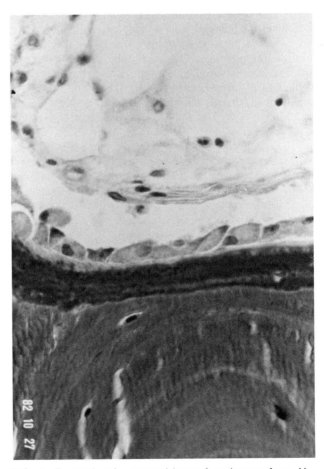

FIG. 1. Example of a normal bone forming surface. Unmineralized osteoid is covered with plump osteoblasts.

HANDLING THE SPECIMENS

The biopsy core specimen should be placed in 70% ethanol immediately following removal. It can be stored for very long times in this solution without deterioration, but it should not be removed in <48 hr in order to ensure proper fixation. The specimen can then be dehydrated, defatted, embedded, and sectioned using one of the published methods (6). Methyl methacrylate is used as the embedding agent in the author's laboratory, but several hard plastics are available and seem to work well. Five μm sections should be cut for light microscopy and 10 μm sections for fluorescence microscopy. A number of stains can be used as previously described (6), and unstained sections should be used with epifluorescence to analyze the fluorochrome labels.

The basic measurements performed at the microscope (2) are trabecular bone volume, bone surface, eroded surface, osteoid surface, mineralized surface, wall thickness, osteoid thickness, and mineral apposition rate. These data can be obtained using a microscope with integrating eyepiece reticule or with camera lucida and drawing tablet. Other important variables can be calculated from these primary data.

INDICATIONS FOR BONE BIOPSY

The first criterion for choosing a diagnostic procedure in clinical medicine is that it establish a diagnosis that will help in a treatment decision. The second is to give information on prognosis. In addition, the risk, discomfort, and expense should be appropriate to the importance of the information to be obtained. In the case of transilial bone biopsy, the list of indications is yet under development and can be expected to expand as more experience is gained and as more of the clinical disorders of bone metabolism become amenable to treatment (Fig. 2).

One impediment to widespread use of the biopsy is that access to it remains limited. Most pathology laboratories are not equipped to handle nondecalcified bone specimens or perform histomorphometry. Nevertheless, Table 1 is offered as if the technology for processing the specimens is available to anyone who desires it.

Postmenopausal Osteoporosis

There are certain situations where bone biopsy is initiated in these patients although it is not indicated in all of

TABLE 1. *Tentative Indications for Transilial Bone Biopsy*

Postmenopausal osteoporosis
Vitamin D-resistant rickets (various forms)
Renal osteodystrophy
Nutritional rickets and osteomalacia
Bone disease associated with chronic GI disease
Bone disease associated with GI surgery
Anticonvulsant osteomalacia
Primary hyperparathyroidism

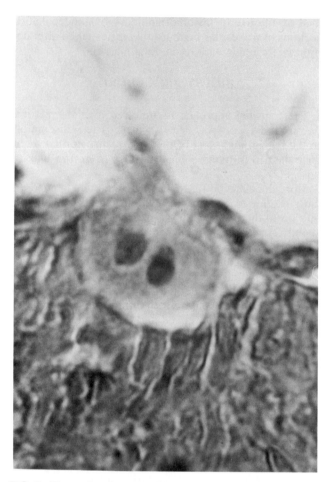

FIG. 2. Example of a normal bone resorbing surface. Multinucleated osteoclasts are located in a Howship's lacuna.

them. For example, it is necessary for most treatment trials in order to be certain that confounding diagnoses are ruled out and to learn whether patients with different remodeling characteristics respond differently to the treatment. The biopsy can be repeated and compared with baseline thus allowing some prediction as to success of the treatment and helping to understand the mechanism of the response before waiting the entire length of time required to detect a bone mass response. In some trials bone biopsy is mandatory in order to determine safety of a test drug that is known or suspected of suppressing remodeling (Fig. 3).

Every new treatment that is tested should be accompanied by bone biopsy until a decision on efficacy can be made. Some treatments can be predicted to fail based on the appearance of the biopsies during treatment. An example would be continuous treatment using an agent that markedly inhibited activation of remodeling and/or impaired bone formation in those remodeling sites undergoing bone formation at the time the agent was introduced. An agent that exhibits these findings on biopsy during treatment might harm the mechanical strength of the skeleton rather than improve it. This problem could be detected earlier by biopsy after fluorochrome labeling than with other technology.

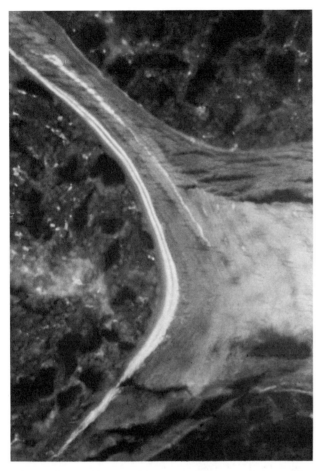

FIG. 3. Mineralizing surface containing two tetracycline labels given on a 3-14-3:5 schedule. One label is tetracycline hydrochloride, and the other is demeclocycline.

The incidence and prevalence of postmenopausal osteoporosis are very high in modern societies (7), and the technology for performing analysis of nondecalcified bone specimens is very limited. It is clearly unrealistic and probably not necessary for every patient with postmenopausal osteoporosis to undergo transilial bone biopsy with tetracycline labeling, because in most cases confounding diagnoses can be ruled out by clinical and clinical biochemical methods. Experimental treatments are administered in centers that usually have the requisite technology and bone biopsy may well be performed. One should be skeptical of trials of new agents or regimens in which transilial bone biopsy coupled with tetracycline labeling is not performed.

Vitamin D-Resistant Rickets

Of course there are many variants of this general syndrome, and a description of the identifying characteristics of each of the known variants is contained in Chapters 68 and 69. Several recent reviews are available for the reader who is interested (8).

These patients present as disorders in growth and development. In the case of a spontaneous mutation, when a family history is not present, bone biopsy may be necessary to make the diagnosis. In patients from families with a known diagnosis and in the follow-up of nonfamilial cases, serial biopsies can be valuable in judging the success of treatment and evaluating the effect of changes in treatment. The evaluation of new treatments requires the use of the biopsy.

Renal Osteodystrophy

This provides the most important diagnostic use of the transilial bone biopsy. Treatment decisions often depend on the results of the biopsy. The most dramatic example is the evaluation of hypercalcemia with bone pain and fractures in patients on chronic dialysis. If the biopsy shows predominantly osteitis fibrosa with brisk bone turnover, then partial parathyroidectomy may be indicated. On the other hand, if the biopsy shows little turnover (little or no fluorochrome label) and extensive aluminum deposits, then treatment with a chelating agent is indicated and parathyroidectomy is contraindicated. The biopsy can also help determine the extent of vitamin D deprivation indicated by the adequacy of vitamin D treatment.

Nutritional Rickets and Osteomalacia

This is very uncommon in the developed world, and thus the call for biopsy to evaluate this is relatively rare. Nevertheless, the problem may be present in occult form among the elderly that reside in nursing homes, retirement centers, or in their own homes and do not get sufficient exposure to sunlight. There has been uncertainty about the biochemical definition of nutritional vitamin D deficiency, and thus the bone biopsy may be a more sensitive way to make the diagnosis (see Chapter 65). In the author's experience, careful histomorphometric analysis and comparison with a valid data base from age- and sex-matched normals (2) are surprisingly sensitive when the measurements of osteoid seam width, osteoid surface, and appositional rate are combined to calculate mineralization lag time (9). It is important to emphasize that simple measurement of osteoid seam width alone is not sufficient to determine whether osteomalacia or "hypovitaminosis D osteopathy" (10) is present.

Bone Disease Associated with GI Disease

The prototype for this category is malabsorption syndrome of any type such as with pancreatic insufficiency or celiac sprue (see Chapter 66). The predominant picture on bone biopsy is osteomalacia, however, the bone loss is proportionally greater than what is seen in "pure" vitamin D deficiency. The lesion seems to be due to both vitamin D and calcium deficiency, the latter due to the combined effects of calcium malabsorption and excessive endogenous fecal calcium losses. Bone biopsy can determine the presence and severity of osteomalacia and response to treatments.

Bone disease can complicate chronic bowel disease such as ulcerative colitis or regional enteritis. The bone biopsy may be the only reliable method of documenting the presence of bone disease in some patients before symptoms develop or before radiographic or biochemical findings develop.

Bone Disease Associated with GI Surgery

Many patients with a history of GI surgery, including gastrectomy and bowel resection, can present with symptoms of musculoskeletal pain, reduced bone mass, and fracture (see Chapter 66). Bone biopsy can be used to document the presence of vitamin D deficiency and distinguish it from the joint and connective tissue disorders that may accompany GI surgery.

Anticonvulsant Osteomalacia

Long-term anticonvulsant therapy, particularly in elderly patients, may cause musculoskeletal pain (11) and vertebral and hip fractures (see Chapters 51 and 72). In addition to osteopenia, patients often have a mineralization defect that produces prolonged mineralization lag time and accumulation of unmineralized osteoid. Transilial bone biopsy may be the only method of discovering this lesion that may require changing the anticonvulsant therapy or adding treatment with one of the vitamin D preparations.

AVAILABILITY OF BONE HISTOMORPHOMETRY

Currently, sufficient laboratory facilities are not available to process biopsies from every patient who seeks medical attention for osteoporosis. However, the procedure of obtaining the specimen is not difficult, and specimens can be mailed to one of the centers now performing bone histomorphometry. It is strongly urged that a physician who contemplates performing the biopsy contact the center ahead of time to obtain explicit instructions on the patient's history, the fluorochrome labeling schedule, performance of the biopsy, fixing solution, and mailing. It should also be made clear that most centers require 4 weeks or more to report the results from a specimen.

REFERENCES

1. Parfitt AM: The cellular basis of bone remodeling: The quantum concept reexamined in light of recent advances in the cell biology of bone. *Calc Tiss Int* 36:S37–S45, 1986
2. Recker RR, Kimmel DB, Parfitt AM, Davies KM, Keshawarz N, Hinders S: Static and tetracycline-based bone histomorphometric data from 34 normal postmenopausal females. *J Bone Min Res* 3:133–144, 1988
3. Frost HM: Tetracycline-based histological analysis of bone remodeling. *Calc Tiss Res* 3:211–239, 1969
4. Rao DS: Practical approach to biopsy. In: Recker RR (ed) *Bone Histomorphometry: Techniques and Interpretation*. CRC Press, Boca Raton, Florida, pp 3–11, 1983
5. Frost HM: Bone histomorphometry: Correction of the labeling "escape error." In: Recker RR (ed) *Bone Histomorphometry: Techniques and Interpretation*. CRC Press, Boca Raton, Florida, pp 133–142, 1983
6. Baron R, Vignery A, Neff L, Silvergate A, Santa Maria A: Processing of undecalcified bone specimens for bone histomorphometry. In: Recker RR (ed) *Bone Histomorphometry: Techniques and Interpretation*. CRC Press, Boca Raton, Florida, pp 13–36, 1983
7. Riggs BL, Melton LJ: Involutional osteoporosis. N Engl J Med 314:1676–1684, 1986
8. Peacock M: Osteomalacia and rickets. In: Nordin BEC (ed) *Metabolic Bone and Stone Diseases*. Churchill Livingstone, London, pp 71–111, 1986
9. Parfitt AM, Drezner MK, Glorieux FH, Kanis JA, Malluche H, Meunier PJ, Ott SM, Recker RR: Histomorphometry: Standardization of nomenclature, symbols and units. *J Bone Min Res* 2: 595–610, 1987
10. Rao DS, Villanueva AR, Mathews M, Pumo B, Frame B, Kleerekoper M, Parfitt AM: Histologic evolution of vitamin D-depletion in patients with intestinal malabsorption or dietary deficiency. In: Frame B, Potts JT (eds) *Clinical Disorders of Bone and Mineral Metabolism*. Excerpta Medica, Amsterdam, pp 224–226, 1983
11. Kragstrup J, Melsen F, Mosekilde L: Reduced wall thickness of completed remodeling sites in iliac trabecular bone following anticonvulsant therapy. *Metab Bone Dis Rel Res* 4:181–185, 1982

SECTION IV

Disorders of Serum Minerals

28. Hypercalcemia: Pathogenesis, Clinical Manifestations, and Differential Diagnosis

Elizabeth Shane, M.D.

Department of Medicine, College of Physicians and Surgeons, Columbia University, New York, New York

The clinical presentation of hypercalcemia may vary from a mild asymptomatic biochemical abnormality detected during routine screening to a life-threatening medical emergency. The pathogenesis, clinical manifestations, differential diagnosis, and management of hypercalcemia will be discussed.

PATHOGENESIS

The concentration of calcium in the extracellular fluid is critical for many physiological processes. Under normal circumstances, the range is remarkably constant, between 8.5–10.5 mg/dL (2.1–2.5 mM). The exact normal ranges vary slightly depending on the laboratory. Approximately half the total serum calcium is bound to plasma proteins, primarily albumin. The remaining half circulates as free calcium ion. It is only this ionized portion of the total serum calcium that is physiologically important, regulating neuromuscular contractility, the process of coagulation, as well as a variety of other cellular activities. A small component of the total calcium is complexed to anions such as citrate or sulfate.

In a variety of chronic illnesses, a substantial reduction in the serum albumin concentration may lower the total serum calcium concentration, whereas ionized calcium concentrations remain normal. A simple correction for hypoalbuminemia is made by adding 0.8 mg/dL to the total serum calcium concentration for every 1.0 g/dL by which the serum albumin concentration is lower than 4.0 g/dL. Thus, a patient with a total serum calcium of 10.5 mg/dL and a serum albumin level of 2.0 g/dL has a corrected total serum calcium of 12.1 mg/dL. Conversely, falsely elevated serum calcium levels may be observed, usually the result of an elevation of the serum albumin due to dehydration or hemoconcentration during venipuncture. A similar maneuver can be performed to correct the serum calcium in this situation, except that the correction factor must be subtracted from the serum calcium level. In contrast to changes in the serum albumin concentration, which affect the total measurement but not the ionized level, alterations in pH affect the ionized calcium concentration. Acidosis increases the ionized calcium by decreasing the binding of calcium ions to albumin, whereas alkalosis decreases the ionized calcium by enhancing binding of calcium ions to albumin. Measurement of total serum calcium is usually adequate for most situations, but in complex cases (changes in both albumin *and* pH) a direct measurement of the ionized calcium can be helpful.

Under normal circumstances, the plasma calcium concentration reflects a balance between the flux of calcium into the extracellular fluid from the gastrointestinal tract, the skeleton, and the kidney, and the flux of calcium out of the extracellular fluid into the skeleton and the urine. Hypercalcemia develops when the rate of calcium entry into the blood compartment is greater than its rate of removal. This occurs most commonly when accelerated osteoclastic bone resorption or, less frequently, when excessive GI calcium absorption delivers quantities of calcium into the blood that exceeds the elimination capacity of the kidney and the capacity of the skeleton to reclaim it. Less commonly, normal rates of calcium entry into the extracellular fluid may result in hypercalcemia if the processes of renal excretion or bone mineralization are impaired.

Accelerated bone resorption by osteoclasts, multinucleated bone resorbing cells, is the primary pathogenetic mechanism in most instances of hypercalcemia (1). Osteoclasts may be stimulated to resorb bone by parathyroid hormone (PTH), PTH-related protein (PTHRP), and 1,25-dihydroxyvitamin D, all of which have been shown to cause hypercalcemia (2,3). A number of cytokines (interleukin 1α, interleukin 1β, tumor necrosis factor-α, lymphotoxin, and transforming growth factor-α) also stimulate osteoclastic bone resorption, but their ability to cause hypercalcemia in human disease has not been definitively established (4). Excessive GI absorption of calcium is a much less common cause of hypercalcemia, although it may play a role in hypercalcemic states characterized by excess vitamin D, such as lymphoma or vitamin D intoxication. Whether the primary cause of the hypercalcemia is accelerated bone resorption or excessive GI tract absorption of calcium, the kidney is the primary defender against a rise in the serum calcium. Thus, hypercalcemia is usually preceded by hypercalciuria; it is only when the capacity of the kidney to excrete calcium has been exceeded that the patient becomes hypercalcemic (5).

Several other factors may contribute to the pathogenesis of hypercalcemia. In addition to stimulating osteoclast-mediated bone resorption, both PTH and PTHRP also increase reabsorption of calcium from the distal tubule, thus interfering with the ability of the kidneys to clear the filtered calcium load. Hypercalcemia per se, interferes with the action of antidiuretic hormone on the distal tubule causing a form of nephrogenic diabetes insipidus that results in polyuria. The thirst mechanism may not be fully operative due to the nausea and vomiting that frequently accompany hypercalcemia; thus urinary fluid losses may not be replaced, and dehydration may ensue. The resulting reduction in the extracellular fluid volume and associated reduction in the glomerular filtration rate exacerbates the hypercalcemia. Finally, immobilization may also contribute to hypercalcemia.

CLINICAL MANIFESTATIONS

The clinical presentation of the hypercalcemic patient (6) may involve several organ systems (Table 1). The signs and symptoms tend to be similar regardless of the etiology of the hypercalcemia. Because an optimal extracellular calcium concentration is necessary for normal neurological function, symptoms of neurological dysfunction often predominate in hypercalcemic states. The patient or family members may notice subtle changes in the ability to concentrate or an increased sleep requirement. With increasing severity of the hypercalcemia, symptoms may gradually progress to depression, confusion, and even coma. Muscle weakness is common.

Gastrointestinal symptoms are often prominent with constipation, anorexia, nausea, and vomiting present in varying degree. Pancreatitis and peptic ulcer disease are unusual but have also been reported. They are somewhat more common if the hypercalcemia is due to primary hyperparathyroidism than to other causes of hypercalcemia.

Polyuria, due to the impaired concentrating ability of the distal nephron, is common, particularly during the early phases. Polydipsia is also usually present. The combination of polyuria and diminished fluid intake due to GI symptoms may lead to severe dehydration. Nephrolithiasis occurs in patients with primary hyperparathyroidism (15–20% in recent series) but along with nephrocalcinosis, may also develop in patients with hypercalcemia due to other causes, particularly when the hypercalcemia is chronic.

Hypercalcemia increases the rate of cardiac repolarization. Thus shortening of the Q-T interval is observed commonly on the electrocardiogram. Bradycardia and first degree A-V block, as well as other arrhythmias, may occur. Caution should be exercised when treating the hypercalcemic patient with digitalis, because increased sensitivity to this drug has been observed.

Although in general, the presence or absence of symptoms correlates with the degree of elevation of the serum calcium and with the rapidity of its rise, there is much individual variation in this regard. Certain patients will be quite symptomatic, with moderate hypercalcemia of 12.0–14.0 mg/dL. Others may show no overt symptomatology. The latter situation occurs most often in the setting of chronic hypercalcemia and in other circumstances should prompt one to measure the ionized calcium level to be certain of the diagnosis. In general, patients do not begin to show clinical features of hypercalcemia until the total calcium concentration exceeds 12 mg/dL. Patients are almost invariably symptomatic above 14 mg/dL.

TABLE 1. *Differential diagnosis of hypercalcemia*

Most Common
  Primary hyperparathyroidism
  Malignant disease
    Parathyroid hormone-related protein (carcinoma of lung, esophagus, head and neck, renal cell, ovary, and bladder)
    Ectopic production of 1,25-dihydroxyvitamin D (lymphoma)
    Lytic bone metastases (multiple myeloma and breast carcinoma)
    Other factor(s) produced locally or ectopically
Uncommon
  Endocrine disorders
    Thyrotoxicosis
  Granulomatous diseases
    Sarcoidosis
  Drug-induced
    Vitamin D
    Thiazide diuretics
    Lithium
    Estrogens and antiestrogens
    Androgens (breast cancer therapy)
    Aminophylline
    Vitamin A
    Aluminum intoxication (in chronic renal failure)
  Miscellaneous
    Immobilization
    Renal failure (acute and chronic)
    Total parenteral nutrition
Rare
  Endocrine disorders
    Pheochromocytoma
    Vasoactive intestinal polypeptide-producing tumor
    Familial hypocalciuric hypercalcemia
  Granulomatous diseases (1,25-dihydroxyvitamin D excess)
    Tuberculosis
    Histoplasmosis
    Coccidioidomycosis
    Leprosy
  Miscellaneous
    Milk-alkali syndrome
    Hypophosphatasia

DIFFERENTIAL DIAGNOSIS

Detection of an elevated serum calcium requires that the etiology be established. The many causes of hypercalcemia are listed in Chapter 43, Table 1, and most will be covered separately in subsequent chapters. However, certain general principles that apply to the differential diagnosis of hypercalcemia are covered here.

Malignancy and primary hyperparathyroidism are by far the most common causes of hypercalcemia, accounting for ~90% of hypercalcemic patients (6). Differentiating between these two diagnoses is generally not difficult on clinical grounds alone. The vast majority of patients with primary hyperparathyroidism have relatively mild hypercalcemia, within 1.0 mg/dL above the upper limits of normal and usually <12.0 mg/dL. They are often asymptomatic. By review of past records, the hypercalcemia can be shown to have been present for months to years before. When symptoms of hypercalcemia are present, they tend to be chronic, such as nephrolithiasis. In contrast, patients with hypercalcemia of malignancy are more often ill and are more likely to manifest the classic signs and symptoms of an elevated serum calcium. In general, the malignancy itself is readily apparent and presents little diagnostic challenge to the physician. Less commonly, occult malignancy may present with hypercalcemia or the patient with primary hyperparathyroidism may present with moderate elevation (12–14 mg/dL) of the serum calcium that is associated with symptoms or with the acute onset of severe hypercalcemia (parathyroid crisis). Such cases are a greater diagnostic problem.

The availability of reliable assays for intact PTH based upon double antibody techniques (two-site, immunoradiometric, or immunochemiluminescent assays) has been of great diagnostic value in the evaluation of the hypercalcemic patient. The majority of patients with primary hyperparathyroidism have intact PTH levels that are frankly elevated. Patients with hypercalcemia of malignancy virtually always demonstrate suppressed or undetectable levels of intact PTH. It is distinctly unusual for a patient with malignancy (excepting parathyroid cancer) to show elevated levels of PTH. When this occurs two possibilities exist: the patient may have concomitant primary hyperparathyroidism or the malignancy itself may be secreting PTH, an uncommon event.

In most patients with malignancy-associated hypercalcemia, the hypercalcemia is due to secretion of PTHRP by the tumor (2). Commercial assays for PTHRP are now available that, when elevated, can prove helpful in the diagnosis of hypercalcemia of malignancy. However, the assays are still in their developmental phase, and a negative result does not exclude the diagnosis. Moreover, certain tumors cause hypercalcemia by mechanisms independent of PTHRP. Some secrete other bone resorbing substances, whereas others are capable of converting 25-hydroxyvitamin D to 1,25-dihydroxyvitamin D. Local bone resorbing effects of tumors such as breast cancer also may be involved.

Hypercalcemia from causes other than malignancy or primary hyperparathyroidism may also occur. A thorough history and physical examination are invaluable in arriving at the correct diagnosis. Each of the etiologies listed in Table 1 is covered in one of the other chapters in this section and thus will not be considered herein.

REFERENCES

1. Attie MF: Treatment of hypercalcemia. *Endocrinol Metab Clin North Am* 18:807–828, 1989
2. Halloran BP, Nissenson BA (eds): *Parathyroid Hormone-Related Protein: Normal Physiology and Its Role in Cancer.* CRC Press, Boca Raton, Florida, 1992
3. Adams JS, Fernandez M, Gacad MA, et al.: Vitamin-D metabolite-mediated hypercalcemia and hypercalciuria in patients with AIDS and non-AIDS associated lymphoma. *Blood* 73:235–239, 1989
4. Mundy GR: Hypercalcemic factors other than parathyroid hormone-related protein. *Endocrinol Metab Clin North Am* 18: 795–805, 1989
5. Harinck HIJ, Bijvoet OLM, Plantingh AST, et al.: Role of bone and kidney in tumor-induced hypercalcemia and its treatment with bisphosphonate and sodium chloride. *Am J Med* 82: 1133–1142, 1987
6. Stewart AF, Broadus AE: Mineral metabolism. In: Felig P, Baxter JP, Broadus AE, Frohman LA (eds) *Endocrinology and Metabolism.* McGraw-Hill, New York, pp 1376–1421, 1987

29. Primary Hyperparathyroidism

John P. Bilezikian, M.D.

Departments of Medicine and Pharmacology, College of Physicians and Surgeons, Columbia University, New York, New York

Primary hyperparathyroidism is a very common cause of hypercalcemia, ranking equally in incidence with the hypercalcemias associated with malignant diseases. In this chapter, the clinical presentation, diagnostic evaluation, and therapy of primary hyperparathyroidism are considered.

Among the endocrine disorders, primary hyperparathyroidism ranks as a relatively common disease, with estimates of incidence as high as 1 in 500 to 1 in 1000 (1). Perhaps only diabetes mellitus and hyperthyroidism are more common endocrine diseases. The high visibility of primary hyperparathyroidism in the population today marks a dramatic change from several generations ago when it was considered a rare disorder. The increase in incidence is due primarily to the widespread use of the autoanalyzer gratuitously providing serum calcium determinations when a serum chemistry profile is ordered for another reason (2). In this regard, hypercalcemia is typically discovered when the patient is being evaluated for a set of complaints completely unrelated to hypercalcemia.

Primary hyperparathyroidism occurs at all ages but is most frequent in the sixth decade of life. Women are affected more often than men by a ratio of 3:2. When found in children, an unusual event, it might be a component of one of several endocrinopathies with a genetic basis such as multiple endocrine neoplasia, type I or II (Chapter 31).

The hallmarks of primary hyperparathyroidism are hypercalcemia occurring in association with elevated levels of parathyroid hormone. The disease is caused by a benign, solitary adenoma 80% of the time. The adenoma is a collection of chief cells surrounded by a rim of normal tissue at the outer perimeter of gland. The remaining three parathyroid glands are normal. Primary hyperparathyroidism may also be due to a pathological process characterized by hyperplasia of all four parathyroid glands. Four-gland parathyroid hyperplasia is seen in 15–20% of patients with primary hyperparathyroidism. It may occur sporadically, but more likely the multiglandular disease is associated with multiple endocrine neoplasia, types I or II (Chapter 31). A very rare presentation of primary hyperparathyroidism is parathyroid carcinoma, occurring in fewer than 1% of patients (3). The diagnosis of parathyroid carcinoma can be exceedingly difficult to make unless gross local or distant metastases are found. Pathological examination of the malignant tissue might show mitoses, vascular invasion, capsule invasion, and fibrous trabeculae.

The pathophysiology of primary hyperparathyroidism relates to the loss of normal feedback control of parathyroid hormone secretion by extracellular calcium. Under virtually all other hypercalcemic conditions, the parathyroid gland is suppressed and parathyroid hormone levels are low. Why the parathyroid cell loses its normal sensitivity to calcium is unknown but in adenomas, this appears to be the major mechanism. In primary hyperparathyroidism due to hyperplasia of the parathyroid glands, the "set point" for calcium is not changed for a given parathyroid cell but the increased number of cells per se gives rise to the hypercalcemia.

The underlying cause of primary hyperparathyroidism is not known. A history of childhood external neck irradiation is noteworthy but is unlikely to be causative in the majority of patients. The clonal origin of most parathyroid adenomas suggests a defect at the level of the gene controlling the regulation and/or expression of parathyroid hormone. Two patients with primary hyperparathyroidism have been discovered in whom the parathyroid hormone gene was shown to be rearranged (4). It is possible that this kind of gene rearrangement is responsible for the altered growth properties of the abnormal parathyroid cell. So far, however, the number of patients shown to have this gene rearrangement is too small to make any assumptions regarding the relative importance of this potential etiological factor.

SIGNS AND SYMPTOMS

Primary hyperparathyroidism is associated classically with two major sites of potential complications: the bones and the kidneys. At skeletal sites, particularly the long bones endowed with a composition predominantly cortical in nature, excess parathyroid hormone can lead to a condition called osteitis fibrosa cystica. Subperiosteal resorption of the distal phalanges, distal tapering of the clavicles, a "salt-and-pepper" appearance of the skull, bone cysts and brown tumors of the long bones are all manifestations of hyperparathyroid bone disease. Despite the fact that the skeleton is a major potential site of involvement, primary hyperparathyroidism is only rarely associated with overt evidence for bone disease.

The kidney may show manifestations of primary hyperparathyroidism in the form of renal stones (nephrolithia-sis) or diffuse deposition of calcium-phosphate complexes in the parenchyma (nephrocalcinosis). Similar to the reduced incidence of overt bone disease in primary hyperparathyroidism, nephrolithiasis or nephrocalcinosis is seen in only ~20% of patients today. In the absence of these renal manifestations, primary hyperparathyroidism may be associated with excessive urinary calcium excretion (>250 mg daily).

Other potential complications of primary hyperparathyroidism are a syndrome of muscle weakness and easy fatiguability best accounted for by neuromuscular dysfunction due to the hyperparathyroid state (5). Peptic ulcer disease and pancreatitis are seen as GI manifestations although a direct pathophysiological link between these complications and primary hyperparathyroidism is not certain. Similarly, the association between primary hyperparathyroidism and hypertension does not enjoy a clear pathophysiological basis. Other problems that rarely may be associated with primary hyperparathyroidism are gout and pseudogout, anemia, and depression.

CLINICAL FORMS OF PRIMARY HYPERPARATHYROIDISM

The most common clinical form of primary hyperparathyroidism is mild, asymptomatic hypercalcemia with calcium levels within 1 mg/dL above the upper limits of normal. Often, these patients do not have specific complaints and do not show evidence for any target organ complications. If specific complications are present, renal stone disease is the one most likely to be seen. Rarely, a patient will demonstrate serum calcium levels in the life-threatening range, so-called acute primary hyperparathyroidism or parathyroid crisis. These patients are invariably symptomatic of hypercalcemia (6).

There are a number of other unusual clinical presentations of primary hyperparathyroidism. Familial forms, include the multiple endocrine neoplasias, types I and II, familial primary hyperparathyroidism not associated with any other endocrine disorder, familial cystic parathyroid adenomatosis, and neonatal primary hyperparathyroidism (Chapter 32).

EVALUATION AND DIAGNOSIS OF PRIMARY HYPERPARATHYROIDISM

The diagnosis of primary hyperparathyroidism depends on laboratory tests. The history and physical examination rarely give any specific indications of primary hyperparathyroidism. The salient chemical feature of the disease is hypercalcemia. It is required for diagnosis and virtually always present. Occasionally, patients with mild hypercalcemia may be found to have a normal serum calcium, but the vast majority of serum calcium measurements will be elevated. The serum phosphorus is usually in the lower range of normal and in approximately one-third of patients, it may be frankly low. The serum alkaline phosphatase may be elevated when bone disease is present. The actions of parathyroid hormone to alter acid-base handling in the kidney may lead in some patients to a mild hyperchloremia and metabolic acidosis. Urinary calcium excretion is elevated in ~25% of patients. Phosphaturia may also be observed in some patients. The circulating 1,25-dihydroxyvitamin D concentration is elevated in some patients with primary hyperparathyroidism (7), although it is of little diagnostic value, as elevated levels of this active vitamin D metabolite are seen in a variety of other hypercalcemic conditions such as sarcoidosis, other granulomatous disease, and some lymphomas (8,9).

The measurement of parathyroid hormone is the most specific way of making the diagnosis of primary hyperparathyroidism. In the presence of hypercalcemia, an elevated level of parathyroid hormone virtually establishes the diagnosis. In >90% of patients with primary hyperparathyroidism, the parathyroid hormone level will be elevated. Moreover, it is distinctly unusual for the other causes of hypercalcemia to be associated with elevated concentrations of parathyroid hormone. Thus, the assay for parathyroid hormone helps also to rule out the other causes of hypercalcemia. The most useful radioimmunoassays are those that recognize the carboxyterminal or midmolecule portions of the parathyroid hormone molecule (10). The immunoradiometric assay for parathyroid hormone recognizes intact hormone and has replaced many of the useful radioimmunoassays as the "gold standard" (11). The usefulness of the assays for parathyroid hormone in the differential diagnosis of hypercalcemia is due to refinements in measurement techniques (such as the immunoradiometric assay technique), as well as appreciation of the fact that the most common other cause of hypercalcemia, namely hypercalcemia of malignancy, is associated with suppressed levels of hormone. This is true even for the syndrome of humoral hypercalcemia of malignancy (Chapter 33) in which assays for parathyroid hormone-related peptide do not cross-react with assays for parathyroid hormone. The only hypercalcemic disorders in which the parathyroid hormone level might be elevated are those related to lithium or thiazide diuretic use (Chapter 36). It is relatively easy to exclude either of these two possibilities by history. If it is possible that the patient has either of these two drug-related hypercalcemias, the only way to make the diagnosis of primary hyperparathyroidism is to withdraw the thiazide or the lithium and to confirm the hypercalcemia with high calcium and parathyroid hormone levels 2–3 months later.

TREATMENT OF PRIMARY HYPERPARATHYROIDISM

Surgery. Primary hyperparathyroidism is a curable disease with successful removal of the parathyroid adenoma. When primary hyperparathyroidism was routinely associated with signs and symptoms, surgery was performed regularly. Now, however, the typical patient does not have signs or symptoms. It is thus not apparent who among the many patients with this disorder are surgical candidates (12). In the absence of the kind of predictive information that would indicate who is at risk for the complications of this disease, a set of guidelines has been used by many endocrinologists who are often in the position of giving advice about the advisability of surgery. If the serum calcium is >1 mg/dL above the upper limit of normal, it is the impression that this kind of patient is at greater risk for developing the complications of primary hyperparathyroidism. If the patient has any complications of primary hyperparathyroidism (e.g., overt bone disease and nephrolithiasis), surgery is generally considered even if the serum calcium may not be impressively high. Another surgical guideline is met by the patient who survives an episode of acute primary hyperparathyroidism characterized by life-threatening hypercalcemia. Hypercalciuria, >250 mg (women) or 300 mg (men) daily, is another general indication for surgery. Recent widespread use of bone densitometry shows a relatively selective effect of mild, asymptomatic primary hyperparathyroidism to involve compact (or cortical) bone. The site of most concern is the distal radius. Patients with asymptomatic primary hyperparathyroidism in whom bone mineral densitometry of the distal radius is <2 SD below age- and sex-associated control values become another group in which surgery is recommended. Finally, it is the impression that the relatively young patient with primary hyperparathyroidism is at greater risk over the long-term simply because the young patient is likely to live longer and be exposed for a greater period of time to the hyperparathyroid state. These guidelines for surgery are not absolute and are tempered both by the physician and the patient. Some physicians will recommend surgery for all patients with primary hyperparathyroidism; other physicians will not recommend surgery unless clear-cut complications of primary hyperparathyroidism are present. The patient enters into this therapeutic dialogue as well. Some patients cannot tolerate the idea of living with a curable disease and will seek surgery in the absence of any of the aforementioned guidelines. Other patients with coexisting medical problems may not wish to face the risk of surgery even though surgical indications are present.

Parathyroid surgery requires expertise. The glands are notoriously variable in location requiring knowledge by the surgeon of typical ectopic sites such as intrathyroidal, retroesophageal, the lateral neck and, of course, the mediastinum. The surgeon must also be aware of the proper operation to perform. In the case of the adenoma, the other glands are ascertained to be normal but not removed. In the case of multiglandular disease, the approach is to remove all tissue save for a remnant that is left *in situ* or transplanted to the forearm.

Postoperatively, the patient may experience a brief period of transient hypocalcemia during which time the normal but suppressed parathyroid glands regain their sensitivity to calcium. It has been shown recently that normal parathyroid glands regain their sensitivity to calcium within the first few days after surgery (13). If overt skeletal disease is present, there may be a prolonged period of hypocalcemia characterized by rapid deposition of calcium and phosphate into bones (Hungry Bone syndrome). A more permanent complication of parathyroid surgery is hypoparathyroidism. Sometimes, the hypoparathyroid state does not become apparent until years after parathyroid surgery. Late-term postsurgical hypoparathyroidism may be due to final compromise of a parathyroid blood supply that had become marginal at the time of the initial neck operation. Another permanent complication of parathyroid surgery is recurrent laryngeal nerve damage with hoarseness and reduced voice volume.

In the patient who has not had previous neck surgery, an experienced parathyroid surgeon will find the abnormal parathyroid gland(s) well over 90% of the time. Thus, for this kind of patient, the value of preoperative localization tests is dubious. On the other hand, for patients who have undergone previous neck surgery, preoperative localization can be extremely useful. Noninvasive tests center around ultrasonography, computed tomography, magnetic resonance imaging, and scintigraphy. No one test is superior and each has ~60% true-positive and 15% false-negative rates (14). It is recommended, thus, that when noninvasive tests are used in patients with previous neck surgery, localization be sought by two of these approaches before concluding with confidence that preoperative localization has been achieved. Although these noninvasive tests have not yet achieved individually the sensitivity and specificity desired, they are replacing invasive testing with arteriography and selective venous catheterization of the neck (15).

Medical Management. If patients with primary hyperparathyroidism are not to undergo parathyroid surgery, a set of general medical guidelines is recommended (16). Adequate hydration and ambulation are always encouraged. Thiazide diuretics are always avoided because they may lead to worsening hypercalcemia. Dietary intake of calcium should be moderate. There is no good evidence that patients with primary hyperparathyroidism show significant fluctuations of their serum calcium as a function of dietary calcium intake. High calcium intakes should be avoided, however, especially in patients whose 1,25-dihydroxyvitamin D level is elevated. Low calcium diets should also be avoided because they could theoretically lead to further stimulation of parathyroid hormone secretion.

In the medical management of primary hyperparathyroidism, we still lack an effective and safe therapeutic agent. Oral phosphate will lower the serum calcium in patients with primary hyperparathyroidism by ~0.5–1 mg/dL. Phosphate appears to act by three mechanisms: interference with absorption of dietary calcium, inhibition of bone resorption, and inhibition of renal production of 1,25-dihydroxyvitamin D. Phosphate, however, is not used widely as a therapy for primary hyperparathyroidism, because of the danger of metastatic calcification in soft tissue as a result of increasing the calcium phosphate product. Moreover, oral phosphate leads to further elevation of parathyroid hormone levels, an unwanted therapeutic consequence (17).

In postmenopausal women, estrogen therapy has been advocated (18,19). The rationale for estrogen use in primary hyperparathyroidism is based on the known antagonism by estrogen of parathyroid hormone-mediated bone resorption. Experience with this potential therapy is not great enough to know how effective it actually is in this disorder. Even though calcium levels do decline after estrogen administration, parathyroid hormone levels do not change.

A final therapeutic possibility in primary hyperparathyroidism is the use of bisphosphonates. Several earlier studies documented the usefulness of dichloromethylene bisphosphonate (20), an agent not available in the United States. The only oral formulation for bisphosphonate that is available, etidronate, is not effective in this condition. Newer bisphosphonates are being developed and it is likely that oral formulations of these newer agents will be shown to be effective in primary hyperparathyroidism.

REFERENCES

1. Bilezikian JP: Hyperparathyroidism. In Stein JH (ed) *Internal Medicine*, 2nd ed. Little-Brown, Boston, pp 2372–2378, 1990
2. Heath H III, Hodgson SF, Kennedy MA: Primary hyperparathyroidism: Incidence, morbidity, and potential economic impact in a community. *N Engl J Med* 302:189, 1980
3. Shane E, Bilezikian JP: Parathyroid carcinoma. In Williams CJ, Krikorian JC, Green MR, Raghavan D (eds) *Textbook of Uncommon Cancer*. New York, John Wiley, pp 763–771, 1988
4. Arnold A, Kim HG, Gaz RD, Eddy RL, Fukushima R, Byers MG, Shows TB, Kronenberg HM: Molecular cloning and chromosomal mapping of DNA rearranged with the parathyroid hormone gene in a parathyroid adenoma. *J Clin Invest* 83:2034–2040, 1989
5. Patten BM, Bilezikian JP, Mallette LE, Prince A, Engle WK, Aurbach GD: The neuromuscular disease of primary hyperparathyroidism. *Ann Intern Med* 80:182–194, 1974
6. Fitzpatrick LA, Bilezikian JP: Acute primary hyperparathyroidism. *Am J Med* 82:275–282, 1987
7. Broadus AE, Horst RL, Lang R, Littledike ET, Rasmussen H: The importance of circulating, 1,25-dihydroxyvitamin D in the pathogenesis of hypercalciuria and renal-stone formation in primary hyperparathyroidism. *N Engl J Med* 302:421–426, 1980
8. Breslau NA, McGuire JL, Zerwekh JE, Frenkel EP, Pak CYC: Hypercalcemia associated with increased calcitriol levels in three patients with lymphoma. *Ann Intern Med* 100:1–6, 1984
9. Barbour GL, Coburn JW, Slatopolsky E, Norman AW, Horst RL: Hypercalcemia in an anephric patient with sarcoidosis: Evidence for extrarenal generation of 1,25-dihydroxyvitamin D. *N Engl J Med* 305:440–443, 1981
10. Mallette LE, Tumna SN, Berger RD, Kirkland JL: Radioimmunoassay for the middle region of human parathyroid hormone using an homologous antiserum with a carboxy-terminal fragment of bovine parathyroid hormone as radioligand. *J Clin Endocrinol Metab* 54:1017–1024, 1982
11. Nussbaum SR, Zahradnik RJ, Lavigne JR, Brennan GL, Nozawa-Ung K, Kim LY, Keutmann HT, Wang C, Potts JT Jr, Segre GV: Highly sensitive two-site immunoradiometric assay of parathyrin and its clinical utility in evaluating patients with hypercalcemia. *Clin Chem* 33:1364–1367, 1987
12. Potts JT Jr, Fradkin JE, Aurbach GD, Bilezikian JP, Raisz LG (eds): Proceedings of the NIH Consensus Development Conference on Diagnosis and Management of Asymptomatic Primary Hyperparathyroidism. *J Bone Miner Res* 6(suppl 2): 51–66, 1991
13. Brasier AR, Wang C, Nussbaum SR: Recovery of parathyroid hormone secretion after parathyroid adenomectomy. *J Clin Endocrinol Metab* 61:495–500, 1988
14. Doppman JL, Miller DL: Localization of parathyroid tumors in patients with asymptomatic primary hyperparathyroidism. *J Bone Miner Res* 2(suppl 2):S153–S158, 1991
15. Mallette LE, Gomez L, Fisher RG: Parathyroid angiography: A review of current knowledge and guidelines for clinical application. *Endocrine Rev* 2:124–135, 1981
16. Shane E: Medical management of asymptomatic primary hyperparathyroidism. *J Bone Miner Res* 6(suppl 2):S131–S134, 1991
17. Broadus AE, Magee JSI, Mallette LE, Horst RL, Lang R, Jen-

sen RG, Gertner JM, Baron R: A detailed evaluation of oral phosphate therapy in selected patients with primary hyperparathyroidism. *J Clin Endocrinol Metabol* 56:953–961, 1983

18. Marcus R, Madvig P, Crim M, Pont A, Kosek J: Conjugated estrogens in the treatment of postmenopausal women with hyperparathyroidism. *Ann Intern Med* 100:633–640, 1984

19. Selby PL, Peacock M: Ethinyl estradiol and norethindrone in the treatment of primary hyperparathyroidism in postmenopausal women. *N Engl J Med* 314:1481–1485, 1986

20. Shane E, Baquiran DC, Bilezikian JP: Effects of dichlormethylene diphosphonate on serum and urine calcium in primary hyperparathyroidism. *Ann Intern Med* 95:23–27, 1981

30. Tertiary Hyperparathyroidism and Refractory Secondary Hyperparathyroidism

Susan C. Galbraith, M.D. and L. Darryl Quarles, M.D.

Department of Medicine, Division of Nephrology, Duke University Medical Center, Durham, North Carolina

All hyperparathyroid disorders are characterized by elevated circulating levels of parathyroid hormone (PTH) that arise from augmented PTH production/secretion per cell and/or from an expanded number of functioning PTH-producing cells. The variable underlying pathophysiology of increased PTH secretion permits subclassification of hyperparathyroidism (HPT) into primary and secondary disorders. Primary HPT (see Chapter 29) is characterized functionally by abnormal synthesis and secretion of PTH in excess of calcium homeostatic needs and morphologically by adenomatous transformation or diffuse hyperplasia of PTH-secreting cells. Secondary HPT, in contrast, is an acquired disorder representing a normal physiological response to perturbations in calcium metabolism. Prolonged abnormalities in calcium metabolism can lead to overexpression of secondary compensatory adjustments made by the parathyroid gland and ultimately lead to states of apparent autonomous PTH secretion. Traditionally, *tertiary* HPT is a term used to describe patients with sustained secondary HPT who develop elevated levels of serum calcium. The term *refractory secondary HPT* defines a second subset of patients with severe secondary HPT without hypercalcemia that display nonsuppressible PTH secretion after correcting the inciting metabolic abnormalities. In both tertiary and refractory secondary HPT, the parathyroid gland has reached a hyperfunctioning state that no longer responds appropriately to physiologic regulation.

PARATHYROID HORMONE/1,25-DIHYDROXYVITAMIN D AXIS

The hormonal actions of PTH increase serum calcium levels by mobilizing osseous calcium stores, enhancing reabsorption of calcium in the distal renal tubule, and increasing production of 1,25-dihydroxyvitamin D_3 [$1,25(OH)_2D_3$] in the kidney. 1,25-Dihydroxyvitamin D_3, in turn, enhances calcium uptake by the intestine, enhances the osseous effects of PTH, and directly modulates PTH gland activity (see Chapters 7 and 16) (1). Overall, the amount of PTH released into the circulation by the parathyroid gland is determined by the rate of PTH secretion, the rate of PTH synthesis, and the number of functioning parathyroid-producing cells. Change in extracellular calcium concentration is the most important acute modulator of PTH secretion. More persistent changes in serum calcium levels affect cellular PTH synthesis at the level of prepro-PTH gene transcription. The actions of extracellular calcium are mediated by parallel increases in intracellular calcium, which act as a second messenger in control of PTH secretion and production. In contrast, $1,25(OH)_2D_3$ has no acute effects on PTH secretion, but displays potent suppressive effects on PTH synthesis at the level of gene transcription. The effects of $1,25(OH)_2D_3$ are mediated via classical cytosolic steroid receptor mechanisms. 1,25-Dihydroxyvitamin D_3 also may have nongenomic effects on intracellular calcium concentrations, but the clinical significance of this pathway in the regulation of PTH secretion and synthesis is not clear. In addition, parathyroid-secreting cells display a basal, nonsuppressible component of PTH production.

The factors controlling parathyroid cell proliferation are less well defined. Although hypocalcemia was felt to be the primary stimulus for parathyroid hyperplasia by early investigators, more recent studies emphasize the importance of vitamin D. 1,25-Dihydroxyvitamin D_3 deficiency is sufficient to stimulate parathyroid gland hyperplasia in normocalcemic dogs, and administration of calcitriol can prevent parathyroid gland hyperplasia in animal models of secondary HPT (1–4). *In vitro* studies have shown that, whereas changes in ambient calcium levels modulate the secretion of PTH in bovine parathyroid cells, these changes do not effect cell number and DNA synthesis. In contrast, vitamin D has a marked inhibitory effect on cellular proliferation in culture. Furthermore, vitamin D, but not calcium, downregulates expression of protooncogenes associated with cellular proliferation in parathyroid tissue and other cell models (5). The frequent association of vitamin D deficiency and hypocalcemia in many subjects with parathyroid hyperplasia (particularly those with uremia), however, makes the separation of the two effects on glandular proliferation difficult to accomplish *in vivo*.

Pathogenesis of "Tertiary"/Refractory Hyperparathyroidism

There are several changes in the parathyroid gland at the tissue, cellular, or molecular level that potentially explain this refractory state of HPT. These include alterations of cellular function that result in dysregulated PTH secretion/production as well as an abnormal number of parathyroid cells. Additionally, noncorrectable end-organ resistance to PTH actions may lead to persistent HPT in spite of calcium and vitamin D treatment.

Role of Increased Gland Size. The most direct explanation for "tertiary"/refractory secondary HPT is an increased number of parathyroid cells that exhibit a nonsuppressible basal component of PTH secretion. The idea that the mass of parathyroid cells may be an important factor in a PTH hypersecretory state is supported experimentally by studies showing that excessive amounts of normal parathyroid tissue implanted into rats produces hypercalcemia (6) and by the findings of persistent low levels of PTH secretion in normal calves that were made profoundly hypercalcemic (7). These studies suggest that an increased number of cells secreting basal amounts of PTH can overcome the normal homeostatic mechanisms controlling steady-state serum PTH levels. Moreover, this increased number of PTH-secreting cells have a long life span with a limited ability to involute (undergo apoptosis), resulting in persistently increased cell numbers (8). The process of cellular hypertrophy (enlargement of individual cells) that precedes hyperplasia in the chronically stimulated gland may also contributes to excess PTH secretion and parathyroid gland enlargement (1). Hyperplasia, however, is predominantly responsible for the marked increase in gland size observed in refractory hyperparathyroid disorders (8). In a recently published series describing the histologic features of 128 parathyroid glands taken from patients with tertiary HPT (all with chronic renal insufficiency), the average weight of a single gland in this series was 25 times the weight of a normal parathyroid gland (9). The parathyroid glands of subjects with secondary HPT, although uniformly enlarged and hyperplastic, are usually smaller than those from patients with tertiary HPT (9).

Phenotypic Alterations of the Parathyroid Gland in Tertiary Hyperparathyroidism. A nodular histologic pattern is frequently found in patients with tertiary HPT. These histologic changes, which superficially resemble adenomatous transformation, may represent clonal selection of abnormal PTH-secreting cells due to prolonged stimulus for parathyroid cell replication. Nodular hyperplastic gland mass tends to be greater than diffusely hyperplastic glands, and nodules are more common in the glands of patients with tertiary than secondary HPT (9). Furthermore, nodular hyperplastic tissue has altered regulation of PTH secretion compared with diffuse hyperplastic tissue, displaying a degree of insensitivity to calcium that resembles regulatory characteristics of primary adenomas (10–12). Immunohistochemical studies also provide evidence of homogeneity of the cells within a nodule suggesting that a single nodule may result from a monoclonal proliferation of a single parathyroid cell (13). Acquired clonal transformation is also supported by recent studies showing molecular defects similar to those found in parathyroid adenomas and multiple endocrine neoplasia-associated hyperplasia (14) in parathyroid tissues obtained from patients with tertiary HPT (15–17).

Although morphological, molecular, and functional similarities between nodular tertiary hyperplasia and primary adenomatous tissue suggest important *in vivo* homologies, the behavior is fundamentally different for nodular hyperplastic tissue of tertiary HPT and primary adenoma or hyperplasia. The difference between behavior of autotransplanted adenomatous tissue and that of tertiary hyperplastic tissue should be noted, with surgeons achieving good results in tertiary HPT patients with drastic reduction in tissue volume (18). An autotransplanted adenoma as reported by Brennan et al. (19), however, continues to secrete autonomously increased levels of PTH resulting in continuing clinical HPT. It should also be noted that adenomas are rarely found at parathyroid exploration in patients with presumed tertiary HPT.

Role of Dysregulated Parathyroid Hormone Production. Although abnormalities in cell number and control of proliferation are important components of tertiary HPT, abnormalities in control of PTH secretion also appear to play an important role. Ultrastructural studies of hyperplastic glands derived from patients with tertiary HPT reveal evidence of increased cellular machinery for production and secretion of hormone as well as an increased number of cells (7,20). Likewise, molecular studies in animal models note an increase in PTH mRNA content per cell consistent with increased PTH synthesis contributing to the hyperparathyroid state (21,22). PTH cells in tertiary HPT, however, do not differ in their maximal-stimulated PTH release from normal cells (23). Rather, as noted previously, tissues derived from hyperplastic glands display a relative insensitivity to the suppressive effects of calcium as reflected by an increased "setpoint" (23,24). The calcium setpoint in parathyroid tissue derived from tertiary HPT is intermediate between that of normal and adenomatous glands. In patients with secondary/tertiary HPT the alteration in setpoint, however, is not uniform between patients with similar pathology, between glands removed from the same patient, or even between cells from the same gland (23).

Studies investigating the mechanism of calcium setpoint aberration have suggested a role for vitamin D deficiency and downregulation of vitamin D receptor number. Indeed, vitamin D-deficient rats are unable to modulate PTH mRNA levels in response to alterations of ambient calcium (21). Likewise, a change in calcium setpoint has been seen in a population of vitamin D-deficient uremic patients with normal serum calcium levels (25). The concentration of vitamin D receptors in the parathyroid tissue of dialysis patients is reduced (26). A reduction of receptors could account for the decreased effect of vitamin D both on direct PTH suppression and on the parathyroid cell's response to ambient calcium concentration. Abnormalities in vitamin D receptor number is not sufficient to explain refractory HPT, because correction of both vitamin D deficiency and abnormalities in vitamin D receptor number by renal transplantation fails to cure "tertiary/refractory" HPT in a significant percentage of patients (26). Moreover, administration of vitamin D, which has been found to upregulate receptor gene expression in the parathyroid *in vivo* (27), is ineffective in suppressing PTH in uremic subjects with refractory HPT. Although the exact molecular mechanisms of tertiary/refractory hyperparathyroidism remain to be defined, a combination of increased quantity of functioning parathyroid tissue coupled with dysregulated control of PTH secretion and production combine to produce a state where PTH production exceeds physiological needs.

CLINICAL CONDITIONS ASSOCIATED WITH TERTIARY/REFRACTORY SECONDARY HYPERPARATHYROIDISM

Refractory HPT has been observed in most chronic disorders of calcium and $1,25(OH)_2D_3$ metabolism, including those that are associated with endstage renal disease (ESRD), nutritional vitamin D deficiency, high-dose phosphate treatment of chronic hypophosphatemia disorders, various vitamin D-resistant/dependent states, and certain liver/biliary diseases.

Endstage Renal Disease. The vast majority of patients seen with tertiary HPT have ESRD. The uremic state presents multiple stimuli to the parathyroid gland that result in eventual hyperplasia and nonsuppressible PTH release. These include hyperphosphatemia, $1,25(OH)_2D_3$ deficiency, downregulation of $1,25(OH)_2D_3$ receptors, altered "setpoint," and hypocalcemia. The development of tertiary HPT in ESRD patients is related to duration of ESRD requiring dialysis. Tertiary HPT may be clinically manifest by the presence of elevated PTH levels with characteristic high-turnover metabolic bone disease, refractory hyperphosphatemia, or hypercalcemia. In recent studies we found that intact PTH measurements by the immunoradiometric assay is an accurate measure of HPT presence and severity in subjects with ESRD on hemodialysis (28). Consistent with end-organ resistance to PTH, the presence of HPT is defined by a circulating level of intact PTH of ~185 pg/mL—roughly threefold greater than the upper limit of normal for PTH in normal individuals (65 pg/mL) (28). Moreover, refractory HPT (subjects that failed to normalize serum PTH levels after intensive medical therapy with calcium, calcitriol, and phosphate binders) were characterized by an average intact PTH level of 1,512 pg/mL (Table 1), which was identical to serum PTH values (1,586 pg/mL) of patients who previously had undergone parathyroidectomy for refractory HPT. Finally, in related studies we found that the degree of PTH suppression in chronic hemodialysis patients was correlated with gland size as estimated by magnetic resonance imaging or high-resolution ultrasound (Fig. 1). These studies are consistent with the notion that uremic secondary hyperparathyroidism is a heterogeneous disorder with variable suppressible PTH levels that are related, in part, to the degree of parathyroid gland hyperplasia.

Renal transplantation often unmasks refractory HPT in patients with preexisting severe secondary HPT of long

TABLE 1. *Relationship between degree of serum intact parathyroid hormone (PTH) elevation and therapeutic response*

	Serum intact PTH (pg/mL)	
	Mean	Range
Responsive[a] (*n* = 11)	752	214–1,594
Refractory		
Calcitriol failures (*n* = 9)	1512[b]	932–2,259
Parathyroidectomy (*n* = 7)	1586[b]	807–2,461

[a] Hemodialysis patients who achieved serum intact PTH < 200 pg/mL after treatment with combinations of calcitriol and calcium carbonate.

[b] Significantly different from responsive subjects at *p* < 0.05.

duration. Indeed, hypercalcemia has been reported to occur in as many as one-third of successfully transplanted subjects (29,30). Although the metabolic abnormalities of uremia are largely corrected by successful renal transplantation, the restoration of $1,25(OH)_2D_3$ production by the renal allograft and amelioration of end-organ resistance to PTH may increase the susceptibility to hypercalcemia during the slow involution of PTH hypersecreting glands. Autopsy specimens taken from transplant patients dying from nonrenal disease without clinically evident

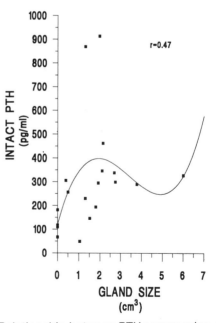

FIG. 1. Relationship between PTH suppression and estimated parathyroid gland size in chronic maintenance hemodialysis patients. Twenty subjects with ESRD were maintained on thrice weekly hemodialysis with 2.5 mEq/L calcium dialysate for 6 weeks before evaluating suppression of PTH by performing hemodialysis with a 3.5 mEq/L dialysis bath. The maximally suppressed serum PTH value derived from such dynamic suppression was correlated with gland volume as estimated by magnetic resonance scanning or high-resolution ultrasound.

HPT confirm that parathyroid gland hyperplasia does not rapidly resolve, even with the nearly normal metabolic milieu resulting from transplantation (31). In addition, the degree of elevation of PTH following hypocalcemic stimulation is correlated with the residual parathyroid gland volume in renal transplant subjects (32). Resolution of soft tissue calcification and overly aggressive treatment of hypophosphatemia with high-dose phosphate may contribute to the persistence of HPT. Glucocorticoids might also contribute to persistent HPT in the posttransplant period through actions to decrease gut calcium absorption and thereby increase PTH secretion. On the other hand, occasionally hypercalcemia may not be manifest until after the dose of prednisone has been tapered, suggesting that the effects of glucocorticoids on calcium metabolism may occasionally mask the clinical expression of PTH excess in renal transplant patients.

In two large surgical series ~65% of patients with posttransplant HPT had spontaneous resolution, mostly within 1–3 years but rarely as late as 7 years postoperatively. Parathyroidectomy is required in <6% of renal transplant patients (31,33).

Vitamin D-Resistant/Dependent States. Large doses of oral phosphorous used to treat children with X-linked hypophosphatemia rickets can result in chronic stimulation of PTH secretion via lowering of the serum-ionized calcium. A subset of these patients appear to develop tertiary HPT associated with diffuse parathyroid gland hyperplasia. Occasionally, parathyroid ademonas are observed. It is not clear whether adenomas represent concurrence of primary HPT or monoclonal expansion derived from diffuse hyperplasia. In any event, subtotal parathyroidectomy and more recently total parathyroidectomy with autotransplantation have been effectively used to decrease functional parathyroid mass in these children (34).

Vitamin D-Deficient States. Chronic vitamin D deficiency has been shown to result in refractory HPT. Detailed studies of a cohort of vitamin D-deficient Asian vegetarians revealed inability to suppress PTH levels completely, even after a full year of therapy with calcium and calcitriol (35). The duration of parathyroid stimulation may be essential to development of a nonsuppressible state, because treatment of vitamin D-deficient children with calcium and vitamin D typically results in rapid normalization of elevated PTH levels (36). Unlike that associated with ESRD and treatment of hypophosphatemic disorders, the HPT of chronic dietary vitamin D deficiency is mild to moderate.

Hepatobiliary Disorders. A similar etiology for PTH hypersecretion has been postulated in patients with primary biliary cirrhosis, a disease state characterized by low 25(OH)D and 1.25(OH)$_2$D$_3$ levels (secondary to inability of the liver to convert vitamin D effectively to 25(OH)D via vitamin D 25-hydroxylase). A group of patients with primary biliary cirrhosis who had been adequately supplemented with calcium and 1,25(OH)$_2$D$_3$ were found to have an average PTH level significantly higher than normal controls. Thirty percent of the patients had a PTH level above the normal range (37). Again, severe hypercalcemia was absent, and other clinical manifestations of HPT were not severe enough to warrant parathyroidectomy in this group of patients.

THERAPY

In general, surgical treatment is indicated in symptomatic patients with nonsuppressible serum PTH levels. Symptoms may include those related to hypercalcemia, hyperparathyroid bone disease, nephrocalcinosis, and/or nephrolithiasis. In ESRD patients, intractable pruritus, severe hyperphosphatemia, calciphylaxis, and soft tissue calcification may be additional indications. In renal transplant patients with persistent HPT, serum calcium levels >12.5 mg/dL after 1 year or progressive and unexplained renal insufficiency are usual indications for parathyroidectomy. Patients with milder forms of tertiary/refractory HPT, similar to asymptomatic primary HPT, are often managed expectantly. There are, however, no controlled studies that evaluate the risk of conservative management of asymptomatic refractory HPT.

It is clear that the original suggestion that high-dose intravenous calcitriol administration might effectively accomplish a "medical" parathyroidectomy of secondary HPT (38) has not been substantiated by controlled studies (39). Indeed, recent studies suggest that pharmacologic calcitriol therapy, regardless of route of administration, is poorly tolerated—50% of subjects developed hypercalcemia and 75% developed hyperphosphatemia (39). Approximately 50% of the subjects with ESRD with secondary HPT failed to attain "normal" serum intact PTH levels (<200 pg/mL). About one-third of these patients were completely refractory to high-dose calcitriol therapy.

Cure of tertiary/refractory HPT requires surgical interventions designed to "debulk" the parathyroid gland. Early approaches used subtotal parathyroidectomy that reduced parathyroid mass by ~⅞'s. With this procedure, some patients remained hyperparathyroid, requiring a second neck exploration for further tissue removal. In 1975 Wells and Gunnells at our institution published experience with total parathyroidectomy and autografting of parathyroid tissue fragments into the muscle of the forearm (18). The advantages of the procedure are lower failure rates and ability to reduce further parathyroid mass without further neck exploration. The disadvantage of the procedure is the occasional induction of hypoparathyroidism. This approach has proven to be successful in many patient types and is generally thought to be the procedure of choice in treatment of most forms of tertiary HPT (18). The exception to this may be the renal transplant patient with HPT. In transplant patients, in order to minimize the risk of hypoparathyroidism, some clinicians prefer subtotal parathyroidectomy.

REFERENCES

1. Silver J: Regulation of parathyroid hormone synthesis and secretion. In: Coe FL, Favus MJ (eds) *Disorders of Bone and Mineral Metabolism.* Raven Press, New York, pp 83–105, 1992

2. Hendy GN, Stotland MA, Grunbaum D, Fraher LJ, Loveridge N, Goltzman D: Characteristics of secondary hyperparathyroidism in vitamin D-deficient dogs. *Am J Physiol* 256:E765–E772, 1989

3. Szabo A, Merke J, Beier E, Mall G, Ritz E: 1,25(OH)₂ vitamin D₃ inhibits parathyroid cell proliferation in experimental uremia. *Kid Int* 35:1049–1056, 1989

4. Nygren P, Larsson R, Johansson H, Ljunghall S, Rastad J, Akerstrom G: 1,25(OH)₂D₃ inhibits hormone secretion and proliferation but not functional dedifferentiation of cultured bovine parathyroid cells. *Calcif Tissue Int* 43:213–218, 1988

5. Kremer R, Bolivar I, Goltzman D, Hendy GN: Influence of calcium and 1,25-dihydroxycholecalciferol on proliferation and proto-oncogene expression in primary cultures of bovine parathyroid cells. *Endocrinology* 125:935–941, 1989

6. Gittes RF, Radde IC: Experimental model for hyperparathyroidism: Effect of excessive numbers of transplanted isologous parathyroid glands. *J Urol* 95:595–603, 1966

7. Mayer GP, Habener JF, Potts JT Jr: Parathyroid hormone secretion in vivo: Demonstration of a calcium-independent, nonsuppressible component of secretion. *J Clin Invest* 57:678–683, 1976

8. Parfitt AM: Hypercalcemic hyperparathyroidism following renal transplantation: Differential diagnosis, management, and implications for cell population control in the parathyroid gland. *Miner Electrolyte Metab* 8:92–112, 1982

9. Krause MW, Hedinger CE: Pathologic study of parathyroid glands in tertiary hyperparathyroidism. *Hum Pathol* 16:772–784, 1985

10. Rudberg C, Akerstrom G, Ljunghall S, et al.: Regulation of parathyroid hormone release in primary and secondary hyperparathyroidism-studies in vivo and in vitro. *Acta Endocrinol* 101:408–413, 1982

11. Rudberg C, Grimelius L, Johansson H, et al.: Alteration in density, morphology and parathyroid hormone release of dispersed parathyroid cells from patients with hyperparathyroidism. *Acta Path Microbiol Immunol Scand* 94:253–261, 1986

12. Wallfelt C, Larsson, R, Gylfe E, Ljunghall S, Rastad J, Akerstrom G: Secretory disturbance in hyperplastic parathyroid nodules of uremic hyperparathyroidism: Implication for parathyroid autotransplantation. *World J Surg* 12:431–438, 1988

13. Oka T, Yoshioka T, Shrestha GR, et al: Immunohistochemical study of nodular hyperplastic parathyroid glands in patients with secondary hyperparathyroidism. *Virchows Archiv A Pathol Anat* 413:53–60, 1988

14. Arnold A, Brown M, Urena P, Drueke T, Sarfati E: X-inactivation analysis of clonality in primary and secondary parathyroid hyperplasia (abstract). *J Bone Min Res* 7:S153, 1992

15. Arnold A, Staunton CE, Kim HG, Gaz RD, Kronenberg HM: Monoclonality and abnormal parathyroid hormone genes in parathyroid adenomas. *N Engl J Med* 318:658–662, 1988

16. Friedman E, Sakaguchi K, Bale AE, et al.: Clonality of parathyroid tumors in familial multiple endocrine neoplasia type I. *N Engl J Med* 321:213–218, 1989

17. Thakker RV, Bouloux P, Wooding C, et al.: Association of parathyroid tumors in multiple endocrine neoplasia type I with loss of alleles on chromosome 11. *N Engl Med* 321:218–324, 1989

18. Wells SA, Gunnells JC, Shelburne JD, Schneider AB, Sherwood LM: Transplantation of the parathyroid glands in man: Clinical indications and results. *Surgery* 78:34–44, 1975

19. Brennan MF, Brown EM, Marx SJ, et al.: Recurrent hyperparathyroidism from an autotransplanted parathyroid adenoma. *N Engl J Med* 299:1057–1059, 1978

20. Svensson O, Wernerson A, Reinholt FP: Effect of calcium depletion on the rat parathyroids. *Bone Miner* 3:259–269, 1988

21. Naveh-Many T, Silver J: Regulation of parathyroid hormone gene expression by hypocalcemia, hypercalcemia, and vitamin D in the rat. *J Clin Invest* 86:1313–1319, 1990

22. Fukagawa M, Kaname S-Y, Igarashi T, Ogata E, Kurokawa K: Regulation of parathyroid hormone synthesis in chronic renal failure in rats. *Kid Int* 39:874–881, 1991

23. Brown EM, Wilson RE, Eastman RC, Pallotta J, Marynick SP: Abnormal regulation of parathyroid hormone release by calcium in secondary hyperparathyroidism due to chronic renal failure. *J Clin Endocrinol Metab* 54:172–179, 1982

24. Wallfelt C, Gylfe E, Larsson R, Ljunghall S, Rastad J, Akerstrom G: Relationship between external and cytoplasmic calcium concentrations, parathyroid hormone release and weight of parathyroid glands in human hyperparathyroidism. *J Endocrinol* 116:457–464, 1988

25. Lopez-Hilker S, Galceran T, Chan Y-L, Rapp N, Martin KJ, Slatpolsky E: Hypocalcemia may not be essential for the development of secondary hyperparathyroidism in chronic renal failure. *J Clin Invest* 78:1097–1102, 1986

26. Korkor AB: Reduced binding of [³H]1,25-dihydroxyvitamin D₃ in the parathyroid glands of patients with renal failure. *N Engl J Med* 316:1573–1577, 1987

27. Naveh-Many T, Marx R, Keshet E, Pike JW, Silver J: Regulation of 1,25-dihydroxyvitamin D₃ receptor gene expression by 1,25-dihydroxyvitamin D₃ in the parathyroid in vivo. *J Clin Invest* 86:1968–1975, 1990

28. Quarles LD, Lobaugh B, Murphy G: Intact parathyroid hormone overestimates the presence and severity of parathyroid-mediated osseous abnormalities in uremia. *J Clin Endocrinol Metab* 75:145–150, 1992

29. David DS, Sakai S, Brennan BL, et al.: Hypercalcemia after renal transplantation: Long-term follow-up data. *N Engl J Med* 289:398–401, 1973

30. Cundy T, Kanis JA, Heynen G, Morris PJ, Oliver DO: Calcium metabolism and hyperparathyroidism after renal transplantation. *Quart J Med* 205:67–78, 1983

31. Diethelm AG, Edwards RP, Whelchel JD: The natural history and surgical treatment of hypercalcemia before and after renal transplantation. *Surgery* 154:481–490, 1982

32. McCarron DA, Muther RS, Lenfesty B, Bennet WM: Parathyroid function in persistent hyperparathyroidism: Relationship to gland size. *Kidney Int* 22:662–670, 1982

33. D'Alesandro AM, Melzer JS, Pirsch JD, et al.: Tertiary hyperparathyroidism after renal transplantation: Operative indications. *Surgery* 106:1049–1056, 1989

34. Kinder BK, Rasmussen H: New applications of total parathyroidectomy and autotransplantation: Use in proximal renal tubular dysfunction. *World J Surg* 9:156–164, 1985

35. Dandona P, Mohiuddin J, Weerakoon JW, Freedman DB, Fonseca V, Healey T: Persistence of parathyroid hypersecretion after vitamin D treatment in Asian vegetarians. *J Clin Endocrinol Metab* 59:535–537, 1984

36. Joffe BI, Hackeng WH, Seftel HC, Hartdegen RG: Parathyroid hormone concentrations in nutritional rickets. *Clin Sci* 42:113–116, 1972

37. Fonseca V, Epstein O, Gill DS, et al.: Hyperparathyroidism and low serum osteocalcin despite vitamin D replacement in primary biliary cirrhosis. *J Clin Endocrinol Metab* 64:873–877, 1987

38. Slatopolsky E, Weerts C, Thielan J, Horst R, Harter M, Martin KJ: Marked suppression of secondary hyperparathyroidism by intravenous administration of 1,25-dihydroxy-cholecalciferol in uremic patients. *J Clin Invest* 74:2136–2143, 1984

39. Yohay DA, Lobaugh B, Bartholomay D, Quarles LD: Intensive calcitriol therapy for secondary hyperparathyroidism in maintenance hemodialysis patients: Intolerance due to hyperphosphatemia (abstract). *J Bone Min Res* 7:S297, 1992

31. Familial Hyperparathyroid Syndromes

*Jozsef Szabo, M.D., †Sundeep Khosla, M.D., and *Hunter Heath III, M.D.

*Division of Endocrinology, Metabolism, and Diabetes, University of Utah,
Salt Lake City, Utah, and †Division of Endocrinology, Mayo Clinic,
Rochester, Minnesota

The medical literature suggests that 1–10% of patients with primary hyperparathyroidism (HPT) are from kindreds having one of the "familial multiple endocrine adenomatosis" or "multiple endocrine neoplasia" (MEN) syndromes. These are associated with hyperplasia and/or tumor formation of different endocrine glands. In addition, there is also a syndrome of familial HPT, as an isolated phenomenon without hyperfunction of other glands. Another important hereditary disorder, familial benign hypercalcemia [(FBH) or familial hypocalciuric hypercalcemia] is discussed in Chapter 32. Table 1 compares the features of the syndromes which are discussed in detail below.

MULTIPLE ENDOCRINE NEOPLASIA-TYPE 1 (WERMER'S SYNDROME)

The familial occurrence of parathyroid, anterior pituitary, and pancreatic tumors was first recognized as a distinct syndrome by Wermer in 1954; today it is referred to as MEN-type 1 (MEN-1). He described a family in which the father and 4 of 9 siblings were affected, and postulated an autosomal dominant mode of inheritance with a high degree of penetrance. The pancreatic tumors were frequently accompanied by gastric and duodenal ulcers. Since the original description, other anomalies have also been noted in these kindreds, including carcinoid tumors of the bronchi and duodenum, as well as subcutaneous and visceral lipomas. Less well-established as part of the syndrome is the presence of adrenal cortical adenomas and/or follicular adenomas of the thyroid.

The *most common feature* of MEN-1 is HPT, which is almost always present (>95%). The clinical presentation of HPT associated with MEN-1 resembles that of nonfamilial or sporadic HPT, except for equal sex ratios in the former and a preponderance of female patients in the latter. The diagnosis of HPT is supported, as in the nonfamilial cases, by the finding of an elevated serum calcium level, hypophosphatemia and an inappropriately elevated serum parathyroid hormone level. In general, patients with MEN-1 are younger at the time of diagnosis than patients with sporadic HPT. In fact, childhood and even neonatal cases have been noted.

The only *definitive therapy for HPT* in MEN-1, as in the sporadic cases, is surgical. The indications for surgery are largely the same as for sporadic cases: significant bone disease, active nephrolithiasis, change of mental status, or serum calcium above an arbitrary value, usually 11.0–11.5 mg/dL (2.75–2.88 mmol/L). Given the younger average age of MEN-1 patients, however, surgical intervention is generally undertaken fairly early in the course of the disease.

The *surgical approach* to patients with HPT as part of the MEN-1 syndrome is dictated by the underlying pathology in the parathyroid glands. Although solitary adenomas have been noted, most authorities now agree that HPT in MEN-1 is a multiglandular disorder, with enlargement and hyperplasia of all four parathyroids. The importance of recognizing four-gland hyperplasia in MEN-1, however, is that resection of a single gland or even less than three glands frequently leads to persistent or recurrent hypercalcemia. In one study, 70% of patients with HPT and MEN-1 had remission of hypercalcemia after removal of three or more glands, whereas only 34% had remission of the hypercalcemia after resection of 2½ glands or less.

Most centers now perform a subtotal parathyroidectomy in patients with MEN-1, resecting 3½ glands and leaving about 50 mg of viable tissue. To avoid persistent hypercalcemia or permanent postoperative hypoparathyroidism, some surgeons perform total parathyroidectomy with autotransplantation of the parathyroid tissue into forearm muscles. They reason that, in these patients, recurrent HPT will not require a second neck exploration. However, graft-dependent recurrent hypercalcemia may occur and be difficult to manage. Regardless of the approach, close follow-up of these patients is mandatory; management of their parathyroid disease can be frustrating.

Patients with MEN-1 also develop *neoplasms of the pancreas and pituitary*. The pancreatic lesions are usually islet cell tumors, in two-thirds of cases secreting excess gastrin, leading to Zollinger–Ellison syndrome with acid hypersecretion and recurrent ulceration. Approximately one-third of the islet cell tumors in MEN-1 hypersecrete insulin, leading to fasting hypoglycemia. In a minority of cases, the islet cell tumors may secrete a variety of other substances, including vasoactive intestinal peptide, prostaglandins, glucagon, pancreatic polypeptide, ACTH, and serotonin.

The pituitary tumors in patients with MEN-1 were thought initially to be largely nonfunctional, although an increasing number are now being recognized as prolactinomas. These tumors may also secrete growth hormone, leading to acromegaly. In a minority of cases, there is hypersecretion of ACTH resulting in Cushing's disease.

In a recent necropsy study of 33 patients with MEN-1, one-third of them had benign enlargement of the adrenal gland. The histopathology included diffuse and nodular cortical hypertrophy, cortical hyperplasia, adenomas, and a single case of adrenocortical carcinoma. Surprisingly,

TABLE 1. *Characteristics of familial hyperparathyroid syndromes*

Feature	MEN-1	MEN-2a	MEN-2b (or 3)	Familial hyperparathyroidism
Hyperparathyroidism	>95%	Histologically up to 50%; only ~10% frankly hypercalcemic	Rare	100%
Pancreatic tumors	30–80%	—	—	—
Pituitary adenomas	15–50%	—	—	—
Medullary carcinoma of the thyroid	—	100%	100%	—
Pheochromocytoma or adrenal medullary hyperplasia	—	Up to 50%	Up to 50%	—
Alimentary tract ganglioneuromatosis (mucosal neuromas); marfanoid habitus	—	—	100%	—
Adrenocortical hyperplasia	<33%	—	—	—
Lichen amyloidosis	—	Described	—	—
Inheritance	Autosomal dominant	Autosomal dominant	Autosomal dominant/ sporadic	Autosomal dominant Autosomal recessive (1 report)

24 of the 33 patients had pancreatic endocrine tumors. The pituitary-independent adrenal hyperplasia in these 33 patients did not seem to be a primary lesion in MEN-1, but perhaps could be related to the pancreatic malignant tumor.

Multiple endocrine neoplasia-type 1 has been mapped to the long arm of chromosome 11 (11q13). Based on the autosomal dominant mode of inheritance, offspring of MEN-1 patients have a 50% risk of inheriting the gene. Because MEN-1–associated lesions develop slowly, risk cannot be excluded as late as age 35 years for persons at risk of being gene carriers, despite extensive biochemical testing, including serum calcium, glucose, gastrin, and serum prolactin assays. Once a patient has been identified with the MEN-1 syndrome, it is important to screen family members. Genetic linkage testing has become feasible, and often can be used for informed genetic counseling in MEN-1 families. There is not a test for MEN-1 in an individual; whole families must be tested. The search for the actual MEN-1 gene is still an area of intense research.

MULTIPLE ENDOCRINE NEOPLASIA-TYPE 2a (SIPPLE'S SYNDROME)

Multiple endocrine neoplasia-type 2a (MEN-2a) syndrome is characterized by medullary carcinoma of the thyroid, pheochromocytoma, and parathyroid hyperplasia (Table 1). Originally described by Sipple in 1961, this syndrome is also inherited as an autosomal-dominant trait.

The dominant feature of the MEN-2a syndrome is *medullary carcinoma of the thyroid*, which can occasionally lead to death from metastatic disease. Early detection and therapy is facilitated by the measurement of plasma calcitonin after infusion of calcium or pentagastrin. Once hypercalcitoninemia is detected in persons with other affected relatives, early total thyroidectomy is generally warranted.

The other major feature of MEN-2a is *pheochromocy-*

toma, present in up to 50% of patients (Table 1), and which may precede or follow detection of thyroid cancer. In contrast to sporadic pheochromocytoma, the tumor in MEN-2a is virtually always bilateral and often requires bilateral total adrenalectomy. Unrecognized pheochromocytoma can be lethal during surgical procedures, so this lesion should be diagnosed and treated before neck exploration. Indeed, patients with MEN-2a are far more likely to die from pheochromocytoma than medullary thyroid carcinoma.

Hyperparathyroidism is less common and milder in MEN-2a than in MEN-1, but also results from parathyroid hyperplasia.

In 1989 a cutaneous manifestation termed *"lichen amyloidosis"* was reported in two families with MEN-2a, and in a short time several more families with identical lesions were described. These pruritic, pigmented cutaneous lesions are unilateral, localized to the upper back, and contain amyloid. A French report in 1992 described three members of a MEN-2a family with upper back lesions that were associated with local paroxysmal pain and hyperesthesia. Biopsies from these individuals did not contain amyloid. The authors felt these lesions were a form of dorsal neuropathy that could be an early clinical marker of the MEN-2a syndrome.

The gene for MEN-2a has been localized by linkage analysis to the centromeric region of chromosome 10. Current intensive research raises hopes for cloning of the gene in the near future. The combination of genetic linkage testing and calcitonin assay in MEN-2a families enables us to estimate risks with greater than 90% accuracy.

Current *laboratory screening for relatives* of MEN-2a patients is directed first at detecting medullary carcinoma of the thyroid, by measuring plasma calcitonin levels after pentagastrin or calcium infusion, and at diagnosing pheochromocytoma with the usual catecholamine assays and imaging studies. Fully affected persons may ultimately have had total thyroidectomy, bilateral adrenalectomy, and subtotal parathyroidectomy.

MULTIPLE ENDOCRINE NEOPLASIA-TYPE 2b

Multiple endocrine neoplasia-type 2b (MEN-2b) (sometimes referred to as MEN-3) resembles MEN-2a in that medullary carcinoma of the thyroid and pheochromocytomas are features of both, and the gene for MEN-2b also maps to the same region of chromosome 10 as that for MEN-2a. Although subtle histologic parathyroid hyperplasia may occur, clinical or laboratory evidence of HPT is rare. The most serious problems are aggressive medullary thyroid carcinoma and bilateral pheochromocytomas. These patients also have a characteristic marfanoid body habitus and alimentary tract ganglioneuromatosis, with disfiguring masses in the lips, buccal mucosa, and tongue that progress with age. Routine screening for thyroid and adrenal tumors resembles that for MEN-2a. However, the ganglioneuromas identify clearly the affected person. Most cases of MEN-2b are sporadic, but the gene is transmissible.

FAMILIAL-ISOLATED PRIMARY HYPERPARATHYROIDISM

The existence of familial HPT as a disorder distinct from the MEN-1 syndrome has been a subject of some debate for years. Kindreds have been described with familial hypercalcemia and no other endocrine abnormalities. Several of these were subsequently reclassified as MEN-1 families when associated anomalies surfaced, and other families were later reclassified as having FBH.

A family followed for 20 years in Denmark was described. Apart from HPT, no clinical or biochemical evidence of MEN-1 or MEN-2 syndromes was observed. Linkage analysis showed that the isolated form of familial HPT was linked to the 11q13 locus. This suggests that the gene responsible for this isolated form of HPT is probably identical to the MEN-1 gene, and may represent an allelic variant.

One kindred has been described with apparent autosomal-recessive inheritance of HPT and recurrent large parathyroid adenomas. Other kindreds have been reported with familial cystic adenomas and fibrous tumors of the maxilla and mandibles.

Thus, the genetic syndromes encompassing HPT as a manifestation are numerous and varied, and may require careful attention to accurate diagnosis and proper choice of therapy.

SELECTED REFERENCES

1. Goldsmith RE, Sizemore GW, Chen IW, Zalme E, Altemeir WA: Familial hyperparathyroidism. Description of a large kindred with physiologic observations and a review of the literature. *Ann Intern Med* 84:36–43, 1976
2. Law WM Jr, Heath H III: Familial benign hypercalcemia (hypocalciuric hypercalcemia). Clinical and pathogenetic studies in 21 families. *Ann Intern Med* 102:511–519, 1985
3. Marx SJ, Vinik AI, Santen RJ, Floyd JC Jr, Mills JL, Green J III: Multiple endocrine neoplasia type I: Assessment of laboratory tests to screen for the gene in a large kindred. *Medicine* 65:226–241, 1986
4. Schimke RN: Genetic aspects of multiple endocrine neoplasia. *Ann Rev Med* 35:25–31, 1984
5. Sizemore GW, Heath H III, Carney JA: Multiple endocrine neoplasia, type 2. *Clin Endocrinol Metab* 9:299–315, 1980
6. Skogseid B, Larsson C, Lindgren PG, Kvanta E, Rastad J, Theodorsson E, Wide L, Wilander E, Oberg K: Clinical and genetic features of adrenocortical lesions in multiple endocrine neoplasia type 1. *J Clin Endocrinol Metab* 75:76–81, 1992
7. Larsson C, Shepherd J, Nakamura Y, Blomberg C, Weber G, Werelius B, Hayward N, Teh B, Tokino T, Seizinger B, Skogseid B, Oberg K, Nordenskjold M: Predictive testing for multiple endocrine neoplasia type 1 using DNA polymorphisms. *J Clin Invest* 89:1334–1349, 1992
8. Kousseff BG, Espinoza C, Zamore GA: Sipple syndrome with lichen amyloidosis as a paracrinopathy: Pleiotropy, heterogeneity, or a contiguous gene? *J Am Acad Dermatol* 25:651–657, 1991
9. Chabre O, Labat-Moleur F, Berthod F, Tarel V, Stoebner P, Sobol H, Bachelot I: Atteinte cutanée associée à la neoplasie endocrinienne multiple de type 2A (syndrome de Sipple): Un marqueur clinique precoce. *La Presse Med* 21:299–303, 1992
10. Lichter JB, Wu J, Genel M, Flynn SD, Pakstis AJ, Kidd JR, Kidd KK: Presymptomatic testing using DNA markers for individuals at risk for familial multiple endocrine neoplasia 2A. *J Clin Endocrinol Metab* 74:368–373, 1992
11. Kassem M, Xu C, Brask S, Eriksen EF, Mosekilde L, Kruse T: Familial isolated primary hyperparathyroidism. *J Bone Min Res* 7(suppl 1):S249, 1992

32. Familial Hypocalciuric Hypercalcemia

Stephen J. Marx, M.D.

Mineral Metabolism Section, National Institute of Diabetes and Digestive and Kidney Diseases, National Institutes of Health, Bethesda, Maryland

Familial hypocalciuric hypercalcemia (FHH) (also termed familial benign hypercalcemia) is an autosomal dominant trait characterized by moderate hypercalcemia and relative hypocalciuria (i.e. urine calcium that is low considering the simultaneous hypercalcemia) with high penetrance for both of these features throughout life (1,2).

CLINICAL FEATURES

Symptoms and Signs. Patients with FHH are usually asymptomatic. Occasionally they note easy fatigability, weakness, thought disturbances, or polydipsia. Although these symptoms are also common in typical primary hyperparathyroidism, they are less common and less severe in FHH. There seems to be an increased incidence of relapsing pancreatitis (1,3), and this can occasionally be severe and life-threatening. There may be an increased incidence of gallstones, diabetes mellitus, and myocardial infarction (1,2). The rate of nephrolithiasis or of peptic ulcer disease is the same as in a normal population.

Radiographs and Indices of Bone Function. Radiographs are usually normal. Nephrocalcinosis has the same incidence as in a normal population. There is an increased incidence of chondrocalcinosis (usually clinically silent) and premature vascular calcification (1). Bone turnover measured by indices of bone formation (serum bone gla-protein and or serum alkaline phosphatase) or of bone resorption (urine hydroxproline to creatinine ratio) is mildly increased (4). Mean bone mass is normal, and there is not increased susceptibility to fracture (2,4).

Serum Electrolytes. Serum calcium in gene carriers is elevated throughout life. Typically the degree of elevation decreases modestly from infancy to old age (1). The degree of elevation is similar to that in typical primary hyperparathyroidism. Both free and bound calcium are increased with a normal ratio of free-to-bound calcium (5). Serum magnesium is typically in the high range of normal or modestly elevated, and serum phosphate is modestly depressed.

Renal Function Indices. Creatinine clearance is generally normal. Urinary excretion of calcium is normal, with affected and unaffected family members showing a similar distribution of values. The normal urinary calcium in the face of hypercalcemia reflects increased renal tubular resorption of calcium (i.e., relative hypocalciuria). The renal tubular resorption of magnesium is also modestly increased. Because calcium excretion depends heavily on glomerular filtration rate, total calcium excretion is not a useful index to distinguish FHH from typical primary hyperparathyroidism. The ratio of calcium clearance to creatinine clearance

$$Cl_{Ca}/Cl_{Cr} = [Ca_u*V/Ca_s]/[Cr_u*V/Cr_s] =$$

$$[Ca_u*Cr_s]/[Cr_u*Ca_s]$$

(where Ca is total calcium, Cr is creatinine, CL is renal clearance, V is volume, u is urine, and s is serum) corrects for most of the variation from glomerular filtration. The clearance ratio in FHH is typically one-third of that in typical primary hyperparathyroidism, and a cutoff value at 0.01 (note that the clearance ratio has no units) is helpful for this distinction in a patient with hypercalcemia.

Parathyroid Function Indices. Biochemical testing of parathyroid function, including serum PTH and 1,25-dihydroxyvitamin D [1,25(OH)$_2$D] is usually normal, with modest elevations in 5–10% of cases (6,7). The normal parathyroid function indices in the presence of lifelong hypercalcemia are inappropriate and indicative of a specific role for the parathyroids in maintenance of hypercalcemia. There is often mild parathyroid gland hyperplasia (evident only by careful measurement of gland size) (8,9).

Response to Parathyroidectomy. Subtotal parathyroidectomy results in only very transient lowering of serum calcium with restoration of hypercalcemia within a week

(2). Familial hypocalciuric hypercalcemia (FHH) has been a common cause of unsuccessful parathyroidectomy, accounting for 10% of unsuccessful operations in several large series during the 1970s, before wider recognition of the implications of this diagnosis (10). Total parathyroidectomy in FHH leads to decreased production of 1,25(OH)$_2$D, hypocalcemia, and features of chronic hypoparathyroidism. In several FHH cases deliberate total parathyroidectomy has been attempted without induction of hypocalcemia; presumably, small amounts of residual parathyroid tissue were sufficient to sustain hypercalcemia.

GENETICS OF FAMILIAL HYPOCALCIURIC HYPERCALCEMIA AND RELATION TO NEONATAL SEVERE PRIMARY HYPERPARATHYROIDISM

There is virtually 100% penetrance for hypercalcemia at all ages among heterozygotes for the FHH gene (1). The hypercalcemia has been documented in the first week of life (11). The degree of hypercalcemia shows clustering within kindreds, with several kindreds showing very modest hypercalcemia and several showing rather severe hypercalcemia (12.5–14 mg/dL) in all affected members (1,12). Genetic linkage analysis in eight families has indicated that a gene for FHH is on the long arm of chromosome 3 (13,14). In one large kindred the FHH trait was linked to the short arm of chromosome 19 (14).

The prevalence of FHH has not been established, but it is probably similar to that for familial multiple endocrine neoplasia-type I; each of these diseases may account for about 2% of cases with asymptomatic hypercalcemia.

Neonatal severe primary hyperparathyroidism is an unusual state of life-threatening severe hypercalcemia with massive hyperplasia of all parathyroid glands. Most of these neonates have had FHH in one or both parents (12,15). Some cases clearly reflect a double-dose of FHH genes (15). Other cases may result from an FHH heterozygote having gestated in a normocalcemic (i.e., FHH-negative) mother, who caused superimposed intrauterine secondary hyperparathyroidism (16,17). The maternal contribution to neonatal hyperparathyroidism in this latter setting may be self-limited.

PATHOPHYSIOLOGY

Biochemical testing has established that the parathyroid gland functions abnormally in FHH (see above). A surgically decreased gland mass can maintain the same calcium level by increasing hormone secretion rate per cell. Parathyroid function shows features expected from a selective and mild increase in glandular "setpoint" for calcium suppression of PTH secretion. "Setpoint" was measured in parathyroid cells from a neonate presumed to have a double-dose of FHH genes (18); these cells showed a setpoint higher than ever seen in any parathyroid adenoma. Depending on definition, FHH can therefore be labeled as a form of "primary hyperparathyroidism." We prefer to consider it an atypical form of primary hyperparathyroidism in distinct contrast to the more typical form associated with hypercalciuria, nephrolithiasis, markedly increased gland mass, clear elevations of plasma PTH, and generally excellent response to subtotal parathyroidectomy.

In addition to the disturbance presumed to be intrinsic to the parathyroids in FHH, there is also a disturbance intrinsic to the kidneys. The tubular reabsorption of calcium, normally regulated by parathyroid hormone, remains strikingly increased even after total parathyroidectomy in FHH (19).

Thus FHH is associated with abnormalities in cellular interaction with extracellular calcium at two organs: the parathyroid and the kidney. The molecular basis for this is not known, nor is it clear whether calcium interactions are abnormal in any other organs. Increased activity of erythrocyte calcium-ATPase in FHH was reported (20,21), but a second laboratory could not reproduce this finding (22).

MANAGEMENT

Intervention in the Typical Case of Familial Hypocalciuric Hypercalcemia. Because of the generally benign course and the lack of response to subtotal parathyroidectomy, virtually all patients should be advised against parathyroidectomy. Attempts to regulate serum calcium with medications (diuretics, estrogens, and phosphates) have not changed serum calcium. Familial hypocalciuric hypercalcemia is compatible with survival into the 80s, and it is uncertain whether there is any decrease in average life expectancy.

Indications for Parathyroidectomy. In rare situations (1) neonatal severe primary hyperparathyroidism resulting from a double dose of FHH gene; 2) adult with relapsing pancreatitis; and 3) child or adult with serum calcium persistently above 14 mg/dL] parathyroidectomy may be necessary. Attempted total parathyroidectomy is recommended in these unusual situations. Several patients have had parathyroidectomy with fresh parathyroid autografts; most have developed graft-dependent recurrent hypercalcemia.

"Sporadic" Hypocalciuric Hypercalcemia. Without a positive family history the decision about management of sporadic hypocalciuric hypercalcemia is difficult. Because there is a wide range of urine calcium values in FHH and in parathyroid adenoma, an occasional patient with parathyroid adenoma will show a very low calcium-to-creatinine clearance ratio. And occasionally a patient with FHH may show a high ratio. Coexistence FHH and idiopathic hypercalciuria has been clearly documented in at least one case (1). "Sporadic" hypocalciuric hypercalcemia should generally be managed as typical FHH. In time the underlying diagnosis may become evident; low morbidity in such patients should be anticipated for the same reasons that morbidity is low in FHH. The FHH gene(s) will probably be identified in the near future (13);

screening such a sporadic patient for mutation could then be useful.

Pregnancy. Pregnancy in an FHH carrier or in the spouse of an FHH carrier requires special understanding, because of possible antagonism between fetal and maternal calcium regulation. The affected offspring of a carrier should show asymptomatic hypercalcemia. The unaffected offspring of a carrier may show symptomatic hypocalcemia from parathyroid suppression. The affected offspring of an unaffected mother may show rather severe neonatal hypercalcemia because of intrauterine secondary hyperparathyroidism; this will usually evolve into asymptomatic hypercalcemia without parathyroidectomy.

Family Screening. Because of the high penetrance for expression of hypercalcemia in FHH carriers, accurate genetic assignments can usually be made from one determination of total calcium (or preferably ionized or albumin-adjusted calcium). Family screening is particularly valuable to avoid unnecessary parathyroidectomy should hypercalcemia be otherwise recognized incidental to blood testing for routine care. In unusual circumstances (i.e. when blood calcium tests are inconclusive) genetic linkage may give a reliable diagnosis.

CONCLUSIONS

Familial hypocalciuric hypercalcemia is a rather common cause of asymptomatic hypercalcemia, particularly when the hypercalcemia presents at early ages. The diagnosis requires alertness to urinary calcium, but the diagnosis cannot currently be established without family testing and recognition of the disorder in first-degree relatives. In the past FHH was a common cause of unsuccessful parathyroidectomy. Although mild symptoms similar to those in typical primary hyperparathyroidism are quite common, virtually all patients should be followed without any intervention.

REFERENCES

1. Marx SJ, Attie MF, Levine MA, Spiegel AM, Downs RW Jr, Lasker RD: The hypocalciuric or benign variant of familial hypercalcemia: Clinical and biochemical features in fifteen kindreds. *Medicine* 60:397–412, 1981
2. Law WM Jr, Heath H III: Familial benign hypercalcemia (hypocalciuric hypercalcemia): Clinical and pathogenetic studies in 21 families. *Ann Intern Med* 102:511–519, 1985
3. Davies M, Klimiuk PS, Adams PH, Lumb GA, Anderson DC: Familial hypocalciuric hypercalcemia and acute pancreatitis. *Br Med J* 282:1029–1031, 1981
4. Kristiansen JH, Rodbro P, Christiansen C, Johansen J, Jensen JT: Familial hypocalciuric hypercalcemia. III. Bone mineral metabolism. *Clin Endocrinol* 26:713–716, 1987
5. Marx SJ, Spiegel AM, Brown EM, Koehler JO, Gardner DG, Brennan MF, Aurbach GD: Divalent cation metabolism. Familial hypocalciuric hypercalcemia versus typical primary hyperparathyroidism. *Am J Med* 65:235–242, 1978
6. Firek AF, Kao PC, Heath H III: Plasma intact parathyroid hormone (PTH) and PTH-related peptide in familial benign hypercalcemia: Greater responsiveness to endogenous PTH than in primary hyperparathyroidism. *J Clin Endocrinol Metab* 72:541–546, 1991

7. Kristiansen JH, Rodbro P, Christiansen C, Brochner MJ, Carl J: Familial hypocalciuric hypercalcemia. II. Intestinal calcium absorption and vitamin D metabolism. *Clin Endocrinol* 23: 511–515, 1985

8. Thorgeirsson U, Costa J, Marx SJ: The parathyroid glands in familial hypocalciuric hypercalcemia. *Hum Pathol* 12:229–237, 1981

9. Law WM Jr, Carney JA, Heath H III: Parathyroid glands in familial benign hypercalcemia (familial hypocalciuric hypercalcemia). *Am J Med* 76:1021–1026, 1984

10. Marx SJ, Stock JL, Attie MF, Downs RW Jr, Gardner DG, Brown EM, Spiegel AM, Doppman JL, Brennan MF: Familial hypocalciuric hypercalcemia: Recognition among patients referred after unsuccessful parathyroid exploration. *Ann Intern Med* 92:351–356 1980

11. Orwoll E, Silbert J, McClung M: Asymptomatic neonatal familial hypercalcemia. *Pediatrics* 69:109–111, 1982

12. Marx SJ, Fraser D, Rapoport A: Familial hypocalciuric hypercalcemia. Mild expression of the gene in heterozygotes and severe expression in homozygotes. *Am J Med* 78:15–22, 1985

13. Chou Y-HW, Brown EM, Levi T, Crowe G, Atkinson AB, Arnqvist H, Toss G, Fuleihan GEH, Seidman JG, Seidman CE: The gene responsible for familial hypocalciuric hypercalcemia maps to chromosome 3q in four unrelated families. *Nature Genet* 1: 295–300, 1992

14. Heath H III, Jackson CE, Otterud B, Leppart MF: Familial benign hypercalcemia (FBH) phenotype results from mutations at two distant loci on chromosomes 3q and 19p. *Clin Res* 41:270A, 1993

15. Marx SJ, Attie MF, Spiegel AM, Levine MA, Lasker RD, Fox M: An association between neonatal severe primary hyperparathyroidism and familial hypocalciuric hypercalcemia in three kindreds. *N Engl J Med* 306:257–264, 1982

15. Eftekhari F, Yousefzadeh DK: Primary infantile hyperparathyroidism: Clinical, laboratory, and radiographic features in 21 cases. *Skeletal Radiol* 8:201–208, 1982

16. Page LA, Haddow JE: Self-limited neonatal hyperparathyroidism in familial hypocalciuric hypercalcemia. *J Pediatr* 111: 261–264, 1987

17. Marx SJ, Lasker RD, Brown EM, Fitzpatrick LA, Sweezey NB, Goldbloom RB, Gillis DA, Cole DE: Secretory dysfunction in parathyroid cells from a neonate with severe primary hyperparathyroidism. *J Clin Endocrinol Metab* 62:445–449, 1986

18. Attie MF, Gill JR Jr, Stock JL, Spiegel AM, Downs RW Jr, Levine MA, Marx SJ: Urinary calcium excretion in familial hypocalciuric hypercalcemia. Persistence of relative hypocalciuria after induction of hypoparathyroidism. *J Clin Invest* 72:667–676, 1983

19. Hoare SF, Paterson CR: Familial benign hypercalcaemia: A possible abnormality in calcium transport by erythrocytes. *Eur J Clin Invest* 14:428–430, 1984

20. Mole PA, Paterson CR: Calcium-ATPase activity in erythrocyte ghosts from patients with familial benign hypercalcaemia. *Scan J Clin Lab Invest* 45:349–353, 1985

21. Donahue HJ, Penniston JT, Heath H III: Kinetics of erythrocyte plasma membrane (Ca^{2+},Mg^{2+}) ATPase in familial benign hypercalcemia. *J Clin Endocrinol Metab* 68:893–897, 1989

33. Humoral Hypercalcemia of Malignancy

Andrew F. Stewart, M.D.

Department of Endocrinology, West Haven Veterans Affairs Medical Center, West Haven, Connecticut, and Yale University School of Medicine, New Haven, Connecticut

The term humoral hypercalcemia of malignancy, or HHM, in broad terms describes a clinical syndrome characterized by hypercalcemia that is caused by secretion by a cancer of a circulating calcemic factor. The tumor typically has limited or no skeletal involvement. The term describes a classic endocrine system, with the tumor being the "secretory gland" and the "target organs" being the skeleton and the kidney. The term can be used in a general sense to describe the production by tumors of any humoral calcemic factor. However, as currently used, the term HHM describes a very specific clinical syndrome that is due to the production of parathyroid hormone-related protein (PTHrP) (see chapters 11 and 20). These patients comprise the large majority of patients with humorally mediated hypercalcemia. Several recent detailed reviews of the syndrome are listed at the end of this section.

The syndrome was first described in 1941. The patient in question had a renal carcinoma with a solitary skeletal metastasis. Subsequent studies in the 1950s and 1960s documented the "humoral" nature of the syndrome by demonstrating that: 1) typical patients had little or no skeletal tumor involvement, and 2) the hypercalcemia and other biochemical abnormalities reversed when the tumor was resected or treated. Evidence provided in the 1960s and 1970s suggested that the responsible factor was prostaglandin E_2, a vitamin D-like sterol,

or PTH. It is now clear that none of these is responsible.

From a clinical standpoint patients with HHM have advanced disease with tumors that are usually obvious clinically and, therefore, carry a poor prognosis. Exceptions to this rule include small, well-differentiated endocrine tumors such a pheochromocytomas or islet cell tumors. In contrast to patients with hypercalcemia due to skeletal involvement with cancer (see Chapter 34) who typically have breast cancer, multiple myeloma or lymphomas, patients with HHM most often have squamous carcinomas (lung, esophagus, cervix, vulva, skin, head, and neck). Other tumor types commonly associated with HHM are renal, bladder, and ovarian carcinomas. Breast carcinomas may cause either typical HHM or may lead to hypercalcemia through skeletal metastatic involvement. Finally, the subset of hypercalcemic patients with lymphomas due to the human T-cell leukemia virus-I appears to have classic biochemical HHM. Patients with HHM account for up to 80% of patients with malignancy-associated hypercalcemia. Certain common tumors (e.g., colon, prostate, thyroid, oat cell, and gastric carcinomas) rarely cause hypercalcemia of any type.

Biochemically and histologically patients with HHM share certain features with patients with primary hyperparathyroidism (HPT), and differ in other respects (Table 1 and Fig. 1). Both groups of patients have a humoral

TABLE 1. *Similarities and differences between patients with primary hyperparathyroidism (HPT) and humoral hypercalcemia of malignancy (HHM)*

	HPT	HHM
Humorally-mediated hypercalcemia	+	+
Hypophosphatemia	+	+
Phosphaturia	+	+
Nephrogenous cAMP elevation	+	+
Increased osteoclastic bone resorption	+	+
Increased renal calcium reabsorption	+	±
Increased plasma 1,25-dihydroxyvitamin D	+	−
Increased osteoblastic bone formation	+	−
Increased circulating immunoreactive parathyroid hormone	+	−
Increased circulating immunoreactive parathyroid hormone-related protein	−	+
Hypercalcemia due primarily to effects on kidney and GI tract	+	−
Hypercalcemia due primarily to bone resorption	−	+

syndrome, both are hypercalcemic, and both are hypophosphatemic and display reductions in the renal tubular phosphorus threshold. Both groups display increased nephrogenous or urinary cAMP excretion, indicating an interaction of the respective humoral mediator with proximal tubular PTH receptors. Both groups display increases in osteoclastic bone resorption when bone is examined histologically (Fig. 2).

In contrast, patients with HHM differ from those with HPT in several important respects (Fig. 1 and Table 1). Parathyroid hormone is a potent stimulus for distal tubular calcium reabsorption, and patients with HPT therefore display only modest hypercalciuria. In contrast, most patients with HHM demonstrate marked increases in calcium excretion, apparently reflecting a weaker effect of PTHrP on distal tubular calcium reabsorption. Parathyroid hormone is also a potent stimulus for the renal production of 1,25-dihydroxyvitamin D [1,25(OH)₂D]. Patients with HPT therefore often demonstrate increases in circulating 1,25(OH)₂D and a resultant increase in calcium

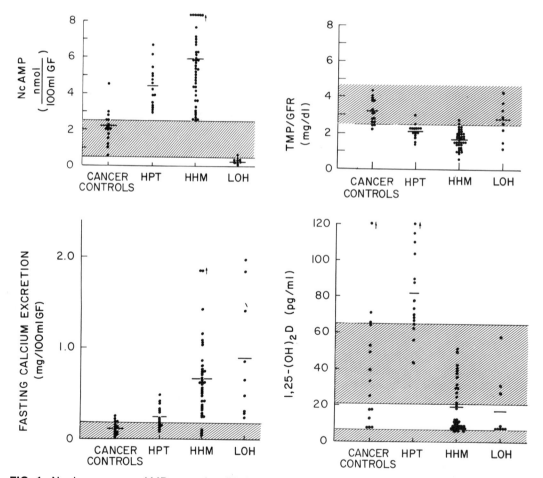

FIG. 1. Nephrogenous cAMP excretion (NcAMP), renal tubular maximum for phosphorus (TmP/GFR), fasting calcium excretion, and plasma 1,25(OH)₂D values in normocalcemic patients with cancer (cancer controls), patients with primary HPT, with HHM, and with hypercalcemia due to bone metastases or "local osteolytic hypercalcemia" (LOH), as defined in Chapter 34. (From Stewart AF, Horst R, Deftos LJ, Cadman EC, Lang R, Broadus AE: Biochemical evaluation of patients with cancer-associated hypercalcemia: Evidence for humoral and nonhumoral groups. *N Engl J Med* 303:1377–1383, 1980.)

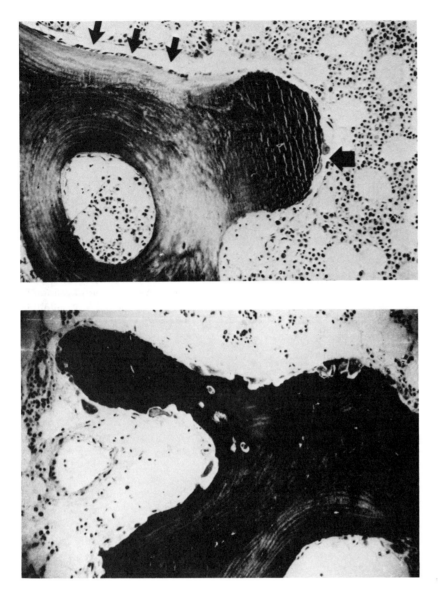

FIG. 2. Comparison of bone histology in a patient with HPT *(top)* and HHM *(bottom).* In both groups osteoclastic activity is accelerated, although it is higher in HHM than in HPT. In HPT, osteoblastic activity and osteoid are increased, but both are markedly decreased in HHM. It is this "uncoupling" of formation from resorption in HHM that plays the major role in causing hypercalcemia.

absorption by the intestine. In contrast, patients with HHM display reductions in 1,25(OH)$_2$D values and in intestinal calcium absorption. The physiology underlying this observation is uncertain since N-terminal PTHrPs *in vitro* and *in vivo* stimulate renal 1αOHase, the enzyme that synthesizes 1,25(OH)$_2$D. Osteoblastic bone formation is increased and coupled to the increased bone resorption rate in patients with HPT (Fig. 2). In patients with HHM osteoblastic bone formation, however, is reduced and is therefore dissociated or "uncoupled" from the increased osteoclastic bone resorption (Fig. 2). The reason for this "uncoupling" is also unclear, because synthetic N-terminal PTHrPs *in vitro* and *in vivo* in animals stimulate osteoblastic activity. Of course, immunoreactive PTH concentrations in plasma are elevated in patients with HPT but are normal or suppressed, depending primarily on the assay used, in patients with HHM (Fig. 3). Conversely, as shown in Fig. 4, immunoreactive PTHrP values are elevated in HHM, but are normal in patients with HPT. Preliminary studies have suggested that immu-

noreactive PTHrP concentration may be useful in monitoring responses to surgery, chemotherapy, or radiotherapy in patients in whom levels are elevated before therapy.

Hypercalcemia in patients with HHM has both skeletal and renal components. The skeletal component, as noted previously, reflects increased osteoclast activity and uncoupling of osteoblasts from osteoclasts. The renal component reflects variable increases in distal tubular calcium reabsorption. Equally or more importantly, patients with HHM are usually volume-depleted as a result of their hypercalcemia with resultant inability to concentrate the urine, and as a result of poor oral fluid intake. The volume depletion leads to a reduction in the filtered load of calcium and a reduction in the fractional excretion of calcium.

Therapy of HHM is discussed in more detail in Chapter 41, but should include measures aimed at 1) reducing the tumor burden, 2) reducing osteoclastic bone resorption, and 3) augmenting renal calcium clearance.

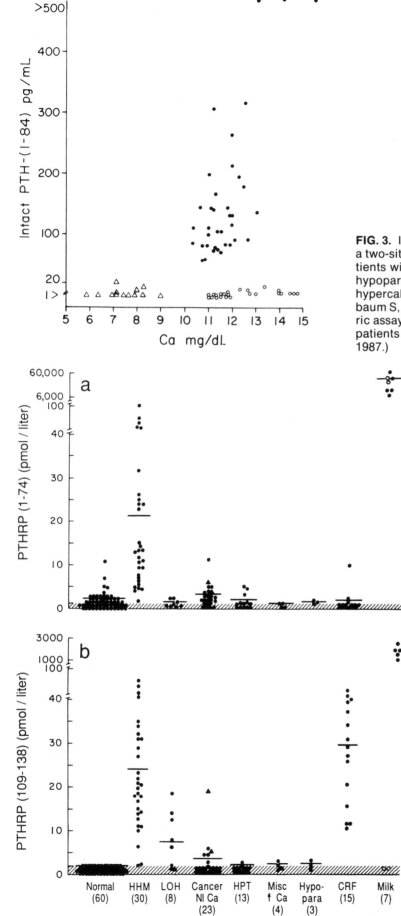

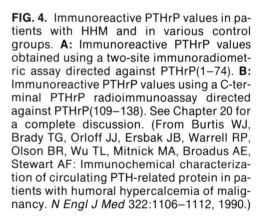

FIG. 3. Immunoreactive PTH concentration of PTH using a two-site immunoradiometric assay for PTH(1–84) in patients with primary HPT (*closed circles*), in patients with hypoparathyroidism (*open triangles*), and in patients with hypercalcemia of malignancy *(open circles)*. (From Nussbaum S, et al.: Highly sensitive two-site immunoradiometric assay of parathyrin and its clinical utility in evaluating patients with hypercalcemia. *Clin Chem* 33:1364–1367, 1987.)

FIG. 4. Immunoreactive PTHrP values in patients with HHM and in various control groups. **A:** Immunoreactive PTHrP values obtained using a two-site immunoradiometric assay directed against PTHrP(1–74). **B:** Immunoreactive PTHrP values using a C-terminal PTHrP radioimmunoassay directed against PTHrP(109–138). See Chapter 20 for a complete discussion. (From Burtis WJ, Brady TG, Orloff JJ, Ersbak JB, Warrell RP, Olson BR, Wu TL, Mitnick MA, Broadus AE, Stewart AF: Immunochemical characterization of circulating PTH-related protein in patients with humoral hypercalcemia of malignancy. *N Engl J Med* 322:1106–1112, 1990.)

SELECTED REFERENCES

1. Massachusetts General Hospital: Case records of the Massachusetts General Hospital (Case 27461). *N Engl J Med* 225:789–791, 1941
2. Rodman JS, Sherwood LM: Disorders of bone and mineral in malignancy. In Avioli LV, Krone SM (eds) *Metabolic Bone Disease*, vol 2. Academic Press, New York, pp 555–631, 1987
3. Skrabanek P, McPartlin J, Powell D: Tumor hypercalcemia and ectopic hyperparathyroidism. *Medicine* 59:262–282, 1980
4. Stewart AF, Horst R, Deftos LJ, Cadman EC, Lang R, Broadus AE: Biochemical evaluation of patients with cancer-associated hypercalcemia: Evidence for humoral and non-humoral groups. *N Engl J Med* 303:1377–1383, 1980
5. Stewart AF, Vignery A, Silverglate A, Ravin ND, LiVolsi V, Broadus AE, Baron R: Quantitative bone histomorphometry in humoral hypercalcemia of malignancy. *J Clin Endocrinol Metab* 55:219–227, 1982
6. Godsall JW, Burtis WJ, Insogna KL, Broadus AE, Stewart AF: *Nephrogenous Cyclic AMP, Adenylate Cyclase-Stimulating Activity, and the Humoral Hypercalcemia of Malignancy. Recent Progress in Hormone Research.* Greep RO (ed). Academic Press, Boca Raton, Florida, pp 705–750, 1986
7. Bonjour J-P, Phillipe J, Guelpa G, Bisetti A, Rizzoli R, Jung A, Rosini S, Kanis JA: Bone and renal components of hypercalcemia in malignancy and responses to a single infusion of clodronate. *Bone* 9:123–130, 1988
8. Nussbaum SR, Zahradnik RJ, Lavigne JR, Brennan GL, Nozawa-Ung K, Kim LY, Keutmann H, Wang CA, Nohs JT, Segre GV: Highly sensitive two-site immunoradiometric assay of parathyrin and its clinical utility in evaluating patients with hypercalcemia. *Clin Chem* 33:1364–1367, 1987
9. Burtis WJ, Brady TG, Orloff JJ, Ersbak JB, Warrell RP, Olson BR, Wu TL, Mitnick MA, Broadus AE, Stewart AF: Immunochemical characterization of circulating PTH-related protein in patients with humoral hypercalcemia of malignancy. *N Engl J Med* 322:1106–1112, 1990

34. Hypercalcemia in Hematologic Malignancies and in Solid Tumors Associated with Extensive Localized Bone Destruction

Gregory R. Mundy, M.D.

Departments of Medicine and Endocrinology, University of Texas Health Science Center, San Antonio, Texas

HYPERCALCEMIA AND BONE DESTRUCTION IN MYELOMA

Almost all patients with myeloma have extensive bone destruction. Bone destruction may occur either as discrete local lesions or diffuse involvement throughout the axial skeleton. This increased bone resorption is responsible for a number of disabling features, including susceptibility to pathological fracture, intractable bone pain and, in some patients, hypercalcemia. Approximately 80% of patients with myeloma present with a chief complaint of bone pain. Hypercalcemia occurs in 20–40% patients at some time during the course of the disease.

The bone destruction that occurs in myeloma is due to an increase in the activity of osteoclasts. Myeloma cells in the marrow cavity produce cytokines that activate adjacent endosteal osteoclasts to resorb bone. This was first recognized by observations on cultured human myeloma cells, which were found to release local factors that stimulate osteoclast activity (1,2). It has been found that the bone-resorbing cytokine lymphotoxin is produced by cultured human myeloma cells (3). This cytokine is produced normally by activated T-lymphocytes. It is a member of the same family of immune cell products as tumor necrosis factor and interleukin-1, both of which are produced by cells in the monocyte-macrophage lineage. Lymphotoxin seems to have overlapping biological properties with those of tumor necrosis factor, and binds to the same receptor. Tumor necrosis factor is thought to be the major

mediator of the systemic effects of endotoxic shock. In bone, these cytokines stimulate osteoclast precursors to replicate, but also stimulate the differentiation of committed osteoclast precursors into mature cells. In addition to these actions, they act on mature multinucleated cells to cause them to form resorption lacunae (4,5). Thus lymphotoxin acts at all sites in the formation, differentiation, and activation of the osteoclast. Lymphotoxin is not the only bone resorbing cytokine that may be involved in myeloma (3). Interleukin-6 and interleukin-1 have also been implicated in enhanced bone resorption and hypercalcemia in myeloma (6,7), and it is possible that all three of these cytokines may play a pathophysiologic role in the bone destruction in myeloma.

Although essentially all patients with myeloma develop extensive bone destruction, <40% become hypercalcemic. Moreover, there is not a close correlation between the extent of bone destruction and the development of hypercalcemia (8). The explanation is that increased bone resorption is most likely to lead to hypercalcemia in those patients with impaired glomerular filtration. Impairment of glomerular filtration decreases the kidney's capacity to excrete calcium and clear it from the circulation. Impairment of glomerular filtration is common in patients with myeloma (9) for a number of reasons. Probably the most important is the development of Bence Jones nephropathy, also called "myeloma kidney." In this circumstance, free light chain fragments of immunoglobulin molecules (Bence Jones proteins) are filtered by the glomerulus, but impair both glomerular and tubular function. Patients with myeloma may also develop azotemia due to recurrent infections, uric acid nephropathy, and amyloidosis.

Because the mechanisms responsible for hypercalcemia are different in patients with myeloma from patients with other types of malignancy, there are subtle differences in laboratory tests at the time of diagnosis. Because renal function is impaired, many patients with myeloma have increased serum phosphorus rather than a decreased serum phosphorus, which is common with other types of malignancy. In addition, serum alkaline phosphatase, a marker of osteoblast activity, is usually not increased in patients with myeloma because there is little active new bone formation. For similar reasons, bone scans may also be negative. The reason for the decrease in osteoblast activity in patients with myeloma is not known.

Treatment of myeloma patients with hypercalcemia may be difficult because of the impairment in glomerular filtration. Agents that are nephrotoxic should be avoided if possible. For example, plicamycin (also called mithramycin) is not an ideal therapeutic agent for hypercalcemia in myeloma because it is directly nephrotoxic and is dependent on the kidneys for its elimination. As a consequence, its use will often be associated with toxicity. Parenteral pamidronate (a bisphosphonate) and gallium nitrate are both extremely effective in this situation, although there is more experience with pamidronate. Pamidronate can be expected to reverse hypercalcemia in essentially all patients with myeloma. However, caution should be used with these agents in patients with severe impaired renal function. Hypercalcemia in many patients with myeloma responds well to treatment of the primary disease with alkylating agents and corticosteroids (10). Corticosteroids themselves are more frequently useful in the treatment of hypercalcemia in myeloma than they are in other malignancies. The combination of calcitonin and corticosteroids is usually effective in myeloma and may be useful particularly in those cases where glomerular filtration is impaired, because neither agent is nephrotoxic. It is generally not advisable to treat an osteopenic patient with corticosteroids, although in myeloma the prognosis for the patient is usually so poor once hypercalcemia has developed that the objectives of therapy are usually to keep the patient symptom-free from hypercalcemia in the remaining months left to live, and corticosteroids may be very effective in this regard.

For patients with myeloma who have intractable bone pain, radiation therapy is recommended if the pain is localized. It can be dramatically effective in relieving symptoms.

HYPERCALCEMIA ASSOCIATED WITH LYMPHOMAS

Occasional patients with various lymphomas develop hypercalcemia (11). This can occur in Hodgkin's disease, in B-cell lymphomas, in T-cell lymphomas, and in Burkitt's lymphoma. In T-cell lymphomas, it is frequently associated with the human T-cell lymphotrophic virus-type I (HTLV-I). This is a recently described oncogenic type C retrovirus that is related to the AIDS virus, infects

certain T-cells, and results in a lymphoproliferative T-cell disorder (12). The cause of hypercalcemia and bone destruction in these lymphomas has not been well characterized. In most cases, it is probably due to a bone-resorbing lymphokine produced by the neoplastic lymphoid cells. These lymphokines have not yet been identified. In a few patients, it may be due, at least in part, to increased 1,25-dihydroxyvitamin D production by the lymphoid cells. Several patients with different types of lymphoma and hypercalcemia have been found to have increased serum 1,25-dihydroxyvitamin D concentrations (13). When measured, this has been associated with increased absorption of calcium from the intestine. Lymphoid cells transformed by inoculation with HTLV-I virus develop the capacity to synthesize 1,25-dihydroxyvitamin D (14). However, there has been controversy about the relative frequency of increased serum 1,25-dihydroxyvitamin D in patients with hypercalcemia associated with lymphoproliferative disorders. One group in California has reported that half of their patients have increased serum 1,25-dihydroxyvitamin D concentrations (15). In contrast, in Japan where hypercalcemia associated with HTLV-lymphoproliferative disorders is common, serum 1,25-dihydroxyvitamin D is not increased but production of the parathyroid hormone-related protein by neoplastic cells has been clearly demonstrated (16). Hypercalcemia also occurs occasionally in other hematologic malignancies such as chronic lymphocytic leukemia, acute leukemia, and chronic myelogenous leukemia, particularly during acute blast transformation. However, the association of hypercalcemia with these disorders is unusual enough that these patients should be carefully evaluated for another cause of hypercalcemia. In most patients, if another cause is present, this other cause will be primary hyperparathyroidism.

HYPERCALCEMIA IN SOLID TUMORS ASSOCIATED WITH EXTENSIVE LOCALIZED BONE DESTRUCTION

Solid tumors frequently spread to involve the skeleton, and when they do so the bone lesions are usually destructive or osteolytic (for a more detailed review, see ref. 17). Approximately one-third to one-half of all tumors spread to bone. Bone is the third most common site of metastasis of solid tumors after the liver and the lung. However, there is a distinct pattern of tumor cell metastasis to bone. Common tumors such as lung, breast, and prostate cancer frequently metastasize to bone, and bone metastases are present in nearly all patients with advanced breast or prostate cancer.

There are two distinct types of tumor metastases: osteoblastic metastases and osteolytic metastases. Osteolytic metastases are much more common and more significant as a clinical problem. Lytic metastases are usually destructive and are much more liable to be associated with pathologic fracture and hypercalcemia.

Osteolytic bone metastasis is one of the most feared complications of malignancy. The consequences for the patient include intractable bone pain at the site of the metastasis, pathological fracture following trivial injury, nerve compression syndromes due to obstruction of fora-mena (the most serious example is spinal cord compression), and hypercalcemia, when bone destruction is great enough. Once tumor cells are housed in the skeleton, curative therapy is no longer possible in most patients and only palliative therapy is available.

Tumor cells metastasize most frequently to the axial skeleton. It is clear that there are important features not just of the tumor cell that metastasizes (the seed), but also of the skeleton (the soil) that determines the likelihood that bone metastases will occur with any tumor. These factors are only now being determined.

Because hypercalcemia of breast cancer is associated with extensive bone metastasis in the majority of patients, understanding the mechanism for tumor cell migration to bone should clarify the mechanisms by which breast cancer cells cause bone destruction. Tumor cells spread to bone after being shed from the primary tumor. Release from the primary site is probably associated with the production of proteolytic enzymes by the cancer cells that cause the cells to detach one from another. Once tumor cells enter the circulation, they traverse vascular organs, including the red bone marrow. Within the bone marrow cavity, they migrate through wide-channeled sinusoids to the endosteal bone surface.

The migration of tumor cells from the bloodstream to the endosteal surfaces of bone is a multistep process that involves a number of distinct steps (18) (Fig. 1). These steps include 1) attachment to the basement membrane, probably via the basement membrane glycoprotein laminin and laminin receptors on the tumor cell surface; 2) production of proteolytic enzymes by tumor cells, which disrupt the basement membrane and allow tumor cells access to the organ stroma; 3) directed migration of tumor cells via chemotactic processes through the basement membrane; and 4) production of mediators that activate

osteoclasts at the bone surface. These processes are now being unraveled by both *in vitro* and *in vivo* techniques. Some facts have become apparent. For example, it has recently been shown that 1) laminin receptors on tumor cells are important for metastasis to form and antagonists of laminin may block the metastatic process to bone; 2) metastatic tumor cells in the bone microenvironment show different properties from the same tumor cells at the primary site (e.g., they may produce parathyroid hormone-related protein in bone but not at the primary site); 3) it is likely that the bone-derived factors stored in bone and released locally when bone is resorbed may alter function of tumor cells in the bone microenvironment; 4) tumor cells can be stimulated to migrate unidirectionally in response to the products of resorbing bone cultures (19), as well as to fragments of type-I collagen (20), which is the most abundant protein in the bone matrix (possibly breast cancer cells are attracted by these mechanisms to sites of relatively active bone turnover, where they form a nidus that eventually becomes an osteolytic deposit); and 5) inhibitors of osteoclastic bone resorption can inhibit progression of the metastatic process (e.g., it has recently been shown that bisphosphonates may inhibit the formation of fresh metastases).

Because bone metastasis is such an important complication of the most common tumors that affect humans, namely lung cancer and breast cancer, understanding the cellular events involved and devising therapeutic strategies to prevent new metastasis and inhibit continued growth of established metastases are very important therapeutic goals for cancer management.

The principles of treatment of patients with metastatic bone disease and hypercalcemia are the same as those for other patients with hypercalcemia of malignancy (21) (see Chapter 41).

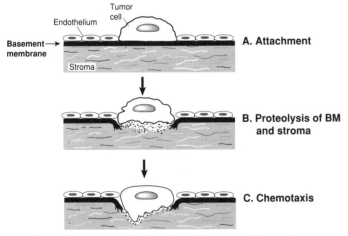

FIG. 1. Stepwise progression of tumor cells as they traverse basement membranes (BM) to migrate to the bone surface. Liotta (18) proposed that this involves a multistep process, including **(A)** attachment of the tumor cell to the basement membrane, **(B)** disruption of the basement membrane by tumor cell production of proteolytic enzymes, and **(C)** unilateral migration (chemotaxis) of tumor cells through the disrupted membrane to the underlying tissue stroma with eventual access to the bone surface (see text for details).

REFERENCES

1. Mundy GR, Raisz LG, Cooper RA, Schechter GP, Salmon SE: Evidence for the secretion of an osteoclast stimulating factor in myeloma. *N Engl J Med* 291:1041–1046, 1974
2. Mundy GR, Bertolini DB: Bone destruction and hypercalcemia in plasma cell myeloma. *Sem Oncol* 13:291–299, 1986
3. Garrett RI, Durie BGM, Nedwin GE, et al.: Production of the bone resorbing cytokine lymphotoxin by cultured human myeloma cells. *N Engl J Med* 317:526–532, 1987
4. Thomson BM, Saklatvala J, Chambers TJ: Osteoblasts mediate interleukin-1 stimulation of bone resorption by rat osteoclasts. *J Exp Med* 164:104–112, 1986
5. Thomson BM, Mundy GR, Chambers TJ: Tumor necrosis factors alpha and beta induce osteoblastic cells to stimulate osteoclastic bone resorption. *J Immunol* 138:775–779, 1987
6. Bataille R, Jourdan M, Zhang Xue-Guang, et al.: Serum levels of interleukin-6, a potent myeloma cell growth factor as a reflection of disease severity in plasma cell dyscrasias. *J Clin Invest* 84:2008–2011, 1989
7. Cozzolino F, Torcia M, Aldinucci D, et al.: Production of interleukin-1 by bone marrow myeloma cells. *Blood* 74:387–390, 1989
8. Durie BGM, Salmon SE, Mundy GR: Relation of osteoclast activating factor production to the extent of bone disease in multiple myeloma. *Br J Haematol* 47:21–30, 1981
9. Harinck HIJ, Bijvoet OLM, Plantingh AST: Role of bone and kidney in tumor-induced hypercalcemia and its treatment with bisphosphonate and sodium chloride. *Am J Med* 82:1113–1142, 1987

10. Binstock ML, Mundy GR: Effects of calcitonin and glucocorticoids in combination with hypercalcemia of malignancy. *Ann Intern Med* 93:269–272, 1980

11. Canellos GP: Hypercalcemia in malignant lymphoma and leukemia. *Ann NY Acad Sci* 230:240–246, 1974

12. Bunn PA, Schechter GP, Jaffe E, et al.: Clinical course of retrovirus-associated adult T-cell lymphoma in the United States. *N Engl J Med* 309:247–264, 1983

13. Breslau NA, McGuire JL, Zerwekh JE, Frenkel EP, Pak CYC: Hypercalcemia associated with increased serum calcitriol levels in three patients with lymphoma. *Ann Intern Med* 100:107, 1984

14. Fetchick DA, Bertolini DR, Sarin PS, Weintraub ST, Mundy GR, Dunn JD: Production of 1,25 dihydroxyvitamin D by human T-cell lymphotrophic virus-I transformed lymphocytes. *J Clin Invest* 78:592–596, 1986

15. Adams JS, Fernandez M, Gacad MA, et al.: Vitamin D metabolite-mediated hypercalcemia and hypercalciuria in patients with AIDS- and non-AIDS-associated lymphoma. *Blood* 73:235–239, 1989

16. Motokura T, Fukumoto S, Matsumoto T, et al.: Parathyroid hormone related protein in adult T-cell leukemia-lymphoma. *Ann Intern Med* 111:484–488, 1989

17. Mundy GR, Martin TJ (eds): Physiology and pharmacology of bone. In: *Handbook of Experimental Pharmacology.* Springer, New York, 1993

18. Liotta LA: Tumor invasion: Role of the extracellular matrix. *Cancer Res* 46:1–7, 1986

19. Orr W, Varani J, Gondek MD, Ward PA, Mundy GR: Chemotactic responses of tumor cells to products of resorbing bone. *Science* 203:176–179, 1979

20. Mundy GR, DeMartino S, Rowe DW: Collagen and collagen fragments are chemotactic for tumor cells. *J Clin Invest* 68:1102–1105, 1981

21. Mundy GR, Martin TJ: The hypercalcemia of malignancy: Pathogenesis and treatment. *Metabolism* 31:1247–1277, 1982

35. Unusual Causes of Malignancy-Associated Hypercalcemia

Andrew F. Stewart, M.D.

Department of Endocrinology, West Haven Veterans Affairs Medical Center, West Haven, Connecticut and Yale University School of Medicine, New Haven, Connecticut

The two broad categories of malignancy-associated hypercalcemia described in Chapters 33 and 34 comprise the vast majority of patients with cancer and hypercalcemia. It should, however, be clear that other mechanisms, although uncommon, may be encountered in occasional patients. For example, patients with clearly humorally mediated hypercalcemic syndromes (i.e., hypercalcemia that is reversed by tumor resection) have been reported, which do not fit into the humoral hypercalcemia of malignancy biochemical categorization described in Chapter 33. The humoral mediator in these patients is unknown. Rare patients with renal carcinomas have been described who appear to have bona fide tumor secretion of prostaglandin E_2 as a cause.

It is important to emphasize that patients with cancer may develop hypercalcemia due to other coexisting conditions such as primary hyperparathyroidism, tuberculosis, sarcoidosis, immobilization, and calcium-containing hyperalimentation solutions. These causes should be actively sought and corrected.

In addition to these poorly characterized syndromes, there are two types of malignancy-associated hypercalcemia, although rare, have been well characterized and are interesting mechanistically. These are discussed briefly.

1,25-DIHYDROXYVITAMIN D-SECRETING LYMPHOMAS

Breslau et al. (1) and Rosenthal et al. (2) have described a total of seven patients with malignancy lymphomas in whom circulating concentrations of 1,25-dihydroxyvitamin D [$1,25(OH)_2D$] were found to be elevated, in some cases strikingly so. This is in contrast to findings in other types of malignancy-associated hypercalcemia. No evidence for a role for either parathyroid hormone (PTH) or PTH-related protein production could be found. Resection or therapy of the lymphomas reversed the hypercalcemia and reversed the elevations in plasma $1,25(OH)_2D$. No unifying histologic theme was present among the lymphomas. Rather, lymphomas of several different subcategories are included in this group. The $1,25(OH)_2D$ elevations and hypercalcemia were corrected with glucocorticoid therapy. This syndrome appears to be the malignant counterpart of sarcoidosis (Chapter 37) with malignant lymphocytes and/or macrophages converting diet- and sun-derived 25-hydroxyvitamin D to $1,25(OH)_2D$.

ECTOPIC HYPERPARATHYROIDISM

From the 1940s through the 1970s, what is now called HHM (Chapter 33) was thought to be caused by ectopic secretion by tumors of PTH. In the 1980s, it became clear that HHM was caused by PTH-related protein, and "ectopic hyperparathyroidism" was viewed as rare or nonexistent. At the time of this writing, three cases of what can be considered authentic ectopic hyperparathyroidism have been described, including small cell carcinomas of the lung and ovary, and a clear cell carcinoma of the ovary. Immunoreactive PTH was found to be elevated in modern, sensitive, specific immunoassays and reversed, together with hypercalcemia, with tumor resection. Parathyroid adenomas were not identified, but a gradient of PTH across one of the tumors was demonstrated. The tumors contained mRNA encoding PTH. In one case, ovarian tumor expression of PTH was shown to be due to both gene amplification and gene rearrangement in tumor cells in the upstream region of one allele of the PTH gene. Parathyroid hormone-related protein mRNA was absent in two of the three tumors but was present in the third. Thus, it is now clear that true ectopic hyperparathyroidism can occur but that is exceedingly rare.

SELECTED REFERENCES

1. Breslau NA, McGuire JL, Zerwekh JE, Frenkel ED, Pak CYC: Hypercalcemia associated with increased serum calcitriol levels in three patients with lymphoma. *Ann Intern Med* 100:1–7, 1984

2. Rosenthal NR, Insogna KL, Godsall JW, Smalldone L, Waldron JA, Stewart AF: Elevations in circulating $1,25(OH)_2D$ in three patients with lymphoma-associated hypercalcemia. *J Clin Endocrinol Metab* 60:29–33, 1985

3. Yoshimoto K, Yamasaki R, Sakai H, Tezuka U, Takahashi M, Iizuka M, Sekiya T, Saito S: Ectopic production of PTH by small cell lung cancer in a patient with hypercalcemia. *J Clin Endocrinol Metab* 68:976–981, 1989

4. Nussbaum SR, Gaz RD, Arnold A: Hypercalcemia and ectopic secretion of parathyroid hormone by an ovarian carcinoma with rearrangement of the gene for PTH. *N Engl J Med* 323:1324–1328, 1990

5. Strewler GJ, Budayr AA, Bruce RJ, Clark OH, Nissenson RA: Secretion of authentic PTH by a malignant tumor. *Clin Res* 38:462A, 1990

36. Hypercalcemia Resulting from Medications

Andrew F. Stewart, M.D.

Department of Endocrinology, West Haven Veterans Affairs Medical Center, West Haven, Connecticut, and Yale University School of Medicine, New Haven, Connecticut

Hypercalcemia is regularly encountered in patients receiving the medications noted in Table 1. Overdosage with vitamin D or its analogs (25-hydroxyvitamin D; 1,25-dihydroxyvitamin D; and dihydrotachysterol) may lead to severe hypercalcemia. The recommended daily allowance for vitamin D is 400 U/day. The amount of vitamin D required to produce hypercalcemia is in excess of 50,000 U/week. Thus, hypercalcemia occurs not from over-the-counter multivitamin overdose but from prescribed vitamin D doses, usually used in the treatment of osteoporosis, hypoparathyroidism, malabsorption, or renal osteodystrophy. The vitamin D analogs described are also prescription drugs and frequently cause hypercalcemia when used in excessive doses. The hypercalcemia that occurs in this setting has gastrointestinal, renal, and skeletal components and responds to withdrawal of the vitamin D compound, volume expansion, and calciuresis. Occasionally glucocorticoid treatment is required. The biologic half-life of vitamin D is very long (weeks to months), whereas, that of its metabolites is relatively short (hours to days).

Vitamin A in large doses (150,000 IU/day) may cause hypercalcemia. Vitamin A-induced hypercalcemia was a medical curiosity limited to occasional intentional drug overdoses and to Arctic explorers who consumed sled-dog and polar bear liver. More recently, however, the widespread use of vitamin A analogs such as *cis*-retinoic acid for the treatment of acne and other dermatologic disorders has been associated with the occasional occurrence of hypercalcemia. The hypercalcemia appears to result from osteoclast-mediated bone resorption.

Estrogens and antiestrogens cause hypercalcemia in approximately 30% of patients when used to treat breast cancer, which is metastatic to the skeleton. The physiologic basis of this "estrogen-" or "antiestrogen-flare" is unknown. It has been associated with subsequent tumor regression when the offending drug can be continued. The hypercalcemia appears to be skeletal in origin, responsive to hydration and glucocorticoids, and self-limiting.

Lithium carbonate in doses of 900–1,500 mg/day has been reported to cause hypercalcemia in approximately 5% of patients receiving the drug. There is no clear consensus as to the mechanism, with some studies, suggesting an upward resetting of the parathyroid gland setpoint for calcium suppression of parathyroid hormone secretion and others indicating that the hypercalcemia is independent of parathyroid function. Except in patients where lithium treatment may have unmasked previously mild primary hyperparathyroidism, the hypercalcemia will resolve if lithium therapy is discontinued.

Thiazide diuretics regularly cause hypercalcemia. The hypercalcemia appears to be largely renal in origin in that thiazide diuretics limit renal calcium excretion and enhance calcium reabsorption in the distal tubule. On the other hand, it has been reported that thiazide diuretics may cause hypercalcemia in anephric patients, suggesting that extrarenal effects of thiazides may be important. Hypercalcemia reverses rapidly with discontinuation of the offending drug. The thiazide effect on the kidney has been used in the treatment of hypoparathyroidism and renal nephrolithasis due to renal calcium wasting.

Aminophylline and its derivatives have been reported to cause hypercalcemia. This has usually been in the setting of an asthmatic patient receiving a loading dose of theophylline that raised serum theophylline levels above the therapeutic range. Serum calcium values become normal when patients are placed on maintenance therapy and serum theophylline levels fall into the therapeutic range. Theophylline-induced hypercalcemia is typically mild. Its mechanism is not known.

TABLE 1. *Medications associated with hypercalcemia*

Medication
Vitamin D and analogs (1)
Vitamin A and analogs (2)
Estrogens and antiestrogens (3,4)
Lithium carbonate (5)
Thiazide diuretics (6)
Aminophylline (7)

SELECTED REFERENCES

1. Haussler MR, McCain TA: Basic and clinical concepts related to vitamin D metabolism and action. *N Engl J Med* 297:974–1041, 1977

2. Valente JD, Elias AN, Weinstein GD: Hypercalcemia associated with oral isotretinoin in the treatment of severe acne. *JAMA* 250:1899, 1983
3. Legha SS, Powell K, Buzdar AU, Blumen-Schein GR: Tamoxifen-induced hypercalcemia in breast cancer. *Cancer* 47:2803, 1981
4. Valentin-Opran A, Eilon G, Saez S, Mundy GR: Estrogens and antiestrogens stimulate release of bone-resorbing activity in cultured human breast cancer cells. *J Clin Invest* 75:726, 1985
5. Speigal AM, Rudorfer MV, Marx SJ, Linnoila M: The effect of short-term lithium administration of suppressibility of parathyroid hormone secretion by calcium *in vivo*. *J Clin Endocrinol Metab* 59:354, 1984
6. Porter RH, Cox BG, Heaney D, Hostetter TH, Stinebaugh BJ, Suki WN: Treatment of hypoparathyroid patients with chlorthalidone. *N Engl J Med* 298:577, 1978
7. McPherson ML, Prince SR, Atamer E, Maxwell DB, Ross-Clunis, Estep H: Theophylline-induced hypercalcemia. *Ann Intern Med* 105:52–54, 1986

37. Hypercalcemia Due to Granuloma-Forming Disorders

John S. Adams, M.D.

Division of Endocrinology and Metabolism, Cedars-Sinai Medical Center, and University of California-Los Angeles School of Medicine, Los Angeles, California

PATHOGENESIS

The association of dysregulated calcium homeostasis and granulomatous disease was established in 1939 by the work of Harrell and Fisher (1). With the advent of automated serum chemistry testing, more recent studies indicate that mild to severe hypercalcemia is detected in ~10% of patients with sarcoidosis, whereas up to 50% of patients will become hypercalciuric at some time during the course of their disease (2). Vitamin D was implicated in the pathogenesis of abnormal calcium metabolism after it was appreciated that patients with sarcoidosis who had hypercalcemia or hypercalciuria (or both) absorbed high fractions of dietary calcium and that normocalcemic patients were prone to hypercalcemia after receiving small amounts of vitamin D or ultraviolet light (3). It has been proposed that bone resorption is an important contributor to the pathogenesis of hypercalciuria and hypercalcemia (4). This proposition was based on the observations that a diet low in calcium seldom induces a normocalcemic state in sarcoidosis patients with moderate to severe hypercalcemia, and that urinary calcium excretion often exceeds dietary calcium intake. Recent studies (5,6) have demonstrated that generalized, accelerated trabecular bone loss occurs in sarcoid patients before institution of steroid therapy. Rizzato et al. (6) showed that: 1) bone mass was significantly decreased in patients with active sarcoidosis; 2) bone loss was most marked in patients with hypercalcemia and/or hypercalciuria; and 3) bone loss was most prominent in postmenopausal females with longstanding disease.

For many years these and similar clinical observations suggested that hypercalcemia and/or hypercalciuria in patients with sarcoidosis resulted from a heightened sensitivity to the biologic effects of vitamin D. However, the discovery that a high proportion of these patients had elevated circulating concentrations of 1,25-dihydroxyvitamin D [1,25(OH)$_2$D] indicated that the endogenous overproduction of an active vitamin D metabolite was the etiology of disordered calcium regulation in this disease. More recently, high serum 1,25(OH)$_2$D concentrations have been reported in hypercalcemic patients with other granulomatous diseases and in patients harboring lymphoproliferative neoplasms (Table 1); in all of these disorders there is a presumed extrarenal source for the hormone.

There are three major lines of clinical evidence suggesting that the endogenous extrarenal synthesis of 1,25-(OH)$_2$D in some hypercalcemic/hypercalciuric patients with granulomatous disease and lymphoma is not subject to normal, physiological regulatory influences (15). First, hypercalcemic patients possess a frankly high or inappropriately elevated serum 1,25(OH)$_2$D concentration, although their serum immunoreactive parathyroid hormone levels are suppressed and serum phosphorus concentrations are relatively elevated. If 1,25(OH)$_2$D synthesis was under the trophic control of parathyroid hormone and phosphorus then 1,25(OH)$_2$D concentrations should be low. Second, unlike normal individuals whose serum 1,25(OH)$_2$D concentrations are not influenced by small-to-moderate increments in circulating 25-hydroxyvitamin D (25OHD) concentrations, the serum 1,25(OH)$_2$D concentration in patients with active sarcoidosis is exquisitely

TABLE 1. *Human disease associated with 1,25-dihydroxyvitamin D-mediated hypercalcemia/hypercalciuria*

Granuloma-Forming Diseases
   Sarcoidosis (7)
   Tuberculosis (8)
   Silicone-induced granulomatosis (9)
   Disseminated candidiasis (10)
   Leprosy (11)
Malignant Lymphoproliferative Disease
   B-Cell lymphoma (12)
   Hodgkins disease (12,13)
   Lymphomatoid granulomatosis (14)

References are in parentheses.

sensitive to an increase in the availability of substrate. Third, serum calcium and $1,25(OH)_2D$ concentrations are positively correlated to indices of disease activity; sarcoidosis patients with widespread disease and high serum angiotensin converting enzyme activity are more likely to be hypercalciuric or frankly hypercalcemic (16–18).

CELLULAR SOURCE OF ACTIVE VITAMIN D METABOLITES

The sentinel report of Barbour et al. (19) proved the source of $1,25(OH)_2D$ to be extrarenal in sarcoidosis. These investigators described an anephric patient with sarcoidosis, hypercalcemia, and a high serum $1,25(OH)_2D$ concentration. The elevated $1,25(OH)_2D$ concentration in patients with sarcoidosis is now known to result from increased production of $1,25(OH)_2D$ by the macrophage (7,20), a prominent constituent of the sarcoid granuloma. Synthesis of $1,25(OH)_2D_3$ from $25OHD_3$ has been demonstrated *in vitro* by alveolar macrophages from hypercalcemic patients with sarcoidosis and by granulomatous tissue. The salient properties of the macrophage $25OHD$ 1-hydroxylation reaction *in vitro* are depicted in Table 2. Although similar to the authentic renal $25OHD$-1-hydroxylase in terms of kinetics and substrate specificity (21), the factors that exert a regulatory influence on the synthetic reaction in the kidney and sarcoid macrophage vary considerably. The sarcoid macrophage 1-hydroxylation reaction is immune to the stimulatory effects of parathyroid hormone, but is very sensitive to stimulation by interferon-gamma (IFN-γ), a lymphokine produced by activated lymphocytes, and modulators of the lymphokine's postreceptor signal transduction pathway (22). The macrophage hydroxylation reaction is very sensitive to inhibition by glucocorticoid, chloroquine and related analogs, and the cytochrome P-450 inhibitor ketoconazole, but is refractory to inhibition by 1,25-dihydroxyvitamin D (21–24). The renal enzyme, on the other hand, is relatively insensitive to inhibition by glucocorticoids (25), but is downregulated by $1,25(OH)_2D$. It is postulated that these differences are more a reflection of the cell in which the hydroxylase is expressed than a difference in the enzyme that catalyzes the reaction. This question cannot be resolved until the responsible enzymes from the macrophage and kidney are structurally characterized.

IMMUNOACTIVITY OF 1,25-DIHYDROXYVITAMIN D

1,25-Dihydroxyvitamin D is known to exert a potent immunoinhibitory effect on activated human lymphocytes *in vitro*. These actions include inhibition of lymphocyte proliferation, lymphokine production, and immunoglobulin synthesis (26). It is suggested (27,28) that $1,25(OH)_2D$ produced by the macrophage in granulomatous diseases exerts a paracrine immunoinhibitory effect on neighboring, activated lymphocytes that express receptors for the hormone and that this acts to slow an otherwise "overzealous" immune response that may be detrimental to the host. Despite the theoretical attractiveness of this model, there are few data to support a role for $1,25(OH)_2D$ playing a paracrine immunoinhibitory role *in vivo* (29).

TREATMENT OF HYPERCALCEMIA/HYPERCALCIURIA

The most important factor in the successful management of disordered vitamin D metabolism of sarcoidosis is recognition of patients at risk. Those at risk include patients with: 1) indices of active, widespread disease (i.e., elevated serum angiotensin converting enzyme levels, diffuse infiltrative pulmonary disease); 2) preexistent hypercalciuria; 3) a previous history of hypercalcemia or hypercalciuria; 4) diets enriched in vitamin D and calcium; and 5) a recent history of sunlight exposure or treatment with vitamin D. All patients with active sarcoidosis should be screened for hypercalciuria. On a timed, fasting urine collection, a fractional urinary calcium excretion rate exceeding 0.16 mg calcium/100 ml glomerular filtrate is considered hypercalciuria. If the fractional urinary calcium excretion rate is elevated, serum $25OHD$ and $1,25(OH)_2D$ concentrations should be determined to judge the efficacy of therapy. Because hypercalciuria frequently precedes the development of overt hypercalcemia, the occurrence of either is an indication for interventive therapy.

Glucocorticoids (40–60 mg prednisone or equivalent daily) are the mainstay of therapy of disordered calcium homeostasis resulting from the endogenous overproduction of active vitamin D metabolites. Institution of glucocorticoid therapy results in a prompt decrease in the

TABLE 2. *Characteristics of the sarcoid macrophage 25-hydroxyvitamin D_1-hydroxylation reaction*

Side chain-substituted secosteroid substrates preferred[a]
High affinity for substrate (50–100 nM)[a]
Not inhibited by product 1,25-dihydroxyvitamin D_3
Not accompanied by a 24-hydroxylase
Stimulated by interferon-γ, calcium ionophore, and leukotriene C_4
Inhibited by glucocorticoid, chloroquine, and ketoconazole

[a] Similar to the renal 1-hydroxylase.

circulating 1,25(OH)$_2$D concentration (within 3 days), presumably by inhibition of the macrophage hydroxylation reaction. Normalization of the serum or urine calcium usually occurs within a matter of days (17). Failure to normalize the serum calcium after 10 days of therapy suggests the coexistence of another hypercalcemic process (i.e., hyperparathyroidism or humoral hypercalcemia of malignancy). Obviously, the dietary intake of calcium and vitamin D should be limited in such patients as should sunlight (UV light) exposure. After a hypercalcemic episode, urinary calcium excretion rates should be monitored intermittently in order to detect recurrence. Glucocorticoids also appear to be effective in the management of vitamin D-mediated hypercalcemia or hypercalciuria in other granulomatous diseases and lymphoma. It should be pointed out, however, the number of such patients so treated is few. Chloroquine and its hydroxy-analog (hydroxychloroquine) (23,30) and ketoconazole (24) are also capable of reducing the serum 1,25(OH)$_2$D and calcium concentration in patients with sarcoidosis. Because of the limited experience with these drugs as antihypercalcemic agents, they should be limited to patients in whom steroid therapy is unsuccessful or contraindicated. The utility of the newer bisphosphonates in blocking bone resorption and decreasing serum and urine calcium levels in hypercalcemic/hypercalciuric patients with sarcoidosis is unknown.

REFERENCES

1. Harrell GT, Fisher S: Blood chemical changes in Boeck's sarcoid with particular reference to protein, calcium and phosphatase values. *J Clin Invest* 18:687–693, 1939
2. Studdy PR, Bird R, Neville E, James DG: Biochemical findings in sarcoidosis. *J Clin Pathol* 33:528–533, 1980
3. Bell NH, Gill JR Jr, Barter FC: On the abnormal calcium absorption in sarcoidosis: Evidence for increased sensitivity to vitamin D. *Am J Med* 36:500–513, 1964
4. Fallon MD, Perry HM III, Teitelbaum SL: Skeletal sarcoidosis with osteopenia. *Metab Bone Dis Res* 3:171–174, 1981
5. Vergnon GM, Chappard D, Mounier D, et al.: Phosphocalcic metabolism, bone quantitative histomorphometry and clinical activity in 10 cases of sarcoidosis. In: Grassi C, Rizzato G, Pozzi E (eds) *Sarcoidosis and Other Granulomatous Disorders.* Elsevier, Amsterdam, pp 499–502, 1988
6. Rizzato G, Montemurro L, Fraioli P: Bone mineral content in sarcoidosis. *Sem Resp Med* 13:411–423, 1992
7. Adams JS, Singer FR, Gacad MA, et al.: Isolation and structural identification of 1,25-dihydroxyvitamin D$_3$ produced by cultured alveolar macrophages in sarcoidosis. *J Clin Endocrinol Metab* 60:960–966, 1985
8. Gkonos PJ, London R, Hendler ED: Hypercalcemia and elevated 1,25-dihydroxyvitamin D levels in a patient with end-stage renal disease and active tuberculosis. *N Engl J Med* 311:1683–1685, 1984
9. Kozeny GA, Barbato AL, Bansal VK, Vertuno LL, Hano JE: Hypercalcemia associated with silicone-induced granulomas. *N Engl J Med* 311:1103–1105, 1984
10. Kantarijian HM, Saad MF, Estey EH, Sellin RV, Samaan NA: Hypercalcemia in disseminated candidiasis. *Am J Med* 74:721–724, 1983
11. Hoffman VH, Korzeniowski OM: Leprosy, hypercalcemia, and elevated serum calcitriol levels. *Ann Intern Med* 105:890–891, 1986
12. Adams JS, Fernandez M, Gacad MA, et al.: Vitamin D metabolite-mediated hypercalcemia and hypercalciuria patients with AIDS- and non-AIDS-associated lymphoma. *Blood* 73:235–239, 1989
13. Breslau NA, McGuire JL, Zerwekh JE, et al.: Hypercalcemia associated with increased serum calcitriol levels in three patients with lymphoma. *Ann Intern Med* 100:1–7, 1984
14. Schienman SJ, Kelberman MW, Tatum AH, Zamkoff KW: Hypercalcemia with excess serum 1,25-dihydroxyvitamin D in lymphomatoid granulomatosis/angiocentric lymphoma. *Am J Med Sci* 301:178–181, 1991
15. DeLuca HF, Schnoes HK: Vitamin D: Recent advances. *Ann Rev Biochem* 52:411–439, 1983
16. Sandler LM, Wineals CG, Fraher LJ, Clemens TL, Smith R, O'Riordan JLH: Studies of the hypercalcaemia of sarcoidosis: Effects of steroids and exogenous vitamin D$_3$ on the circulating concentration of 1,25-dihydroxyvitamin D$_3$. *Q J Med* 53:165–180, 1984
17. Meyrier A, Valeyre D, Bouillon R, Paillard F, Battesti J-P, Georges R: Resorptive versus absorptive hypercalciuria in sarcoidosis: correlations with 25-hydroxyvitamin D$_3$ and 1,25-dihydroxyvitamin D$_3$ and parameters of disease activity. *Q J Med* 54:269–281, 1985
18. Adams JS, Gacad MA, Anders AA, et al.: Biochemical indicators of disordered vitamin D and calcium homeostasis in sarcoidosis. *Sarcoidosis* 3:1–6, 1986
19. Barbour GL, Coburn JW, Slatopolsky E, Norman AW, Horst RL: Hypercalcemia in an anephric patient with sarcoidosis: Evidence for extrarenal generation of 1,25-dihydroxyvitamin D. *N Engl J Med* 305:440–443, 1981
20. Insogna KL, Dreyer BE, Mitnick M, Ellison AF, Broadus AE: Enhanced production rate of 1,25-dihydroxyvitamin D in sarcoidosis. *J Clin Endocrinol Metab* 66:72–75, 1988
21. Adams JS, Gacad MA: Characterization of 1α-hydroxylation of vitamin D$_3$ sterols by cultured alveolar macrophages from patients with sarcoidosis. *J Exp Med* 161:755–765, 1985
22. Adams JS, Gacad MA, Diz MM, Nadler JL: A role for endogenous arachidonate metabolites in the regulated expression of the 25-hydroxyvitamin D-1-hydroxylation reaction in cultured alveolar macrophages from patients with sarcoidosis. *J Clin Endocrinol Metab* 70:595–600, 1990
23. Adams JS, Diz MM, Sharma OP: Effective reduction in the serum 1,25-dihydroxyvitamin D and calcium concentration in sarcoidosis-associated hypercalcemia with short-course chloroquine therapy. *Ann Intern Med* 111:437–438, 1989
24. Adams JS, Sharma OP, Diz MM, Endres DB: Ketoconazole decreases the serum 1,25-dihydroxyvitamin D and calcium concentration in sarcoidosis-associated hypercalcemia. *J Clin Endocrinol Metab* 70:1090–1095, 1990
25. Henry HL: Effect of dexamethasone on 25-hydroxyvitamin D$_3$ metabolism by chick kidney cell cultures. *Endocrinology* 118:1134–1138, 1986
26. Rigby WFC: The immunobiology of vitamin D. *Immunol Today* 9:54–58, 1988
27. Holick MF, Adams JS: Vitamin D metabolism and biological function. In: Avioli LV, Krane SM (eds): *Metabolic Bone Disease, 2nd ed.* W.B. Saunders, Philadelphia, pp 155–195, 1990
28. Adams JS: Hypercalcemia and hypercalciuria. *Sem Resp Med* 13:402–410, 1992
29. Barnes PF, Modlin RL, Bickle DD, Adams JS: Transpleural gradient of 1,25-dihydroxyvitamin D in tuberculous pleuritis. *J Clin Invest* 83:1527–1532, 1989
30. O'Leary TJ, Jones G, Yip A, et al.: The effects of chloroquine on serum 1,25-dihydroxyvitamin D and calcium metabolism in sarcoidosis. *N Engl J Med* 315:727–730, 1986

38. The Milk-Alkali Syndrome

Thomas P. Jacobs, M.D.

Department of Medicine, Columbia University, College of Physicians and Surgeons, New York, New York

In 1915 Sippy introduced a new diet for patients with peptic ulcers consisting of large amounts of milk and absorbable alkaline salts of calcium and magnesium. Soon afterward a toxic syndrome was described consisting of headache, nausea, neuromuscular irritability, arthralgias, weakness, and lethargy in association with azotemia and systemic alkalosis—all largely reversible with discontinuation of the ulcer regimen (1). Hypercalcemia with normal or reduced urine calcium excretion was subsequently found to be a constant feature of what came to be known as the "milk-alkali syndrome," the association of hypercalcemia, metabolic alkalosis, and renal impairment following acute or chronic ingestion of calcium with absorbable alkali, usually calcium carbonate. Risk factors for this condition include renal impairment, vomiting or gastric aspiration, thiazide diuretic use, and possibly an intrinsic inability to reduce fractional absorption of ingested calcium. Orwoll (2) has suggested a likely pathogenesis of this syndrome, in which the renal excretion of both calcium and alkali is each inhibited by the other. Discontinuing ingestion of the offending agent and correction of fluid and electrolyte abnormalities usually returns the patient to good health, but some are left with renal dysfunction due to nephrocalcinosis. The incidence of this condition appeared to be decreasing following the introduction of nonabsorbable antacids and H_2-blockers for the treatment of peptic ulcer disease, but there have been recent reports describing larger numbers of cases occurring in association with calcium carbonate prescribed for skeletal preservation (3).

REFERENCES

1. Hardt LL, Rivers AB: Toxic manifestations following the alkaline treatment of peptic ulcer. *Arch Intern Med* 31:171–180, 1923
2. Orwoll ES: The milk-alkali syndrome: Current concepts. *Ann Intern Med* 97:242–248, 1982
3. Kapener P, Langsdorf L, Marcus R, Kraemer FB, Hoffman AR: Milk-alkali syndrome in patients treated with calcium carbonate after cardiac transplantation. *Arch Intern Med* 146:1965–1968, 1986

39. Immobilization

Andrew F. Stewart, M.D.

Department of Endocrinology, West Haven Veterans Affairs Medical Center, West Haven, Connecticut, and Yale University School of Medicine, New Haven, Connecticut

Weightlessness (as occurs in space flight) and complete, prolonged immobilization (as occurs with voluntary complete bedrest, orthopedic casting or traction, or spinal cord injury or other neurologic disorder) regularly leads to accelerated bone resorption and hypercalcemia in individuals whose underlying rate of bone turnover is high. These individuals include children, adolescents, and young adults, patients with primary hyperparathyroidism, secondary hyperparathyroidism (as occurs in renal failure), patients with Paget's disease of bone (Chapter 82), and patients with early, mild, or "subclinical" instances of malignancy-associated hypercalcemia. Hypercalcemia develops within days to weeks of the onset of bedrest, and is associated with: 1) uncoupling of bone cell activity (i.e., increases in osteoclastic bone resorption and decreases in osteoblastic bone formation); 2) hypercalciuria leading to both upper and lower urinary tract nephrolithasis; and 3) if the condition is allowed to continue, osteopenia. The osteoclastic bone resorption, hypercalciuria, and hypercalcemia promptly reverse with the resumption of normal weight-bearing. Passive range of motion exercises are ineffective. Circulating parathyroid hormone and 1,25-dihydroxyvitamin D levels are reduced as is urinary cAMP excretion. Preliminary evidence suggests that treatment with diphosphonates may reverse or diminish immobilization-induced hypercalcemia and osteopenia. The mechanism responsible for immobilization-induced bone resorption remains speculative.

SELECTED REFERENCES

1. Stewart AF, Adler M, Byers CM, Segre GV, Broadus AE: Calcium homeostasis in immobilization: An example of resorptive hypercalciuria. *N Engl J Med* 306:1136–1140, 1982
2. Bergstrom WH: Hypercalciuria and hypercalcemia complicating immobilization. *Am J Dis Child* 132:553–554, 1978

40. Hypercalcemic Syndromes in Infants and Children

Craig B. Langman, M.D.

Department of Pediatrics, Northwestern University and Mineral Metabolism
Laboratory, Division of Nephrology, Children's Memorial Hospital,
Chicago, Illinois

Blood-ionized calcium levels in normal infants and young children are similar to those of adults with a mean ± 2 SDs = 1.21 ± 0.13 mM. In neonates, the normal blood ionized calcium level is dependent on postnatal age (1). In the first 72 hr after birth, there is a significant decrease in blood-ionized calcium level in term newborns from 1.4 to 1.2 mM; the decrease is exaggerated in preterm neonates.

Chronic hypercalcemia in young infants and children may not be associated with the usual signs and symptoms described in this section. Rather, the predominant manifestation of hypercalcemia is "failure to thrive" in which linear growth arrest and lack of appropriate weight gain occur. Additional features of chronic hypercalcemia in children includes nonspecific symptoms of irritability, abdominal pain, and anorexia. Acute hypercalcemia is very uncommon in infants and children; when it occurs, its manifestations are similar to those of older children and adults.

WILLIAMS'S SYNDROME

Williams et al. (2) described a syndrome in infants with supravalvular aortic stenosis and peculiar ("elfin-like") facies; hypercalcemia during the first year of life was also noted (3). However, the severe elevations in serum calcium initially described have failed to appear with equal frequency in subsequent series of such infants. Other series of children who have the cardiac lesion have failed to demonstrate the associated facial dysmorphism. It is thought that there exists a spectrum of infants with some or all of the above abnormalities, and a scoring system has been described to assign suspected infants as lying within or outside of the syndrome classification (4).

Two-thirds of infants with Williams's syndrome have been small for gestational age and many are born past their expected date of confinement. The facial abnormalities consist of structural asymmetry, temporal depression, flat malae with full cheeks, microcephaly, epicanthal folds, lacy or stellate irises, a short nose, long philtrum, arched upper lip with full lower lip, and small, maloccluded teeth. The vocal tone is often hoarse. Neurologic manifestations include hypotonia, hyperreflexia, and mild-to-moderate motor retardation. The personality of affected children has been described as "cocktail party," in that they are unusually friendly to strangers. Other vascular abnormalities have been described in addition to supravalvular aortic stenosis, including other congenital heart defects, and many peripheral organ arterial stenoses (renal, mesen-teric, and celiac). Hypertension may be present in infancy in a minority of children but increases in incidence after the first decade of life.

Hypercalcemia, if initially present, rarely persists to the end of the first year of life and generally disappears spontaneously. Despite the rarity of chronic hypercalcemia, persistent hypercalciuria is not uncommon. Additionally, many of the signs and symptoms of hypercalcemia mentioned previously and in the introduction to this section have been noted in these infants. The long-term prognosis for patients with Williams's syndrome seems to depend on the features other than the level of blood calcium, such as the level of mental retardation and the clinical significance of the cardiovascular abnormalities.

The pathogenesis of the disorder is unknown, although many studies have focused on disordered control of vitamin D metabolism. Previous studies of affected children have demonstrated increased circulating levels of 25-hydroxyvitamin D after vitamin D administration (5), increased levels of calcitriol (1,25-dihydroxyvitamin D) during periods of hypercalcemia (6), but not during normocalcemia (7,8), or diminished levels of calcitonin during calcium infusions (9). Although excess administration of vitamin D to pregnant rabbits may produce a clinical picture not dissimilar to Williams's syndrome, the overwhelming majority of children with Williams's syndrome are not the result of maternal vitamin D intoxication.

IDIOPATHIC INFANTILE HYPERCALCEMIA

Lightwood (10) reported a series of infants with severe hypercalcemia in the early 1950s in England. Epidemiologic investigations have revealed that the majority of affected infants were born to mothers ingesting foods heavily fortified with Vitamin D. The incidence of the disease declined dramatically with reduction of vitamin D supplementation. Other cases have been described without previous exposure to excessive maternal vitamin D intake and the incidence of idiopathic infantile hypercalcemia (IIH) has remained fixed over the past 20 years. Affected infants have polyuria, increased thirst, and the general manifestations of hypercalcemia previously noted. Severely affected neonates may have cardiac lesions similar to those seen in Williams's syndrome and even manifest the dysmorphic features of those infants and children. The distinction between the two syndromes remains problematic (11). Other clinical manifestations include chronic arterial hypertension, strabismus, inguinal hernias, musculoskeletal abnormalities (disordered posture and mild kyphosis), and bony abnormalities (radioulnar synostosis and dislocated patella). Hyperacusis is present in the majority of affected children with IIH but not Williams's syndrome and is persistent.

As in Williams's syndrome, disordered vitamin D metabolism with increased vitamin D sensitivity with respect to gastrointestinal transport of calcium has been posited as the cause of this disorder (12), although the data are conflicting.

We have recently identified seven consecutive children with IIH in whom the presence of an elevated level of N-terminal parathyroid hormone-related protein (PTHrP) was demonstrated at the time of hypercalcemia (13). Further, in five of those children who achieved normocalcemia, the levels of PTHrP normalized or were unmeasurably low, and in one child with persistent hypercalcemia, the level of PTHrP remained elevated. No other nonmalignant disorder of childhood that we have examined, including two children with hypercalcemia from Williams's syndrome, have had elevated levels of PTHrP.

In distinction to the hypercalcemia of Williams's syndrome, the level of blood calcium in IIH remains elevated for a prolonged period in affected children. Therapy includes the use of glucocorticoids to reduce gastrointestinal absorption of calcium, as well as the avoidance of vitamin D and excess dietary calcium.

FAMILIAL HYPOCALCIURIC HYPERCALCEMIA

This disorder is also called familial benign hypercalcemia and has been recognized since 1972 (14) as a cause of elevated total and serum ionized calcium. The onset of the change in calcium is commonly before age 10 and has been described in newborns (15). However, in distinction to primary hyperparathyroidism, circulating levels of parathyroid hormone, phosphate, and calcitriol tend to be normal. Serum magnesium is also elevated. Renal clearances of calcium and magnesium are generally reduced. Overt clinical manifestations are generally uncommon and not those described for hypercalcemia with the exception of fatigue and weakness. Renal function is preserved and there is a noted absence of either hypertension or nephrolithiasis (16,17). The hypercalcemia is lifelong in the majority of affected individuals. The hypercalcemia is not cured by parathyroidectomy, although abnormalities of parathyroid histology have been reported in patients with the disorder. The pathogenesis of the disorder is unknown but may involve a generalized cellular defect in calcium transport.

NEONATAL PRIMARY HYPERPARATHYROIDISM

Primary hyperparathyroidism is uncommon in neonates and children (18), with <100 cases reported to date. Additionally, only 20% of cases occur in children <10 years of age. Hypercalcemia in the first decade of life may more likely be due to other disorders discussed previously. The presenting clinical manifestations have been weakness,

anorexia, and irritability, which are seen in a multitude of pediatric disorders. The association with other endocrine disorders occurs with decreased frequency in young children with primary hyperparathyroidism. Histologic examination of the parathyroid glands demonstrates that 20–40% of affected children may have hyperplasia rather than the more typical adenoma in older individuals.

MISCELLANEOUS DISORDERS

Subcutaneous Fat Necrosis. Michael et al. (19) reported the association of significant birth trauma with fat necrosis in two small-for-gestational age infants who subsequently developed severe hypercalcemia (serum calcium > 15 mg/dL) and violaceous discolorations in pressure sites. Histologic examination of the affected pressure sites in such patients demonstrates both an inflammatory, mononuclear cell infiltrate and crystals that contain calcium. We have also noted hypercalcemia in several children with subcutaneous fat necrosis associated with major trauma or disseminated varicella. The mechanism of the hypercalcemia is unknown but may be related to mildly elevated levels of 1,25-dihydroxyvitamin D or excess prostaglandin E production. The prognosis for infants and children with subcutaneous fat necrosis depends on the duration of the hypercalcemia. Reductions in serum calcium have been noted with the use of exogenous corticosteroids, saline, and furosemide diuresis, and the avoidance of excess dietary calcium and vitamin D. Recurrence of hypercalcemia has not been seen.

Hypophosphatasia. This disorder is discussed in detail in Chapter 70 and is mentioned only for completeness here. Severe infantile hypophosphatasia is associated with markedly elevated serum calcium levels and a reduction in circulating alkaline phosphatase, increase in urinary phosphoethanolamine, and elevated serum pyridoxal-5 phosphate concentrations.

Sarcoidosis (20) (see Chapter 37). Thirty to 50% of children with this autoimmune disorder manifest hypercalcemia and an additional 20–30% demonstrate hypercalciuria with normocalcemia. Many of the presenting manifestations of children with sarcoid may be related to the presence of hypercalcemia.

Limb Fracture (21) (see Chapter 39). Isolated weight-bearing limb fracture, which requires immobilization for even several days, may be associated with elevated blood-ionized calcium levels and hypercalciuria in young children and adolescents. Although prolonged immobilization itself commonly produces hypercalcemia and hypercalciuria, the occurrence after short-term bedrest in children probably reflects their more rapid skeletal turnover.

Vitamin D (Metabolite) Therapy (22) (see Chapter 36). Children with renal osteodystrophy are commonly treated with calcitriol and develop hypercalcemia once every 12–15 treatment months. 25-Hydroxyvitamin D_3 therapy of children with renal osteodystrophy is associated with a slight decrease in the incidence of hypercalcemia. Children with hypocalcemic disorders treated with 1,25-dihydroxyvitamin D_3 therapy develop hypercalcemia at one-third the frequency of children with renal osteodystrophy treated with any vitamin D metabolite. Treatment with the parent vitamin D compound is associated with the production of hypercalcemia similar to the rate produced with calcitriol. However, the hypercalcemia associated with vitamin D is prolonged four- to sixfold in comparison to hypercalcemia with metabolite therapy.

Jansen Syndrome (23). This disorder presents in neonates with hypercalcemia and skeletal radiographs that resemble a rachitic condition. It is a form of metaphyseal dysplasia, and after infancy, the radiographic condition evolves into a more typical picture, with mottled calcifications in the distal end of the long bones. These areas represent patches of partially calcified cartilage protruding into the diaphyseal portion of bone. The skull and spine may be affected also.

The hypercalcemia appears to be lifelong. Its mechanism remains uncertain, but intrinsic hyperparathyroidism or extrarenal production of 1,25-dihydroxyvitamin D does not occur. We have measured the serum level of PTHrP and found it to be undetectable (<2 pM).

REFERENCES

1. Specker BL, Lichtenstein P, Mimouni F, Gormley C, Tsang RC: Calcium-regulating hormones and minerals from birth to 18 months of age: A cross-sectional study. II. Effects of sex, race, age, season, and diet on serum minerals, parathyroid hormone and calcitonin. *Pediatrics* 77:891–896, 1986
2. Williams JCP, Barratt-Boyes BG, Lowe JB: Supravalvular aortic stenosis. *Circulation* 24:1311–1316, 1961
3. Black JA, Bonham Carter RE: Association between aortic stenosis and facies of severe infantile hypercalcemia. *Lancet* 2: 745–748, 1963
4. Preus M: The Williams's syndrome: Objective definition and diagnosis. *Clin Genet* 25:422–428, 1984
5. Taylor AB, Stern PH, Bell NH: Abnormal regulation of circulating 25OHD in the Williams's syndrome. *N Engl J Med* 306: 972–975, 1982
6. Garabedian M, Jacqz E, Guillozo H, Grimberg R, Guillot M, Gadnadoux M-F, Broyer M, Lenoir G, Balsan S: Increased plasma 1,25(OH)$_2$D$_3$ concentrations in infants with hypercalcemia and an elfin facies. *N Engl J Med* 312:948–952, 1985
7. Martin NDT, Snodgrass GJAI, Makin HLJ, Cohen RD: Letter to the editor. *N Engl J Med* 313:888–889, 1986
8. Chesney RW, DeLuca HF, Gertner JM, Genel M: Letter to the editor. *N Engl J Med* 313:889–890, 1986
9. Culler FL, Jones KL, Deftos LJ: Impaired calcitonin secretion in patients with Williams's syndrome. *J Pediatr* 107:720–723, 1985
10. Lightwood RL: Idiopathic hypercalcemia with failure to thrive. *Arch Dis Child* 27:302–303, 1952
11. Martin NDT, Snodgrass GJAI, Cohen RD: Idiopathic infantile hypercalcemia—A continuing enigma. *Arch Dis Child* 59: 605–613, 1984
12. Aarskog D, Asknes L, Markstead T: Vitamin D metabolism in idiopathic infantile hypercalcemia. *Am J Dis Child* 135: 1021–1025, 1981
13. Langman CB, Budayr AA, Sailer DE, Strewler GJ: Nonmalignant expression of parathyroid hormone-related protein is responsible for idiopathic infantile hypercalcemia. *J Bone Miner Res* 7:593, 1992
14. Foley TP Jr, Harrison HC, Arnaud CD, Harrison HE: Familial benign hypercalcemia. *J Pediatr* 81:1060–1067, 1972
15. Marx SJ, Attie MF, Spiegel AM, Levine MA, Lasker RD, Fox M: An association between neonatal severe primary hyperparathyroidism and familial hypocalciuric hypercalcemia. *N Engl J Med* 306:257–264, 1982
16. Marx SJ, Attie MF, Levine MD, Spiegel AM, Downs RW Jr, Lasker RD: The hypocalciuric or benign variant of familial hypercalcemia: Clinical and biochemical features in fifteen kindreds. *Medicine* 60:397–412, 1981
17. Law WM Jr, Heath H III: Familial benign hypercalcemia (hypocalciuric hypercalcemia) clinical and pathogenetic studies in 21 families. *Ann Intern Med* 102:511–519, 1985
18. Bernulf J, Hall K, Sjogren I, Werner I: Primary hyperparathyroidism in children. *Acta Pediatr Scand* 59:249–258, 1970
19. Michael AF, Hong R, West CD: Hypercalcemia in infancy. *Am J Dis Child* 104:235–244, 1962
20. Jasper PL, Denny FW: Sarcoidosis in children. *J Pediatr* 73: 499–512, 1968
21. Rosen JF, Wolin DA, Finberg L: Immobilization hypercalcemia after single limb fractures in children and adolescents. *Am J Dis Child* 132:560–564, 1978
22. Chan JCM, Young RB, Alon U, Manunes P: Hypercalcemia in children with disorders of calcium and phosphate metabolism during long-term treatment with 1,25(OH)2D3. *Pediatrics* 72: 225–233, 1983
23. Frame B, Poznanski AK: Conditions that may be confused with rickets. In: Deluca HF, Anast CN (eds) *Pediatric Diseases Related to Calcium*. Elsevier, New York, pp 269–289, 1980

41. Endocrine Causes of Hypercalcemia Other Than Primary Hyperparathyroidism

Andrew F. Stewart, M.D.

Department of Endocrinology, West Haven Veterans Affairs Medical Center, West Haven, Connecticut, and Yale University School of Medicine, New Haven, Connecticut

THYROTOXICOSIS

Mild hypercalcemia (serum calcium values of 10.5–11.5 mg/dL) frequently accompanies thyrotoxicosis. Although coexisting hyperparathyroidism has proved to be the cause of hypercalcemia in some of these patients, it is clear that thyrotoxicosis alone can lead to hypercalcemia, a scenario that has been reported to occur in up to 50% of hyperthyroid patients. Renal calcium reabsorption and circulating 1,25-dihydroxyvitamin D values have been reported to be reduced in such patients, reflecting suppression of parathyroid function. Bone turnover and resorption are increased. Thus, hypercalcemia is believed to result from thyroxine and triiodothyronine-induced bone resorption, a phenomenon which, over the long-term, would appear to account at least in part for the osteopenia associated with thyrotoxicosis. Hypercalcemia may respond to therapy with β-adrenergic antagonists. Establishment of a diagnosis of hyperthyroidism as the cause of hypercalcemia requires that hypercalcemia reverse with therapy of the thyrotoxicosis.

PHEOCHROMOCYTOMA

Hypercalcemia, at times severe, has been reported to occur in patients with pheochromocytoma. In most instances, hypercalcemia results from primary hyperparathyroidism due to parathyroid hyperplasia coexisting with the pheochromocytoma as manifestations of the multiple endocrine neoplasia syndrome Type IIa (Chapter 31). Occasionally, however, hypercalcemia reverses following adrenalectomy for the pheochromocytoma, an observation that suggests that the hypercalcemia resulted from the secretion by the pheochromocytoma of a circulating factor that stimulates bone resorption or that induces hyperparathyroidism. Some evidence, albeit weak, suggests that catecholamines may play these roles. More recently, however, pheochromocytomas have been demonstrated to produce parathyroid hormone-related protein (see Chapters 11 and 33). Pheochromocytomas should be suspected and excluded prior to parathyroidectomy in all hypertensive patients with hyperparathyroidism.

ADDISON'S DISEASE

Hypercalcemia has been reported to occur in patients with adrenal insufficiency, typically during Addisonian crisis. The majority of such reports are in the older literature, and the pathophysiology has not been thoroughly evaluated. Hypercalcemia may simply reflect hemoconcentration and volume contraction. Hypercalcemia responds to volume expansion and glucocorticoids.

ISLET TUMORS OF THE PANCREAS

Islet cell tumors may secrete parathyroid hormone-related protein (see Chapters 11 and 33) or may occur with parathyroid gland hyperplasia as a feature of the multiple endocrine neoplasia type I syndrome (Chapter 31). Interestingly, however, 90% of patients with islet cell tumors that secrete vasoactive intestinal polypeptide (VIP) develop hypercalcemia. These "VIP-omas" are manifested clinically by the WDHA syndrome: severe watery diarrhea ("pancreatic cholera"), hypokalemia, and achlorhydria. The mechanism responsible for hypercalcemia is unknown.

SELECTED REFERENCES

1. Peerenboom H, Keck E, Kruskemper GL, Strohmeyer G: The defect in intestinal calcium transport in hyperthyroidism and its response to therapy. *J Clin Endocrinol Metab* 59:936–940, 1984
2. Burman KD, Monchick JM, Earll JM, Wartofski L: Ionized and total serum calcium and parathyroid hormone in hyperthyroidism. *Ann Intern Med* 84:668–671, 1976
3. Ross DS, Nussbaum SR: Reciprocal changes in parathyroid hormone and thyroid function after radioiodine treatment of hyperthyroidism. *J Clin Endocrinol Metals* 68:1216–1219, 1989
4. Rude RK, Oldham SB, Singer FR, Nicoloff JT: Treatment of thyrotoxic hypercalcemia with propranolol. *N Engl J Med* 294: 431–433, 1976
5. Stewart AF, Hoecker J, Segre GV, Mallette LE, Amatruda T, Vignery A: Hypercalcemia in pheochromocytoma: Evidence for a novel mechanism. *Ann Intern Med* 102:776–779, 1985
6. Muls E, Bouillon R, Boelaert J, Lamberigts G, Van Imschoot S, Daneels R, DeMoor P: Etiology of hypercalcemia in a patient with Addison's disease. *Calcif Tiss Int* 34:523–526, 1982

42. Management of Hypercalcemia

Elizabeth Shane, M.D.

Department of Medicine, College of Physicians and Surgeons, Columbia University, New York, New York

The decision to institute therapy for the hypercalcemic patient depends to a major extent on the level of the serum calcium and the presence or absence of clinical manifestations of an elevated serum calcium. In general, patients with mild hypercalcemia (<12.0 mg/dL) do not have symptoms of hypercalcemia and do not derive significant clinical benefit from normalization of their serum calcium. Thus, immediate intervention is not usually necessary. In contrast, when the serum calcium is greater than 14.0 mg/dL, therapy should be initiated regardless of whether or not the patient has signs or symptoms of hypercalcemia. Moderate elevation of the serum calcium (12.0–14.0 mg/dL) should be treated aggressively if the patient demonstrates clinical signs or symptoms consistent with hypercalcemia. However, if such a patient is asymptomatic, a more conservative approach may be appropriate. It is also important to consider the underlying cause of the hypercalcemia when deciding whether therapy is necessary and the type of therapy to institute. For example, a patient with acute primary hyperparathyroidism, a completely curable condition, would warrant more aggressive treatment than a patient with diffuse metastatic cancer and a poor prognosis. Another difficult situation arises in the patient with a serum calcium that is not within the range

TABLE 1. *Management of hypercalcemia*

General
  Hydration
  Saline diuresis
  Loop diuretics
  Dialysis
  Mobilization
Specific
  Plicamycin (mithramycin)
  Bisphosphonates
    Etidronate
    Pamidronate
    Clodronate
  Calcitonin
  Gallium nitrate
  Therapy of underlying etiology

one would usually treat aggressively (<12.0 mg/dL), yet who has an altered mental status or other symptoms that could conceivably be ascribed to their hypercalcemic state. In such situations, it is important to consider other potential causes for the symptoms before instituting therapy.

The management of hypercalcemia is outlined in Table 1. When the serum calcium exceeds 12.0 mg/dL and signs and symptoms are present, a series of general measures is instituted. Most of these therapeutic maneuvers tend to lower serum calcium by increasing urinary calcium excretion (1,2). Dehydration, due to the pathophysiologic events induced by the hypercalcemia (anorexia, nausea, vomiting, defective urinary concentrating mechanism and polyuria) is very common. Hydration with normal saline, to correct the extracellular fluid deficit, is central to the early management of hypercalcemia from any cause. Restoration of the volume deficit can usually be achieved by the continuous infusion of 3–4 L of 0.9% sodium chloride over a 24- to 48-hr period. This manuever generally lowers the serum calcium by ~1.5–2.5 mg/dL. Hydration with saline enhances urinary calcium excretion by increasing glomerular filtration of calcium and decreasing both proximal and distal tubular reabsorption of sodium and calcium. However, saline hydration alone does not usually establish normocalcemia unless the calcium concentration is only modestly elevated. Moreover, this form of therapy must obviously be used with caution in elderly patients or in others with compromised cardiovascular or renal function.

Under certain circumstances a loop diuretic, such as furosemide or ethacrynic acid, may be added to saline hydration in the therapy of hypercalcemia. Loop diuretics act on the thick ascending limb of Henle to inhibit both sodium and calcium reabsorption. Thus the use of such agents enhances urinary calcium losses, increases the likelihood of normalization of the serum calcium level, and mitigates against the dangers of hypernatremia and volume overload that may accompany the use of intravenous saline. Only *after* extracellular fluid volume has been replenished, small doses of furosemide (10–20 mg) may be administered as necessary to control clinical manifestations of volume excess. Overzealous use of loop diuretics

before intravascular volume has been restored can worsen hypercalcemia by exacerbating volume depletion. Hypokalemia and other electrolyte abnormalities can ensue. Intensive therapy with large doses of furosemide (80–100 mg every 1–2 hr) and replacement of fluid and electrolytes based on measured urinary losses is rarely indicated. It must be emphasized that thiazide diuretics are contraindicated in this setting because they invariably decrease renal calcium excretion and worsen hypercalcemia.

Dialysis, another general measure, is usually reserved for the severely hypercalcemic patient. Peritoneal or hemodialysis with a low calcium dialysate will lower serum calcium rapidly in those patients who are refractory to other measures or who have renal insufficiency. Finally the patient should be mobilized as soon as clinically feasible to minimize the negative calcium balance that accompanies immobilization.

Specific approaches to the hypercalcemic patient are based on the underlying pathophysiology. Excessive mobilization of calcium from the skeleton due to an accelerated rate of bone resorption is the most common and important factor in the pathogenesis of hypercalcemia in the majority of patients. Numerous pharmacologic agents are available now that specifically block osteoclast-mediated bone resorption and effectively lower serum calcium in most hypercalcemic patients (Table 1).

Plicamycin, previously called mithramycin, is a cytotoxic antibiotic that blocks RNA synthesis in osteoclasts and therefore inhibits bone resorption. When administered intravenously in a dose of 15–25 μg/kg over a period of 4–6 hr, plicamycin effectively lowers elevated calcium levels in most patients. The serum calcium usually begins to decline ~12 hr after administration and generally reaches its nadir within 48–72 hr. Often a single dose may be sufficient to achieve normocalcemia. However, if necessary, the dose may be repeated several times at 24- to 48-hr intervals. The duration of the normocalcemia depends on the intensity of underlying bone resorption and may vary from days to weeks. Plicamycin has considerable toxicity (bone marrow, renal, hepatic); it may be associated with transient elevation of transaminases and/or serum creatinine, proteinuria, and thrombocytopenia, particularly when repeated administrations (more than three or four) are required. These toxicities make this drug of limited usefulness in the setting of chronic hypercalcemia. However, in the severely hypercalcemic patient, when serum calcium requires rapid correction, plicamycin is a major drug of choice.

Inorganic pyrophosphates are naturally occurring inhibitors of bone resorption. Bisphosphonates are analogs of pyrophosphate that are resistant to phosphatases. These drugs are bone-seeking compounds that bind to hydroxyapatite and prevent its dissolution. Osteoclast function is impaired after exposure to bisphosphonates, and these drugs have enjoyed increasing use in disorders characterized by excessive bone resorption. Gastrointestinal absorption of bisphosphonates is very poor and therefore intravenous administration is necessary when they are used to treat hypercalcemia. Two bisphosphonates, etidronate and pamidronate, are currently approved for use in the United States. Another effective bisphosphonate, clodronate, is widely available in Europe and the United Kingdom, but is unavailable in the United States. A new generation of more potent bisphosphonates, including alendronate, risedronate, and aminobutane bisphosphonate, show promise and are currently under investigation.

Etidronate is administered by intravenous infusion at a daily dose of 7.5 mg/kg over 2–4 hr. Generally, the serum calcium begins to decline during the second day of therapy and reaches its nadir by the seventh day. If the serum calcium falls to near normal levels or into the normal range before completion of 3 days of therapy, the standard approved duration of therapy, the drug should be withheld. Administration of the drug for up to 7 days (either consecutive or interrupted) (9) or as a single 24-hr infusion at a dose of 20–25 mg/kg (10) is more efficacious, but these approaches are not "officially" approved. Intravenous etidronate is safe and well-tolerated. The oral use of etidronate to prevent recurrent hypercalcemia is of limited effectiveness and may be complicated by osteomalacia when administered chronically.

Pamidronate is a more potent bisphosphonate (1). It too is effective for the treatment of hypercalcemia. Pamidronate, given as a single 24-hr infusion of 90 mg or in lower doses (30–60 mg) daily for 3 days is safe and effective. The time course of the decrease in serum calcium is similar to etidronate. Pamidronate may cause transient fever and myalgias during the day following the infusion. Pretreatment with acetaminophen ameliorates these side effects in the majority of patients. Occasionally, transient leukopenia may develop. Mild, usually asymptomatic, hypocalcemia may occur in some patients. The duration of the hypocalcemic effect of both etidronate and pamidronate is variable, but may range from several days to several weeks.

Calcitonin is a polypeptide hormone that is secreted by the parafollicular C-cells of the thyroid gland. Salmon calcitonin is the most potent and frequently used form of the drug. Calcitonin should theoretically be an ideal agent to treat hypercalcemia, because it inhibits osteoclastic bone resorption, increases urinary calcium excretion, and has an excellent safety profile. Moreover, calcitonin has the most rapid onset of action of the available calcium-lowering drugs, causing the serum calcium to fall within a few hours of administration. The usual dose ranges from 4 to 8 U/kg administered by intramuscular or subcutaneous injection every 6–8 hr. Unfortunately, the hypocalcemic effect of calcitonin is transient and not as potent as plicamycin or the bisphosphonates. The serum calcium concentration usually declines by <2 mg/dL and may begin to rise again within 24 hr, despite continued therapy. Calcitonin given in combination with bisphosphonates or plicamycin appears to achieve a more rapid and greater decrease in the serum calcium than when either drug is administered by itself. Used in this way, calcitonin may have a role at the outset of therapy in severe instances of hypercalcemia, when it is desirable to lower the serum calcium more rapidly than can be accomplished with either plicamycin or a bisphosphonate alone (1).

Gallium nitrate, originally studied as a therapeutic agent for cancer, has recently been approved by the Food and Drug Administration for the therapy of hypercalcemia. Although its precise mechanism of action is uncertain, it appears to adsorb to hydroxyapatite crystals (1). It may inhibit bone resorption by reducing crystal solubility rather than by directly affecting the osteoclast. When administered as a continuous 5-day infusion at a dose of 200 mg/m^2/day, it has been reported to normalize the serum calcium in a majority of patients. The rate of fall of the serum calcium was rather slow in that a normal level was not reached until the end of the 5-day infusion, and the nadir was not achieved until 3 days later. Gallium nitrate causes elevation of the serum creatinine that may be potentiated by volume depletion and concomitant administration of other nephrotoxic drugs. Its use is contraindicated in renal insufficiency and when other nephrotoxic agents are being used. It may also be associated with reduction in the serum phosphate and hemoglobin concentration. A wider experience is needed with this agent.

Glucocorticoid therapy has been used for many years to treat hypercalcemia, particularly when due to hematologic malignancies such as lymphoma and multiple myeloma. Glucocorticoids are also effective in situations in which the hypercalcemia is mediated by the actions of 1,25dihydroxyvitamin D such as vitamin D toxicity or granulomatous diseases. Glucocorticoids are seldom effective in patients with solid tumors or primary hyperparathyroidism and are rarely used in those situations. The usual dose is 200–300 mg of intravenous hydrocortisone, or its equivalent, daily for 3–5 days.

Intravenous phosphate was used in the past to lower serum calcium in hypercalcemic patients. However, intravenous phosphate is accompanied by a substantial risk of precipitation of calcium-phosphate complexes leading to severe organ damage and even death. This form of therapy should rarely be necessary today and is not recommended.

Therapy of the underlying etiology of the hypercalcemia should not be neglected, because specific therapy may be the most effective approach to the problem. Finally, patients with widespread metastatic disease, in whom no further specific antitumor chemotherapy is to be given, may be approached with the realization that reduction of the serum calcium per se will achieve little in the long run. In these circumstances, sometimes the best approach is to resist specific measures to reduce the serum calcium and to make the patient as comfortable as possible.

SELECTED REFERENCES

1. Bilezikian JP: Management of acute hypercalcemia. *N Engl J Med* 326:1196–1203, 1992
2. Shane EJ, Bilezikian JP: Disorders of calcium, phosphate and magnesium metabolism. In: Askanazi J, Starker PM, Weissman C (eds) *Fluid and Electrolyte Management in Critical Care.* Butterworth, London, pp 337–353, 1986
3. Jacobs TP, Gordon AC, Silverberg SJ, et al.: Neoplastic hypercalcemia: Physiologic response to intravenous etidronate disodium. *Am J Med* 82(suppl 2A):42–50, 1987
4. Flores JF, Singer FR, Rude RK: Twenty-four hour infusion of etidronate for hypercalcemia of malignancy. *Miner Elect Metab* 1993 (in press)

43. Hypocalcemia: Pathogenesis, Differential Diagnosis, and Management

Elizabeth Shane, M.D.

Department of Medicine, College of Physicians and Surgeons, Columbia University, New York, New York

Hypocalcemia is encountered commonly in medical practice. Like hypercalcemia, hypocalcemia varies in its clinical presentation from an asymptomatic biochemical abnormality to a severe life-threatening condition.

PATHOGENESIS AND DIFFERENTIAL DIAGNOSIS

The concentration of calcium in the extracellular fluid is critical for many physiological processes. Under normal circumstances, the range is kept remarkably constant, between 8.5–10.5 mg/dL (2.1–2.5 mM). The exact normal ranges vary slightly depending on the laboratory. Approximately half the total serum calcium is bound to plasma proteins, primarily albumin. A small component is complexed to anions such as citrate or sulfate. The remaining half circulates as free calcium ion. It is only this ionized portion of the total serum calcium that is physiologically important, regulating neuromuscular contractility, the activity of many enzymes, the process of coagulation, as well as a variety of other cellular activities.

In many chronic illnesses, substantial reductions may occur in the serum albumin concentration that may lower total serum calcium concentration while the ionized calcium concentration remains normal. A simple correction for hypalbuminemia can be made by adding 0.8 mg/dL to the total serum calcium for every 1.0 g/dL by which the serum albumin is lower than 4.0 g/dL. Thus, a patient with a serum calcium of 7.8 mg/dL and a serum albumin of 2.0 mg/dL, has a corrected total serum calcium of 9.4 mg/dL. In contrast to changes in the serum albumin that affect the total but not the ionized calcium level, alterations in pH affect the ionized calcium concentration without altering the total calcium level. Acidosis increases the ionized calcium by decreasing the binding of calcium ions to albumin, whereas alkalosis decreases the ionized calcium by enhancing binding of calcium ions to albumin. Measurement of total serum calcium is usually adequate for most clinical situations, but in complex cases direct measurement of the ionized calcium should be performed.

The parathyroid glands are extremely sensitive to small changes in the serumionized calcium level. Parathyroid hormone, through its acute effects on bone resorption and renal calcium reabsorption in the distal tubule, is responsible for the minute-to-minute regulation of the serum calcium level. Adjustments in intestinal calcium absorption via parathyroid hormone-stimulated renal 1,25-dihydroxyvitamin D production require 24–48 hr to become maximal and therefore come into play only when the hypocalcemic stimulus is of a more chronic nature. Hypocal-cemia occurs when there is a failure of or incomplete compensation by the parathyroid hormone-controlled homeostatic mechanisms that defend against a hypocalcemic stimulus (Chapter 7). The principal causes of hypocalcemia include hypoparathyroidism, deficiency or abnormal metabolism of vitamin D, hypomagnesemia, and acute or chronic renal failure. In general, the hypocalcemic state may be classified according to whether it is associated with inappropriately low levels of parathyroid hormone (hypoparathyroid states; Table 1) or whether parathyroid hormone levels are elevated, indicating normal parathyroid gland responsiveness to the low serum calcium (secondary hyperparathyroid states; Table 2).

Idiopathic hypoparathyroidism is manifested by hypocalcemia and coexistent low or absent parathyroid hormone levels. It most often occurs as part of an autoimmune syndrome associated with deficient function of one or more endocrine glands (adrenals, thyroid, and ovaries), pernicious anemia, alopecia, vitiligo, and mucocutaneous candidiasis. This disorder is often familial, and its inheritance appears to be autosomal recessive. Familial hypoparathyroidism may also occur as an isolated defect, the mode of inheritance varying in each kindred. Rarely, congenital aplasia of the parathyroid glands may occur, usually in conjunction with defective development of the thymus (DiGeorge's syndrome). Postsurgical hypoparathyroidism, transient or permanent, may develop following neck surgery for thyroid disease due to inadvertent removal of or trauma to the parathyroid glands or their vascular supply. The widespread use of radioactive iodine to treat thyrotoxicosis has decreased the frequency of this occurrence. Neck exploration for primary hyperparathyroidism is now the most frequent situation in which postsurgical hypoparathyroidism occurs. Severe and prolonged hypocalcemia frequently develops after parathyroid surgery for osteitis fibrosis due to chronic renal insufficiency. In this situation, the relative hypoparathyroidism induced by the surgical procedure is complicated by deposition of available calcium into the healing bony lesions (hungry bone syndrome). Severe magnesium deficiency is a rather common cause of hypocalcemia. The normal serum magnesium level is 1.8–3.0 mg/dL (0.8–1.2 mmol/L). In general, the serum magnesium is <1.0 mg/dL (0.4 mmol/L) when hypocalcemia is due to hypomagnesemia. At least two pathogenetic mechanisms have been implicated. Impaired secretion of parathyroid hormone resulting in absolute or relative hypoparathyroidism is present in the vast majority of patients with hypocalcemia secondary to hypomagnesemia. Increased resistance to the action of parathyroid hormone at bone

TABLE 1. *Hypocalcemia due to hypoparathyroidism*

Idiopathic
Postsurgical
Severe hypomagnesemia
After neck irradiation
Infiltrative
   Hemochromatosis
   Thalassemia
   Wilson's disease
   Metastatic carcinoma
DiGeorge's syndrome
Neonatal hypocalcemia

and kidney has also been demonstrated in some patients with severe hypomagnesemia (Chapter 47). A number of less common causes of hypoparathyroidism due to parathyroid hormone deficiency are listed in Table 1.

Hypocalcemia may also complicate a large number of primary disorders (Table 2) in patients who have intrinsically normal parathyroid glands. In these conditions the fall in serum calcium caused by the underlying disease process results in a compensatory increase in parathyroid hormone secretion. This state of "secondary hyperparathyroidism" has the effect of raising the serum calcium, frequently into the low-normal range, by enhancing bone resorption, renal tubular calcium reabsorption and, where possible, gastrointestinal calcium absorption. The most common causes of hypocalcemia with normal parathyroid function (nonhypoparathyroid hypocalcemia) are related to the deficiencies in vitamin D and/or its active metabolites (Chapter 49) that accompany a large number of gastrointestinal or renal diseases. The syndromes of parathyroid hormone resistance (pseudohypoparathyroidism) and vitamin D resistance, also accompanied by secondary hyperparathyroidism, are reviewed in Chapters 46 and 49, respectively. Other causes of hypocalcemia include acute pancreatitis (Chapter 48), osteoblastic metastases, multi-

TABLE 2. *Nonhypoparathyroid hypocalcemia*

Vitamin D deficiency
   Lack of sunlight exposure
   Dietary lack
   Malabsorption
   Upper GI tract surgery
   Liver disease
   Renal disease
   Anticonvulsants
   Vitamin D-dependent rickets, type I
Parathyroid hormone resistance
   Pseudohypoparathyroidism
   Hypomagnesemia
Vitamin D resistance
   Vitamin D-resistant rickets
   Vitamin D-dependent rickets, type II
   Familial vitamin D resistance
Miscellaneous
   Acute pancreatitis
   Osteoblastic metastases
   Multiple citrated blood transfusions
   Acute rhabdomyolysis

ple transfusions of citrated blood, and acute rhabdomyolysis. In each of these situations, when the secondary hyperparathyroidism is insufficient to compensate for the hypocalcemic stimulus, hypocalcemia ensues.

CLINICAL FEATURES OF HYPOCALCEMIA

The signs and symptoms of acute hypocalcemia (Table 3) are primarily due to enhanced neuromuscular irritability. Sensations of numbness and tingling involving the fingertips, toes, and circumoral region are early symptoms. Increased neuromuscular irritability may be demonstrated at the bedside by eliciting Chvostek's sign or Trousseau's sign. Chvostek's sign is twitching of the circumoral muscles in response to gently tapping the facial nerve just anterior to the ear. It should be noted that ~10% of normal individuals will demonstrate a slight twitch in response to this maneuver. Trousseau's sign is carpal spasm elicited by inflation of a blood pressure cuff to 20 mm Hg above the patient's systolic blood pressure for 3 min. The classic response—flexion of the wrist and metacarpophalangeal joints, extension of the interphalangeal joints, and adduction of the digits—reflects the heightened irritability of the nerves due to ischemia in the region of the cuff. A positive Trousseau's sign is rare in the absence of significant hypocalcemia.

Muscle cramps are often experienced by hypocalcemic patients. They most commonly involve the lower back, legs, and feet. In severe or acute hypocalcemia, the muscle cramps may progress to spontaneous carpopedal spasm (tetany). Laryngospasm or bronchospasm may also develop. Seizures of all types (syncopal episodes, petit mal, grand mal, and focal) may occur whether the hypocalcemia is acute or chronic. Other central nervous system manifestations include irritability, impaired intellectual capacity, and personality disturbances. Severe hypocalcemia may be accompanied by prolongation of the Q-T interval on the electrocardiogram and rarely, congestive heart failure; both manifestations are reversible with correction of the hypocalcemia. Although the presence of symptoms primarily reflects the degree of the hypocalcemia, a rapid rate of fall of the serum calcium and/or the concomitant presence of alkalosis, which enhances binding of ionized calcium to albumin, may also be associated with more severe signs and symptoms.

Patients with chronic hypocalcemia due to idiopathic hypoparathyroidism or pseudohypoparathyroidism may

TABLE 3. *Clinical features of hypocalcemia*

Neuromuscular irritability
Paresthesias
Chvostek's sign
Trousseau's sign
Laryngospasm
Bronchospasm
Tetany
Seizures
Prolonged Q-T interval on EKG

also have calcification of the basal ganglia and extrapyramidal neurological symptoms. Subcapsular cataracts and abnormal dentition are also common in such patients (Chapters 45 and 46).

MANAGEMENT OF ACUTE HYPOCALCEMIA

Management of acute hypocalcemia will be considered in this chapter. Therapy of chronic hypocalcemia is discussed in Chapters 45, 46, and 49.

The decision to treat the patient with hypocalcemia depends on the severity of the hypocalcemia, the rapidity with which it developed, and the presence or absence of clinical signs and symptoms. At one end of the spectrum, an asymptomatic patient with mild hypocalcemia (7.5–8.5 mg/dL or 1.9–2.1 mmol/L) may warrant cautious observation and require only oral calcium supplements (250–500 mg elemental calcium every 6 hr). In contrast, a patient with tetany, a sign of severe hypocalcemia, must be treated aggressively with intravenous calcium administration. Serum calcium levels of <7.5 mg/dL (1.9 mmol/L) or any level in a patient with symptoms, require parenteral calcium therapy.

The mainstay of therapy for acute symptomatic hypocalcemia is intravenous administration of calcium salts. Calcium should be administered with caution in digitalized patients, because sensitivity to the adverse effects of digitalis, particularly arrhythmias, is increased by hypercalcemia. Calcium gluconate (90 mg elemental calcium/10 mL ampule) is preferred over calcium chloride (272 mg elemental calcium/10 mL ampule), because it is less irritating to the veins. Initially, 1 to 2 ampules of calcium gluconate diluted in 50–100 mL of 5% dextrose (180 mg of elemental calcium) should be infused over 5–10 min. This procedure should be repeated as necessary to control symptomatic hypocalcemia. Persistent or less severe hypocalcemia may be managed by administration of more dilute calcium solutions over longer periods. In general, 15 mg/kg of elemental calcium infused over 4–6 hr will raise the serum calcium by 2–3 mg/dL (0.5–0.75 mmol/L). One practical approach is to initiate therapy with 10 ampules of calcium gluconate in 1 L of 5% dextrose infused at a rate of 50 mL/hr (45 mg of elemental calcium/hr); the rate of the infusion then may be titrated to maintain the serum calcium in the low normal range. In situations when volume is of concern, the concentration of the solution may be increased. However, solutions of >200 mg/100 mL of elemental calcium (more than 2 ampules of calcium gluconate/100 mL) should be avoided because of the propensity for irritation of veins and, in the event of extravasation, soft tissues. If hypocalcemia is likely to persist, therapy should be initiated early with oral calcium supplements (1–2 g elemental calcium) and 1,25-dihydroxyvitamin D (0.5–1.0 μg) daily.

The hypomagnesemic patient who is also hypocalcemic will require treatment of the hypomagnesemia before the hypocalcemia will resolve. Moreover, in the acutely hypocalcemic patient in whom magnesium deficiency is clinically likely, it is appropriate to add magnesium to the treatment regimen while awaiting laboratory confirmation of hypomagnesemia.

SELECTED REFERENCES

1. Shane EJ, Bilezikian JP: Disorders of calcium, phosphate and magnesium metabolism. In: Askanazi J, Starker PM, Weissman C (eds) *Fluid and Electrolyte Management in Critical Care*. Butterworth, London, pp 337–353, 1986
2. Stewart AF, Broadus AE: Mineral metabolism. In: Felig P, Baxter JP, Broadus AE, Frohman LA (eds) *Endocrinology and Metabolism*. McGraw-Hill, New York, pp 1422–1433, 1987
3. Nagant de Deuxchaisnes C, Krane SM: Hypoparathyroidism. In: Avioli LV, Krane SM (eds) *Metabolic Bone Disease*. Academic Press, New York, pp 217–445, 1978

44. Protein Binding Abnormalities

Ethel S. Siris, M.D.

Department of Medicine, College of Physicians and Surgeons, Columbia University, New York, New York

Calcium appears in the circulation in three major fractions. About 45–50% of the total serum calcium is in the ionized form, Ca^{2+}, and this fraction represents the biologically active component of total calcium measurement. Another 8% of total serum calcium is complexed to organic and inorganic acids (e.g., citrate, phosphate, and sulfate). This complexed portion, like the ionized calcium, is diffusible or ultrafilterable. Finally, there is the protein-bound fraction of calcium, present in amounts approximately equal to the ionized calcium. This protein-bound component of total calcium is not biologically active, but provides a reservoir of available calcium should a need for increased ionized calcium arise. Binding of calcium to protein can vary according to ionized calcium concentrations, and dissociation of calcium from albumin (to which 80% of this component of calcium is bound) or globulin (to which 20% is bound) can occur.

The protein-bound component of total serum calcium

can also provide the clinician with some confusion as to the true circulating ionized calcium value in states of hypo- or hyperproteinemia. Hypoalbuminemia due to chronic illness, nephrotic syndrome, liver disease, etc. will lower total serum calcium while no change in ionized calcium occurs. Volume contraction, with its associated hyperalbuminemia, may lead to elevations in total, but not ionized, serum calcium. Similarly, increases in globulin, particularly large increases in IgG in rare patients with multiple myeloma, will occasionally raise the total serum calcium above normal. Such a patient would typically have a total (but not ionized) serum calcium that is frankly elevated without symptoms of hypercalcemia. Hydration

and saline diuresis would fail to normalize the total serum calcium. A measurement of ionized calcium would be normal. Protein electrophoresis would show a homogeneous γ-globulin spike with a quantitative increase in γ-globulin as well.

SELECTED REFERENCE

1. Merlini G, Fitzpatrick L, Siris ES, Bilezikian JP, Birken S, Beychok S, Osserman EF: A human myeloma immunoglobulin G binding four moles of calcium associated with asymptomatic hypercalcemia. *J Clin Immunol* 4:185–196, 1984

45. Hypoparathyroidism

Louis M. Sherwood, M.D.

Medical and Scientific Affairs, Merck Human Health Division, West Point, Pennsylvania, and Albert Einstein College of Medicine Bronx, New York

Hypoparathyroidism usually presents as a rare, sporadic, or familial disorder or, more commonly, as a postoperative disorder. Functional hypoparathyroidism may also result from magnesium deficiency (usually associated with alcoholism) or resistance to the effects of parathyroid hormone (PTH). Idiopathic and postsurgical hypoparathyroidism will be described in this chapter.

SURGICAL HYPOPARATHYROIDISM

The most common cause of hypoparathyroidism is that associated with extensive thyroid or repeated neck surgery. This was much more common in the early part of this century than it is today, and in various series it is usually <5% (and often only 1–2%). It is much more likely to occur in patients who have had total thyroidectomy for thyroid cancer or in patients who have had recurrent parathyroid surgery for parathyroid hyperplasia or a persistent parathyroid adenoma. Hypocalcemia that is transient following parathyroid surgery is usually reversible and requires little or no treatment. More prolonged hypocalcemia presenting weeks to even years after neck surgery suggests a permanent hypoparathyroid condition and should be treated like idiopathic hypoparathyroidism. Patients with postsurgical hypoparathyroidism may require higher doses of vitamin D derivatives for effective management of the hypocalcemia. The surgical procedure and disease, as well as the skill of the surgeon, are important factors in determining the potential risk. In patients with nonmalignant disease, transplantation of the parathyroid glands to the sternocleidomastoid or brachioradialis muscle (in the forearm) is quite successful. It is also possible to freeze a normal parathyroid gland under liquid nitrogen and dimethylsulfoxide and transplant it into the patient at a later date if necessary. It is better to prevent postsurgical

hypoparathyroidism than to be forced to treat it. Partial hypoparathyroidism has been observed in a small number of patients who have received extensive radiation to the neck and mediastinum.

IDIOPATHIC HYPOPARATHYROIDISM

This is a rare disorder characterized by absent or decreased secretion of PTH from hypoplastic parathyroid glands and is associated with hypocalcemia and hyperphosphatemia. Although it has been suggested that an abnormal PTH or inhibitor may be present in some cases, molecular studies so far have not established any clear pattern.

Fewer than 200 patients had been described in the medical literature up to the early 1960s, but routine screening of serum calcium since that time has suggested that it may not be quite so unusual.

Classification

Because the disease is uncommon and may present at different ages, it has been somewhat difficult to classify.
Early Childhood Onset. The DiGeorge syndrome is due to congenital abnormalities in the third and fourth branchial pouches and includes both hypoparathyroidism and cellular immune deficiency. As the parathyroid glands and thymus are both derived from the third and fourth branchial pouches, such clinical consequences would be anticipated. Parathyroid glands in this disorder may be absent, hypoplastic, or ectopic.
Later Onset. It is more common for idiopathic hypoparathyroidism to present beyond the early childhood phase, and this may occur between 5 and 10 years of age or even much later in life. This more common form of the

disease may be associated with other endocrine deficiency states such as hypoadrenalism, gonadal failure, diabetes, and moniliasis. In this setting, the hypoparathyroidism is presumed to be autoimmune in origin because of the autoimmune nature of the endocrinopathies. Isolated hypoparathyroidism may be a different disorder than the one associated with polyendocrine deficiencies.

Familial Form. Early-onset hypoparathyroidism has been reported in a few families in which males, but not females, had male siblings who were affected. It has been suggested that this might be due either to a sex-linked recessive or autosomal dominant mode of transmission. Only a minority of late-onset patients with isolated hypoparathyroidism are familial. About 50% of the patients with polyendocrine disorders are familial, but the inheritance seems to be autosomal recessive in these cases. In any one family, various members may have a variety of different endocrine deficiencies. There are recent reports of patients from consanguinous marriages with a syndrome of developmental delay and dysmorphic features associated with hypoparathyroidism.

Natural History

Because the diseases in this group are relatively uncommon, little is known about natural history, and the fate of the patients will depend on the organs affected. In the past, mortality rate in infants with the DiGeorge syndrome was significant (~30–35%), but the use of thymic transplantation has improved the outlook. Children with isolated hypoparathyroidism may remain undiagnosed for many years although dental examinations may result in earlier diagnosis. The onset of clinical hypoparathyroidism is usually earlier in patients with multiple endocrine deficiency disorders and tends to average 7–8 years.

In patients with multiple endocrine deficiencies, there is frequently a sequence in the appearance of the disorders. The first clinical manifestation is often moniliasis, followed years later by hypoparathyroidism, and then at a later age, adrenal insufficiency. Although the sequence may vary, moniliasis almost always precedes other manifestations. The combination of hypoparathyroidism, adrenal insufficiency, and moniliasis is known as the HAM syndrome. The clinical presentation of adrenal insufficiency may manifest itself only in improvement of the hypoparathyroidism with requirements for smaller doses of calcium supplements and vitamin D. Therapy of the adrenal insufficiency may worsen the hypocalcemia. Pernicious anemia or diabetes usually develops later than hypoparathyroidism. A few patients have had a normal serum calcium documented for some years before the development of hypoparathyroidism.

Antibodies directed against the parathyroid gland are present in 33% of patients with isolated disease and 41% with hypoparathyroidism and associated endocrine deficiencies. As with all autoimmune diseases, the relationship of the antibody to the disease is unclear in terms of etiology. Parathyroid antibodies have also been detected in patients with adrenal insufficiency and Hashimoto's thyroiditis, as well as in occasional normal individuals. When hypoparathyroidism was present with adrenal insufficiency, 53% of patients had adrenal antibodies, but antibodies were present in only 11% of patients with hypoparathyroidism without adrenal insufficiency.

Pathophysiology

Varying pathology may be found. The parathyroid glands may be absent, aplastic or hypoplastic, rudimentary, or totally replaced by fat. In occasional patients, the gland is ectopic and found fused with the thymus or in the pharynx. Some patients have had lymphocytic infiltration of the parathyroids that is consistent with an autoimmune etiology.

Hypocalcemia and hyperphosphatemia are characteristic of hypoparathyroidism. Because of the hypocalcemia and low filtered load, urinary calcium excretion is decreased, even though the absence of PTH decreases renal tubular reabsorption of calcium. The clearance of phosphate is also decreased, making hyperphosphatemia a common finding. The deficiency of PTH causes diminished bone resorption and a decrease in 1α-hydroxylase activity in the kidney. The latter is further diminished by the hyperphosphatemia. The low levels of serum 1,25-dihydroxyvitamin D_3 [$1,25(OH)_2D_3$] result in reduced intestinal calcium absorption as well as decreased bone resorption. The reduced intestinal calcium absorption together with the lowered renal threshold for calcium and, to a lesser extent, decreased bone resorption, produce the hypocalcemia.

Clinical Features

Clinical signs and symptoms (vide supra) are caused by the decreased levels of calcium in the circulation and include seizures and overt or latent tetany (Chvostek's and Trousseau's signs). Other features include dental abnormalities that may be present both in idiopathic hypoparathyroidism and in pseudohypoparathyroidism. These may include pitting and defects due to hypoplasia of the enamel, defects in dentin, shortened premolar roots, and delayed eruption of the teeth. There may be thickening of the lamina dura. These teeth are also more prone to caries, and occasional patients may be edentulous. Alopecia, coarse hair, and dry skin, as well as cataracts, have also been described. Mental retardation may be found in some cases. Subcutaneous calcifications that may be present in pseudohypoparathyroidism are not present in the idiopathic disorder. Rare clinical manifestations include pseudopapilledema and cardiomyopathy due to hypocalcemia.

Other endocrine deficiencies and moniliasis may occur. The latter is quite common in the DiGeorge syndrome (about two-thirds of patients), whereas only 15% of isolated cases have moniliasis. It may affect the skin, mucosal surfaces of the mouth and vagina, as well as the nails. Moniliasis is often intractable, even in the absence of hypocalcemia, and may have some relationship to genetic predisposition or impairment in immune function. Adrenal insufficiency is present in 10% of patients with hypoparathyroidism.

Laboratory Abnormalities

The plasma calcium is usually lower than that present in pseudohypoparathyroidism and may average 6–7 mg/dL, whereas the serum P levels may vary from 6–9 mg/dL. Alkaline phosphatase is normal, but indices of bone turnover such as hydroxyproline clearance are decreased. In assays of PTH that can discriminate normal and hypoparathyroid levels, the values are usually undetectable or low, and the levels of $1,25(OH)_2D_3$ are also low. Urinary cAMP and phosphorus excretion are diminished but increase dramatically after the administration of PTH (Ellsworth–Howard test; see Chapter 46 on pseudohypoparathyroidism). The renal threshold for calcium excretion is decreased due to the absence of PTH. Calcification of the basal ganglia and other sites in the brain may be present on skull x-rays or CT scans and lead after many years to neurologic manifestations. EEG abnormalities are common.

Diagnosis

There is often a delay in the diagnosis of hypoparathyroidism, but the condition can readily be diagnosed if the possibility is considered. In most patients with clinical symptoms such as tetany or even seizures, a low serum calcium should suggest this diagnosis. The clinical presentation of tetany in the absence of alkalosis, and the laboratory findings of a decreased serum calcium and increased phosphate (in the absence of renal insufficiency), support strongly the diagnosis of primary hypoparathyroidism. Radiographic bone findings are usually normal, and these together with a normal alkaline phosphatase and the abnormalities in the teeth provide further support. The usual differential diagnosis is from pseudohypoparathyroidism. In the latter disorder, the presence of phenotypic abnormalities is helpful in supporting the diagnosis. In patients in whom the differential diagnosis is difficult, the Ellsworth–Howard test (Appendix) and the values of PTH in the serum of hypocalcemic patients can usually resolve any difficulties.

Treatment

The objectives of therapy are to restore serum calcium to levels high enough to prevent complications of hypocalcemia but not high enough to lead to hypercalcemia. In general, the serum calcium should be kept at or below the lower end of normal (8.0–9.2 mg/dL) to prevent hypercalciuria. Regular monitoring at 3- to 6-month intervals may be necessary, because spontaneous changes occasionally occur. Once a patient is controlled at a satisfactory level of serum calcium and an appropriate therapeutic dose of a vitamin D derivative established, substitution of other agents may produce toxicity. If it is necessary to change treatment, it is better to use ~30% less of the theoretical equivalent of the new drug and then monitor and adjust dose until the desired level of serum and urine calcium is reached.

Calcium supplements are generally used, and it is important to add to the diet at least 1 g/day elemental calcium. Milk and cheese products (that are high in phosphate content) should be avoided. One g of calcium is present in 2.5 g calcium carbonate, 5 g calcium citrate, 8 g calcium lactate, or 10 g calcium gluconate. Although calcium gluconate is generally more palatable than the rest, it is also much more expensive. Calcium carbonate preparations are plentiful and inexpensive. It is also essential to keep serum phosphorus levels somewhat reduced to prevent soft tissue calcification. If necessary, phosphate-binding antacids may be used. In some cases, the use of thiazide diuretics has enhanced the elevation of serum calcium that may result from treatment with calcium supplements and/or vitamin D, because they increase tubular reabsorption of calcium and decrease urinary calcium. Mild disease may be managed occasionally with calcium and thiazide diuretics alone.

There are now a wide variety of choices for therapy with vitamin D (see Appendix V). This may vary from 25–100,000 U (1.25–5 mg/day) of vitamin D_3 (cholecalciferol) or D_2 (ergocalciferol), which is the least expensive form of therapy. It also has the longest duration of action and can result in prolonged toxicity. More recently, there has been widespread use of other metabolites that includes 25-hydroxyvitamin D_3 (25–200 μg/day), as well as $1,25(OH)_2D_3$ (0.25–2.0 μg/day). Although dihydrotachysterol has been used extensively in the past (at doses of 0.2–1.2 mg/day), it is less frequently utilized now.

SELECTED REFERENCES

1. Ahn TG et al.: Familial isolated hypoparathyroidism: A molecular genetic analysis of 8 families with 23 affected persons. *Medicine* 65:73–81, 1986
2. Bell NH: Vitamin D endocrine system. *J Clin Invest* 76:1–5, 1985
3. Burckhardt P: Idiopathic hypoparathyroidism and autoimmunity. *Hormone Res* 16:304–309, 1982
4. Haussler MR, Cordy PE: Metabolites and analogues of vitamin D: Which for what? *JAMA* 247:841–844, 1982
5. Illum F, Dupont E: Prevalence of CT-detected calcification in the basal ganglia in idiopathic hypoparathyroidism and pseudohypoparathyroidism. *Neuroradiology* 27:32–37, 1985
6. Mallette L: Synthetic human parathyroid hormone 1–34 fragment for diagnostic testing. *Ann Intern Med* 109:800–802, 1988
7. Muric A, Levine MA: Analysis of the preopPTH gene by denaturing gradient gel electrophoresis in familial isolated hypoparathyroidism. *J Clin Endocrin Metab* 74:509–516, 1992
8. Nusynowitz ML, Frame B, Kolb FO: The spectrum of the hypoparathyroid states: A classification based on physiologic principles. *Medicine* 55:105–121, 1976
9. Okano O, Furukawa Y, Morii H, Fujita T: Comparative efficacy of various vitamin D metabolites in the treatment of various types of hypoparathyroidism. *J Clin Endocrinol Metab* 55:238–243, 1982
10. Porter RH, Cox BG, Heaney D, Hostetter TH, Stinebaugh BJ, Suki WN: Treatment of hypoparathyroid patients with chlorthalidone. *N Engl J Med* 298:577–581, 1978
11. Porat A, Sherwood LM: Disorders of mineral homeostasis and bone. In: Kohler PO (ed) *Clinical Endocrinology*. John Wiley and Sons, New York, pp 376–426, 1986
12. Zaloga GP, Chernow B: Hypocalcemia in critical illness. *JAMA* 256:1924–1929, 1986

46. Parathyroid Hormone Resistance Syndromes

Michael A. Levine, M.D.

*Department of Medicine, The Johns Hopkins University School of Medicine,
Baltimore, Maryland*

The term *pseudohypoparathyroidism* (PHP) describes a heterogeneous syndrome characterized by biochemical hypoparathyroidism (i.e., hypocalcemia and hyperphosphatemia), increased plasma levels of parathyroid hormone (PTH), and peripheral unresponsiveness to the biological actions of PTH. Thus PHP differs substantially and fundamentally from true hypoparathyroidism; in contrast to the latter condition, PHP is characterized by excessive PTH secretion and hyperplasia of the parathyroid glands.

In the initial description of PHP, Fuller Albright and his associates (1) focused on the failure of patients with this syndrome to show either a calcemic or a phosphaturic response to administered parathyroid extract. These observations provided the basis for the hypothesis that biochemical hypoparathyroidism in PHP was due not to a deficiency of PTH but rather to resistance of the target organs, bone and kidney, to the biological actions of PTH.

PTH activates its target cells by binding to specific receptors located on the external surface of the cell plasma membrane. Interaction of PTH with its receptor triggers G proteins that activate signal effector systems that generate intracellular second messengers that then mediate the multiple distal effects of PTH. These second messengers include cAMP (2,3), inositol 1,4,5-trisphosphate and diacylglycerol (4,5), and cytosolic calcium (6–9). The best-characterized mediator of PTH action is cAMP, which rapidly activates protein kinase A (10). The relevant target proteins that are phosphorylated by protein kinase A and the precise mode(s) of action of these proteins remain uncharacterized, although proteins that activate genes responsive to cAMP and ion channel proteins are strong candidates. The intracellular accumulation of cAMP produces a biochemical chain reaction that begins with activation of protein kinase A and phosphorylation of specific protein substrates, and ultimately concludes with expression of the physiologic response to agonist recognition by the cell (Fig. 1). In contrast to the well-recognized biologic effects of cAMP in PTH target tissues, the physiological importance of metabolites phosphotidylinositol and intracellular calcium as PTH-induced second messengers has not yet been established.

PATHOGENESIS OF PSEUDOHYPOPARATHYROIDISM

Characterization of the molecular basis for PHP commenced with the observation that cAMP mediates many of the actions of PTH on kidney and bone, and that administration of biologically active PTH to normal subjects leads to a significant increase in the urinary excretion of nephrogenous cAMP (11). The PTH infusion test remains the most reliable test available for the diagnosis of PHP and enables distinction between the several variants of the syndrome (Fig. 2). Thus, patients with PHP type I fail to show an appropriate increase in urinary excretion of both cAMP and phosphate (11), whereas subjects with the less common type II form show a normal increase in urinary cAMP excretion but have an impaired phosphaturic response (12).

Pseudohypoparathyroidism Type I

The blunted nephrogenous cAMP response to exogenous PTH in subjects with PHP type I first suggested that PTH resistance is caused by a defect in the adenylyl cyclase complex that produces cAMP in renal tubule cells. Recent studies (reviewed in ref. 13) have shown that the hormone-sensitive adenylyl cyclase system is far more complex than originally suspected, consisting of at least three membrane-bound proteins (Fig. 1). Adenylyl cyclase is regulated by hormones and neurotransmitters that bind to specific *receptors* that are predicted to have seven transmembrane segments (14). Receptors that result in stimulation (R_s) of adenylyl cyclase include those for β-adrenergic agonists, PTH, ACTH, gonadotropins, glucagon, and many others. Adenylyl cyclase activity is also under inhibitory control by such agents as somatostatin, α_2-adrenergic and muscarinic agonists, and opioids. These ligands bind to specific inhibitory receptors (R_i). Receptors communicate with the actual *catalyst* of adenylyl cyclase through their interaction with a pair of homologous *guanine nucleotide-binding* signal transducing proteins (G proteins), one of which (G_s) mediates stimulation of adenylyl cyclase activity, whereas the other (G_i) regulates inhibition of enzyme activity.

G Proteins and Hormone-Sensitive Signal Transduction

The G proteins are members of a superfamily of guanine triphosphate (GTP)-binding proteins that includes *ras* and *ras*-like proteins, soluble proteins that are involved in protein synthesis and elongation, and cytoskeletal proteins such as tubulin. The G proteins couple cell-surface receptors to their second-messenger signal generation systems, and thereby regulate activity of intracellular effector enzymes and ion channels (15,16). G proteins share a heterotrimeric structure composed of α, β, and γ subunits. At least 20 G protein α chains associate with a smaller pool of β- (>4) and γ-subunits (>7) (17). The Gα subunit contains the guanine nucleotide-binding site, has intrinsic

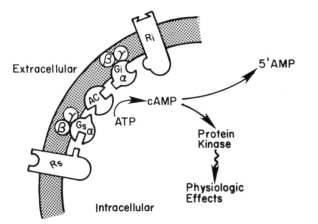

FIG. 1. Schematic outline of the adenylyl cyclase system. H_s and H_i denote stimulatory and inhibitory ligands, respectively; R_s and R_i denote stimulatory and inhibitory receptors; and G_s and G_i denote the stimulatory and inhibitory guanine nucleotide-binding regulatory proteins. C denotes the catalytic unit of adenylyl cyclase. The subunit structure of the G proteins and their interactions with the catalytic unit are described in the text.

GTPase activity, and is thought to confer functional specificity on each G protein, allowing it to discriminate among multiple receptors and effectors (for review see ref. (17). The Gβ and Gγ subunits associate specifically to form distinct dimers (18) that differ in their ability to couple α subunits to receptors or to modulate effectors (19).

The G proteins share a common mechanism of action, acting as "molecular switches" in which "on" and "off" states are regulated by a GTPase cycle. When an agonist binds to its receptor, a conformational change is transmitted to the G protein that facilitates exchange of tightly

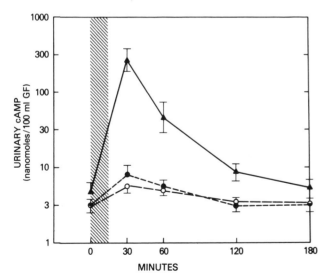

FIG. 2. cAMP excretion in urine in response to the intravenous administration of bovine parathyroid extract (300 USP units) from 9:00–9:15 AM. The peak response in normals (▲) is 50- to 100-fold times basal. Patients with PHP type Ia (●) or PHP type Ib (○) show only a 2- to 5-fold response.

bound guanine diphosphate (GDP) for GTP. Binding of GTP to the α chain activates the G protein and leads to dissociation of the βγ dimer. The GTP-bound form of the α-chain is typically the effector-modulating moiety, although βγ dimers may influence activity of some effectors (e.g., adenylyl cyclase). Interaction of the α subunit with an effector is terminated when GTP is hydrolyzed to GDP. The α chain subsequently reassociates with its βγ dimer to reassemble a heterotrimeric G protein that is able to couple to a receptor and thereby undergo another round of the GTPase cycle. Receptors that are coupled to G proteins show high affinity for agonists; binding of GTP to the G protein leads to dissociation of the G protein from its receptor and thereby lowers receptor affinity for agonist. Once activated, a single receptor molecule can interact with several G proteins, each of which will then be able to activate multiple effector molecules. Thus, receptors not only transmit extracellular signals, but also provide a basis for amplification of the signal.

At least six forms of mammalian adenylyl cyclase with estimated molecular weights of approximately 120 to 150 kDa have been identified by molecular cloning (20). Portions of the catalytic domains of these molecules show significant (50–92% sequence identity) structural conservation. The adenylyl cyclases can be distinguished by their tissue distribution and by their responses to βγ dimers and calcium-calmodulin. The type I adenylyl cyclase is expressed exclusively in the brain (21), and the type III adenylyl cyclase is expressed primarily in olfactory neuroepithelium (22). Both of these adenylyl cyclases are stimulated by calcium-calmodulin. By contrast, other forms of adenylyl cyclase are insensitive to calcium-calmodulin, and are expressed in the heart [types V (23) and VI (24)] or the lung [type II (25)] as well as the brain. A type IV adenylyl cyclase is widely expressed in liver, kidney, heart, lung, and other tissues (26). It is likely that additional forms of adenylyl cyclase exist.

All forms of adenylyl cyclase are stimulated by $G_s\alpha$ and the diterpene forskolin and inhibited by $G_i\alpha$. Activity of some forms of adenylyl cyclase is also modulated by G protein βγ dimers. In the presence of activated $G_s\alpha$, adenylyl cyclase activity may be stimulated (types II and IV), inhibited (type I), or unaffected (type III) by βγ subunits (19,27). Thus, tissue-specific patterns of hormone responsiveness (i.e., cAMP generation) can be determined not only by the types of receptors present on the cell surface, but also by the types of adenylyl cyclase expressed in the cell.

Pseudohypoparathyroidism Type Ia

Albright's original description of PHP emphasized PTH resistance as the biochemical hallmark of this disorder. Resistance to PTH alone would be consistent with a defect in the cell surface receptor specific for PTH. However, some patients with PHP type I display resistance to multiple hormones, including PTH, thyroid-stimulating hormone, gonadotropins, and glucagon, whose effects are mediated by cAMP (28). In addition, these patients have a peculiar constellation of somatic characteristics collec-

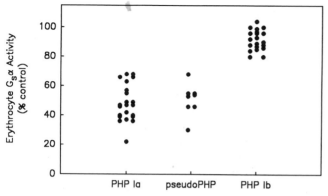

FIG. 3. $G_s\alpha$ activity in PHP type I and pseudoPHP. $G_s\alpha$ activity was measured in erythrocyte membrane extracts by complementation with membranes from S49 cyc⁻ cells, which genetically lack $G_s\alpha$. The resultant adenylyl cyclase activity is expressed as a percentage of that of a control membrane preparation consisting of pooled erythrocyte membranes from several normal subjects.

tively referred to as Albright hereditary osteodystrophy (AHO) and comprising subcutaneous ossifications, brachydactyly, obesity, round facies, and short stature (1). These patients, referred to as PHP type Ia, have an approximately 50% reduction in $G_s\alpha$ activity in plasma membranes from multiple cell types (29) (Fig. 3). In most of these subjects, there is a similar 50% reduction in amounts of both $G_s\alpha$ mRNA (30,31) and protein (32). A generalized deficiency of $G_s\alpha$ may reduce the ability of many hormones and neurotransmitters to activate adenylyl cyclase and thereby produce hormone resistance.

Some subjects with AHO do not manifest biochemical evidence of hormone resistance and have a normal urinary cAMP response to PTH (11,33). This normocalcemic variant of AHO has been termed *pseudopseudohypoparathyroidism* (34) (pseudoPHP) to call attention to the physical similarity (AHO) yet metabolic dissimilarity (normal hormone responsiveness) of this disorder to PHP. PseudoPHP is genetically related to PHP. Early clinical observations of AHO kindreds in which several affected members had only AHO (i.e., pseudoPHP), whereas others had PTH resistance as well (i.e., PHP) first suggested that the two disorders might reflect variability in expression of a single genetic lesion. Further support for this view derives from recent studies indicating that within a given kindred, subjects with either pseudoPHP or PHP type Ia have equivalent functional $G_s\alpha$ deficiency (30,33). It therefore seems reasonable to use the term AHO to simplify description of this syndrome, and to acknowledge the common clinical and biochemical characteristics that patients with PHP type Ia and pseudoPHP share.

The inheritance of $G_s\alpha$ deficiency in patients with AHO (33,35) first led to the speculation that the primary defect in this disorder involves the $G_s\alpha$ gene. The primary structure of the human $G_s\alpha$ protein has been deduced from characterization of complementary (36) and genomic (37) DNA clones. The human gene is composed of 13 exons

and 12 introns (Fig. 4) (37), and has been mapped to chromosome 20q13.2 → q13.3 in man (38). The observation that patients with AHO have reduced (30,31) or normal (30) levels of $G_s\alpha$ mRNA has suggested that $G_s\alpha$ deficiency might arise from a variety of genetic mutations. Heterozygous mutations of the $G_s\alpha$ gene that lead to reduced mRNA and/or functional protein have been identified in subjects with AHO (39,40), thus providing molecular confirmation that transmission of $G_s\alpha$ gene defects accounts for the autosomal dominant inheritance of AHO. Distinct $G_s\alpha$ mutations have been found in each kindred studied, implying that new and independent mutations must sustain the disorder (Fig. 4).

These studies provide a molecular basis for $G_s\alpha$ deficiency, but they do not explain the striking variability in biochemical and clinical phenotype. Why do some $G_s\alpha$-coupled pathways show reduced hormone responsiveness (e.g., PTH, thyroid-stimulating hormone, and gonadotropins), whereas other pathways are clinically unaffected (ACTH in the adrenal and vasopressin in the renal medulla). Perhaps even more intriguing is the paradox of why some subjects with $G_s\alpha$ deficiency have hormone resistance (PHP type Ia), whereas others do not (pseudoPHP). These observations suggest that $G_s\alpha$ deficiency may be necessary but not sufficient to cause hormone resistance. Perhaps variability in other components of the signal transduction pathway (i.e., adenylyl cyclase) may explain why identical defects in $G_s\alpha$ can have such variable consequences in different tissues or in different individuals.

In AHO, inherited $G_s\alpha$ gene mutations reduce expression or function of $G_s\alpha$ protein. By contrast, in the McCune–Albright syndrome, somatic mutations in the $G_s\alpha$ gene enhance activity of the protein (41,42). These mutations lead to constitutive activation of adenylyl cyclase, and produce proliferation and autonomous hyperfunction of hormonally responsive cells. Identification of contrasting defects in the same gene as the basis for these two syndromes, which may be the reverse of one another, confirms the clinical importance of G protein defects as a basis for human disease.

Pseudohypoparathyroidism Type Ib

Some subjects with PHP type I lack features of AHO. These patients typically show hormone resistance that is limited to PTH target organs (Fig. 1) and have normal $G_s\alpha$ activity (Fig. 3) (28). This variant, termed PHP type Ib, may be due to a defect in the receptor for PTH (43). Although patients with PHP type Ib fail to show a nephrogenous cAMP response to PTH, they often manifest skeletal lesions similar to those that occur in patients with hyperparathyroidism (44). These observations have suggested that at least one intracellular signaling pathway coupled to the PTH receptor may be intact in patients with PHP type Ib.

The molecular basis for reduced PTH receptor activity in PHP type Ib has not been clearly defined. The recent cloning of cDNAs encoding an opossum kidney PTH receptor (45) and a rat bone PTH receptor (46) indicates

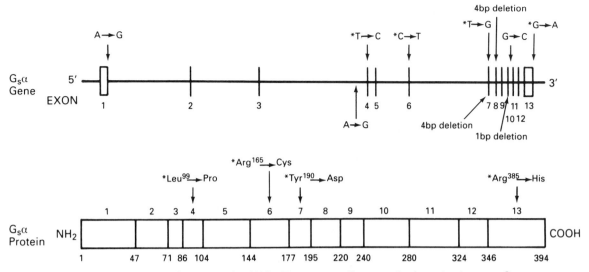

FIG. 4. Mutations in the $G_s\alpha$ gene in AHO. The upper diagram depicts the human $G_s\alpha$ gene, which spans over 20-kilobase pairs and contains 13 exons and 12 introns. Ten distinct mutations have been identified in affected members of ten unrelated families. The mutation in exon 1 eliminates the initiator methionine codon and prevents synthesis of a normal $G_s\alpha$ protein (39). The four base-pair deletions in exon 7 (57) and exon 8 (58), and the one base-pair deletion in exon 10 all shift the normal reading frame and prevent normal mRNA and/or protein synthesis. Mutations in intron 3 and at the donor splice junction between exon 10 and intron 10 cause splicing abnormalities that prevent normal mRNA synthesis (40). The four mutations indicated with an *asterisk* represent missense mutations (58–60); the resultant amino acid substitutions are indicated in the schematic diagram of the $G_s\alpha$ protein at the bottom of the figure. Some of these mutations may prevent normal protein synthesis by altering protein secondary structure, but the arg → his substitution in exon 13 appears to encode an altered protein that cannot couple normally to receptors (59).

that this receptor is a member of the superfamily of seven transmembrane segments receptors that are coupled by G proteins to intracellular signal effector molecules. Agonist binding to the cloned PTH receptor expressed in COS-7 cells leads to stimulation of adenylyl cyclase and activation of phospholipase C (46), suggesting that a single PTH receptor can couple efficiently to two *divergent* G proteins (e.g., G_s and a G protein linked to phospholipase C). Thus, defects that uncouple the PTH receptor from adenylyl cyclase but leave intact the ability of the receptor to activate other signal transduction pathways may explain the clinical observations noted above.

Pseudohypoparathyroidism Type Ic

In a few patients with PHP type I resistance to multiple hormones occurs in the absence of a demonstrable defect in G_s or G_i (28,47). The nature of the lesion in such patients is unclear, but it could be related to some other general component of the receptor-adenylyl cyclase system, such as the catalytic unit (48). Alternatively, these patients could have functional defects of G_s (or G_i) that do not become apparent in the assays presently available.

Pseudohypoparathyroidism Type II

Pseudohypoparathyroidism type II is a heterogeneous disorder without a clear genetic or familial basis. In these

patients renal resistance to PTH is manifested by a reduced phosphaturic response to administration of PTH, despite a normal increase in urinary cAMP excretion (12). These observations suggest that the PTH receptor-adenylyl cyclase complex functions normally to increase cAMP in response to PTH, and are consistent with a model in which PTH resistance arises from an inability of intracellular cAMP to initiate the chain of metabolic events that result in the ultimate expression of PTH action.

Although no supportive data are yet available, a defective cAMP-dependent protein kinase A has been proposed (12). Alternatively, the defect in PHP type II may not reside in the generation of an intracellular cAMP response, but rather in other PTH-sensitive signal transduction pathways that lead to increased concentrations of the intracellular second messengers inositol 1,4,5-trisphosphate and diacylglycerol (4,5) and cytosolic calcium (6–9).

A Parathyroid Hormone Inhibitor as a Cause of Parathyroid Hormone Resistance

Several studies have reported an apparent dissociation between plasma levels of endogenous immunoreactive and bioactive PTH in patients with PHP type I. Despite high circulating levels of immunoreactive PTH, the levels of bioactive PTH in many patients with PHP type I have been found to be within the normal range when measured with highly sensitive renal (49) and metatarsal (50) cytochemical bioassay systems. Furthermore, plasma from many of these patients has been shown to diminish the biological activity of exogenous PTH in these *in vitro* bioassays (51). Currently, the nature of this putative inhibitor or antagonist remains unknown. The observation that prolonged hypercalcemia can remove or reduce significantly the level of inhibitory activity in the plasma of patients with PHP has suggested that the parathyroid gland may be the source of the inhibitor. In addition, analysis of circulating PTH immunoactivity after fractionation of patient plasma by reversed-phase high-performance liquid chromatography has disclosed the presence of aberrant forms of immunoreactive PTH in many of these patients (52). Although it is conceivable that a PTH inhibitor may cause PTH resistance in some patients with PHP, it is more likely that circulating antagonists of PTH action arise as a consequence of the sustained secondary hyperparathyroidism that results from the primary biochemical defect.

DIAGNOSIS OF PSEUDOHYPOPARATHYROIDISM

The biochemical hallmark of PHP is failure of the PTH target organ, the kidney, to respond to PTH. Accordingly, a diagnosis of PHP should be considered in an individual with biochemical hypoparathyroidism (i.e., hypocalcemia and hyperphosphatemia) who has an elevated plasma concentration of immunoreactive PTH. Additional evidence of PHP is provided by the presence of AHO. Because reduced serum concentrations of magnesium have been reported to impair target organ responsiveness to PTH, it is important first to exclude hypomagnesemia in these subjects.

The classical tests for PHP, the Ellsworth–Howard test and later modifications by Chase, Melson, and Aurbach (11), involved the administration of 200–300 USP units of purified bovine PTH or parathyroid extract. Although these preparations are no longer available, the synthetic human PTH(1–34) peptide has recently been approved for human use, and several protocols for its use in the differential diagnosis of hypoparathyroidism have been developed (53–55). The patient should be fasting, supine except for voiding, and hydrated (250 ml of water hourly from 6:00 AM to noon). Two control urine specimens are collected before 9:00 AM. Synthetic human PTH(1–34) peptide (30 μg, 100 Units) is administered intravenously from 9:00–9:15 AM, and experimental urine specimens are collected from 9:00–9:30, 9:30–10:00, 10:00–11:00, and 11:00–12:00. Blood samples should be obtained at 9:00 and 11:00 AM for measurement of serum creatinine and phosphorous concentrations. Urine samples are analyzed for cAMP, phosphorous, and creatinine concentrations, and results are expressed as nanomoles of cAMP/100 ml glomerular filtration and thymidine monophosphate/glomerular filtration rate. Normal subjects and patients with hormonopenic hypoparathyroidism usually display a 10- to 20-fold increase in urinary cAMP excretion, whereas patients with PHP type I (types Ia and Ib), regardless of

their serum calcium concentration, will show a markedly blunted response (Fig. 2). Thus, this test can distinguish patients with so-called "normocalcemic" PHP (i.e., patients with PTH resistance who are able to maintain normal serum calcium levels without treatment) from subjects with pseudoPHP (who will have a normal urinary cAMP response to PTH(11,33)). Recent studies indicate that measurement of plasma cAMP (55) or plasma 1,25-dihydroxyvitamin D (56) after infusion of human PTH(1–34) may also differentiate PHP type I from other causes of hypoparathyroidism. Further testing (e.g., $G_s\alpha$ protein or gene analysis) is indicated only to confirm the diagnosis of PHP type Ia.

The diagnosis of PHP type II, a much rarer entity, is less straightforward. Documentation of elevated serum PTH and basal urinary (or nephrogenous) cAMP is a prerequisite for a definitive diagnosis of PHP type II (12). These subjects have a normal urinary cAMP response to infusion of PTH, but characteristically fail to show a phosphaturic response. Unfortunately, interpretation of the phosphaturic response to PTH is often complicated by random variations in phosphate clearance, and it is sometimes not possible to classify a phosphaturic response as normal or subnormal regardless of the criteria used. More perplexing yet is the observation that biochemical findings that resemble PHP type II have been found in patients with various forms of vitamin D deficiency. In these patients, marked hypocalcemia is accompanied by hyperphosphatemia due presumably to an acquired dissociation between the amount of cAMP generated in the renal tubule and its effect on phosphate clearance.

TREATMENT

The basic principles of treatment of hypocalcemia in PHP are essentially those outlined for the treatment of hormonopenic hypoparathyroidism. Therapy is directed at maintaining a low- to midnormal serum calcium concentration and thereby controlling symptoms of tetany while avoiding hypercalciuria. Happily, the risk of treatment-related hypercalciuria is far less for patients with PHP than for individuals with hypoparathyroidism.

Patients with PHP type Ia will frequently manifest resistance to other hormones in addition to PTH and may display clinical evidence of hypothyroidism or gonadal dysfunction. The basic principles used in the treatment of primary hypothyroidism apply to therapy of hypothyroidism in patients with PHP type Ia, as do approaches for the evaluation and treatment of hypogonadism.

REFERENCES

1. Albright F, Burnett CH, Smith PH: Pseudohypoparathyroidism: An example of "Seabright-Bantam syndrome." *Endocrinology* 30:922–932, 1942
2. Melson GL, Chase LR, Aurbach GD: Parathyroid hormone-sensitive adenyl cyclase in isolated renal tubules. *Endocrinology* 86:511–518, 1970
3. Chase LR, Fedak SA, Aurbach GD: Activation of skeletal ade-

nyl cyclase by parathyroid hormone in vitro. *Endocrinology* 84: 761–768, 1969

4. Civitelli R, Reid IR, Westbrook S, Avioli LV, Hruska KA: PTH elevates inositol polyphosphates and diacylglycerol in a rat osteoblast-like cell line. *Am J Physiol* 255:E660–E667, 1988

5. Dunlay R, Hruska K: PTH receptor coupling to phospholipase C is an alternate pathway of signal transduction in bone and kidney. *Am J Physiol* 258:F223–F231, 1990

6. Gupta A, Martin KJ, Miyauchi A, Hruska KA: Regulation of cytosolic calcium by parathyroid hormone and oscillations of cytosolic calcium in fibroblasts from normal and pseudohypoparathyroid patients. *Endocrinology* 128:2825–2836, 1991

7. Civitelli R, Martin TJ, Fausto A, Gunsten SL, Hruska KA, Avioli LV: Parathyroid hormone-related peptide transiently increases cytosolic calcium in osteoblast-like cells: Comparison with parathyroid hormone. *Endocrinology* 125:1204–1210, 1989

8. Reid IR, Civitelli R, Halstead LR, Avioli LV, Hruska KA: Parathyroid hormone acutely elevates intracellular calcium in osteoblastlike cells. *Am J Physiol* 253:E45–E51, 1987

9. Yamaguchi DT, Hahn TJ, Iida-Klein A, Kleeman CR, Muallem S: Parathyroid hormone-activated calcium channels in an osteoblast-like clonal osteosarcoma cell line. *J Biol Chem* 262: 7711–7718, 1987

10. Bringhurst FR, Zajac JD, Daggett AS, Skurat RN, Kronenberg HM: Inhibition of parathyroid hormone responsiveness in clonal osteoblastic cells expressing a mutant form of 3′,5′-cyclic adenosine monophosphate-dependent protein kinase. *Mol Endocrinol* 3:60–67, 1989

11. Chase LR, Melson GL, Aurbach GD: Pseudohypoparathyroidism: Defective excretion of 3′,5′-AMP in response to parathyroid hormone. *J Clin Invest* 48:1832–1844, 1969

12. Drezner MK, Neelon FA, Lebovitz HE: Pseudohypoparathyroidism type II: A possible defect in the reception of the cyclic AMP signal. *N Engl J Med* 280:1056–1060, 1973

13. Smigel MD, Ferguson KM, Gilman AG: Control of adenylate cyclase activity by G proteins. *Adv Cyclic Nucleotide Protein Phosphorylation Res* 19:103–111, 1985

14. Dohlman HG, Thorner J, Caron MG, Lefkowitz RJ: Model systems for the study of seven-transmembrane-segment receptors. *Annu Rev Biochem* 60:653–688, 1991

15. Johnson GL, Dhanasekaran N: The G-protein family and their interaction with receptors. *Endocr Rev* 10:317–331, 1989

16. Spiegel AM, Shenker A, Weinstein LS: Receptor-effector coupling by G proteins: Implications for normal and abnormal signal transduction. *Endocr Rev* 13:536–565, 1992

17. Simon MI, Strathmann MP, Gautam N: Diversity of G proteins in signal transduction. *Science* 252:802–808, 1991

18. Schmidt CJ, Thomas TC, Levine MA, Neer EJ: Specificity of G protein beta and gamma subunit interactions. *J Biol Chem* 267:13807–13810, 1992

19. Tang WJ, Gilman AG: Type-specific regulation of adenylyl cyclase by G protein beta gamma subunits. *Science* 254:1500–1503, 1991

20. Tang WJ, Gilman AG: Adenylyl cyclases. *Cell* 70:869–872, 1992

21. Krupinski J, Coussen F, Bakalyar HA, et al.: Adenylyl cyclase amino acid sequence: Possible channel- or transporter-like structure. *Science* 244:1558–1564, 1989

22. Bakalyar HA, Reed RR: Identification of a specialized adenylyl cyclase that may mediate odorant detection. *Science* 250: 1403–1406, 1990

23. Ishikawa Y, Katsushika S, Chen L, Halnon NJ, Kawabe J, Homcy CJ: Isolation and characterization of a novel cardiac adenylylcyclase cDNA. *J Biol Chem* 267:13553–13557, 1992

24. Katsushika S, Chen L, Kawabe J, et al.: Cloning and characterization of a sixth adenylyl cyclase isoform: Types V and VI constitute a subgroup within the mammalian adenylyl cyclase family. *Proc Natl Acad Sci USA* 89:8774–8778, 1992

25. Feinstein PG, Schrader KA, Bakalyar HA, et al.: Molecular cloning and characterization of a Ca²⁺/calmodulin-insensitive adenylyl cyclase from rat brain. *Proc Natl Acad Sci USA* 88: 10173–10177, 1991

26. Gao BN, Gilman AG: Cloning and expression of a widely distributed (type IV) adenylyl cyclase. *Proc Natl Acad Sci USA* 88: 10178–10182, 1991

27. Federman AD, Conklin BR, Schrader KA, Reed RR, Bourne HR: Hormonal stimulation of adenylyl cyclase through Gi-protein beta gamma subunits. *Nature* 356:159–161, 1992

28. Levine MA, Downs RW Jr, Moses AM, et al.: Resistance to multiple hormones in patients with pseudohypoparathyroidism. Association with deficient activity of guanine nucleotide regulatory protein. *Am J Med* 74:545–556, 1983

29. Levine MA, Aurbach GD: Pseudohypoparathyroidism. In DeGroot LJ (ed) *Endocrinology*. W.B. Saunders, Philadelphia, pp 1065–1079, 1989

30. Levine MA, Ahn TG, Klupt SF, et al.: Genetic deficiency of the alpha subunit of the guanine nucleotide-binding protein Gs as the molecular basis for Albright hereditary osteodystrophy. *Proc Natl Acad Sci USA* 85:617–621, 1988

31. Carter A, Bardin C, Collins R, Simons C, Bray P, Spiegel A: Reduced expression of multiple forms of the alpha subunit of the stimulatory GTP-binding protein in pseudohypoparathyroidism type Ia. *Proc Natl Acad Sci USA* 84:7266–7269, 1987

32. Patten JL, Levine MA: Immunochemical analysis of the alpha-subunit of the stimulatory G-protein of adenylyl cyclase in patients with Albright's hereditary osteodystrophy. *J Clin Endocrinol Metab* 71:1208–1214, 1990

33. Levine MA, Jap TS, Mauseth RS, Downs RW, Spiegel AM: Activity of the stimulatory guanine nucleotide-binding protein is reduced in erythrocytes from patients with pseudohypoparathyroidism and pseudopseudohypoparathyroidism: Biochemical, endocrine, and genetic analysis of Albright's hereditary osteodystrophy in six kindreds. *J Clin Endocrinol Metab* 62: 497–502, 1986

34. Albright F, Forbes AP, Henneman PH: Pseudopseudohypoparathyroidism. *Trans Assoc Am Physicians* 65:337–350, 1952

35. Van Dop C, Bourne HR, Neer RM: Father to son transmission of decreased Ns activity in pseudohypoparathyroidism type Ia. *J Clin Endocrinol Metab* 59:825–828, 1984

36. Bray P, Carter A, Guo V, et al.: Human cDNA clones for an alpha subunit of Gi signal-transduction protein. *Proc Natl Acad Sci USA* 84:5115–5119, 1987

37. Kozasa T, Itoh H, Tsukamoto T, Kaziro Y: Isolation and characterization of the human Gs alpha gene. *Proc Natl Acad Sci USA* 85:2081–2085, 1988

38. Levine MA, Modi WS, Obrien SJ: Mapping of the gene encoding the alpha subunit of the stimulatory G protein of adenylyl cyclase (GNAS1) to 20q13.2 → q13.3 in human by in situ hybridization. *Genomics* 11:478–479, 1991

39. Patten JL, Johns DR, Valle D, et al.: Mutation in the gene encoding the stimulatory G protein of adenylate cyclase in Albright's hereditary osteodystrophy. *N Engl J Med* 322:1412–1419, 1990

40. Weinstein LS, Gejman PV, Friedman E, et al.: Mutations of the Gs alpha-subunit gene in Albright hereditary osteodystrophy detected by denaturing gradient gel electrophoresis. *Proc Natl Acad Sci USA* 87:8287–8290, 1990

41. Schwindinger WF, Francomano CA, Levine MA: Identification of a mutation in the gene encoding the alpha subunit of the stimulatory G protein of adenylyl cyclase in McCune-Albright syndrome. *Proc Natl Acad Sci USA* 89:5152–5156, 1992

42. Weinstein LS, Shenker A, Gejman PV, Merino MJ, Friedman E, Spiegel AM: Activating mutations of the stimulatory G protein in the McCune-Albright syndrome. *N Engl J Med* 325:1688–1695, 1991

43. Silve C, Santora A, Breslau N, Moses A, Spiegel A: Selective resistance to parathyroid hormone in cultured skin fibroblasts from patients with pseudohypoparathyroidism type Ib. *J Clin Endocrinol Metab* 62:640–644, 1986

44. Kidd GS, Schaaf M, Adler RA, Lassman MN, Wray HL: Skeletal responsiveness in pseudohypoparathyroidism: A spectrum of clinical disease. *Am J Med* 68:772–781, 1980

45. Juppner H, Abou Samra AB, Freeman M, et al.: A G protein-linked receptor for parathyroid hormone and parathyroid hormone-related peptide. *Science* 254:1024–1026, 1991

46. Abou Samra AB, Juppner H, Force T, et al.: Expression cloning of a common receptor for parathyroid hormone and parathyroid hormone-related peptide from rat osteoblast-like cells: A single receptor stimulates intracellular accumulation of both cAMP and

inositol trisphosphates and increases intracellular free calcium. *Proc Natl Acad Sci USA* 89:2732–2736, 1992

47. Farfel Z, Brothers VM, Brickman AS, Conte F, Neer R, Bourne HR: Pseudohypoparathyroidism: Inheritance of deficient receptor-cyclase coupling activity. *Proc Natl Acad Sci USA* 78: 3098–3102, 1981

48. Barrett D, Breslau NA, Wax MB, Molinoff PB, Downs RW Jr: New form of pseudohypoparathyroidism with abnormal catalytic adenylate cyclase. *Am J Physiol* 257:E277–E283, 1989

49. De Deuxchaisnes CN, Fischer JA, Dambacher MA, et al.: Dissociation of parathyroid hormone bioactivity and immunoreactivity in pseudohypoparathyroidism type I. *J Clin Endocrinol Metab* 53:1105–1109, 1981

50. Bradbeer JN, Dunham J, Fischer JA, Nagant De Deuxchaisnes C, Loveridge N: The metatarsal cytochemical bioassay of parathyroid hormone: Validation, specificity, and application to the study of pseudohypoparathyroidism type I. *J Clin Endocrinol Metab* 67:1237–1243, 1988

51. Loveridge N, Fischer JA, Nagant De Deuxchaisnes C, et al.: Inhibition of cytochemical bioactivity of parathyroid hormone by plasma in pseudohypoparathyroidism type I. *J Clin Endocrinol Metab* 54:1274–1275, 1982

52. Mitchell J, Goltzman D: Examination of circulating parathyroid hormone in pseudohypoparathyroidism. *J Clin Endocrinol Metab* 61:328–334, 1985

53. Mallette LE: Synthetic human parathyroid hormone 1-34 fragment for diagnostic testing. *Ann Intern Med* 109:800–804, 1988

54. Mallette LE, Kirkland JL, Gagel RF, Law WM Jr, Heath H III: Synthetic human parathyroid hormone-(1–34) for the study of pseudohypoparathyroidism. *J Clin Endocrinol Metab* 67: 964–972, 1988

55. Yamamoto M, Furukawa Y, Konagaya Y, et al.: Human PTH(1–34) infusion test in differential diagnosis of various types of hypoparathyroidism: An attempt to establish a standard clinical test. *Bone Miner* 6:199–212, 1989

56. Miura R, Yumita S, Yoshinaga K, Furukawa Y: Response of plasma 1,25-dihydroxyvitamin D in the human PTH(1–34) infusion test: An improved index for the diagnosis of idiopathic hypoparathyroidism and pseudohypoparathyroidism. *Calcif Tissue Int* 46:309–313, 1990

57. Weinstein LS, Gejman PV, De Mazancourt P, American N, Spiegel AM: A heterozygous 4-bp deletion mutation in the $G_s\alpha$ gene (GNAS 1) in a patient with Albright hereditary osteodystrophy. *Genomics* 13:1319–1321, 1992

58. Miric A, Vechio JD, Levine MA: Heterozygous mutations in the gene encoding the alpha subunit of the stimulatory G protein of adenylyl cyclase in Albright hereditary osteodystrophy. *J Clin Endocrinol Metab* 1993 (in press)

59. Schwindinger WF, Miric A, Levine MA: Identification of a novel missense mutation in the gene encoding the alpha subunit of the stimulatory G protein of adenylyl cyclase in a subject with Albright hereditary osteodystrophy. *Program and Abstracts*, 74th Annual Meeting of the Endocrine Society, Abstract 35, 1992

60. Miric A, Levine MA: Mutations within the gene encoding the stimulatory G-protein of adenylyl cyclase as the basis for Albright hereditary osteodystrophy. In: Milligan G, Wakelam M (eds) *G Proteins: Signal Transduction and Disease*. Academic Press, San Diego, pp 29–46, 1992

47. Hypocalcemia Due to Magnesium Deficiency

Robert K. Rude, M.D.

Department of Medicine, University of Southern California, Los Angeles, California

Magnesium deficiency is a commonly encountered clinical problem. In large city hospitals 10% of admitted patients are hypomagnesemic, whereas up to 65% of patients in medical intensive care units may be hypomagnesemic. Hypocalcemia is a common manifestation of moderate to severe magnesium deficiency. The hypocalcemia may be a major contributing factor in the increased neuromuscular excitability often present in magnesium deficient patients.

PATHOGENESIS

The pathogenesis of hypomagnesemia is multifactorial. In normal subjects, an acute change in the serum magnesium concentration will affect parathyroid hormone (PTH) secretion. That is, an acute fall in serum magnesium stimulates PTH secretion while hypermagnesemia inhibits PTH secretion. During chronic and severe magnesium deficiency, however, PTH secretion is impaired. The majority of patients will have serum concentrations of immunoreactive parathyroid hormone (iPTH) that are undetectable or inappropriately normal for the degree of hypocalcemia. Some patients, however, may have iPTH levels above the normal range that may reflect early magnesium depletion. Regardless of the basal circulating iPTH concentration, an acute injection of magnesium stimulates PTH secretion as illustrated in Fig. 1. Impaired PTH secretion therefore appears to be a major factor in hypomagnesemia-induced hypocalcemia.

Hypocalcemia in the presence of normal or elevated iPTH concentrations also suggests end-organ resistance to PTH. Patients with hypocalcemia due to magnesium deficiency have both renal and skeletal resistance to exogenously administered PTH as manifested by subnormal urinary cAMP and phosphate excretion and diminished calcemic response. This renal and skeletal resistance to PTH is reversed following several days of magnesium therapy. The basis for the defect in PTH secretion and PTH end-organ resistance is not known. Because cAMP appears to be important in PTH secretion and mediating PTH effects in kidney and bone, it has been postulated that there may be a defect in the adenylate cyclase complex. Magnesium is necessary for cAMP formation as substrate (MgATP) as well as being an allosteric activator of adenylate cyclase.

Clinically, patients with hypocalcemia due to magnesium deficiency are resistant not only to PTH, but also to parenteral calcium and vitamin D therapy. The vitamin D resistance may be due to impaired metabolism of vita-

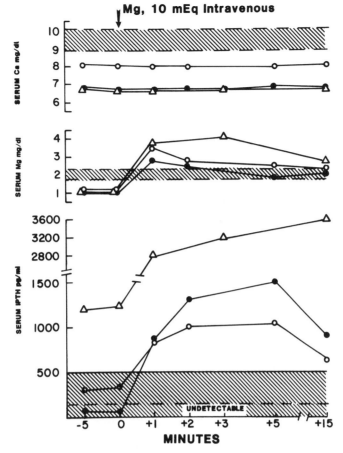

FIG. 1. Effect of an intravenous injection of 10 mEq magnesium on the serum concentration of calcium, magnesium, and iPTH in hypocalcemic magnesium-deficient patients with undetectable (●), normal (○), or elevated (△), levels of iPTH. *Shaded area* represents the range of normal for assay. *Broken line* for the iPTH assay represents the level of detectability. The magnesium injection resulted in a marked rise in PTH secretion within 1 min in all three patients.

min D, as serum concentrations of 1,25-dihydroxyvitamin D are low.

DIAGNOSIS OF MAGNESIUM DEFICIENCY

Because vitamin D and calcium therapy are relatively ineffective in correcting the hypocalcemia, there must be a high index of suspicion for the presence of magnesium deficiency. Patients with magnesium deficiency severe enough to result in hypocalcemia are usually significantly hypomagnesemic (serum magnesium concentration <1.5 mEq/L). However, occasionally, patients may have normal serum magnesium concentrations. This reflects the fact that magnesium is principally an intracellular cation with <1% of the body's magnesium in the extracellular fluid. Magnesium deficiency in the presence of a normal serum magnesium concentration has been demonstrated by measuring intracellular magnesium (in lymphocytes or muscle biopsy), or by whole-body retention of infused magnesium (Chapter 54). Therefore, hypocalcemic patients who are at risk for magnesium deficiency, but who have normal serum magnesium levels, should receive a trial of magnesium therapy.

THERAPY

An effective therapeutic regimen is the administration of $MgSO_4 \cdot 7H_2O$ either intramuscularly or intravenously. A 50% solution is available for intramuscular injection in 2 ml ampules. A dose of 16 mEq magnesium intramuscularly three times daily is usually effective in normalizing serum calcium. Because injections may be painful, a continuous intravenous infusion of 48 mEq magnesium/24 hr may be preferable.

Therapy must be continued for several days. Despite the fact that PTH secretion increases within minutes after beginning magnesium administration, the serum calcium concentration may not return to normal for 3–7 days. This probably reflects slow restoration of intracellular magnesium. During this period of therapy, serum magnesium concentration may be normal, but the total body deficit may not yet be corrected. Magnesium should be continued until the clinical and biochemical manifestations of magnesium deficiency are resolved. If the patient has excessive ongoing magnesium losses (e.g., diarrhea), therapy may be continued longer. Therapy with magnesium should be modified if renal failure is present (serum creatinine > 2.0 mg/dL). In such cases the recommended dose of MgSO$_4$ should be reduced by 50% and serum magnesium concentration monitored daily to avoid hypermagnesemia and magnesium intoxication.

SELECTED REFERENCES

1. Rude RK, Singer FR: Magnesium deficiency and excess. *Ann Rev Med* 32:245–259, 1981
2. Flink E: Magnesium deficiency: Etiology and clinical spectrum. *Acta Med Scand* 647:125, 1981
3. Wong ET, Rude RK, Singer FR: A high prevalence of hypomagnesemia in hospitalized patients. *Am J Clin Pathol* 79:348–352, 1983
4. Ryzen E, Wagers PW, Singer FR, Rude RK: Magnesium deficiency in a medical ICU population. *Crit Care Med* 13:19–21, 1985
5. Rude RK, Oldham SB, Sharp CF, Singer FR: Parathyroid hormone secretion in magnesium deficiency. *J Clin Endocrinol Metab* 47:800–806, 1978
6. Rude RK, Oldham SB, Singer FR: Functional hypoparathyroidism and parathyroid hormone end-organ resistance in human magnesium deficiency. *Clin Endocrinol* 5:209–224, 1976
7. Rude RK, Adams JS, Ryzen E, Endres DB, Niimi H, Horst RL, Haddad JG Jr, Singer FR: Low serum concentrations of 1,25-dihydroxyvitamin D in human magnesium deficiency. *J Clin Endocrinol Metab* 761:933–940, 1985
8. Ryzen E, Elbaum N, Singer FR, Rude RK: Parenteral magnesium tolerance testing in the evaluation of magnesium deficiency. *Magnesium* 4:137–147, 1985
9. Rude RK, Oldham SB: Hypocalcemia of Mg deficiency: Altered modulation of adenylate cyclase by Mg^{++} and Ca^{++} may result in impaired PTH secretion and PTH end-organ resistance. In: Altura BM, Aurbach J, Seelig JS (eds) *Magnesium in Cellular Processes and Medicine*. Karger, Basel, pp 183–195, 1987

48. Hypocalcemia Due to Pancreatitis

Andrew F. Stewart, M.D.

Department of Endocrinology, West Haven Veterans Affairs Medical Center, West Haven, Connecticut, and Yale University School of Medicine, New Haven, Connecticut

Hypocalcemia and tetany were first recorded in patients with pancreatitis in the early 1940s. Langerhans had observed in 1890 that the white deposits in the retroperitoneum ("fat necrosis") associated with pancreatitis were, in fact, insoluble calcium soaps or complexes of calcium and free fatty acids (FFAs). It is now believed that FFAs are generated by the action of pancreatic lipase, released from the damaged pancreas, on retroperitoneal and omental fat (triglyceride) to release their component FFAs into the peritoneum. These in turn avidly chelate calcium, removing it from extracellular fluid. Other mechanisms may be responsible for hypocalcemia in individual instances of pancreatitis-induced hypocalcemia. Hypoalbuminemia regularly occurs in patients with pancreatitis and leads to a reduction in total (but not ionized) serum calcium. Hypomagnesemia resulting from poor oral intake, alcohol use, and/or vomiting is common in pancreatitis and may lead to hypocalcemia (see Chapter 47). It has also been postulated that hypocalcemia may result from excessive calcitonin secretion, resulting in turn from excessive pancreatic glucagon release. Support for this possibility is weak. Finally, it has been suggested that pancreatitis may liberate systemic factors, such as proteases that inhibit parathyroid hormone secretion and/or degrade circulating parathyroid hormone. There is no recent support for this possibility.

Clinically, patients with pancreatitis-induced hypocalcemia have severe pancreatitis, and hypocalcemia portends a poor outcome. Hypocalcemia is treated with parenteral calcium and magnesium replacement when indicated. Hypocalcemia due to vitamin D deficiency/malabsorption should be considered and excluded (see Chapters 49 & 66).

SELECTED REFERENCES

1. Stewart AF, Longo W, Kreutter D, Jacob R, Burtis WJ: Hypocalcemia due to calcium soap formation in a patient with a pancreatic fistula. *N Engl J Med* 315:496–498, 1986
2. Dettelbach MA, Deftos LJ, Stewart AF: Intraperitoneal free fatty acids induce severe hypocalcemia in rats. *J Bone Miner Res* 5:1249–1255, 1990

49. Hypocalcemia Due to Vitamin D Disorders

Karl L. Insogna, M.D.

*Department of Internal Medicine, Yale University School of Medicine,
New Haven, Connecticut*

Hypocalcemia as an isolated finding resulting from disordered vitamin D metabolism is rare. Most individuals with abnormalities in either the production or action of vitamin D metabolites present with other findings such as rickets or osteomalacia. The reader is therefore referred to Chapters 65 through 69, which deal with these two clinical entities for a more detailed consideration of the hypocalcemia seen with these disorders. The reader is also referred to Chapters 13 and 21 for more detailed reviews of vitamin D metabolism, chemistry and serum assays.

Abnormalities in vitamin D metabolism can be divided into three broad categories: vitamin D deficiency, acquired or inherited disorders of vitamin D metabolism, and resistance to the actions of vitamin D.

Vitamin D deficiency is unusual because the practice of vitamin D supplementation of dairy products and other foods is common in the United States (see Chapter 65). It can only occur in patients in whom both exposure to UV light and dietary intake of vitamin D are inadequate. Certain subgroups, such as breast-fed infants of strictly vegetarian mothers, continue to be at risk for vitamin D deficiency, however (1). Recent immigrants from the Middle East to Northern latitudes who continue to wear traditional dress—including long garments, hoods, and veils—represent another example. In more moderate stages of vitamin D deficiency, serum calcium concentrations are normal, whereas hypophosphatemia due to secondary hyperparathyroidism may be apparent. In more severe disease, the clinical manifestations of rickets and/or osteomalacia are profound, and hypocalcemia is a more prominent biochemical finding. Serum 25-hydroxyvitamin D (25OHD) levels are important in the diagnosis of patients with nutritional vitamin D deficiency.

Vitamin D malabsorption leading to vitamin D deficiency may occur in patients with one of several gastrointestinal disorders (see Chapter 66). These include nontropical sprue, Crohn's disease, and pancreatic insufficiency. Osteomalacia and hypocalcemia may develop in these patients despite adequate nutritional intake and UV light exposure. The pathogenesis is not entirely clear; 25OHD and 1,25-dihydroxyvitamin D [1,25(OH)$_2$D] both undergo enterohepatic circulation, and it may be that losses due to interruption of this pathway lead to vitamin D deficiency (2). It is also possible that the diseased bowel may be incapable of absorbing vitamin D or responding to 1,25(OH)$_2$D. Circulating 25OHD concentrations are reduced, and hypocalcemia, when present, is usually modest.

Acquired or inherited abnormalities in vitamin D metabolism comprise the next broad group of disorders associated with hypocalcemia. Patients with cholestatic liver disease (see Chapter 66) may develop osteomalacia and secondary hyperparathyroidism as a consequence of reduced hepatic hydroxylation of vitamin D to 25OHD or due to intestinal malabsorption of vitamin D metabolites. Circulating levels of 25OHD are reduced and may be aggravated by poor nutritional intake and inadequate UV light exposure. Hypocalcemia is usually modest in these patients as well.

Patients with advanced renal insufficiency often have hypocalcemia, which is due in part to the low production rates of 1,25(OH)$_2$D (see Chapter 74). Other factors, including hyperphosphatemia and acidosis, contribute to the hypocalcemia in renal failure.

A variety of medications may be associated with acquired disorders of vitamin D metabolism (3) (see Chapter 72). Of these, anticonvulsants are the most frequent medications causing mild hypocalcemia. Accelerated metabolism of 25OHD to more polar inactive metabolites has been suggested as the cause of these abnormalities. Nutritional and other environmental factors may also contribute (4).

Vitamin D-dependent rickets type I (VDDR I) is a rare autosomal recessive disorder presenting in children in which hypocalcemia is a prominent manifestation (see Chapter 67). Clinical features were initially described in 1961 and include profound rickets, hypocalcemia, marked secondary hyperparathyroidism, elevated alkaline phosphatase, and generalized aminoaciduria. The pathogenesis of this disorder appears to be a selective defect in 1α-hydroxylase activity with consequent inability to convert 25OHD to 1,25(OH)$_2$D (5). Thus, patients with this disorder are generally resistant to therapy with vitamin D, but physiological doses of 1,25(OH)$_2$D$_3$ lead to prompt healing of the rachitic lesions and correction of the hypocalcemia.

End-organ resistance to the action of 1,25(OH)$_2$D results in hypocalcemic vitamin D-dependent rickets type II (VDDR II; see Chapter 67). In contrast to hypocalcemic VDDR I, hypocalcemia in VDDR II is accompanied by dramatic elevations in circulating 1,25(OH)$_2$D. The phenotypic features of this autosomal recessive syndrome are similar to those of vitamin D-resistant rickets type I with the additional finding of partial or complete alopecia. The relationship of this finding to the abnormalities in vitamin D function remains unknown. As might be anticipated, a number of molecular defects appear to result in the same phenotypic manifestations. The final common abnormality seems to be an inability of 1,25(OH)$_2$D to induce the usual intracellular events associated with binding to the vitamin D receptor and receptor-hormone complex binding to DNA. Thus, in all cases tested, the normal induction of the enzyme 25OHD 24-hydroxylase by 1,25(OH)$_2$D is absent. Point mutations is the DNA binding domain of the human vitamin D receptor gene have been demonstrated in skin fibroblasts from patients with this syndrome (6).

Although therapy with high dose $1,25(OH)_2D_3$ has been largely unsuccessful in the treatment of VDDR II, it has been reported that prolonged intravenous infusions of calcium may cure the rickets and correct the secondary hyperparathyroidism.

REFERENCES

1. Bachrach S, Fisher J, Parks J: An outbreak of vitamin D deficiency rickets in a susceptible population. *Pediatrics* 64:871–877, 1979

2. Kumar R: Hepatic and intestinal osteodystrophy and the hepatobiliary metabolism of vitamin D. *Ann Intern Med* 98:662–663, 1983
3. Frame B: Hypocalcemia and osteomalacia associated with anticonvulsant therapy. *Ann Intern Med* 74:294–295, 1971
4. Weinstien R, Bryce G, Sappington L, King D, Gallagher B: Decreased serum ionized calcium and normal vitamin D metabolite levels with anticonvulsant drug treatment. *J Clin Endocrinol Metab* 58:1003–1009, 1984
5. Fraser D, Kooh S, Kind P, Holick M, Tanaka Y, Deluca H: Pathogenesis of hereditary vitamin D-dependent rickets. *N Engl J Med* 289:817–822, 1973
6. Hughes M, Malloy P, Kieback D, Kesterson R, Pike J, Feldman D, O'Malley B: Point mutation in the human vitamin D receptor gene associated with hypocalcemic rickets. *Science* 242: 1702–1705, 1988

50. Hypocalcemia Due to Hyperphosphatemia

Karl L. Insogna, M.D.

Department of Internal Medicine, Yale University School of Medicine, New Haven, Connecticut

Since the 1930s it has been appreciated that oral or parenteral phosphorus may lower serum calcium levels. The mechanism whereby phosphorus administration lowers serum calcium remains unknown, however. Herbert et al. (1) showed that phosphate infusion lowered serum calcium in the presence and absence of the parathyroid glands, and changes in fecal and urinary calcium excretion during phosphate administration could not account for the fall in serum calcium. They suggested that the blood calcium phosphorus molar product, when exceeded, leads to spontaneous precipitation of calcium phosphate salts in soft tissues. The [Ca] × [P] product, when estimated from total serum calcium and phosphate concentrations (as mg/dL), normally is <60.

Hyperphosphatemia sufficient to cause hypocalcemia usually has an abrupt onset, is severe in magnitude, and usually occurs in the setting of impaired renal function. Four clinical settings conducive to phosphate-induced hypocalcemia are recognized: excessive enteral or parenteral phosphate administration; the tumor-lysis syndrome; rhabdomyolysis-induced acute renal failure; and the hypocalcemia of advanced renal insufficiency.

Excessive oral or parenteral phosphate administration may cause hypocalcemia by promotion of soft tissue calcification. Soft tissue calcification has been observed during the treatment of hypophosphatemia due to diabetic ketoacidosis and acute alcoholism (2). Adults receiving phosphate-containing enemas and infants fed "humanized" cow milk rich in phosphate (3,4) may also become hypocalcemic. Discontinuation of phosphate usually leads to prompt correction of serum calcium, but chronic phosphate-induced hypocalcemia has been reported to cause secondary hyperparathyroidism.

Hypocalcemia caused by massive tumor lysis results from the release of intracellular phosphate during massive cell destruction. A common setting of the tumor lysis syndrome is during chemotherapy for rapidly proliferating neoplasms such as acute lymphoblastic leukemia in children (5). Under these conditions, hypocalcemia may persist beyond the hyperphosphatemia and may be aggravated by suppressed 1,25-dihydroxyvitamin D [$1,25(OH)_2D$] levels (6). Optimal management of patients with tumor-lysis syndrome may include early use of phosphate binding antacids and $1,25(OH)_2D_3$, although these have not been tested by well-controlled clinical studies.

Rhabdomyolysis-induced acute renal failure may occur with trauma, or drug or alcohol abuse, and is frequently associated with marked hypocalcemia in the early oliguric phase and moderate to severe hypercalcemia in the subsequent polyuric phase (7). The mechanism of the hypocalcemia during rhabdomyolysis may be similar to the tumor-lysis syndrome, as Llach et al. (7) have described hyperphosphatemia and suppressed serum $1,25(OH)_2D_3$ during the initial appearance of hypocalcemia. The appearance of hypercalcemia and high serum $1,25(OH)_2D_3$ levels during the diuretic phase of acute renal failure with rhabdomyolysis may result from the rapid development of secondary hyperparathyroidism during the initial hypocalcemia. Treatment goals include restriction of phosphate intake, and absorption and maintenance of normal serum calcium.

Hypocalcemia may develop during the course of chronic renal failure, and its severity may be aggravated by oral phosphate administration. The hypocalcemia may result for hyperphosphatemia due to reduced renal phosphate clearance by the failing kidney and phosphate-induced suppression of already reduced rates of $1,25(OH)_2D_3$ production. Prevention of secondary hyperparathyroidism may be achieved by early administration of phosphate binding antacids and judicious use of $1,25(OH)_2D_3$.

REFERENCES

1. Herbert L, Lemann J, Petersen J, Lennon E: Studies of the mechanism by which phosphate infusion lowers serum calcium concentration. *J Clin Invest* 45:1886–1894, 1966
2. Chernow B, Rainey T, Georges L, O'Brian J: Iatrogenic hyperphosphatemia: A metabolic consideration in critical care medicine. *Crit Care Med* 9:772–774, 1981
3. Biberstein M, Parker B: Enema-induced hyperphosphatemia. *Am J Med* 79:645–646, 1985
4. Venkaraman P, Tsang R, Greer F, Noguchi A, Laskarzewski P,

Steichen J: Late infantile tetany and secondary hyperparathyroidism in infants fed humanized cow milk formula. *Am J Dis Child* 139:664–668, 1985
5. Zusman T, Brown D, Nesbit M: Hyperphosphatemia, hyperphosphaturia and hypocalcemia in acute lymphoblastic leukemia. *N Engl J Med* 289:1335–1340, 1973
6. Dunlay R, Camp M, Allon M, Fanti P, Malluche H, Llach F: Calcitriol in prolonged hypocalcemia due to the tumor lysis syndrome. *Ann Intern Med* 110:162–164, 1989
7. Llach F, Felsenfeld A, Haussler M: The pathophysiology of altered calcium metabolism in rhabdomyolysis-induced acute renal failure. *N Engl J Med* 305:117–123, 1981

51. Medications That Cause Hypocalcemia

Andrew F. Stewart, M.D.

Department of Endocrinology, West Haven Veterans Affairs Medical Center, West Haven, Connecticut, and Yale University School of Medicine, New Haven, Connecticut

Hypocalcemia may occur as the result of overzealous treatment with medications intended to reverse hypercalcemia and/or excessive bone resorption. Thus *mithramycin* (plicamycin), *calcitonin, diphosphonates*, and oral or parenteral *phosphate* preparations (see Chapter 28) have all been reported to cause hypocalcemia. Hypocalcemia and osteomalacia may occur as the result of prolonged therapy with anticonvulsants such as diphenylhydantoin (phenytoin) or *phenobarbital* (see Chapter 72). *Fluoride* overdosage has been associated with hypocalcemia, possibly due to excessive rates of skeletal mineralization and complexing of calcium by fluoride. Transfusion and plasmapheresis with *citrated blood* has been reported to cause hypocalcemia, particularly in patients receiving exchange transfusions. A recent addition to the list of drugs that may cause hypocalcemia is *radiographic contrast dyes* that may contain the calcium chelator, EDTA, in conjunction with citrate. Chelation of calcium plus dilutional/osmotic effects of these agents are believed to be responsible for the mild hypocalcemia which has

been observed. Finally, foscarnet (trisodium phosphonoformate) used in the treatment of patients with AIDS and opportunistic infections has been reported to cause reductions in total and ionized serum calcium concentrations, perhaps through chelation or complexing of calcium in extracellular fluid.

SELECTED REFERENCES

1. Tofalletti J, Nissenson RA, Endres D, McGarry E, Mogollon G: Influence of continuous infusion of citrate on responses of immuno-reactive PTH, calcium, magnesium components, and other electrolytes in normal adults during plasmapheresis. *J Clin Endocrinol Metab* 60:874–879, 1985
2. Mallette LE, Gomez LS: Systemic hypocalcemia after clinical injection of radiographic contrast media: Amelioration by ommission of calcium chelating agents. *Radiology* 147:677–679, 1982
3. Jacobson MA, Gambertoglio JG, Aweeka FT, Causey DM, Portale AA: Foscarnet-induced hypocalcemia and effects of foscarnet on calcium metabolism. *J Clin Endocrinol Metals* 72:1130–1135, 1991

52. Hypocalcemia in Acute Illness

Robert S. Weinstein, M.D.

Metabolic Bone Disease Laboratory, Section of Metabolic and Endocrine Disease, Department of Medicine, Medical College of Georgia, Augusta, Georgia

Hypocalcemia is found in more than two-thirds of patients admitted to intensive care units (ICUs) and often heralds a fatal outcome (1,2). Acute hypocalcemia may cause circumoral tingling paresthesias, painful muscle cramps, carpopedal spasm, generalized seizures, hoarseness or laryn-

geal stridor due to spasm of the muscles of the glottis, congestive heart failure, refractory hypotension, prolongation of the QTc interval [the measured QT divided by the square root of the RR interval (normal is <0.39 in women and <0.41 in men)], ventricular tachyarrhyth-

TABLE 1. *Causes of acute hypocalcemia*

Renal failure
Magnesium depletion[a]
Alkalosis
Acute pancreatitis (10)
Gram-negative sepsis
Anticonvulsant drug therapy[b] (11)
After neck exploration for thyroid, parathyroid, or laryngeal disease
Hypoparathyroidism
Hungry bones syndrome
Intestinal malabsorption
Vitamin D deficiency[b]
Toxic shock syndrome[c]
Measles
High-dose, prolonged furosemide therapy[d]
Hyperphosphatemia
    Tumor-lysis syndrome[c]
    Rhabdomyolysis[c]
    Malignant hyperthermia
    Excessive use of potassium phosphate salts in diabetic ketoacidosis
    Phosphate-containiang laxatives and enemas
Hypermagnesemia[c]
Burns
Transfusion of citrated blood[e,f] (12)
Plasmapheresis and plateletpheresis (12)
Radiographic contrast media (diatrizoate)[f]
Osteoblastic metastases
Colchicine overdose
Foscarnet antiviral treatment (13)

---

[a] May be accompanied by hypokalemia and often occurs with low-normal levels of serum magnesium.
[b] Especially with elderly, institutionalized, or recluse patients.
[c] Especially with renal insufficiency.
[d] Especially with preexisting disorders of bone and mineral metabolism.
[e] Especially with renal or hepatic disease.
[f] Serum total calcium may not show a decrease.

mias, elevated levels of serum creatinine phosphokinase and lactic dehydrogenase, diarrhea, increased intracranial pressure with papilledema, hyperventilation, apprehension, and acute psychiatric disorders (3,4). Because calcium is an essential ion for the secretion and action of many hormones, hypocalcemia may also be one of the causes of the glucose intolerance typical of patients in the ICU (5). Known causes of acute hypocalcemia are listed in Table 1.

ROLE OF SERUM-IONIZED CALCIUM DETERMINATIONS IN CRITICAL CARE

In critically ill patients, serum-ionized calcium measurements are more useful than total calcium levels (6). Samples must be collected anaerobically in filled red top tubes and the ionized calcium analyzed within 1 hr of venipuncture. The ratio of ionized to total calcium is frequently abnormal in critically ill patients because of hypoalbuminemia, pH abnormalities, fluctuations of the concentration of bicarbonate ions (independent of the effect on pH and calcium binding to proteins), infusions of albumin, heparin or intravenous lipid administration, radiographic contrast media, excessive citrate infusion during rapid blood transfusion, vigorous intravenous fluid therapy, increases in serum free fatty acids that induce increased binding of calcium ions to albumin, hemodialysis, and sepsis that are frequently encountered in these patients (7–9). In spite of attempts to correct the total calcium for these alterations, the ionized calcium fraction cannot be reliably predicted from the total calcium concentration under the above conditions.

CLINICAL APPROACH TO ACUTE HYPOCALCEMIA

First, determine the clinical impact of the hypocalcemia. Symptoms are related not only to the absolute level of ionized calcium, but also to the rate of decline. The threshold for development of symptoms also depends on the serum pH, severity of concomitant hypomagnesemia, hypokalemia and hyponatremia, and administered sedatives and anticonvulsant drugs. Patients that require immediate attention may exhibit a positive Chvostek's sign (indicated by a twitch of the corner of the mouth after tapping over the facial nerve in the parotid area), a positive Trousseau's sign (carpal spasm within 2 min after inflation of an arm sphygmomanometer cuff above systolic blood pressure), severe apprehension, seizures, papilledema, loss of deep tendon reflexes, hypotension, and an EKG showing a prolonged ST segment and QT interval with ventricular arrhythmias. In the ICU, objects in the mouth or bandages over the face and arms can interfere with signs of hypocalcemia. Sudden death can occur when the ionized calcium falls below 2 mg/dL (our normal range is 4.73–5.21). Even without clinical symptoms, an ionized calcium level below 3 mg/dL indicates the need for supplemental calcium.

Second, consider whether hypomagnesemia could be the cause of the hypocalcemia. Severe hypomagnesemia impairs parathyroid hormone secretion and action. Often there is accompanying hypokalemia. Clinical settings for serious hypomagnesemia include ethanol abuse, chronic diarrhea, diuretics, hyperalimentation, posttreatment for diabetic ketoacidosis and after administration of gentamycin, *cis*-platinum, carbenicillin, amphotericin, and cyclosporin. Calcium therapy is still warranted in hypomagnesemic hypocalcemia but magnesium replacement will also be required. If immediate control of seizures or tetanic contractures is needed, 1–2 ampules of 50% magnesium sulfate (8–16 mEq elemental magnesium) may be given intravenously over 15 min. Replacement of a magnesium deficit frequently requires 40 mEq/day. Magnesium therapy should be stopped if the deep tendon reflexes become diminished or if oliguria or hypotension occur. Hypocalcemia may paradoxically occur with extreme hypermagnesemia, almost exclusively due to the administration of magnesium-containing antacids to patients with renal insufficiency or during magnesium treatment of eclampsia.

Third, acute symptomatic hypocalcemia is a medical emergency. One to two ampules of 10% calcium gluconate (90–180 mg elemental calcium) should be given intravenously over 5–10 min to reverse tetany. Aggravation or initiation of arrhythmias may be avoided by this slow administration, especially when digitalis, hypomagnesemia, or hypokalemia is present. Maintenance of the serum calcium may require 10 ampules of 10% calcium gluconate intravenously over 10 hr or until oral therapy is effective. Because therapy may preempt diagnostic efforts, serum samples for calcium-regulating hormones should be obtained before calcium administration. The most effective oral regimen is calcitriol, 0.25–0.50 µg by mouth every 12 hr and calcium carbonate tablets (1 g contains 400 mg elemental calcium), supplying 1.5–3.0 g of elemental calcium/day (in 3–4 divided doses). If there is concurrent severe hyperphosphatemia as may occur with severe rhabdomyolysis, dialysis therapy may be required to improve the hypocalcemias while avoiding precipitation of calcium phosphate salts. The risk of extra-skeletal calcifications is increased with a high serum calcium-phosphorus product. Serum potassium, magnesium, inorganic phosphorus, and creatinine should be monitored during therapy. Normocalcemia is difficult to maintain in patients with hypothyroidism, therefore thyroid function tests should be obtained, especially if there has been previous neck surgery.

REFERENCES

1. Desai TK, Carlson RW, Geheb MA: Prevalence and clinical implications of hypocalcemia in acutely ill patients in a medical intensive care setting. *Am J Med* 84:209–214, 1988

2. Zaloga GP, Chernow B: Hypocalcemia in critical illness. *JAMA* 256:1924–1929, 1986
3. Juan D: Hypocalcemia: Differential diagnosis and mechanisms. *Arch Intern Med* 139:1166–1171, 1979
4. Conner TB, Rosen BL, Blaustein MP, Applefeld MM, Doyle LA: Hypocalcemia precipitating congestive heart failure. *N Engl J Med* 307:869–872, 1982
5. Yasuda K, Hurukawa Y, Okuyama M, Kikuchi M, Yoshinaga K: Glucose tolerance and insulin secretion in patients with parathyroid disorders: Effect of serum calcium on insulin release. *N Engl J Med* 292:501–504, 1975
6. Zaloga GP, Chernow B, Cook D, Snyder R, Clapper M, O'Brian JT: Assessment of calcium homeostasis in the critically ill surgical patient: The diagnostic pitfalls of the McLean-Hastings nomogram. *Ann Surg* 202:587–594, 1985
7. Zaloga GP, Willey S, Tomasic P, Chernow B: Free fatty acids alter calcium binding: A cause for misinterpretation of serum calcium values and hypocalcemia in critical illness. *J Clin Endocrinol Metab* 64:1010–1014, 1987
8. Zaloga GP, Chernow: The multifactorial basis for hypocalcemia during sepsis: Studies of the parathyroid hormone-vitamin D axis. *Ann Intern Med* 107:36–41, 1987
9. Taylor B, Sibbald WJ, Edmonds MW, Holliday RL, Williams C: Ionized hypocalcemia in critically ill patients with sepsis. *Can J Surg* 21:429–433, 1978
10. Stewart AF, Longo W, Kreutter D, Jacob R, Burtis WJ: Hypocalcemia associated with calcium-soap formation in a patient with a pancreatic fistula. *N Engl J Med* 315:496–498, 1986
11. Weinstein RS, Bryce GF, Sappington LJ, King DW, Gallagher BB: Decreased ionized calcium and normal vitamin D metabolic levels with anticonvulsant drug treatment. *J Clin Endocrinol Metab* 58:1003–1009, 1984
12. Toffaletti J, Nissenson R, Endres D, McGarry E, Mogollon G: Influence of continuous infusion of citrate on responses of immunoreactive parathyroid hormone, calcium and magnesium components and other electrolytes in normal adults during plateletpheresis. *J Clin Endocrinol Metab* 60:874–879, 1985
13. Jacobson MA, Gambertoglio JG, Aweeka FT, Causey DM, Portale AA: Foscarnet-induced hypocalcemia and effects of foscarnet on calcium metabolism. *J Clin Endocrinol Metab* 72:1130–1135, 1991

53. Neonatal Hypocalcemia

Thomas O. Carpenter, M.D.

Department of Pediatrics, Yale University School of Medicine, New Haven, Connecticut

CALCIUM METABOLISM IN THE PERINATAL PERIOD

Mineralization of the fetal skeleton is provided for by active calcium transport from mother to fetus across the placenta. The rate of regulation of calcium transport is apparently a calcium pump in the basal membrane (fetus-directed side) of the trophoblast. Evidence in the pregnant ewe suggests that a C-terminal fragment of parathyroid hormone-related peptide may play a role in the regulation of this function. At term the fetus is hypercalcemic, is likely to have elevated circulating calcitonin, and may have low levels of parathyroid hormone (PTH) compared with maternal circulation. An abrupt transition to autonomous regulation of mineral homeostasis occurs at partum. The abundant placental supply of calcium is removed and the circulating calcium level begins to fall, reaching a nadir within the first 4 days of life, and subsequently rising to normal adult levels in the second week of life.

HYPOCALCEMIC SYNDROMES IN THE NEWBORN PERIOD

Manifestations of neonatal hypocalcemia (Table 1) are variable and may not correlate with the magnitude of depression in the circulating ionized calcium level. As in older people, increased neuromuscular excitability (tetany) is a cardinal feature of newborn hypocalcemia. Generalized or focal clonic seizures, jitteriness, irritability, and frequent twitches or jerking of limbs are seen. Hyperacusis and laryngospasm may occur. Nonspecific signs

TABLE 1. *Neonatal hypocalcemia*

	Characteristics	Mechanism
Early	Onset within first 3–4 days of life; seen in infants of diabetic mothers, perinatal asphyxia and preeclampsia	Uncertain; possible exaggerated postnatal calcitonin surge, possible decrease in parathyroid response
Late	Onset days 5–10 of life; seen in winter, in infants of mothers with marginal vitamin D intake; associated with dietary phosphate load	Possible transient parathyroid dysfunction; hypomagnesemia in some cases; calcium malabsorption
Other		
Congenital hypoparathyroidism	Usually presents after first 5 days of life with overt tetany	
"Late-late" hypocalcemia	Presents in prematures at 2–4 months; associated with skeletal hypomineralization and inadequate dietary mineral or vitamin D intake	
Infants of hyperparathyroid mother	May present as late as 1 year of age; mother possibly undiagnosed	
Ionized hypocalcemia	In exchange transfusion with citrated blood products, lipid infusions, or alkalosis	

include apnea, tachycardia, tachypnea, cyanosis, and edema; vomiting has also been reported. Neonatal hypocalcemia may be classified by its time of onset; differences in etiology are suggested by "early"-occurring hypocalcemia as contrasted with that occurring "late."

Early Neonatal Hypocalcemia

Early neonatal hypocalcemia occurs during the first 3 days of life, usually between 24 and 48 hr, and characteristically is seen in premature infants, infants of diabetic mothers, and asphyxiated infants. The premature infant normally has an exaggerated postnatal depression in circulating calcium, dropping lower and earlier than in the term infant. Total calcium levels may drop below 7.0 mg/dL, but the proportional drop in ionized calcium is less, and may explain the lack of symptoms in many prematures with total calcium in this range.

Prematures have been variably reported to show normal, elevated, or impaired secretion of PTH during citrate-induced hypocalcemia. Conflict also exists regarding the action of PTH in the newborn. A several day delay in the phosphaturic effect of PTH in both term and preterm infants has been described; resultant hyperphosphatemia may decrease serum calcium. The premature infant's exaggerated rise in calcitonin may provoke hypocalcemia. A role for vitamin D and its metabolites in early neonatal hypocalcemia is less convincing.

The infant of the diabetic mother (IDM) also demonstrates an exaggerated postnatal drop in the circulating calcium level when compared with other infants of comparable maturity. As in premature infants the decrease is not entirely explained by a fall in ionized calcium concentrations. The pregnant diabetic patient tends to have lower circulating PTH and magnesium levels; the IDM has lower circulating magnesium and PTH, but normal calcitonin. Abnormalities in vitamin D metabolism do not appear to play a role in the development of hypocalcemia in the IDM. Strict maternal glycemic control during pregnancy

results in a decreased incidence of hypocalcemia in the IDM.

Early hypocalcemia occurs in asphyxiated infants; calcitonin response is augmented and PTH levels are elevated. Infants of preeclamptic mothers, and postmature infants with growth retardation develop early hypocalcemia, and are prone to hypomagnesemia.

Late Neonatal Hypocalcemia

The presentation of hypocalcemic tetany between 5 and 10 days of life is termed "late" neonatal hypocalcemia. The incidence of this disorder is greater in full term than in premature infants and is not correlated with birth trauma or asphyxia. Children affected are often being fed cow's milk or cow's milk formula, which may have 3–4 times the phosphate content of human milk. Hyperphosphatemia is associated with late neonatal hypocalcemia and may reflect: 1) inability of the immature kidney to excrete phosphate efficiently; 2) dietary phosphate load; or 3) transiently low levels of circulating PTH. Others have noted an association between late neonatal hypocalcemia and modest maternal vitamin D insufficiency. An increased occurrence of late neonatal hypocalcemia in winter has also been noted.

Hypocalcemia associated with magnesium deficiency may present as late neonatal hypocalcemia. Severe hypomagnesemia (circulating levels <0.8 mg/dL) may occur in congenital defects of intestinal magnesium absorption or renal tubular reabsorption. Transient hypomagnesemia of unknown etiology is associated with a less severe decrease in circulating magnesium (between 0.8–1.4 mg/dL). Hypocalcemia frequently complicates hypomagnesemic states due to impaired secretion of PTH. Impaired PTH responsiveness has also been demonstrated as an inconsistent finding in magnesium deficiency.

Other Causes of Neonatal Hypocalcemia

Symptomatic neonatal hypocalcemia may occur within the first 3 weeks of life in infants born to mothers with hyperparathyroidism. Presentation at 1 year of age has also been reported. Serum phosphate is often >8 mg/dL; symptoms may be exacerbated by feeding cow's milk or other high phosphate formulas. The proposed mechanism for the development of neonatal hypocalcemia in the infant of the hyperparathyroid mother is as follows: maternal hypercalcemia occurs secondary to hyperparathyroidism, resulting in increased calcium delivery to the fetus and fetal hypercalcemia, which inhibits fetal parathyroid secretion. The infant's oversuppressed parathyroid is not able to maintain normal calcium levels postpartum. Hypomagnesemia may be observed in the infant of the hyperparathyroid mother. Maternal hyperparathyroidism has been diagnosed after hypocalcemic infants have been identified.

"Late-late" neonatal hypocalcemia has been used in reference to premature infants who develop hypocalcemia with poor bone mineralization within the first 3–4 months of life. These infants tend to have an inadequate dietary supply of mineral and/or vitamin D.

The previously discussed forms of neonatal hypocalcemia are generally found to be of a transient nature. More rarely hypocalcemia, which is permanent, is detected in the newborn periods and due to congenital hypoparathyroidism. Isolated absence of the parathyroids may be inherited in X-linked or autosomal recessive fashion. Congenital hypoparathyroidism also occurs as the DiGeorge anomaly, classically the triad of hypoparathyroidism, T-cell incompetence due to a partial or absent thymus, and conotruncal heart defects (e.g., tetralogy of Fallot and truncus arteriosus) or aortic arch abnormalities. These structures are derived from the embryologic third and fourth pharyngeal pouches; the usual sporadic occurrence reflects developmental abnormalities of these structures. Other defects may variably occur in this broad spectrum field defect. Familial occurrences have been reported; associations with abnormalities of chromosomes 22 and 10 have been reported. The Kenny–Caffey syndrome is another congenital anomaly associated with hypoparathyroidism, growth retardation, and medullary stenosis of tubular bones.

Decreases in the ionized fraction of the circulating calcium occur in infants undergoing exchange transfusions with citrated blood products or receiving lipid infusions. Citrate and fatty acids form complexes with ionized calcium, reducing the free calcium compartment. Alkalosis secondary to adjustments in ventilatory assistance may provoke a shift of ionized calcium to the protein-bound compartment.

TREATMENT OF NEONATAL HYPOCALCEMIA

Early neonatal hypocalcemia may be asymptomatic, and the necessity of therapy may be questioned in such infants. Most authors recommend that early neonatal hypocalcemia be treated when the circulating concentration of total serum calcium is <5–6 mg/dL (1.25–1.50 mmol/L)

or of ionized calcium <2.5–3 mg/dL (0.62–0.72 mmol/L) in the premature infant and when total serum calcium is <6–7 mg/dL (1.50–1.75 mmol/L) in the term infant. Emergency therapy of acute tetany consists of intravenous (never intramuscular) calcium gluconate (10% solution) given slowly (<1 ml/min). A dose of 1–3 mL will usually arrest convulsions. Doses should generally not exceed 2 mg/kg body weight, and may be repeated up to four times/ 24 hr. After successful management of acute emergencies, maintenance therapy may be achieved by intravenous administration of 20–50 mg of elemental calcium/kg body weight/24 hr. Calcium gluconate is a commonly used oral supplement. Management of late neonatal tetany should include low-phosphate formula such as Similac PM 60/40, in addition to calcium supplements. A calcium:phosphate ratio of 4:1 has been recommended. Monitoring generally reveals that therapy can be discontinued after several weeks.

When hypomagnesemia is a causal feature of the hypocalcemia, magnesium administration may be indicated. Magnesium sulfate is given intravenously using cardiac monitoring or intramuscular as a 50% solution at a dose of 0.1–0.2 mL/kg. One or two doses may treat transient hypomagnesemia: a dose may be repeated after 12–24 hr. Patients with primary defects in magnesium metabolism require long-term oral magnesium supplements.

The place of vitamin D in the management of transient hypocalcemia is less clear. Daily supplementation of 400–800 U of vitamin D has been suggested for all premature infants as a preventative measure. Patients with normal intestinal absorption who develop "late-late" hypocalcemia with vitamin D deficiency rickets should respond within 4 weeks to 1,000–2,000 U of daily oral vitamin D. Such patients should receive a total of at least 40 mg of elemental calcium/kg body weight/day. In the various forms of persistent congenital hypoparathyroidism, long-term treatment with vitamin D (or its therapeutic metabolites) is used.

REFERENCES

1. Hillman LS, Haddad JG: Hypocalcemia and other abnormalities of mineral homeostasis during the neonatal period. In: Heath DA, Marx SJ (eds) *Calcium Disorders*. Clinical Endocrinology. Butterworths International Medical Reviews. Butterworths, London, pp 248–276, 1982
2. Anast CS: Disorders of mineral and bone metabolism. In: Avery ME, Taeusch HW (eds) *Schaeffer's Diseases of the Newborn*, 5th ed. W.B. Saunders, Philadelphia, pp 464–479, 1984
3. Pitkin RM: Calcium metabolism in pregnancy and the perinatal period: A review. *Am J Obstet Gynecol* 151:99–109, 1985
4. Cole DEC, Carpenter TO, Goltzman D: Calcium homeostasis and disorders of bone and mineral metabolism. In: Collu R (ed) *Pediatric Endocrinology, Comprehensive Endocrinology Series*. Raven Press, New York, pp 509–580, 1988
5. Care AD: The placental transfer of calcium. *J Development Physiol* 15:253–257, 1991
6. Root AW: Parathyroid glands, calcium, phosphorus and vitamin D metabolism. In: Hung W (ed) *Clinical Pediatric Endocrinology*. Mosby-Year Book, St. Louis, pp 89–128, 1992

54. Magnesium Deficiency and Hypermagnesemia

Robert K. Rude, M.D.

*Department of Medicine, University of Southern California,
Los Angeles, California*

MAGNESIUM DEFICIENCY

Magnesium (Mg) deficiency is very common. Ten percent of patients admitted to city hospitals are hypomagnesemic and as many as 65% of patients in an intensive care unit may be hypomagnesemic. Hypomagnesemia and/or Mg deficiency is usually due to losses of Mg from either the gastrointestinal tract or the kidney, as outlined in Table 1.

Causes of Magnesium Deficiency

The Mg content of upper intestinal tract fluids is ~1 mEq/L. Vomiting and nasogastric suction therefore may contribute to Mg depletion. The Mg content of diarrheal fluids and fistulous drainage are much higher (up to 15 mEq/L), and consequently Mg depletion is common in acute and chronic diarrhea, regional enteritis, ulcerative colitis, and intestinal and biliary fistulas. Malabsorption syndromes due to nontropical sprue, radiation injury resulting from therapy for disorders such as Whipple's disease and carcinoma of the cervix, and intestinal lymphangiectasia may also result in Mg deficiency. Steatorrhea and resection or bypass of the small bowel, particularly the ileum, often results in Mg loss.

Excessive excretion of Mg into the urine may be the basis of Mg depletion. Renal Mg reabsorption is proportional to tubular fluid flow as well as to sodium and calcium excretion. Therefore, chronic parenteral fluid therapy, particularly with saline, and volume expansion states such as primary aldosteronism, may result in Mg deficiency. Hypercalcemia and hypercalciuria have been shown to decrease renal Mg reabsorption and are probably the cause of renal Mg wasting and hypomagnesemia observed in most hypercalcemic states. Osmotic diuresis due to glucosuria will result in urinary Mg wasting. Diabetes mellitus is probably the most common clinical problem associated with hypomagnesemia. An increasing list of drugs are becoming recognized as causing renal Mg wasting and Mg depletion. Diuretics acting at the loop of Henle such as furosemide and ethacrynic acid have been shown to result in marked Mg wasting. Aminoglycosides have been shown to cause a reversible renal lesion that results in magnesuria and hypomagnesemia. Similarly, amphotericin B therapy has been reported to result in renal Mg wasting. Other renal-Mg-wasting agents include cisplatin and cyclosporin. A rising blood alcohol level has been associated with magnesuria and is one factor contributing to Mg deficiency in chronic alcoholism. Metabolic acidosis due to diabetic ketoacidosis, starvation, or alcoholism also causes renal Mg wasting.

Hypomagnesemia may accompany a number of other disorders. Phosphate depletion has been shown experimentally to result in urinary Mg wasting and hypomagnesemia. Hypomagnesemia may also accompany the "hungry bone" syndrome, a phase of rapid bone mineral accretion in subjects with hyperparathyroidism or hyperthyroidism following surgical treatment. Finally, a chronic renal tubular, glomerular, or interstitial diseases may be associated with renal Mg wasting.

Manifestations of Magnesium Deficiency

Because Mg deficiency is usually secondary to another disease process or to a therapeutic agent, the features of the primary disease process may complicate or mask Mg deficiency. A high index of suspicion is therefore warranted.

Neuromuscular hyperexcitability is often the presenting complaint. Latent tetany, as elicited by positive Chvostek's and Trousseau's signs, or spontaneous carpalpedal spasm may be present. Frank generalized seizures may also occur. Although hypocalcemia may contribute to the neurological signs, hypomagnesemia without hypocalcemia has been reported to result in neuromuscular hyperexcitability. Other signs may include vertigo, ataxia, nystagmus, and athetoid and choreiform movements as well as muscular tremor, fasciculation, wasting, and weakness.

Electrocardiographic abnormalities of Mg deficiency in man include prolonged P-R interval and Q-T interval. Mg deficiency may also result in arrhythmias. Supraventricular arrhythmias including premature atrial complexes, atrial tachycardia, atrial fibrillation, and junctional arrhythmias have been described. Ventricular premature complexes, ventricular tachycardia, and ventricular fibrillation are more serious complications.

Mg deficiency may result in hypocalcemia. Details of this complication of Mg depletion are discussed in Chapter 45. A common laboratory feature of Mg deficiency is hypokalemia. During Mg deficiency there is loss of potassium from the cell with intracellular potassium depletion as well as an inability of the kidney to conserve potassium. Attempts to replete the potassium deficit with potassium therapy alone are not successful without simultaneous Mg therapy. This biochemical feature may be a contributing cause of the electrocardiologic findings and cardiac arrhythmias discussed above.

Diagnosis of Magnesium Deficiency

Measurement of the serum Mg concentration is the most commonly used test to assess Mg status. The normal

TABLE 1. *Common causes of Mg deficiency*

Gastrointestinal Disorders	Renal Loss (continued)
Prolonged nasogastric suction	Drugs
Malabsorption syndromes	Diuretics (furosemide, ethacrynic acid)
Extensive bowel resection or bypass	Aminoglycosides
Acute and chronic diarrhea	Cisplatin
Intestinal and biliary fistulas	Cyclosporin
Renal Loss	Amphotericin B
Chronic parenteral fluid therapy	Metabolic acidosis
	Chronic renal disease
	Endocrine and Metabolic
	Diabetes mellitus
Osmotic diuresis (glucose, urea)	Phosphate depletion
	Primary hyperparathyroidism
Hypercalcemia	Hypoparathyroidism
Alcohol	Primary aldosteronism
	Hungry bone syndrome

serum Mg concentration ranges from 1.5–1.9 mEq/L (1.8–2.2 mg/dL) and a value <1.5 mEq/L usually indicates Mg deficiency. Mg is principally an intracellular cation and < 1% of the body Mg content is in the extracellular fluid compartments. Serum Mg concentration therefore may not reflect the intracellular Mg content. Mg tolerance test (or retention test) appears to be an accurate means of assessing Mg status. Correlations with skeletal muscle Mg content and Mg balance studies have been shown. A suggested protocol for the Mg tolerance test is shown in Table 2.

Therapy

Patients who present with signs and symptoms of Mg deficiency should be treated with Mg. These patients will usually be hypomagnesemic and/or have an abnormal Mg tolerance test. The extent of the total body Mg deficit is impossible to predict, but it may be as high as 200–400 mEq. Under these circumstances parenteral Mg administration is usually indicated. An effective treatment regimen is the administration of 2g $MgSO_4 \cdot 7H_2O$ (16.2 mEq Mg) as a 50% solution every 8 hr intramuscularly. These injections can be painful; a continuous intravenous infusion of 48 mEq over 24 hr may therefore be preferred and is better tolerated. Either regimen will usually result in a normal to slightly elevated serum Mg concentration. The restoration of a normal serum Mg concentration does not indicate repletion of body Mg stores, however, and therapy should be continued for approximately 3–7 days. By this time symptoms should resolve and biochemical abnormalities such as hypocalcemia and hypokalemia should correct. Patients who are hypomagnesemic and have seizures or an acute arrhythmia may be given 8–16 mEq of Mg as an intravenous injection over 5–10 min followed by 48 mEq intravenously/day. Ongoing Mg losses should be monitored during therapy. If the patient continues to lose Mg from the intestine or kidney, therapy may have to be continued for a longer duration. Once repletion has been accomplished, patients usually can maintain a normal Mg status on a regular diet. If repletion is accomplished and the patient cannot eat, a maintenance dose of 8 mEq should be given daily. Patients who have chronic Mg loss from the intestine or kidney may require continued oral Mg supplementation. A daily dose of 300 mg of elemental Mg may be given in divided doses to avoid the cathartic effect of Mg.

Caution should be taken during Mg therapy in patients with any degree of renal failure. If a decrease in glomerular filtration rate exists, the dose of Mg should be halved, and the serum Mg concentration must be monitored daily. If hypermagnesemia ensues, therapy must be stopped.

HYPERMAGNESEMIA

Mg intoxication is not a frequently encountered clinical problem, although mild to moderate elevations in the serum Mg concentration may be seen in as many as 12% of hospitalized patients.

Symptomatic hypermagnesemia is virtually always due to excessive intake or administration of Mg salts. The majority of patients with hypermagnesemia have concomitant renal failure. Hypermagnesemia is usually seen in patients with renal failure who are receiving Mg as an antacid, enema, or infusion. Hypermagnesemia is also sometimes seen in acute renal failure in the setting of rhabomyolysis.

TABLE 2. *Suggested protocol for clinical use of Mg tolerance test*

1. Collect baseline urine (spot or timed) for Mg/creatinine ratio.
2. Infuse 0.2 mEq (2.4 mg) elemental Mg/kg lean body weight in 50 mL 5% D/W over 4 hr.
3. Collect urine (starting with infusion) for Mg and creatinine for 24 hr.
4. Calculate percentage of Mg retained using following formula:

$$\% \text{ Mg retained} = 1 - \frac{\text{Postinfusion 24 hr urine Mg} - \left(\frac{\text{Preinfusion urine Mg/creatinine ratio}}{} \times \frac{\text{Postinfusion urine creatinine}}{}\right)}{\text{Total elemental Mg infused}} \times 100$$

5. Criteria for Mg deficiency

             >50% retention at 24 hr = definite deficiency
             >25% retention at 24 hr = probable deficiency

Large amounts of oral Mg have rarely been reported to cause symptomatic hypermagnesemia in patients with normal renal function. The rectal administration of Mg for purgation may result in hypermagnesemia. Mg is a standard form of therapy for pregnancy induced hypertension (preeclampsia and eclampsia) and may cause Mg intoxication in the mother as well as in the neonate. Ureteral irrigation with hemiacidrin (Renacidin) has been reported to cause symptomatic hypermagnesemia in patients with and without renal failure. Modest elevations in the serum Mg concentration may be seen in familial hypocalcemic hypercalcemia, lithium ingestion, and during volume depletion.

Signs and Symptoms

Neuromuscular symptoms are the most common presenting problem of Mg intoxication. One of the earliest demonstrable effects of hypermagnesemia is the disappearance of the deep tendon reflexes. This is reached at serum Mg concentrations of 4–7 mEq/L. Depressed respiration and apnea due to paralysis of the voluntary musculature may be seen at serum Mg concentrations in excess of 8–10 mEq/L. Somnolence may be observed at levels as low as 3 mEq/L and above.

Moderate elevations in the serum Mg concentration of 3–5 mEq/L result in a mild reduction in blood pressure. High concentrations may result in severe symptomatic hypotension. Mg can also be cardiotoxic. At serum Mg concentrations >5 mEq/L electrocardiographic findings of prolonged P-R intervals as well as increased QRS duration and QT interval are seen. Complete heart block, as well as cardiac arrest, may occur at concentrations >15 mEq/L.

Hypermagnesemia causes a fall in the serum calcium concentration. The hypocalcemia may be related to the suppressive effect of hypermagnesemia on PTH secretion or to hypermagnesemia-induced parathyroid hormone end-organ resistance. A direct effect of Mg on decreasing the serum calcium is suggested by the observation that hypermagnesemia causes hypocalcemia in hypoparathyroid subjects as well.

Other nonspecific manifestations of Mg intoxication include nausea, vomiting, and cutaneous flushing at serum levels of 3–9 mEq/L.

Therapy

The possibility of Mg intoxication should be anticipated in any patient receiving Mg, especially if the patient has a reduction in renal function. Mg therapy should merely be discontinued in patients with mild to moderate elevations in the serum Mg level. Excess Mg will be excreted by the kidney, and any symptoms or signs of Mg intoxication will resolve. Patients with severe Mg intoxication may be treated with intravenous calcium. Calcium will antagonize the toxic effects of Mg. This antagonism is immediate, but transient. The usual dose is an infusion of 100–200 mg of elemental calcium over 5–10 min. If the patient is in renal failure, peritoneal dialysis or hemodialysis against a low dialysis Mg bath will rapidly and effectively lower the serum Mg concentration.

SELECTED REFERENCES

1. Rude RK, Singer FR: Magnesium deficiency and excess. *Ann Rev Med* 32:245–259, 1981
2. Flink E: Magnesium deficiency: etiology and clinical spectrum. *Acta Med Scand* 647:125–137, 1981
3. Ryzen E, Wagers PW, Singer FR, Rude RK: Magnesium deficiency in a medical ICU population. *Crit Care Med* 12:19–21, 1985
4. Ryzen E, Elbaum N, Singer FR, Rude RK: Parenteral magnesium tolerance testing in the evaluation of magnesium deficiency. *Magnesium* 4:137–147, 1985
5. Whang R, Flink EB, Dyckner T, Wester PO, Aikawa JK, Ryan MP: Magnesium depletion as a cause of refractory potassium repletion. *Arch Intern Med* 145:1686–1689, 1985
6. Ryan MP: Diuretics and potassium/magnesium depletion: directions for treatment. *Am J Med* 82(suppl 3A):38–47, 1987
7. Patel R, Savage A: Symptomatic hypomagnesemia associated with gentamicin therapy. *Nephron* 23:50–52, 1979
8. Zaloga GP, Chernow B, Pock A, Wood B, Zaritsky A, Zucker A: Hypomagnesemia is a common complication of aminoglycoside therapy. *Surg Gynecol Obstet* 158:561–565, 1984
9. June CH, Thompson CB, Kennedy MS, Nims J, Thomas ED: Profound hypomagnesemia and renal magnesium wasting associated with the use of cyclosporine for marrow transplantation. *Transplantation* 39:620–624, 1985
10. Dyckner T, Wester PO: Magnesium deficiency contributing to ventricular tachycardia. *Acta Med Scand* 212:89–91, 1982
11. Iseri LT, Fairshter RD, Hardemann JL, Brodsky MA: Magnesium and potassium therapy in multifocal atrial tachycardia. *Am Heart J* 110:789–794, 1985
12. Rasmussen HS, McNair P, Norregard P, Backer V, Lindeneg O, Balslev S. Intravenous magnesium in acute myocardial infarction. *Lancet* 1:234–235, 1986
13. Kafka H, Langevin L, Armstrong PW: Serum magnesium and potassium in acute myocardial infarction: Influence on ventricular arrhythmias. *Arch Intern Med* 147:465–469, 1987
14. Mordes JP: Excess magnesium. *Pharmacol Rev* 29:273–300, 1978
15. Fassler CA, Rodriguez RM, Badesch DB, Stone WJ, Marini JJ: Magnesium toxicity as a cause of hypotension and hypoventilation: Occurrence in patients with normal renal function. *Arch Intern Med* 145:1604–1606, 1985
16. Cholst IN, Steinberg SF, Trooper PJ, Fox HE, Segre GV, Bilezikian JP: The influence of hypermagnesemia on serum calcium and parathyroid hormone levels in human subjects. *N Engl J Med* 310:1221–1225, 1984
17. Slatopolsky E, Mercado A, Morrison A, Yates J, Klahr S: Inhibitory effects of hypermagnesemia on the renal action of parathyroid hormone. *J Clin Invest* 58:1273–1279, 1976
18. Zwanger ML: Hypermagnesemia and perforated viscus. *Ann Emerg Med* 15:1219–1220, 1986

55. Hyperphosphatemia and Hypophosphatemia

Keith A. Hruska, M.D., and Felice Rolnick, M.D.

Renal Division, Jewish Hospital of St. Louis, St. Louis, Missouri

HYPERPHOSPHATEMIA

Serum inorganic phosphorus (Pi) concentrations are generally maintained between 2.5 and 4.5 mg/dL or 0.75 and 1.45 mM. Hyperphosphatemia most frequently results from renal insufficiency and the attendant inability to excrete Pi efficiently. Besides excretory deficiencies related to renal dysfunction, hyperphosphatemia may be the consequence of an increased intake of Pi or translocation of Pi from tissue breakdown into the extracellular fluid. Table 1 lists this and many of the other causes of hyperphosphatemia.

Etiology and Pathogenesis

During the early and middle stages of *chronic renal insufficiency*, phosphate balance is maintained by a progressive reduction in tubular Pi transport leading to increased Pi excretion by the remaining nephrons and a maintenance of normal renal Pi clearance. In advanced renal insufficiency, the fractional excretion of Pi may be as high as 60–90% of the filtered load of phosphate. However, when the number of functional nephrons becomes too diminished (glomerular filtration rate usually <20 mL/min), and dietary intake is constant, Pi balance can no longer be maintained by reductions of tubular reabsorption, and hyperphosphatemia develops. When hyperphosphatemia develops, the filtered load of Pi per nephron increases and Pi excretion rises. As a result, Pi balance and renal excretory rate are reestablished, but at a higher serum Pi level.

Defects in renal excretion of Pi in the absence of renal failure may be primary, as in *pseudohypoparathyroidism* or *tumoral calcinosis*. The latter is usually seen in young black males and is characterized by increased tubular reabsorption of calcium, Pi, and normal parathyroid hormone (PTH) levels. Secondary tubular defects include *hypoparathyroidism* and high blood levels of growth hormone. Serum phosphorus values are normally elevated in children as compared with adults. Finally, certain drugs such as ethanehydroxydiphosphonate (didronel) increase renal Pi reabsorption and lead to hyperphosphatemia.

Hyperphosphatemia can also be the consequence of an *increased intake* or administration of Pi. Intravenous administration of 1–2 g of Pi during the treatment of Pi depletion or hypercalcemia can cause hyperphosphatemia, especially in patients with underlying renal insufficiency. Hyperphosphatemia may also result from overzealous use of oral phosphates or phosphate-containing enemas. Administration of vitamin D and its metabolites in pharmacological doses may be responsible for the development of hyperphosphatemia, although suppression of PTH and

hypercalcemia-induced renal failure are important pathogenetic factors in this setting.

Transcellular shift of Pi from cells into the extracellular fluid compartment may lead to hyperphosphatemia, as seen in conditions associated with increased catabolism or tissue destruction (e.g., systemic infections, fulminant hepatitis, severe hyperthermia, crush injuries, nontraumatic *rhabdomyolysis*, and cytotoxic therapy for hematologic malignancies such as acute lymphoblastic leukemia and Burkitt's lymphoma). In this *"tumor lysis syndrome,"* serum Pi levels typically rise within 1–2 days after initiating treatment. The rising serum Pi concentration often is accompanied by hypocalcemia, hyperuricemia, hyperkalemia, and renal failure.

Patients with *diabetic ketoacidosis* commonly have hyperphosphatemia at the time of presentation despite total body Pi depletion. Insulin, fluid, and acid-base therapy is accompanied by a shift of Pi back into cells and the development of hypophosphatemia. In *lactic acidosis*, hyperphosphatemia likely results from tissue hypoxia with a breakdown of ATP to AMP and Pi. Hyperphosphatemia may be *artifactual* when hemolysis occurs during the collection, storage, or processing of blood samples.

Clinical Consequences of Hyperphosphatemia

The most important short-term consequences of hyperphosphatemia are hypocalcemia and tetany, which occur most commonly in patients with an increased Pi load from any source, exogenous or endogenous. By contrast, soft tissue calcification and secondary hyperparathyroidism are long-term consequences of hyperphosphatemia that occur mainly in patients with renal insufficiency and decreased renal Pi excretion.

Hypocalcemia and Tetany

With rapid elevations of serum Pi, hypocalcemia and tetany may occur with serum Pi concentrations as low as 6 mg/dL, a level that, if reached more slowly, has no detectable effect on serum calcium. Hyperphosphatemia, in addition to its effect on the calcium × phosphate ion product with resultant calcium deposition in soft tissues, also inhibits the activity of 1α-hydroxylase in the kidney, resulting in a lower circulating level of 1,25-dihydroxyvitamin D_3. This further aggravates hypocalcemia by impairing intestinal absorption of calcium and inducing a state of skeletal resistance to the action of PTH.

Phosphate-induced hypocalcemia is common in patients with acute or chronic renal failure, and usually develops slowly. Tetany is uncommon unless a superimposed acid-base disorder produces an abrupt rise in

213

TABLE 1. *Causes of hyperphosphatemia*

Decreased renal phosphate excretion
    Renal insufficiency/failure
        Chronic
        Acute
    Hypoparathyroidism
    Pseudohypoparathyroidism
    Acromegaly
    Diphosphonates
    Tumoral calcinosis
    Children
Increased phosphate entrance to extracellular fluid
    Administration of intravenous, oral, or rectal phosphate
        salts
    Transcellular shifts
        Catabolic states
        Infections
        Fulminant hepatitis
        Hyperthermia
        Crush injuries
        Nontraumatic rhabdomyolysis
        Cytotoxic therapy
        Hemolytic anemia
        Acute leukemia
        Metabolic acidosis
        Respiratory acidosis
        Artifacts

plasma pH that acutely lowers the serum ionized calcium concentration. Profound hypocalcemia and tetany are occasionally observed during the early phase of the "tumor lysis" syndrome and rhabdomyolysis.

Soft Tissue Calcification

Ectopic calcification is usually seen in patients with chronic renal failure. Occasionally, an acute rise in serum Pi (e.g., during Pi treatment for hypercalcemia) may lead to ectopic calcification, especially when the calcium phosphate product exceeds 70. The blood vessels, skin, cornea ("band-keratopathy"), and periarticular tissues are common sites of calcium precipitation.

Secondary Hyperparathyroidism and Renal Osteodystrophy

Hyperphosphatemia due to renal failure also plays a critical role in development of secondary hyperparathyroidism and renal osteodystrophy (see Chapter 80). In patients with advanced renal failure, the enhanced phosphate load from PTH-mediated osteolysis may ultimately become the dominant influence on serum phosphorus levels. This phenomenon may account for the correlation between serum phosphorus levels and the severity of osteitis fibrosa cystica in patients maintained on chronic hemodialysis.

Treatment

Correction of the pathogenetic defect should be the primary aim in the treatment of hyperphosphatemia. In most instances, however, the most effective way to treat hyperphosphatemia is to reduce dietary Pi intake. Bcause Pi is present in almost all foodstuffs, rigid *dietary phosphate restriction* requires a barely palatable diet that few patients can accept. However, dietary Pi can be reduced 600–1000, mg/day with modest protein restriction. A predialysis level of 4.5–5.0 mg/dL is reasonable and allows some room for removal of phosphorus with dialysis, while avoiding severe postdialysis hypophosphatemia. To achieve this, most patients require the addition of *phosphate binders* to reduce intestinal absorption of dietary Pi.

Aluminum hydroxide or aluminum carbonate (30–60 mL of gel or 1–4 tablets, with each meal), when administered to patients with renal failure over the long term, have been shown to result in aluminum toxicity with encephalopathy, osteomalacia, proximal myopathy, and anemia. Therefore, calcium salts have replaced aluminum salts as first line Pi binders. Calcium acetate and aluminum carbonate are equally potent and bind more Pi than equivalent amounts of calcium carbonate or citrate. In general treatment is started with 1 g of calcium carbonate with each meal and gradually increased up to 8–12 g daily. This regimen effectively controls serum Pi in about two-thirds of patients on chronic dialysis. Calcium salts tend to increase serum calcium levels, and if hypercalcemia (>11 mg/dL) develops, calcium carbonate should not be increased further. If hyperphosphatemia persists, the patient should also receive aluminum gels. However, aluminum gels and calcium citrate must not be taken concomitantly because citrate markedly increases the absorption of aluminum. Maximal Pi binding occurs when phosphate binder is taken with a meal rather than 2 hr afterward.

The treatment of chronic hyperphosphatemia secondary to hypoparathyroidism occasionally requires that phosphate binders be added to the other therapeutic agents.

HYPOPHOSPHATEMIA

Hypophosphatemia is defined as an abnormally low concentration of inorganic phosphate in serum or plasma. Hypophosphatemia does not necessarily indicate total body Pi depletion, because only 1% of the total body Pi is found in extracellular fluids. Conversely, serious Pi depletion may exist in the presence of a normal or even elevated serum Pi concentration. Moderate hypophosphatemia, defined as a serum Pi concentration between 2.5 and 1 mg/dL, is not uncommon and is usually not associated with signs or symptoms. Severe hypophosphatemia, defined as serum phosphorus levels below 1.0 mg/dL, is often associated with clinical signs and symptoms that require therapy. Approximately 2% of hospital patients have levels of serum Pi below 2 mg/dL according to some estimates. Hypophosphatemia is encountered more frequently among alcoholic patients, and up to 10% of patients admitted to hospitals because of chronic alcoholism are hypophosphatemic.

TABLE 2. *Causes of moderate hypophosphatemia*

Increased urinary losses
  Hyperparathyroidism
  Malabsorption
  Renal tubular defects
  Renal transplantation
  Abnormalities of vitamin D metabolism
    Vitamin D deficiency
    X-linked hypophosphatemic rickets
    Vitamin D-dependent rickets
  Oncogenic osteomalacia
  Alcohol abuse
  Poorly controlled diabetes mellitus
  Metabolic or respiratory acidosis
  Drugs: calcitonin, diuretics, glucocorticoids, and bicarbonate
  Respiratory alkalosis
  Extracellular fluid volume expansion
Decreased intestinal absorption
  Antacid abuse
  Vitamin D deficiency
  Malabsorption
  Starvation and alcohol abuse
Shifts into cells
  Nutritional repletion
  Respiratory alkalosis
  Recovery from hypothermia
  Recovery from acidosis
  Acute gout
  Gram-negative bacteremia
  Salicylate poisoning
  Glucose
  Fructose
  Glycerol
  Insulin
  Blast crisis in leukemia

Pathogenesis of Hypophosphatemia

Three types of pathophysiologic abnormalities can cause hypophosphatemia and total body Pi depletion: decreased intestinal absorption of Pi, increased urinary losses of this ion, and a shift of Pi from extracellular to intracellular compartments. Combinations of these disturbances are common. The causes and mechanisms of moderate hypophosphatemia are shown in Table 2; the clinical conditions associated with severe hypophosphatemia are shown in Table 3.

TABLE 3. *Causes of severe hypophosphatemia*

Alcohol withdrawal
Nutritional repletion: oral, enteral, and parenteral nutrition
Diabetes/diabetic ketoacidosis
Respiratory alkalosis
Thermal burns
Leukemia
Increased urinary losses
Impaired gastrointestinal absorption

Primary Hyperparathyroidism

This is a common entity in clinical medicine. Parathyroid hormone is secreted in excess of the physiologic needs for mineral homeostasis owing either to adenoma or hyperplasia of the parathyroid glands (see Chapter 29). This results in decreased phosphorus reabsorption by the kidney, and the urinary losses of phosphorus result in hypophosphatemia. The degree of hypophosphatemia varies considerably because mobilization of phosphorus from stimulation of skeletal remodeling, in part, mitigates the hypophosphatemia.

Secondary hyperparathyroidism associated with normal renal function has been observed in patients with gastrointestinal abnormalities resulting in calcium malabsorption will have low levels of serum calcium and phosphorus. In these patients, the hypocalcemia is responsible for increased release of PTH. Decreased intestinal absorption of phosphorus as a result of the primary gastrointestinal disease may contribute to the decrement in the levels of the serum phosphorus. In general, these patients have urinary losses of phosphorus that are out of portion to the hypophosphatemia in contrast to patients with predominant phosphorus malabsorption and no secondary hyperparathyroidism in whom urinary excretion of phosphorus is low.

Renal Tubular Defects

Several conditions characterized by either single or multiple tubular ion transport defects have been characterized in which phosphorus reabsorption is decreased. In the Fanconi syndrome, patients excrete not only increased amount of phosphorus in the urine, but also increased quantities of amino acids, uric acid, and glucose, resulting in hypouricemia and hypophosphatemia. There are other conditions in which an isolated defect in the renal tubular transport of phosphorus has been found, for example, in fructose intolerance, an autosomal recessive disorder. Following renal transplantation, an acquired renal tubular defect may be responsible for the persistence of hypophosphatemia in some patients.

Abnormalities of Vitamin D Metabolism

Vitamin D and its metabolites play an important role in phosphorus homeostasis. Vitamin D promotes intestinal absorption of calcium and phosphorus, and it is necessary to maintain the normal mineralization and remodeling processes of bone. Additionally, vitamin D metabolites have important actions in the control of renal tubular ion transport.

Vitamin D-deficient rickets (when the deficiency occurs in children) or osteomalacia (when the deficiency occurs in adults) may result in severe deformities of the skeleton (see Chapter 67). Hypophosphatemia is the most frequent biochemical alteration associated with this metabolic abnormality.

X-Linked Hypophosphatemic Rickets

This X-linked dominant disorder is characterized by hypophosphatemia, decreased reabsorption of phosphorus by the renal tubule, decreased absorption of calcium and phosphorus from the gastrointestinal tract, and varying degrees of rickets or osteomalacia (see Chapter 69). Patients with this disorder and the murine homologue (Hyp) exhibit normal levels of 1,25-dihydroxycholecalciferol in the face of severe hypophosphatemia. Thus, a defect in the 25-hydroxycholecalciferol 1α-hydroxylase has been documented. 1,25-Dihydroxyvitamin D_3 therapy increases plasma phosphorus by pharmacologic stimulation of phosphorus absorption from the gastrointestinal tract. The defect in renal phosphorus reabsorption is unchanged despite treatment with 1,25-dihydroxyvitamin D_3. Therapeutically, the combination of neutral phosphate supplementation and 1,25-dihydroxycholecalciferol has lead to an improvement in the bone disease of patients and an increase in their plasma phosphorus. However, episodes of hypercalcemia and secondary extraskeletal calcification have limited aggressive therapy.

Vitamin D-Dependent Rickets

This is a recessively inherited form of vitamin D-refractory rickets associated with hypophosphatemia, hypocalcemia, elevated levels of serum alkaline phosphatase, and, sometimes, generalized amino aciduria and severe bone lesions. There are two main forms of the syndrome. Type I is an inborn error in conversion of 25-hydroxyvitamin D to 1,25-dihydroxyvitamin D due to deficiency of the renal 1-hydroxylase enzyme. This condition responds to very large doses of vitamin D_2 and D_3, but to normal doses of 1,25-dihydroxyvitamin D_3. Type II is characterized by an end-organ resistance to 1,25-dihydroxyvitamin D_3 due to an abnormal vitamin D receptor. Plasma levels of 1,25-dihydroxyvitamin D_3 are elevated. Large pharmacologic doses of 1,25-dihydroxyvitamin D_3 are required for treatment of this syndrome.

Osteogenic Osteomalacia

This entity is characterized by hypophosphatemia in association with malignant tumors. The patients exhibit osteomalacia on histomorphologic examination of bone biopsies, renal wasting of phosphorus, and markedly reduced levels of 1,25-dihydroxyvitamin D_3. The abnormalities of vitamin D metabolism have not been carefully elucidated (see Chapter 69).

Alcohol and Alcohol Withdrawal

Alcohol abuse is the most common cause of severe hypophosphatemia (Table 3). Among the factors responsible for Pi depletion in the alcoholic are poor intake, the use of antacids, and vomiting. Ethanol enhances urinary Pi excretion, and marked phosphaturia tends to occur during

episodes of alcoholic ketoacidosis. Because such patients often eat poorly, ketonuria is common. Repeated episodes of ketoacidosis catabolize organic phosphates within cells and cause phosphaturia by mechanisms analogous to those seen in diabetic ketoacidosis. Chronic alcoholism may also cause magnesium deficiency and hypomagnesemia that may, in turn, cause phosphaturia and Pi depletion, especially in skeletal muscle (see Chapter 54).

Nutritional Repletion: Oral, Enteral, and Parenteral Nutrition

Nutritional repletion of the malnourished patient implies the provision of sufficient calories, protein, and other nutrients to allow accelerated tissue accretion. In the course of this process, cellular uptake and utilization of Pi increase. When insufficient amounts of Pi are provided, an acute state of severe hypophosphatemia and intracellular Pi depletion with serious clinical and metabolic consequences can occur. This type of hypophosphatemia has been observed in malnourished patients receiving parental nutrition and following refeeding of prisoners of war.

Diabetes Mellitus

Patients with well-controlled diabetes mellitus do not have excessive losses of phosphate. However, in the presence of hyperglycemia, polyuria and acidosis, Pi is lost through the urine in excessive amounts. In ketoacidosis, intracellular organic components tend to be broken down, releasing large amounts of Pi into the plasma that is subsequently lost in the urine. This process, combined with the enhanced osmotic Pi diuresis secondary to glycosuria, ketonuria, and polyuria, may cause large urinary loses of Pi and subsequent depletion. The plasma Pi is usually normal or slightly elevated in the ketotic patient, in spite of the excessive urinary losses, because of the continuous large shift of Pi from the cells into the plasma. With insulin, fluids, and correction of the ketoacidosis, however, serum and urine Pi may fall sharply. Despite the appearance of hypophosphatemia during treatment, previously well-controlled patients with diabetic ketoacidosis of only a few days duration almost never have serious phosphorus deficiency. Serum Pi rarely falls below 1.0 mg/dL in these patients. Administration of Pi-containing salts does not improve glucose utilization, reduce insulin requirements, or the time for recovery from ketoacidosis. Thus, Pi therapy should be reserved for patients with serum Pi concentration <1.0 mg/dL.

Respiratory Alkalosis

Intense hyperventilation for prolonged periods may depress serum Pi to values below 1.0 mg/dL. This is important in patients with alcoholic withdrawal because of attendant hyperventilation. A similar degree of alkalemia induced by infusion of bicarbonate depresses Pi concentration only mildly. The combined hypophosphatemic effects of respiratory and metabolic alkalosis may be pronounced.

Severe hypophosphatemia is common in patients with extensive burns. It usually appears within several days after the injury. Phosphorus is virtually undetectable in the urine. Hypophosphatemia may result from transductive losses, respiratory alkalosis, or other factors.

Increased Urinary Losses

Abnormalities in tubular handling of phosphate have been implicated in the genesis of severe hypophosphatemia induced by hypokalemia, hypomagnesemia, systemic acidosis, hypothyroidism, X-linked hypophosphatemic rickets (see Chapter 68), hyperparathyroidism (see Chapter 29), and humoral hypercalcemia of malignancy (see Chapter 33). During the recovery phase from severe burns, hypophosphatemia may occur secondary to massive diuresis with phosphaturia. Renal transplantation may be followed by severe phosphaturia and hypophosphatemia due to tubular defects.

Impaired Gastrointestinal Absorption

Severe hypophosphatemia and phosphate depletion may result from vigorous use of oral antacids, which bind phosphate, usually for peptic ulcer disease. Patients so treated may develop osteomalacia and severe skeletal symptoms due to phosphorus deficiency.

Intestinal malabsorption can cause hypophosphatemia and phosphate depletion through malabsorption of Pi, vitamin D, and through increased urinary Pi losses resulting from secondary hyperparathyroidism induced by calcium malabsorption.

Leukemia

Advanced leukemia that is markedly proliferative ("blast crisis"), with total leukocyte counts above 100,000, has been associated with severe hypophosphatemia. This would appear to result from excessive phosphorus uptake into rapidly multiplying cells.

Clinical Effects of Severe Hypophosphatemia

Severe hypophosphatemia with phosphorus deficiency may cause widespread disturbances. There are at least eight well-established effects of severe hypophosphatemia (Table 4). The signs and symptoms of severe

TABLE 4. Consequences of severe hypophosphatemia

Red cell dysfunction	Rhabdomyolysis
Leukocyte dysfunction	Osteomalacia/rickets
Platelet dysfunction	Metabolic acidosis
CNS dysfunction	Cardiomyopathy

hypophosphatemia may be related to a decrease in 2,3-diphosphoglycerate in the red cell. This change is associated with increased affinity of hemoglobin for oxygen and therefore tissue hypoxia. There is also a decrease in tissue content of ATP and consequently, a decrease in the availability of energy-rich phosphate compounds for cell function.

Central Nervous System

Some patients with severe hypophosphatemia display symptoms compatible with metabolic encephalopathy. They may display in sequence, irritability, apprehension, weakness, numbness, paraesthesias, dysarthria, confusion, obtundation, seizures, and coma. In contrast to delirium tremens, the syndrome does not include hallucinations. Patients with very severe hypophosphatemia may show diffuse slowing of the EEG.

Hematopoietic System

A decrease in the red cell content of 2,3-diphosphoglycerate and ATP leads to increased rigidity and in rare instances, hemolysis. Hemolysis is usually provoked by a unusual stress on the metabolic requirements of the red cell, such as severe metabolic acidosis or infection. When hemolysis has occurred, ATP content has invariably been <15% of normal.

Leukocyte/macrophage dysfunction can be demonstrated in vitro using Pi-depleted cells. Suggestion that a predisposition to infection commonly seen in patients on intravenous hyperalimentation may be partly related to hypophosphatemia remains to be proven. Hypophosphatemia impairs granulocyte function by interfering with ATP synthesis.

In experimental hypophosphatemia there is an increase in platelet diameter, suggesting shortened platelet survival and also a marked acceleration of platelet disappearance from the blood. These lead to thrombocytopenia and a reactive megakaryocytosis. In addition there is an impairment of clot retraction and a hemorrhagic tendency, especially involving gut and skin.

Musculoskeletal System

Myopathy and Rhabdomyolysis

Muscle tissue requires large amounts of high energy bonds (ATP and creatine phosphate) and oxygen for contraction, for maintenance of membrane potential, and for other functions. Pi deprivation induces muscle cell injury characterized by a decrease in intracellular Pi and an increase in water, sodium, and chloride. An apparent relationship between hypophosphatemia and alcoholic myopathy has been observed in chronic alcoholism. The muscular clinical manifestations of Pi deficiency syndrome include myalgia, objective weakness, and myopathy, with pathologic findings of intracellular edema and a subnormal resting muscle membrane potential on electromyography. In patients with preexisting Pi deficiency who develop acute hypophosphatemia, rhabdomyolysis may occur. Hypophosphatemia and phosphate deficiency may be associated with creatine phosphokinase elevations in blood.

Bone

Skeletal defects have been reported in association with Pi depletion of different causes. These are discussed in detail in Chapters 65–69, 71, and 73. Suffice it to say here that phosphate depletion is associated with rickets in children and ostemalacia in adults.

Cardiovascular System

Severe hypophosphatemia has been associated with a cardiomyopathy characterized by a low cardiac output, a decreased ventricular ejection velocity, and an elevated left ventricular end-diastolic pressure. A decrease in myocardial content of inorganic phosphorus, ATP, and creatinine phosphate seems to underlie the impairment in myocardial contractibility.

During phosphorus depletion, blood pressure may be low and the pressor response to naturally occurring vasoconstrictor agonists such as norepinephrine or angiotensin II is reduced.

Renal Effects of Hypophosphatemia and Phosphate Depletion

Severe hypophosphatemia and phosphate depletion affect the balance and serum concentrations of various electrolytes. It may produce changes in cardiovascular function as described above; renal hemodynamics affect renal tubular transport processes and induce marked changes in renal cell metabolism. These disturbances are listed in Table 5.

TABLE 5. *Consequences of hypophosphatemia and phosphate depletion on renal function*

Glomerular filtration rate reduction
Metabolic abnormalities
   Reduced cellular inorganic phosphorus, ATP, and phospholipid precursors
   Reduced gluconeogenesis
   Insulin resistance
   Hypoparathyroidism and reduced urinary cAMP
   Increased 1,25-dihydroxyvitamin D_3
Transport abnormalities
   Hypercalciuria
   Reduced proximal tubular Na^+ transport
   Hypermagnesiuria
   Pi retention
   Bicarbonaturia
   Metabolic acidosis
   Reduced glucose transport

Tubular Transport

Calcium

A marked increase in urinary calcium excretion occurs during phosphate depletion proportional to the severity of phosphate depletion and the degree of hypophosphatemia.

Phosphate

Dietary Pi restriction and Pi depletion is associated with enhanced renal tubular reabsorption of Pi. Urinary excretion of Pi declines within hours after the reduction in its dietary intake, and Pi virtually disappears from the urine within 1–2 days. The changes in renal tubular reabsorption of Pi occur before detectable falls in the serum Pi. The adaptation to a reduction in Pi supply is a direct response of the proximal tubule. In addition, the ability of the kidney to conserve Pi produces a resistance to phosphaturic stimuli. Thus, the phosphaturic response to PTH is severely blunted during states of Pi depletion. However, it is also clear that the mechanism of Pi transport stimulated by Pi depletion does not share the regulatory pathways affected by PTH. The adaptation to reduced Pi supply is a separate system for the regulation of renal tubular Pi reabsorption.

Metabolic Acidosis

Severe hypophosphatemia with Pi deficiency may result in metabolic acidosis through three mechanisms. First, severe hypophosphatemia is generally associated with a proportionate reduction of Pi excretion in the urine, thereby limiting hydrogen excretion as a titratable acid. Second, if Pi buffer is inadequate, acid secretion depends on production of ammonia and its conversion to ammonium ion. Ammonia production is severely depressed in Pi deficiency. The third mechanism is that of decreased renal tubular reabsorption of bicarbonate.

Treatment

The appropriate management of hypophosphatemia and Pi depletion requires identification of the underlying causes, treatment with supplemental Pi when necessary, and prevention of recurrence of the problem by correcting the underlying causes. The symptoms and signs of Pi depletion can vary, are nonspecific, and are usually seen in patients with multiple problems such as those encountered in intensive care unit settings. This makes it difficult to identify Pi depletion as the cause of clinical manifestations, and Pi depletion is frequently overlooked.

Mild hypophosphatemia secondary to redistribution, with plasma Pi levels higher than 2 mg/dL, is transient and requires no treatment. In cases of moderate hypophosphatemia, associated with Pi depletion (serum Pi higher than 1.0 mg/dL in adults or 2.0 mg/dL in children), Pi supplementation should be administered in addition to treating the cause of hypophosphatemia. Milk is an excellent source of phosphorus, containing 1 g (33 mM) of inorganic phosphorus per liter. Skimmed milk may be better tolerated than whole milk, especially in children and malnourished patients because of concomitant lactose or fat intolerance. Alternatively Neutraphos® tablets (which contain 250 mg of Pi/tablet as a sodium or potassium salt) may be given. Oral Pi can be given in a dose up to 3 g/day (i.e., 3 tablets of Neutraphos every 6 hr). The serum Pi level rises by as much as 1.5 mg/dL, 60–120 min after ingestion of 1,000 mg of Pi. A phosphosoda enema solution, composed of buffered sodium phosphate, may also be used in a dose of 15–30 mL three or four times daily.

Severe hypophosphatemia with serum levels lower than 0.5 mg/dL occurs only when there is cumulative net loss of more than 3.3 g of Pi. If asymptomatic, oral replacement with a total of 6–10 g of Pi (1–3 g of Pi/day) over a period of a few days is usually sufficient. Presence of symptomatic hypophosphatemia indicates that net Pi deficit exceeds 10 g. In these cases 20 g of Pi is given spread over a period of 1 week (up to 3 g/day). Patients with Pi deficiency tolerate substantially larger doses of oral Pi without side effects, such as diarrhea, than do normal subjects. However, patients with severe symptomatic hypophosphatemia who are unable to eat may be safely treated intravenously with 1 g of Pi delivered in 1 L of fluid over 8–12 hr. This is usually sufficient to raise serum Pi level to 1.0 mg/dL. It is unusual for hypophosphatemia to cause metabolic disturbances at serum Pi >1.0 mg/dL, so full parenteral replacement is neither necessary or desirable.

Treatment with phosphate can result in diarrhea, hyperphosphatemia, hypocalcemia, and hyperkalemia. These side effects can be prevented by careful attention to phosphorus dosages.

Prevention

The most effective approach to hypophosphatemia is prevention of predisposing conditions. Patients on total parenteral nutrition should receive a daily maintenance dose of Pi amounting to 1,000 mg in 24 hr, with increases as required by the clinical and metabolic states. Alcoholic patients and malnourished individuals receiving intravenous fluids, particularly those containing glucose, should receive Pi supplementation, particularly if hypophosphatemia is observed.

ACKNOWLEDGMENTS

This work was supported by the National Institutes of Health Grants AR32087, AR39561, and DK09976, and by a grant from the Shriner's Hospital for Crippled Children.

SELECTED REFERENCES

1. Slatopolsky E, Rutherford WE, Rosenbaum R, Martin K, Hruska K: Hyperphosphatemia. *Clin Nephrol* 7:138, 1977
2. Slatopolsky, E. Weerts C, Lopez-Hilker S, Norwood K, Zink M, Windus D, Delmez J: Calcium carbonate as a phosphate binder in patients with chronic renal failure undergoing dialysis. *N Engl J Med* 315:157, 1986
3. Hercz G, Coburn JW: Prevention of phosphate retention and hyperphosphatemia in uremia. *Kidney Int* 22(suppl):S215, 1987
4. Sheikh MS, Maguire JA, Emmett M, et al.: Reduction of dietary phosphorus absorption by phosphorus binders. *J Clin Invest* 83:66, 1989
5. Fuller TJ, Nichols WW, Brenner BJ, et al.: Reversible depression in myocardial performance in dogs with experimental phosphorus deficiency. *J Clin Invest* 62:1194, 1978
6. Schnitker MA, Mattman P, Bliss TL: A clinical study of malnutrition in Japanese prisoners of war. *Ann Intern Med* 35:69, 1951
7. Silvis SE, Paragos PD Jr: Paresthesias, weakness, seizures and hypophosphatemia in patients receiving hyperalimentation. *Gastroenterology* 62:513, 1972
8. Berner YN, Shike M: Consequences of phosphate imbalance (a review). *Ann Rev Nutr* 8:121, 1988
9. Martin HE, Smith K, Wilson WL: The fluid and electrolyte therapy of severe diabetic acidosis and ketosis: A study of twenty-nine episodes (twenty-six patients). *Am J Med* 24:376, 1958
10. Knochel JP: The clinical status of hypophosphatemia. *N Engl J Med* 313:447, 1985
11. Knochel JP: Hypophosphatemia. In: Massry SG, Glassock RI (eds) *Textbook of Nephrology, 2nd ed.* Williams & Wilkins, Baltimore, MD, pp 347–352, 1989
12. Janson AU, Birnbaum G, Baker FJ: Hypophosphatemia. *Ann Emerg Med* 12:107–116, 1983
13. Slatopolsky E, Hruska K, Klahr S: Disorders of phosphorus, calcium, and magnesium metabolism. In: Schrier RW, Gottschalk CW (eds) *Diseases of the Kidney, vol III, 5th ed.* Little, Brown and Co., Boston, pp 2599–2644, 1993

SECTION V

Metabolic Bone Diseases

56. Evaluation and Treatment of Postmenopausal Osteoporosis

*Michael Kleerekoper, M.D., and †Louis V. Avioli, M.D.

*Bone and Mineral Division, Henry Ford Hospital, Detroit, Michigan, and
†Division of Bone and Mineral Diseases, Washington University School of
Medicine, St. Louis, Missouri

Osteoporosis is a disease characterized by a low bone mass and the development of nontraumatic or atraumatic fractures as a direct result of the low bone mass. A nontraumatic fracture has been arbitrarily defined as one occurring from trauma equal to or less than a fall from a standing height. In the preclinical state, the disease is characterized simply by a low bone mass without fractures. This totally asymptomatic state is often termed osteopenia. Osteoporosis and osteopenia are the most common metabolic bone diseases in the developed countries of the world, whereas osteomalacia may be more prevalent in underdeveloped countries where nutrition is suboptimal. Osteoporotic fractures may affect any part of the skeleton except the skull. Most commonly fractures occur in the distal forearm (Colles' fracture), thoracic and lumbar vertebrae, and proximal femur (hip fracture). The incidence of osteoporotic fractures increases with age, is higher in whites than in blacks, and higher in women than in men. The female to male ratio is ~1.5:1 for the Colles' fracture, 7:1 for the vertebral fracture, and 2:1 for the hip fracture. Because most osteoporotic fractures do not require admission to the hospital, it is difficult to obtain precise figures on the true prevalence of this disease. Almost without exception, a hip fracture requires admission to a hospital, and current estimates indicate that there are ~275,000 new osteoporotic hip fractures each year in the United States. It has been estimated that after menopause a woman's lifetime risk of sustaining an osteoporotic fracture is one in three. Regrettably, despite improvements in surgical techniques and anesthesiology, most hip fractures require surgical intervention on a nonelective basis, and there is a 15–20% excess mortality following an osteoporotic hip fracture. Perhaps more importantly, following such fractures less than one-third of the patients are restored to their prefracture functional state within 12 months of the fracture. Most patients require some form of ambulatory support and many require institutional care. Current estimates indicate that each new case of osteoporotic hip fracture cost ~$40,000 and that the annual expenditure on short-term care following an osteoporotic hip fracture already exceeds $8 billion.

PATHOGENESIS

Once peak adult bone mass has been attained in the third, possibly fourth, decade of life, bone mass at any point in time is the difference between peak adult bone mass and the loss of bone mass that has occurred since this was attained. Because age-related bone loss is a universal phenomenon in humans, any circumstance that limits an individual's ability to maximize peak adult bone mass increases the likelihood of developing osteoporosis later in life. Strategies for maximizing peak adult bone mass have been described in the preceding chapter (Chapter 58).

The excessive bone loss that characterizes the pathogenesis of osteoporosis results from abnormalities in the bone remodeling cycle. This cycle has been discussed in detail in Chapter 6. In brief, bone remodeling is a mechanism for keeping the skeleton "young" by a process of removal of old bone and replacement with new bone. The cycle is initiated by resorption of old bone, recruitment of osteoblasts, deposition of new matrix, and mineralization of that newly deposited matrix. It appears that with each cycle there is a slight, imperceptible deficit in bone formation. The total bone loss is, therefore, a function of the number of cycles in process at any one time. Conditions that increase the rate of activation of the bone remodeling process, increase the proportion of the skeleton undergoing remodeling at any one time, and increase the rate of bone loss. In this circumstance, which is called high-turnover osteoporosis, the deficit per unit of remodeling is apparently constant. Most of the secondary causes of osteoporosis (Table 1) are associated with this increased rate of activation of the remodeling cycle. In the normal aging process, there appears to be a progressive impairment of the signaling between bone resorption and bone formation, such that with every cycle of remodeling, there is an increase in the deficit between resorption and formation because osteoblast recruitment is inefficient. Thus, excessive bone loss can occur even when activation of the skeleton is not increased and, in fact, when activation of the skeleton might be decreased. This gives rise to the concept of low turnover osteoporosis.

CLASSIFICATION OF OSTEOPOROSIS

In addition to describing osteoporosis as being of the high- or low-turnover type, there are several other classification systems for osteoporosis. The first is the classification into primary and secondary, the latter being osteoporosis where a clearly identifiable etiologic mechanism is recognized. Primary osteoporosis is further characterized into postmenopausal and senile. Postmenopausal osteoporosis has been further classified into type I and type II on the basis of the fracture patterns that evolve. Type I osteoporosis has been designated as the osteoporosis predominantly relating to early postmenopausal bone

TABLE 1. *Factors commonly associated with osteopenic and/or osteoporotic syndrome(s)*

Genetic
  White or Asiatic ethnicity
  Positive family history
  Small body frame (<127 lbs)
Lifestyle
  Smoking
  Inactivity
  Nulliparity
  Excessive exercise (producing amenorrhea)
  Early natural menopause
  Late menarche
Nutritional factors
  Milk intolerance
  Lifelong low dietary calcium intake
  Vegetarian dieting
  Excessive alcohol intake
  Consistently high protein intake
Medical disorders
  Anorexia nervosa
  Thyrotoxicosis
  Parathyroid overactivity
  Cushing's syndrome
  Type I diabetes
  Alterations in gastrointestinal and hepatobiliary function
  Occult osteogenesis imperfecta
  Mastocytosis
  Rheumatoid arthritis
  "Transient" osteoporosis
  Prolonged parenteral nutrition
  Prolactinoma
  Hemolytic anemia
Drugs
  Thyroid replacement therapy
  Glucocorticoid drugs
  Anticoagulants
  Chronic lithium therapy
  Chemotherapy (breast cancer or lymphoma)
  Gonadotropin-releasing hormone agonist or antagonist therapy
  Anticonvulsants
  Chronic phosphate binding antacid use
  Extended tetracycline use[a]
  Diuretics producing calciuria[a]
  Phenothiazine derivatives[a]
  Cyclosporin A[a]

[a] Not yet associated with decreased bone mass in humans, although identified as either toxic to bone in animals or as inducing calciuria and/or calcium malabsorption in humans.

loss, where there is an apparent excess loss of cancellous bone with relative sparing of cortical bone, and the clinical syndromes involve Colles' fracture and vertebral fracture. In type II osteoporosis, there is a more concordant loss of both cortical and cancellous bone. The presumed pathogenesis of type II osteoporosis is uncertain, but it is postulated to result from age-related decline in renal production of 1,25-dihydroxyvitamin D with subsequent secondary hyperparathyroidism. It is the hyperparathyroidism that is largely responsible for the excess cortical bone loss. The fracture syndrome associated with type II osteoporosis is the hip fracture.

CLINICAL MANIFESTATIONS OF OSTEOPOROSIS

As has been mentioned previously, osteoporosis without fracture is entirely without symptoms. This does not lessen its importance, because the aim of all therapies should be to prevent even the first fracture, let alone subsequent fractures. When osteoporosis is complicated by the development of an osteoporotic fracture, the symptoms and signs are those related to the fracture itself. Osteoporotic vertebral fractures may represent a unique situation and this will be discussed separately. Primary orthopedic management of peripheral fractures should not be influenced by the fact that the fracture results from osteoporosis. Management consists of immobilization and analgesia. There does not appear to be anything about an osteoporotic fracture that results in delayed fracture union. If delayed fracture union or fracture nonunion complicates an osteoporotic fracture, one needs to look for conditions other than osteoporosis, such as osteomalacia or hyperparathyroidism, that resulted in the bone loss leading to the fracture. Immobilization should be for only a limited period of time sufficient to ensure the primary fracture healing. Longer immobilization would lead to accelerated bone loss and must be avoided. The brittleness of the osteoporotic skeleton may complicate open surgical repair of osteoporotic fractures with limited purchase for pins, plates, screws, nails, etc. Restoration of the prefracture anatomic and functional state is the goal in management of osteoporotic fractures of the appendicular skeleton. Regrettably, with respect to osteoporotic hip fractures, this is not often the outcome that is attained with the excess morbidity and mortality already discussed. In general, this is because surgical repair of an osteoporotic hip fracture is usually a nonelective procedure. Circumstances that appear to increase mortality following a hip fracture are generally related to the overall medical health and nutritional status of the subject sustaining the fracture. Frail, elderly subjects on large numbers of medications with mental impairment have the greatest mortality, and this is particularly so in males compared with females. Of those patients who survive the early operative intervention for an osteoporotic hip fracture, less than one-third are restored to their prefracture functional state, and either require institutionalized care or some form of ambulatory support.

Osteoporotic vertebral fractures are quite different from other osteoporotic fractures. Surveys of spine radiographs in older subjects suggest that many vertebral fractures have occurred in the absence of acute symptoms. If acute symptoms do occur at the time of fracture, these will be manifest by intense pain and limitation of motion. Operative intervention is infrequently required for control of these fractures. However, the principles of immobilization for a short period of time should still hold. The concept of placing the patient with an osteoporotic fracture in a back brace for years is to be decried. Similarly, the acute skeletal pain following an osteoporotic vertebral fracture should dissipate within 4–6 weeks. If skeletal tenderness persists much beyond this, other causes for the fracture (e.g., metastatic disease and multiple myeloma) should be considered. Osteoporotic fractures of the vertebral bodies rarely result in long tract symptoms or signs. Again, if a fracture is complicated by long tract symptoms or signs, causes other than osteoporosis should be considered.

Once a vertebral body has been fractured restoration of normal anatomy is not possible. In fact, refracture of the same vertebrae with further abnormalities of shape and size is often the outcome. Thus, even those vertebral fractures that are not associated with any acute symptoms at the time of fracture give rise to chronic pain, disability, and often obvious deformity. All vertebral fractures are associated with loss of stature: in the thoracic spine this is associated with a progressive increase in the degree of kyphosis and in the lumbar spine this is associated with progressive flattening of the lordotic curve. As the number of vertebrae involved increases and the severity of individual vertebral deformities progress, these anatomic changes become more pronounced. There is gradual loss of the waistline contour, there is protuberance of the abdomen and in severe cases the lower ribs approximate the pelvic rim and ultimately lie within the pelvis. Each of these progressive anatomic deformities is associated with symptoms. The progressive loss of stature results in progressive ''shortening'' of the paraspinal musculature, that is, the paraspinal muscles are actively contracting resulting in the pain of muscle fatigue. This is the major cause of the chronic back pain in spinal osteoporosis. Careful clinical examination reveals that the skeleton (spine) itself is not tender and most patients indicate that the pain is paraspinal. The pain is worse with prolonged standing and often relieved by walking. Following an acute fracture there may be associated paraspinal muscle spasm, but this dissipates with time. The loss of height and the protuberant abdomen are usually not associated with direct symptoms per se, but do give the patient the emotional discomfort of the altered body image. Many patients attempt to wear abdominal flattening girdles or go on weight reduction diets, both of which will be of limited benefit and of potential harm. It is important that the patient be advised of the irreversible nature of these anatomic changes. One common complaint of patients with advanced disease is vague gastrointestinal distress aggravated by eating. This can be alleviated somewhat by having the patient consume frequent smaller meals. This is a particularly vexing problem for patients with chronic airway disease who have osteoporosis as a result of therapy with corticosteroids. In these patients the flattened diaphragm coupled with the shortened spinal column results in marked diminution of the size of their abdominal cavity.

There are several important approaches to the long-term management of patients with these chronic deformities from spinal osteoporosis. Of particular importance is educating the patient to understand the nature of the deformity so that he/she can have realistic expectations concerning body image and the anticipated goals of ther-

apy (relief of pain, restoration of function, maintenance of a reasonable quality of life, and prevention of further fractures). The major focus of therapy should be rehabilitation and analgesia aimed at lessening the chronic back pain. However, caution must be used with analgesics and nonsteroidal antiinflammatories, many of which cause significant constipation. Straining of the stool to relieve the constipation from narcotic analgesics tends to greatly aggravate back pain. In this regard, it is worth noting that many generi calcium preparations also tend to cause vague GI symptoms, including constipation in some patients. It is equally important to instruct the patient adequately in activities of daily living so that he/she bends, lifts, and stoops, in a manner that does not increase strain on the brittle skeleton. Nurses, physical therapists, and occupational therapists become important partners in the management of the patient with spinal osteoporosis. In many regards this nonpharmacologic approach to these patients is far more important than the pharmacologic therapy.

Diagnostic Studies in Osteoporosis

The same diagnostic approach should be taken to patients suspected of having osteoporosis whether or not they have already sustained a vertebral fracture. These studies should only be undertaken once an appropriate history and physical examination have been completed. The history, physical examination, and studies should all be conducted with the aims of determining the extent and severity of disease, the pathogenesis of the bone loss, and the physiology of the skeleton at the time of presentation. Although postmenopausal and senile osteoporosis are the most prevalent forms of the disease, it must be remembered that as many as 20% of women who otherwise appear to have postmenopausal osteoporosis can be shown to have additional etiologic factors above and beyond their age, gender, and ethnic background. Many of these secondary causes of osteoporosis (Table 1) can be suggested from the history and physical examination and appropriate investigations ordered.

If an osteoporotic fracture is suspected it is imperative that radiographs of the appropriate part of the skeleton be taken. However, there is no clear indication for radiographs of the skeleton if fracture is not suspected. All patients suspected of having osteoporosis, with or without fracture, should have measurement of bone mass (see Chapter 26 for details). The one possible exception is the patient with far advanced disease, clinically and radiographically. Because osteoporosis may be the only manifestation of many of the secondary causes listed above, it is appropriate to perform simple screening studies looking for these causes in each patient. Biochemical profile will provide information about renal and hepatic function, primary hyperparathyroidism, and possible malnutrition. Hematologic profile might also provide clues for the presence of myeloma or malnutrition. The precise role of hyperthyroidism, particularly exogenous, in the pathogenesis of accelerated bone loss and osteoporosis remains unresolved. Nonetheless, it would, for the time being at least, seem prudent to obtain a sensitive thyroid-stimulating hormone assay on all patients with documented bone loss. A 24-hr urine collection for measurement of calcium (which should always be accompanied by measurement of creatinine and sodium) will detect patients with hypercalcuria that may be the end result of excess skeletal loss or may contribute to excess skeletal loss. In contrast, a very low urine calcium (<50 mg for 24 hr) may provide a clue to the presence of vitamin D malnutrition or malabsorption (22). Because it is our practice to obtain a 24-hr urine collection on all osteoporotic subjects, we have adopted a policy of measuring 24-hr urine-free cortisol in the same collection to detect occult Cushing's disease, which may have osteoporosis as the only presenting feature. The yield from this is quite small, but it is probably the only way to detect this uncommon disorder. In general, the intensity with which one looks for occult secondary causes of accelerated bone loss should be related to any unusual features of the clinical presentation such as bone loss in a premenopausal woman, a woman very early in the menopause, or in a man without obvious hypogonadism. One should also pay particular attention to patients whose fractures occur at unusual sites.

Calcitropic Hormones and Biochemical Markers of Bone Remodeling

In most cases of osteoporosis there is no indication to measure the calcitropic hormones (parathyroid hormone, calcitriol, or calcitonin) unless there is a specific indication for these measurements based on the above history, physical examination, and biochemical screening. Although there are reports of abnormalities in some of these measurements when compared with published reference ranges, this is not the case when the reference values are appropriately adjusted for age, gender, and ethnic background.

In contrast, it is becoming increasingly important to monitor the biochemical markers of bone remodeling that are discussed in detail in Chapter 22. The control of bone remodeling is detailed in Chapter 6, and the role of abnormalities in the remodeling cycle in the pathogenesis of osteoporosis has been briefly described. It may be useful to make an analogy between turnover abnormalities leading to osteoporosis and abnormalities in the red cell life cycle leading to anemia. High-turnover bone loss with increased resorption and increased, but insufficient formation, would be analogous to hemolytic anemia with increased red cell destruction and increased (but insufficient) red cell formation characterized by the increased reticulocyte count in this type of anemia. Low-turnover bone loss with normal resorption and subnormal formation would be analogous to anemia or chronic disease.

There is increasing evidence that biochemical markers of bone formation and resorption are a useful adjunct to the prediction of future rate of bone loss and the response to therapy. The only serum marker of bone resorption is tartrate-resistant acid phosphatase, a specific gene product of the osteoclasts. A reliable assay for this enzyme is only available in a small number of research laboratories

and to our knowledge few if any reference laboratories. There are, however, several reliable urine markers of the bone resorption process. As bone is resorbed, breakdown products of the skeleton (protein and mineral) enter the circulation and are excreted in the urine. The most readily available of these markers is the urine calcium excretion, both the 24-hr urine calcium and the fasting urine calcium to creatinine ratio. The specificity of these markers can be improved by placing the patient on a low calcium diet for several days before the collection. This is not often very practical. Despite these limitations, in general if the fasting urine calcium to creatinine ratio in a spot sample of the second voided urine is >0.15 (mg/g), it is suggestive of increased endogenous loss of calcium (skeleton). The traditional marker of skeletal protein breakdown has been the urinary hydroxyproline excretion. The 24-hr urine hydroxyproline measurement requires a patient to be on a gelatin-free diet for 48 hr before the urine collection and during the urine collection. This is also impractical in most circumstances. The sensitivity of the results has been improved by obtaining the fasting hydroxyproline to creatinine ratio; values >21 (mg/g) suggest increased endogenous loss of skeleton. Because hydroxyproline is a component of many tissue collagens, this test will always have limited specificity. Assays have been developed for measurement of urinary pyridinoline cross-links of collagen both the lysyl and hydroxylysyl derivatives. These breakdown products of collagen are more specific for bone collagen although not completely so. Deoxypyridinoline cross-links are the more specific, but routine assays for this marker are currently unavailable. There are several reliable serum markers of bone formation. Bone-specific alkaline phosphatase, osteocalcin (bone GLA protein), and the extension peptides of procollagen I are all specific gene products of the osteoblasts, and there are reliable assays available in several reference laboratories. Bone-specific alkaline phosphatase has greater specificity than total alkaline phosphatase in evaluating patients with osteoporosis. (This would not be the case in diseases such as Paget's disease or osteomalacia where the total alkaline phosphatase is generally substantially elevated above normal.)

In summary, the current approach to the evaluation of the osteoporotic patient involves a documentation of bone mass, documentation of fractures if present, a diligent search for secondary causes, and then an evaluation of the biochemistry of skeletal remodeling.

Medical Therapy

At the time of this writing the only drugs approved by the Food and Drug Administration (FDA) for treatment of postmenopausal osteoporosis are estrogen and calcitonin. Although calcitriol and etidronate are both approved by the FDA for use in the United States, osteoporosis is currently not an approved indication. Oral calcium supplements are not subject to FDA regulation, and sodium fluoride as a supplement is also not subject to FDA regulation. In the following sections, we will discuss what is known about each of these possible therapies for postmenopausal osteoporosis.

The primary role for estrogen in the prevention of early postmenopausal bone loss and the subsequent development of osteoporotic fractures has been discussed in detail in Chapter 58. A definitive role for the use of estrogen in established osteoporosis is much less well established. Estrogen is an "antiresorptive" agent in that it inhibits bone resorption by decreasing the frequency of activation of the bone remodeling cycle. Estrogen would be expected to be most efficient if bone remodeling or bone turnover was increased. This is why it is so effective in the early stages of menopause. If an individual patient with established osteoporosis can be shown to have increased bone remodeling, estrogen will be effective in inhibiting remodeling, no matter how long it has been since the patient had her menopause. Thus, estrogen therapy will slow down the rate of bone loss in any estrogen-deficient woman so treated. However, the ability of estrogen to result in any net gain in bone mass is limited, with the best results being a 2–4% annual increase for ~2 years. There are very few studies showing that estrogen reduces the rate of occurrence of new vertebral fractures in patients with established osteoporosis. The usual starting dose is 0.625 mg of conjugated equine estrogen (Premarin®) or 0.05 mg of transdermal estrogen (Estraderm®). Short-term complications of estrogen therapy in women with established osteoporosis include breast tenderness and vaginal bleeding (13). If estrogens are given without progesterone there is increased likelihood of endometrial hyperplasia. The relationship between estrogen therapy and breast cancer is not well established, but most studies would suggest that there is little if any increased risk of breast cancer during the first 10–15 years of therapy. Such long-term studies in established osteoporosis have not been conducted, and, as long as therapy is tolerated, estrogen therapy, once indicated, should be continued indefinitely.

Synthetic salmon calcitonin (Calcimar® and Miacalcin®) is only available in the United States as a subcutaneous injection. Clinical trials with nasal spray calcitonin are in progress. Like estrogen, calcitonin inhibits bone resorption and slows down the rate of bone loss. The ability of calcitonin to increase bone mass is a function of the rate of bone remodeling at the time calcitonin therapy is initiated. In patients with increased bone turnover, the response is better than patients with low turnover (1). Again, a beneficial effect is observed as long as the medication is used, especially in intermittent pulse regimens (1–5). There is increasing evidence that calcitonin has inherent analgesic properties, and many physicians recommend its use in the early postfracture period because of this effect (6). The major side effects of calcitonin are transient flushing of the face and nausea. These side effects are all dose-dependent and virtually disappear with nasal spray formulations. The recommended dose is 100 U subcutaneously daily, but few, if any patients, tolerate this large dose initially. We have found that starting with a dose as low as 25 U subcutaneously three times/week is tolerated by most patients, and the dose can be gradually increased over a period of 2–3 months if needed. Intermittent pulse-dose regimens have also been used with documentation of increased bone mass and decreased fracture incidence (7). Calcitonin is dispensed in a concentration of 200 U/mL. Because most patients use insulin syringes calibrated for a dose of 100 U/mL, it is important that they receive adequate instruction on the amount of solution to inject to achieve the desired dosage. Therapy should be continued for as long as the drug is tolerated (8).

Etidronate (Didronel®), the first bisphosphonate to become clinically available, has been used in several clinical trials to stabilize or increase bone mass and also to possibly reduce vertebral fracture rate (16,19). However, the effect on vertebral fracture rate is still controversial and by no means well established. The major short-term effect of bisphosphonate is nausea (16,19). The treatment regimen for Etidronate is 400 mg orally daily for 2 weeks followed by a 10- to 12-week Etidronate-free period, with a repeat of this 3-month cycle for 2 years. Because this bisphosphonate is poorly absorbed orally and because its absorption is obliterated when given concurrently with calcium, it is important to advise the patient not to ingest any calcium, either as a supplement or in food, for 4 hr before or after ingestion of each tablet. Clinical trials of this therapy used 1,500 mg calcium as a daily supplement during the Etidronate-free periods. It is imperative that Etidronate be used in this rigorous treatment cycle and that the dose not be exceeded in amount or duration. There is evidence from long-term treatment of Paget's disease that large doses or longer duration of therapy with Etidronate may result in a mineralization defect and increased risk of developing osteomalacia and hip fractures. As noted earlier for calcitonin and estrogen, Etidronate is an antiresorptive drug. There is very little formal evidence that its effectiveness is a function of the remodeling at the time therapy is initiated. One can anticipate a gain of 2–4% annually in spinal bone mass.

Although calcitriol (Rocaltrol®) in a dose of 0.25 μg/day has been shown, in one study, to reduce the vertebral fracture rate compared with a group of patients taking calcium alone (21), other clinical trials have not found calcitriol to be effective in this regard. However, because calcitriol is the most potent metabolite (17) of vitamin D, it does increase intestinal calcium absorption, often resulting in hypercalcuria and/or hypercalcemia. Patients should be monitored every 6–8 weeks for development of these biochemical abnormalities, because clinical symptoms and signs of hypercalcuria and hypercalcemia may be very subtle and not clinically evident until irreversible renal damage has occurred. It is unclear what specific effect calcitriol has on bone mass although, in some instances, increments in bone mass of 1–2%/annum have been recorded.

The effect of calcium supplementation on bone mass and vertebral fracture rate in established osteoporotic syndromes is not well studied. Studies that are available suggest that calcium supplementation in perimenopausal females does decrease the rate of bone loss when administered in doses of 1,000–1,500 mg/day, especially in individuals with histories of marginally low calcium intakes (9–13). A combination of calcium supplements and exercise has also proven effective in stabilizing skeletal bone loss rates in postmenopausal female populations. Obviously, it is important to maintain adequate calcium supplement in doses of 1,000–1,500 mg/day, in addition to the active drug during estrogen or calcitonin therapeutic intervals, because it is difficult to mineralize newly formed matrix fully in the absence of adequate calcium.

Sodium fluoride is widely used as a therapy for postmenopausal osteoporosis. In doses between 50–75 mg/day, the increase in spinal bone mass achieved with sodium fluoride approximates 8%/year, twice that seen with either estrogen, calcitonin, or bisphosphonates. However, there is little evidence from properly conducted clinical trials that this increase in bone mass translates to a reduction in vertebral fractures. Moreover, sodium fluoride is associated to a significant degree of gastrointestinal distress and also a painful lower extremity syndrome felt to represent stress factors induced by fluoride. Because of these questions concerning the efficacy of sodium fluoride and its side effects, it cannot be recommended for use in postmenopausal osteoporosis at the present time (23).

There are reports that the prevalence of osteoporotic hip fractures decreases in patients receiving long-term therapy with hydrochlorothiazide (14). This has not been confirmed in all studies. There are however, to our knowledge, no formal studies of thiazide diuretic therapy being prescribed specifically for the treatment of osteoporosis. Until such studies are reported and shown to be effective, thiazide diuretics should not be used as therapy for osteoporosis. However, a case could be made for selecting thiazides as the diuretic of choice in patients with osteoporosis, should diuretic therapy be otherwise indicated. Because thiazides decrease renal excretion of calcium and, uncommonly, may lead to mild hypercalcemia, extreme caution should be used when considering calcitriol therapy in a patient on thiazides or thiazides in a patient on calcitriol. Side effects such as hypomagnesimia, hyperglycemia, hypercholesterolemia, and hypokalemia, preclude advocating this drug as potentially therapeutic for osteoporotic patients who are not hypertensive (15,18).

Newer generations of bisphosphonates, synthetic parathyroid hormone, and various combinations and treatment regimens of these experimental drugs as well as the drugs listed above are currently undergoing extensive clinical trials. At the present time the safety and efficacy of these various drugs and their potential combinations are not well established. Consequently, their use cannot be recommended.

Selecting a Therapy and Monitoring the Response to Therapy

At a minimum, every patient with established osteoporosis with or without fractures should be given supplemental calcium of 1,000–1,500 mg/day. Specific therapy for osteoporosis should be restricted to estrogen and calcitonin, recognizing that these drugs are approved by the FDA for an osteoporosis indication. We would recommend that each patient should have a baseline measurement of biochemical markers of bone remodeling before initiating therapy. The patient should be seen and clinically evaluated 4–6 weeks later to ascertain compliance and possible side effects from therapy. It would also be appropriate to repeat the biochemistry at this time to determine that there is indeed a decrease in the rate of bone remodeling. If there is no satisfactory change in the biochemistry one should consider increasing the dose. If the dose of medication is changed for whatever reason, clinical and biochemical evaluation should be repeated in 4–6 weeks until a satisfactory response is achieved. If there is no response to 3 months of therapy, one should consider a change in medication. Bone mass, which should always be measured at baseline, should be monitored at the end of 6 and 12 months of therapy. A decrease in bone mass of 2% or greater at either of these measurements should prompt a change in therapy, either a change in dose or a change in medication. After a patient has experienced one full year of successful therapy, that is 1 year of therapy with either an increase in bone mass or <2% decrease, monitoring could be restricted to annual measurement of bone mass. At the present time there is no indication that therapy should be discontinued as long as the patient is tolerating the medication and there is no progressive decrement in bone mass. It should be noted that the antifracture efficacy of each of these drugs, during the early therapeutic phase, is not well established, and the occurrence of an osteoporotic fracture within the first 6–12 months of therapy should not be taken as an indication of failed therapy. The patient should be made completely aware of this before initiation of therapy. As far as is known, there are no ill effects of long-term use of calcitonin in the treatment schedule described previously. Cost and convenience become important factors in long-term patient acceptance of these drugs. Because of the potential association between long-term estrogen therapy and development and endometrial and breast cancer, appropriate monitoring for these complications must be continued. Patients need to be instructed in the technique of monthly breast self-examination and must undergo an annual examination by a clinician and an annual mammogram. All episodes of unexplained vaginal bleeding must be fully evaluated by a gynecologist. In women with an intact uterus, progesterone should be given along with estrogen and in a short period of time most patients develop either amenorrhea or a stable, recognizable bleeding pattern that should not give rise to concern or investigation.

It is important to reemphasize that drug therapy only should never be substituted for the common sense approaches to daily living discussed in some detail in earlier sections. This includes emphasizing safety and fall prevention and avoiding drugs such as sedatives, hypnotics, and antihypertensives that might predispose to sedation, ataxia, or postural hypotension. Patients should all be encouraged to become involved in a regular active exercise/rehabilitation program. With appropriate medical, nursing, and rehabilitation care, most patients, except those with the most advanced disease with multiple vertebral compression fractures, can be expected to be restored to reasonable functional health with a good quality of life. Likewise, an anticipated goal of therapy should be to prevent even the first osteoporotic fracture in patients whose therapy is initiated early.

REFERENCES

1. Avioli LV: Heterogeneity of osteoporotic syndromes and the response to calcitonin therapy. *Calcif Tissue Int* 49(suppl 2): S16–19, 1991
2. Rico H, Hernandez ER, Diaz-Mediaville J, et al.: Treatment of multiple myeloma with nasal spray calcitonin: A histomorphometric and biochemical study. *Bone Miner* 8:231–237, 1990
3. Mazzuloi GF, Passeri M, Gennari C, et al.: Effects of salmon calcitonin in postmenopausal osteoporosis: A controlled double-blind clinical study. *Calcif Tissue Int* 38:3–8, 1986
4. Civitelli R, Gonnelli S, Zacchei F, et al.: Bone turnover in postmenopausal osteoporosis. *J Clin Invest* 82:1268–1274, 1988
5. Overgaard K, Riis BJ, Christiansen C, et al.: Effect of calcitonin given intranasally on early postmenopausal bone loss. *Br Med J* 299:477–479, 1989
6. Lyritis GP, Tsakalabos S, Magiasis B, et al.: Analgesic effect of salmon calcitonin on osteoporotic vertebral fractures. Double-blind, placebo-controlled study. *Calcif Tissue Int* 49:369–372, 1991
7. Rico H, et al.: Salmon calcitonin reduces vertebral fracture rate in the postmenopausal crush fracture syndrome. *Bone Miner* 1: 131–138, 1992
8. Overgaard K, Hansen MA, Nielsen V-AH, Riis BJ, Christiansen C: Discontinuous calcitonin treatment of established osteoporosis: Effects of withdrawal of treatment. *Am J Med* 89:1–6, 1990
9. Dawson-Hughes B, Dallal GE, Krall EA, Sadowski L, Sahyoun N, Tannenbau S: Controlled trial of the effect of calcium supplementation on bone density in postmenopausal women. *N Engl J Med* 323:878–883, 1990
10. Dawson-Hughes B: Calcium supplementation and bone loss: A review of controlled clinical trials. *Am J Clin Nutr* 54: 274S–280S, 1991
11. Elders PJM, Netelenbos JC, Lips P, van Ginkel FC, Khoe E, Leeuwenkamp OR, Hackeng WHL, van der Stelt PF: Calcium supplementation reduces vertebral bone loss in perimenopausal women: A controlled trial in 248 women between 46 and 55 years of age. *J Clin Endocrinol Metab* 73:533–540, 1991
12. Licata AA, Jones-Gall DJ: Effect of supplemental calcium on serum and urinary calcium in osteoporotic patients. *J Am Coll Nutr* 11:164–167, 1992
13. Prince RL, Smith M, Dick IM, Price RI, Webb PG, Henderson NK, Harris MM: Prevention of postmenopausal osteoporosis. Comparative study of exercise, calcium supplementation, and hormone replacement therapy. *N Engl J Med* 325:1189–1195, 1991
14. LaCroix AZ, Wienpahl J, White LR, Wallace RB, Scherr PA, George LK, Cornoni-Huntley J, Ostfeld AM: Thiazide diuretic agents and the incidence of hip fracture. *N Engl J Med* 322: 286–290, 1990
15. Martin BJ, Milligan K: Diuretic associated hypomagnesemia in the elderly. *Arch Intern Med* 147:1768–1771, 1987
16. Mautalen CA, Casco CA, Gonzalez D, Ghiringhelli GR, Massironi C, Fromm GA, Plantalech L: Side effects of disodium aminohydroxypropylidenediphosphonate (APD) during treatment of bone diseases. *Br Med J* 288:828–829, 1984
17. Ott SM, Chesnut CH, III: Calcitriol treatment is not effective in postmenopausal osteoporosis. *Ann Intern Med* 110:267–274, 1989
18. Ray WA: Thiazide diuretics and osteoporosis: Time for a clinical trial (editorial)? *Ann Intern Med* 115:64–65, 1991
19. Roux C, Listrat V, Villette B, Lessana-Leibowitch M, Ethgen D, Dougados M, Amor B: Longlasting dermatological lesions after tiludronate therapy. *Calcif Tissue Int* 50:378–380, 1992
20. Swales JD: Magnesium deficiency and diuretics. *Br Med J* 285: 1377–1378, 1982
21. Tilyard MW, Spears GFS, Thompson J, Dovey S: Treatment of postmenopausal osteoporosis with calcitriol or calcium. *N Engl J Med* 326:357–361, 1992
22. Villareal DT, Civitelli R, Chines A, Avioli LV: Subclinical vitamin D deficiency in postmenopausal women with low vertebral bone mass. *J Clin Endocrinol Metab* 72:628–634, 1991
23. Hedlund LR, Gallagher JC: Increased incidences of fractures in osteoporosis patients treated with sodium fluoride. *J Bone Mineral Res* 4:223–225, 1989

57. Radiology of Osteoporosis

Harry K. Genant, M.D.

Department of Radiology, Musculoskeletal Section, Osteoporosis Research Group, University of California, San Francisco, California

Osteoporosis represents the most common form of metabolic bone disease, and its radiologic features are presented herein. The list of processes that are associated with or result in a generalized deficient quantity of bone (osteoporosis) is extensive (see Table 1). Histologically, the end result in each of these disorders is a deficient amount of osseous tissue, although different pathogenic mechanisms may be involved. In essence, the generalized osteoporoses represent a heterogeneous group of conditions encompassing many pathogenetic mechanisms variably associated with low, normal, or increased bone-remodeling states.

Many terms have been employed to describe the radiographic features of diminished bone density such as *osteoporosis, demineralization, undermineralization, deossification,* and *osteopenia*. Osteopenia, meaning poverty of the bone, has become acceptable as a nonspecific, gross descriptive term for generalized or regional rarefaction of the skeleton.

Portions of this chapter have appeared in the following: Vogler JB, Genant HK: Metabolic and endocrine disease. In: Grainger RG, Allison DJ (eds): *Diagnostic Radiology—An Anglo-American Textbook of Imaging*. Churchill Livingstone: London, 1992 (2nd edition), Genant HK, Block JE Postmenopausal and Senile Osteoporosis: Clinical Epidemiology and Detection. In: Viamonte M (ed): *Geriatric Radiology*. Williams & Wilkins: Baltimore, Maryland, 1992, and Genant HK, Vogler JB, Block JE, Radiology of Osteoporosis. In: Riggs BL, Melton LJ (eds): *Osteoporosis: Pathogenesis, Diagnosis and Etiology*. Raven Press: New York, 1992.

PRIMARY OSTEOPOROSIS

Involutional, Postmenopausal, or Senile Osteoporosis

The term, *involutional osteoporosis,* has been used to describe the condition of gradual, progressive bone loss,

TABLE 1. *Disorders associated with radiographic osteoporosis (osteopenia)*

I. Primary Osteoporosis
  1. Involutional osteoporosis (postmenopausal and senile)
  2. Juvenile osteoporosis
II. Secondary Osteoporosis
  A. Endocrine
    1. Adrenal cortex
      Cushing's disease
      Addison's disease
    2. Gonadal disorders
      Hypogonadism
    3. Pituitary
      Acromegaly
      Hypopituitarism
    4. Pancreas
      Diabetes mellitus
    5. Thyroid
      Hyperthyroidism
      Hypothyroidism
    6. Parathyroid
      Hyperparathyroidism
  B. Marrow replacement and expansion
    1. Myeloma
    2. Leukemia
    3. Metastatic disease
    4. Gaucher's disease
    5. Anemias (sickle cell, thalasemia)
  C. Drugs and substances
    1. Corticosteroids
    2. Heparin
    3. Anticonvulsants
    4. Immunosuppressants
    5. Alcohol
  D. Chronic disease
    1. Chronic renal disease
    2. Hepatic insufficiency
    3. GI malabsorption
    4. Chronic inflammatory polyarthropathies
    5. Chronic debility/immobilization
  E. Deficiency states
    1. Vitamin D
    2. Vitamin C (scurvy)
    3. Calcium
    4. Malnutrition
  F. Inborn errors of metabolism
    1. Osteogenesis imperfecta
    2. Homocystinuria

often accompanied by fractures, seen in postmenopausal women and, with increasing age, in both men and women. It has been suggested that this broad category of involutional osteoporosis may represent two distinct syndromes—postmenopausal osteoporosis and senile osteoporosis. Although there is substantial overlap between these two subcategories, it is convenient to discuss them as separate entities because of differing clinical features and proposed pathoetiologies. The separation is based primarily on the different patterns of bone loss and types of fracture that are observed in these two processes.

Postmenopausal osteoporosis (also termed type I osteoporosis) (1) is believed to represent that process occurring in a subset of postmenopausal women, typically between the ages of 50 to 65 years. This group is characterized by accelerated trabecular bone resorption related to estrogen deficiency, and is identified by a fracture pattern that involves predominantly the spine and wrist. Accelerated and disproportionate loss of trabecular bone in these areas structurally weakens the bone and predisposes them to fractures. In senile osteoporosis (or type II osteoporosis) (2), there is a proportionate loss of cortical and trabecular bone, in contrast to the disproportionate loss of trabecular bone in postmenopausal osteoporosis. Senile osteoporosis is characterized by: fractures of the hip, proximal end of the humerus, tibia, and pelvis in elderly women and men usually 75 years of age or older. The etiology of senile osteoporosis is speculative. However, factors that play a role include age-related decrease in bone formation, diminished adrenal function, reduced intestinal calcium absorption, and secondary hyperparathyroidism.

Radiographic-Pathologic Findings

In the normal adult physiologic state, the rates of bone formation and bone resorption are roughly equal (i.e. coupled), allowing the total amount of osseous tissue to remain constant. In osteoporosis (2), this equilibrium is loss such that bone resorption predominates. This is reflected radiographically as various patterns of trabecular and cortical bone resorption ultimately leading to osteopenia.

Trabecular bone resorption in the axial skeleton, particularly in Type I osteoporosis, results in marked thinning and dissolution of transverse trabeculae with relative preservation of the primary trabeculae or those aligned with the axis of stress. In areas in which trabecular bone predominates such as the spine and pelvis, the combination of osteopenia and reinforcement of primary trabeculae may produce a striated bony appearance (Fig. 1). The reinforced primary trabeculae have a sharp appearance in osteoporosis bones, which occasionally aids in distinguishing osteoporosis from osteomalacia. In osteomalacia, the trabeculae may appear indistinct or "fuzzy", a result of irregular resorption from accompanying secondary hyperparathyroidism and from the trabeculae that become coated by a layer of partially unmineralized osteoid. The loss of trabecular bone mass also accentuates the cortical outline, producing the so-called "picture framing" or "empty box" seen in osteoporosis of the vertebral bodies (Fig. 2). The vertebral bodies become weakened and the intervertebral disc may protrude into the adjacent vertebral body. The degree of protrusion varies, ranging from bending and buckling of the endplates, (biconcave appearance) to herniation of disc material into the vertebral body (Schmorl's node formation) (Fig. 3). In more advanced cases complete compression fractures of the vertebral bodies occur (Fig. 4).

Bone loss in the appendicular skeleton is initially most apparent radiographically at the ends of long and tubular bones due to the predominance of cancellous bone in these regions. Endosteal resorption of bone has a prominent role, particularly in type II osteoporosis. The net result of this chronic process, is widening of the medullary canal with thinning of the cortices, which is most pronounced in the appendicular skeleton (Fig. 5). In late

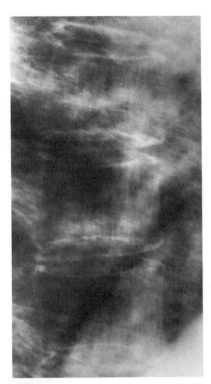

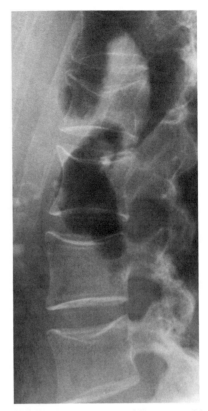

FIG. 1. Moderate postmenopausal osteoporosis of the thoracic spine with overall loss of bone density. The cortices are thinned and the vertebral bodies have a 'striated' appearance due to loss of secondary trabeculae and reinforcement of sharply defined primary trabeculae.

FIG. 3. Moderate osteoporotic fractures with endplate deformities of the lumbar spine due to involutional osteoporosis.

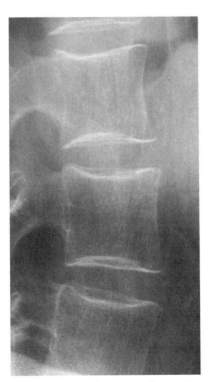

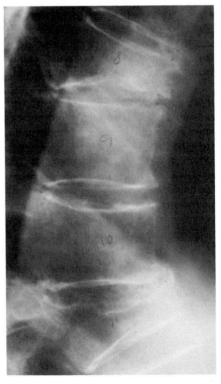

FIG. 2. Due to the loss of trabecular bone, there is accentuation of the cortices resulting in the appearance of 'picture framing' in this patient with postmenopausal osteoporosis.

FIG. 4. Advanced osteoporotic fractures of the thoracic spine. Wedging and compression fractures have occurred as a result of involutional osteoporosis.

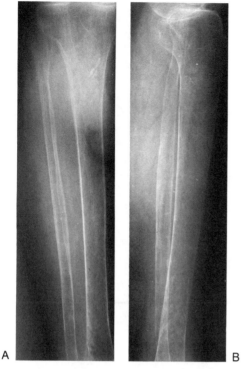

FIG. 5. Advanced involutional osteoporosis of the **(A)** tibia and **(B)** fibula producing marked thinning of the cortices due to chronic endosteal resorption and widening of the medullary space.

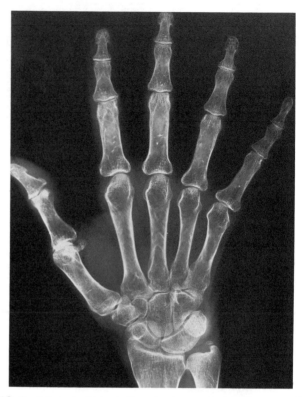

FIG. 6. Advanced involutional osteoporosis with generalized cortical thinning and uniform trabecular resorption.

stages of senile osteoporosis, the cortices are "paper thin" and the endosteal surfaces are smooth (Fig. 6). On the other hand, in rapidly evolving postmenopausal osteoporosis, accelerated endosteal and intracortical bone resorption may be seen and can be directly assessed by high resolution radiographic techniques (Fig. 7).

When there is an overall loss of bone mass and progressive osteopenia, the skeletal system becomes weakened, and fractures occur. These fractures are commonly seen in the vertebral bodies, femoral neck (Fig. 8), femoral intertrochanteric region (Fig. 9), distal radius, ribs, and pelvis. These may be the result of minor trauma or even normal stress on the abnormal bone (insufficiency fracture). Vertebral body and wrist fractures (type I osteoporosis) are generally seen at an earlier age than fractures of the femur (type II osteoporosis). Occasionally, these osteoporotic fractures are not identified on initial radiographs, but are identified by radionuclide bone scan, computed tomography (Fig. 10), magnetic resonance imaging, or by follow-up radiographic studies, as healing occurs. The radiologic appearance in the setting of partial healing, may suggest a metastatic neoplastic process, particularly with fractures of the vertebrae, sacrum, hip, and pelvis (Fig. 11).

Idiopathic Juvenile Osteoporosis

The etiology of this rare disorder (3-4) is not known. Patients prior to puberty, typically present with osteoporosis that is progressive initially and later stabilizes.

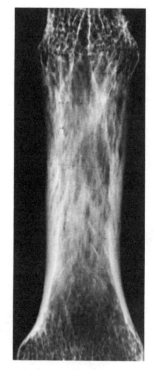

FIG. 7. High resolution radiographs of a proximal phalanx showing endosteal scalloping and intracortical striation indicating aggressive bone resorption in a recently (2 years prior) oophorectomized woman.

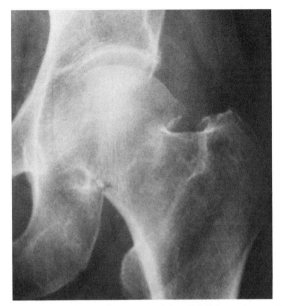

FIG. 8. Femoral neck fracture with mild valgus impaction in a patient with involutional osteoporosis.

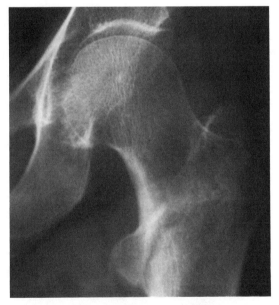

FIG. 9. Minimally displaced intertrochanteric fracture in a patient with late involutional osteoporosis.

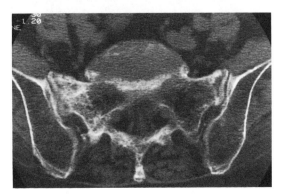

FIG. 10. Insufficiency fractures of the sacral ala due to advanced involutional osteoporosis.

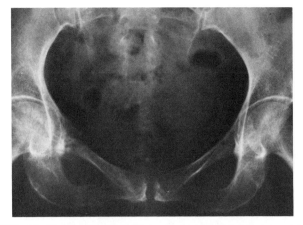

FIG. 11. Pelvic ring insufficiency fractures of right pubic and iscial bones in a patient with involutional osteoporosis. Irregular resorption and reactive callus simulate a neoplastic process.

Radiological-Pathological Considerations

Bone formation is thought to proceed normally while, there is an increase in osteoclastic activity, yielding increased bone resorption (4). This causes a decrease in the quantity of bone (osteoporosis), while the quality of remaining bone is normal. This osteoporosis becomes most evident in the thoracic and lumbar spine with anterior wedging and biconcave deformities (Fig. 12) of the vertebral bodies also found, and the condition should be distinguished from juvenile epiphysitis, or Scheuremann's

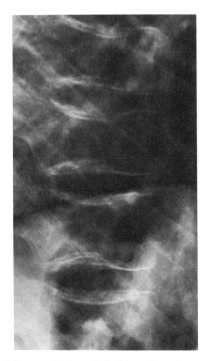

FIG. 12. Advanced idiopathic juvenile osteoporosis with biconcave vertebral deformities.

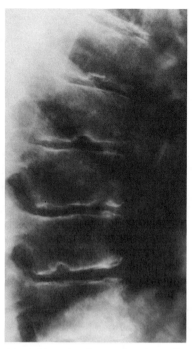

FIG. 13. Scheuermann's disease or juvenile epiphysitis with multiple discrete Schmorl's nodes and mild wedge deformities in the thoracic spine.

disease (Fig. 13). Although fractures may be seen in the diaphysis of long bones, they more characteristically occur at the metaphyses. Presumably this is related to the bony abnormality being more evident at sites of active bone turnover. Slipped capital femoral epiphyses may be seen.

The disorder is usually self-limited; however, if a large amount of osseous tissue is lost, the radiographic appearance may not return to normal. Laboratory values are typically normal and the diagnosis is made by exclusion.

SECONDARY OSTEOPOROSIS

Cushing's Disease (Endogenous and Exogenous)

Cushing's disease (3,5–7), is the result of an excess of adrenocortical steroids. This excess may be endogenous or exogenous. Endogenous Cushing's disease is caused by adrenal hyperplasia in the vast majority of cases, with other less frequent causes being tumors of the adrenal and pituitary glands. Exogenous Cushing's disease, far more common than endogenous, results from excessive corticosteroid medication.

Radiologic-Pathologic Considerations

As in osteoporosis, the equilibrium between bone formation and bone resorption is disrupted such that resorption predominates. Thus, the typical findings of osteoporosis are seen. Wedge, biconcave and compression

fractures are also seen. Histologically, exuberant endosteal callus formation is seen in compressed vertebrae and is manifested radiographically by increased density in the bony tissue adjacent to the vertebral endplate, referred to as marginal condensation (Fig. 14). This excessive callus formation is also evident in fractures involving other bones, including the ribs, which are commonly fractured in Cushing's disease.

Additional findings occasionally seen in Cushing's disease include, a mottled appearance of the skull secondary to osteoporotic involvement. Osteonecrosis, particularly of the femoral heads is not uncommon in the case of exogenous steroid administration, but occurs infrequently in the endogenous cases for unknown reasons (8). Other less common findings seen only in exogenous Cushing's disease are; joint infections, neuropathic–like joints, tendon rupture, delayed skeletal maturation, and decreased osteophyte formation (3).

Osteomalacia

Osteomalacia (3,9) is characterized by defective mineralization of osteoid in mature cortical and cancellous bone. It is a general term describing similar histopathological and radiological changes, which are seen in a large group of diverse disorders. The etiology of osteomalacia in these disorders is also diverse and may or may not be the result of a defect in vitamin D metabolism.

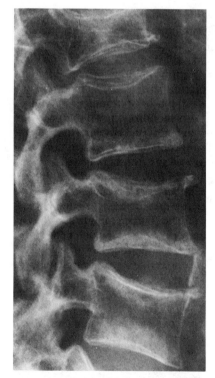

FIG. 14. Exogenous Cushing's disease. A lateral view of the lumbar spine demonstrates osteoporosis and biconcave vertebral bodies. The increased density adjacent to the vertebral endplates called "marginal condensation" is the result of exuberant endosteal callus formation.

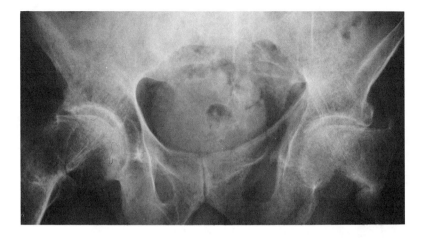

FIG. 15. Advanced osteomalacia showing generalized osteopenia with bending deformities of the proximal femurs accompanied by medial pseudofractures of the femoral necks.

Radiologic-Pathologic Considerations

The prime abnormality in osteomalacia, is the presence of excessive amounts of inadequately mineralized osteoid. This material is seen coating the trabeculae and accounts for the unsharp appearance of these structures.

Focal accumulations of osteoid are seen to occur in compact bone at right angles to the long axis. Radiographically these are known as Looser's zones or pseudofractures and are a distinguishing sign of osteomalacia, although they may occur in Paget disease and rarely in simple osteoporosis (10). The exact etiology of Looser's zones is unclear, although they probably represent partial insufficiency fractures. They are often symmetrical in distribution and are principally seen in the pubic rami and femoral necks (Fig. 15), scapulae, ribs, long bones, and metatarsals. While they may remain unchanged for months or even years, true lateral fractures may develop in these areas since they represent an area of weakened bone.

Intracortical bone resorption or cortical tunnelling, is observed in the tubular and long bones. High resolution magnification techniques demonstrate these findings in the phalanges and metacarpals as a manifestation of the frequently associated secondary hyperparathyroidism (Fig. 16A). The most sensitive, although nonspecific, radiographic abnormality in osteomalacia, is intracortical resorption or tunnelling which is far more common than radiographic pseudofractures.

Radiological thinning and loss of secondary trabeculae occur, resulting in decreased bone density and the coarsened appearance of the trabecular pattern especially in the spine (Fig. 16B). Overall, the bones lose intrinsic strength and bowing of long bones may occur. Scoliosis occasionally develops and the vertebral bodies may assume a biconcave appearance (Fig. 17). Bone "softening" in other areas of the body may result in basilar invagination, protrusio acetabuli, and a triradiate appearance of the pelvis (3).

In some disorders causing osteomalacia, such as those associated with renal osteodystrophy, the massive amounts of osteoid present in the bones can become partially mineralized, typically in the presence of severe secondary hyperparathyroidism with a high serum calcium-phosphorus product. This results in increased bone density particularly in the spine appearing as the "Rugger-Jersey" (11) (Fig. 18). The exact mechanism of osteosclrosis in renal osteodystrophy, however, remains unclear.

Rickets

Like the term osteomalacia, rickets (3) is a general term used to describe the histopathological and radiological changes resulting from a group of diverse disorders. The final common pathway of these disorders is a loss of orderly maturation and mineralization of cartilage cells at the growth plate, resulting in similar pathological and radiological changes. Rickets represents osteomalacia in the growing skeleton.

Radiologic-Pathologic Considerations

The radiological findings at the physeal plate are a reflection of the altered pathophysiology. The normal ordered maturation and mineralization of cartilage cells becomes disrupted. This occurs predominantly in the hypertrophic zone, where the number of chondrocytes is seen to increase and the normal columnar formation of the cells is lost. There is a continued build up of cells resulting in the earliest radiographic finding of widening and lengthening of the growth plate (Fig. 19). Defective mineralization of the chondrocytes in the zone of provisional calcification yields the irregular metaphyseal margins seen on radiographs. Similar defective mineralization occurring in the zones of primary and secondary spongiosa, produces a "frayed" appearance of the metaphyseal trabecular bone. As the cell mass in the hypertrophic zone continues to increase, it protrudes into the weakened metaphyseal region causing cupping and widening of the metaphyses (Fig. 20). While this process is occurring on the metaphyseal side of the growth plate, similar processes are occurring on the epiphyseal side. The defective maturation and mineralization seen here results in an epiphysis, which is osteopenic and has irregular, unsharp borders.

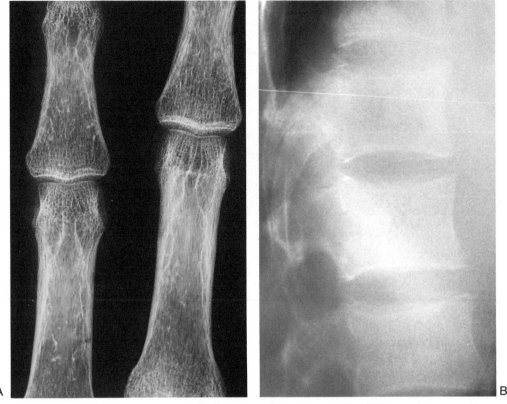

FIG. 16. Osteomalacia secondary to intestinal malabsorption. **(A)** High resolution radiograph of the hand demonstrates osteopenia accompanied by increased intracortical tunneling due to associated secondary hyperparathyroidism. **(B)** Lateral view of the spine in this patient demonstrates osteopenia with indistinct cortical and trabecular outlines. Biconcave deformities of the vertebral bodies are also evident.

In the metaphysis and diaphysis, there is also defective mineralization of osteoid. In these areas, where mature bone is present, the radiographic findings of osteomalacia are produced.

Additional radiographic findings include prominence of the growth plates at the costochondral junctions, producing the *rachitic rosary*. The squared configuration of the skull, occasionally seen, results from excessive osteoid build up, in addition to abnormal remodeling. Because of the weakened nature of the bones, there is often bowing, resulting from normal weight-bearing and muscular stresses. Scoliosis, slipped capital femoral epiphyses, a triradiate configuration of the pelvis, and basilar invagination may also be seen.

Primary Hyperparathyroidism

This disorder stems from a primary defect in the parathyroid glands resulting in an increased secretion of parathyroid hormone (PTH), causing elevation of serum calcium and reduction in serum phosphorus. The serum calcium becomes elevated, in part, by the action of PTH on bone by activation of the osteoclastic system and remodeling of osseous tissue. The resultant bony changes give the radiographic picture of primary hyperparathyroidism (3,11–13).

Radiologic-Pathologic Considerations

One of the effects of the elevated levels of PTH and a hallmark of this disorder, is resorption of bone, *osteitis fibrosa*. The resorption is felt to be the result primarily of stimulation of the osteoclast and occurs at many different sites (intracortical, endosteal, subchondral, subligamentous, and trabecular). Subperiosteal bone resorption, which is most characteristic of hyperparathyroidism (3), is seen in approximately 10% of patients, most commonly on the radial aspect of the middle phalanges of the second and third digits (Fig. 21). Other sites commonly affected include, the phalangeal tufts and the metaphyseal cut–away zones of the medial aspects of the proximal humerus, femur, and tibia.

Cortical striations and intracortical tunnelling due to osteoclastic bone resorption (13) may be seen in over half the patients, and are best detected in the tubular bones of the hands using magnification techniques (Fig. 22).

Erosions involving the sacroiliac joints, symphysis pubis, ligamentous insertions, resorption of the distal or medial ends of the clavicle, and the development of "aggressive" Schmorl's nodes may all be attributed in part to subchondral resorption in these sites of high bone turnover.

In patients with primary hyperparathyroidism, the skull

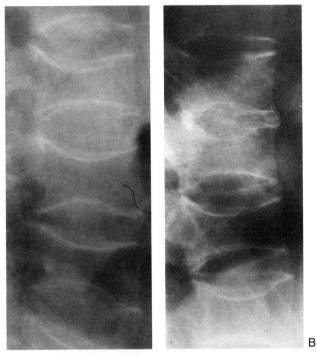

FIG. 17. Lateral views of the lumbar (**A**) and thoracic (**B**) spine in patient with osteomalacia demonstrates moderate osteopenia involving the vertebral bodies. The trabeculae in the vertebral bodies appear indistinct or unsharp, and there is evidence of bone softening with bowing of the endplates.

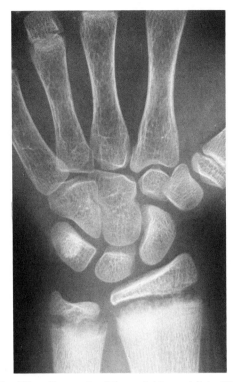

FIG. 19. AP radiograph of the wrist in a child with rickets and osteopenia. Widening of the growth plates of the distal radius and ulna are evident. Also the zone of provisional calcification in both the radius and ulna is indistinct and the metaphyseal margins appear irregular. The cortices of the metacarpals are abnormally thin.

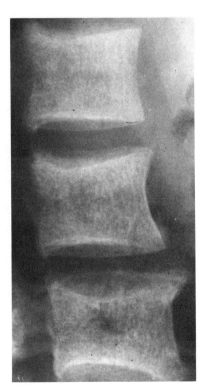

FIG. 18. Lumbar spine in renal osteodystrophy demonstrates mottled subchondral bands of sclerosis, the "Rugger-Jersey" spine.

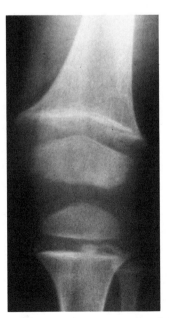

FIG. 20. AP radiograph of the knee in rickets demonstrates diffuse osteopenia. The growth plates have widened and protrude into the weakened metaphyseal region causing cupping and widening of the metaphyses. Note also the irregular, unsharp borders of the femoral epiphysis.

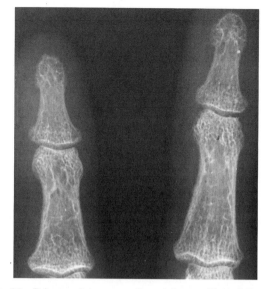

FIG. 21. Primary hyperparathyroidism with subtle subperiosteal bone resorption of the radial aspects of the middle phalanges, and irregular resorption of the tufts.

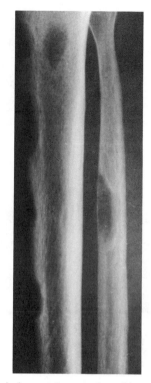

FIG. 23. Multiple brown tumors in primary hyperparathyroidism. Lateral radiograph of the leg in this patient with primary hyperparathyroidism demonstrates multiple brown tumors involving the tibia and fibula. The well-defined lytic appearance of these lesions is characteristic of brown tumors.

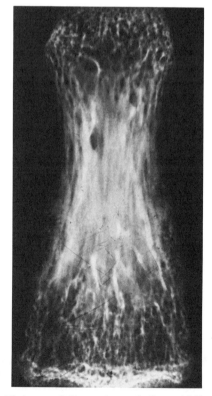

FIG. 22. High resolution view of the middle phalanx shows marked subperiosteal and intracortical bone resorption in primary hyperparathyroidism.

occasionally has a characteristic "pepper-pot" pattern, which results from trabecular resorption and remodeling of the medullary space (3). Erosions of the calcaneus and inferior aspect of the distal clavicles are evidence of subligamentous resorption of these sites.

The combined effect of all these patterns of bone resorption, is osteopenia in the majority of patients. Detection of this osteopenia by noninvasive bone mineral measurement then becomes important for early diagnosis, since very few patients show diagnostic radiographic appearances of hyperparathyroidism on clinical presentation. Rarely, patients may demonstrate diffuse osteosclerosis (11).

Brown tumors (osteoclastomas) represent focal, bone-replacing lesions most often occurring in the metaphyses and diaphyses though epiphyseal involvement may be seen (Fig. 23). They contain collections of giant cells, which are usually responsive to parathyroid hormone since the majority of lesions demonstrate healing with removal of the adenoma. They may occur as solitary lesions or involve multiple bones.

Osteogenesis Imperfecta

Osteogenesis imperfecta (OI) (3,14), is an inherited disorder of connective tissue that is usually transmitted in an autosomal dominant pattern. The exact defect in this disorder is unclear; however, it is felt to be related to abnormal maturation of collagen (mineralized and non-mineralized) (6). The classical clinical triad in this disease is: (1) fragility of the bones, (2) blue sclerae, and (3) deafness. Two forms are recognized: the congenita form, in which life expectancy is usually short, and the tarda form, in which life expectancy is normal.

Radiologic-Pathologic Considerations

The abnormal maturations of collagen seen in this disorder results in a primary defect in bone matrix. This and defective mineralization result in overall loss of bone density involving both the axial and appendicular skeleton. The long bones may either be thin and gracile, as is usually the case in the tarda form, or they may be short and thick, as seen almost exclusively in the congenita form (Fig. 24). Multiple fractures, usually transverse, occur predominantly in the lower extremities, typically producing bowing deformities. This bowing may serve as an indication of the severity of the disease since it tends to correlate with the number of fractures. Avulsion fractures are also common.

Fracture healing is usually normal but may demonstrate exuberant callus and pseudarthrosis. Inevitably, the extremities become shortened which, in part, accounts for

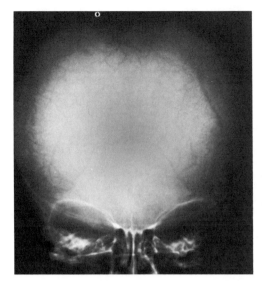

FIG. 25. Osteogenesis imperfecta. Typical skull findings in patients with OI include the presence of numerous unfused ossification centers (wormian bones).

the short stature seen in most cases (14). Premature degenerative changes are often seen involving the joints, primarily from intra-articular fractures and ligamentous laxity.

The skull and axial skeleton also show typical changes. Wormian bones (Fig. 25), enlargement of the paranasal sinuses, platybasia and basilar impression are frequent findings. Severe kyphoscoliosis, biconcave vertebral bodies, wedge-shaped vertebral bodies, triradiate pelvis, and protrusio acetabuli may be present (Fig. 26).

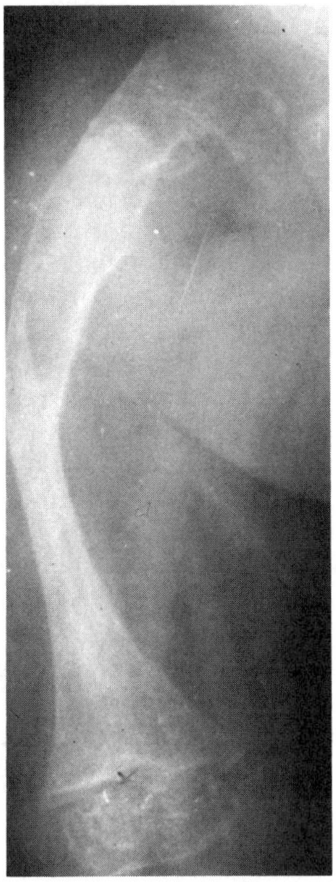

FIG. 24. Osteogenesis imperfecta (congenita form). An AP radiograph of the femur in this infant with OI demonstrates bowing and thickening due to multiple fractures and exuberant callus formation.

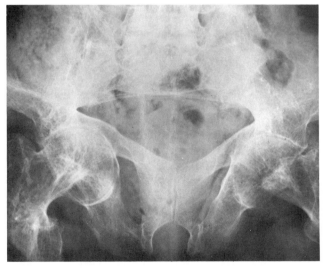

FIG. 26. A 50 year-old woman with osteogenesis imperfecta (tarda form). An AP pelvis radiograph demonstrates diffuse osteopenia. The pelvis has a triradiate configuration and there is bilateral protrusio acetabuli.

REFERENCES

1. Riggs BL, Melton LJ: Evidence for two distinct syndromes of involutional osteoporosis. *Am J Med* 75:899–901, 1983
2. Riggs BL, Melton LJ: Involutional osteoporosis. *N Eng J Med* 314:1676–1685, 1986
3. Resnick D, Niwayama G (eds): *Diagnosis of Bone and Joint Disorders,* (2nd ed.). W.B. Saunders, Philadelphia, PA, 1988
4. Jowsey J, Johnson KA: Juvenile osteoporosis: bone findings in seven patients. *J Pediatr* 81:511–517, 1972
5. Bondy PK: The adrenal cortex. In: Bony PK, Rosenberg LE (eds). *Metabolic Control and Disease, 8th ed.* W.B. Saunders, Philadelphia, PA, 1980, p 1427
6. Jaffe HL: Metabolic, *Degenerative and Inflammatory Diseases of Bones and Joints.* Lea & Febiger, Philadelphia, PA, 1972
7. Sissons HA: The osteoporosis of Cushing's syndrome. *J Bone Joint Surg* 38B:418–433, 1956
8. Madell SH, Freeman LM: Avascular necrosis of bone in Cushing's syndrome. *Radiology* 83:1068–1070, 1964
9. Pitt MJ: Rachitic and osteomalacic syndromes. *Radiol Clin NA* 19:581–599, 1981
10. Perry GM, Weinstein RS, Teitelbaum SL, Avioli LV, Fallon MD: Pseudofractures in the absence of osteomalacia. *Skel Radiol* 8:17–19, 1982
11. Genant HK, Baron JM, Straus FH II, Paloyan E, Jowsey J: Osteosclerosis in primary hyperparathyroidism. *Am J Med* 59:104–113, 1975
12. Genant HK, Heck LL, Lanzl LH, Rossmann K, Horst JV, Paloyan JE: Primary Hyperparathyroidism. A comprehensive study of clinical, biochemical and radiographic manifestations. *Radiology* 109:513–524, 1973
13. Steinbach HL, Gordan GS, Eisenberg E, et al.: Primary hyperparathyroidism: a correlation of roentgen, clinical and pathologic features. *AJR* 86:329–343, 1961
14. King JD, Bobechko WP: Osteogenesis imperfecta. An orthopaedic description and surgical review. *JBJS* 53B:72–89, 1971

58. Prevention of Osteoporosis

Robert Lindsay, M.B.Ch.B., Ph.D., F.R.C.P.

Department of Medicine, Helen Hayes Hospital, Regional Bone Center, West Haverstraw, New York, and Department of Medicine, Columbia University, College of Physicians and Surgeons, New York, New York

An ounce of prevention is worth more than any amount of treatment.

The phenomenon of bone loss that precedes fracture is associated in cancellous bone with alterations in the microarchitecture that include complete loss of trabecular elements, a process that is mostly irreversible. It is clear, therefore, that the most efficient method of tackling these skeletal changes is their prevention. It may be that other strategies that are aimed at reducing the risk of injury among the elderly will also play a role in prevention of fracture, but such strategies are insufficiently developed, apart from some broad generalities, to put into clinical practice at present. The institution of any program of prevention requires most of all that it be safe, at least as much as it requires efficacy. Additionally it should ideally be inexpensive and applicable on a population basis. No such proven strategy for osteoporosis prevention exists. Therefore, there need to be available sufficiently stringent methods both of determining those most at risk, while excluding those who will not require intervention. Although this is also not entirely true for osteoporosis, there are methods that allow risk assessment that can be used in clinical practice and can form the basis for decision making about therapy.

IDENTIFICATION OF "AT-RISK" INDIVIDUALS

Bone loss is an asymptomatic process and in some ways can be considered clinically to be equivalent to hypertension. In each case patients present to the health care system when a complication arises, either fracture, in the case of osteoporosis, or stroke in hypertension. The key is each case is early identification of the patients at greatest risk, targeting those for intervention. For osteoporosis, these clues are divided into "risk factors" and estimates of skeletal status.

Risk Factor Assessment

As in many other disorders of aging a large number of factors (Table 1) have been incriminated in the pathogenesis of fractures among the elderly (1). Some clearly change the onset, duration, or rate of bone loss in individuals, whereas others increase fracture risk by modifying the risk of injury. Yet others may be linked by association that is statistically significant without any cause-and-effect relationship. Only relatively few are of value clinically, and even these suffer from the difficulties inherent in translating epidemiological data into clinical practice. Thus, clinical usefulness of such data is limited by a lack of understanding about the specific effects of each in the individual patient. The most frequently cited risk factors fall into four broad groups (Table 1). Superimposed on these are a variety of sporadic factors that can affect the skeleton, including chronic illness, disuse, and a wide variety of drugs (steroids, diuretics, thyroid hormone, gonadotropin-releasing hormone agonists, dilantin, tetracyclines, aluminum, and methotrexate).

In general, for each patient, the more risk factors present, and the longer the duration of their presence, the greater the risk of future problems (1). Physicians can use the presence of these factors in two ways. First, they can be used to sensitize the patient, and physician, to the like-

TABLE 1. *Proposed risk factors for osteoporosis*

Genetic
  Race
  Sex
  Familial prevalence
Nutritional
  Low calcium intake
  High alcohol
  High caffeine
  High sodium
  High animal protein
Lifestyle
  Cigarette use
  Low physical activity
Endocrine
  Menopausal age (oophorectomy)
  Obesity

lihood of osteoporosis. Second, those risk factors that are amenable to elimination or alteration should be discussed with the patient. Many risk factors also contribute to development of other diseases in organ systems other than bone, and should be discussed in those terms.

Practically, menopause is the usual time when evaluation of the patient for osteoporosis begins, although nutritional and lifestyle habits should be changed as early in life as possible. No combination of these risk factors indicates skeletal status for the individual patient. The analogy is again hypertension for which there is also a list of risk factors, but no assemblage of these predicts an individual patient's blood pressure. Nevertheless, risk factor review is often a useful "initial" approach to the patient.

Skeletal Status

The osteoporotic process is one of loss of bone tissue, which within cancellous bone is accompanied by disruption of the microarchitecture (2). For any individual we do not know whether the peak bone mass or the subsequent rate of loss is more important in determining fracture risk. Several issues support the concept that initial bone mass must be of some significant importance. Peak bone mass is primarily under genetic control and may be the familial factor in osteoporosis risk. Longitudinal data confirm that, because variance in bone mass does not change with age and those who start with less bone tend to track within the same region over time. Fracture prevalence and incidence have been shown to be greater in those with low bone mass at any age. Finally, several studies indicate that low bone mass is predictive of an increased fracture risk (3,4). This suggests that a single measurement of bone mass will provide information that can be used clinically to determine risk of osteoporosis.

Thus, measurement of bone mass plays an important role in evaluation of the asymptomatic patient. For a complete review of the techniques available for bone mass measurement, the reader is referred to Chapter 26. The clinician should learn the use of the techniques available in his/her area. Measurement of bone at any site is of

value, because all seem to predict the risk of *all* fractures equally well. However, if the clinician is interested in the fracture risk at a specific site, then a measurement at that site may be preferable. For most perimenopausal women, therefore, the preferred site is the spine, and the preferred technique, dual energy x-ray absorptiometry (DXA). However, if this technique is not available, the clinician is encouraged to use whichever is available. The analogies in clinical practice are the measurement of blood pressure as a risk assessment for cerebrovascular accident, cholesterol, or lipoprotein fractionation as risk factors for coronary heart disease. The National Osteoporosis Foundation has established clinical guidelines for the use of bone mass measurement (4). For perimenopausal and postmenopausal women bone mass measurement is a useful guide for the requirement of therapy. For patients who have asymptomatic vertebral abnormalities, bone mass measurement allows the diagnosis of osteoporosis to be confirmed or excluded. Women with bone mass in the lowest quartile of the range for young normal individuals would be most likely to benefit from preventative measures. Those with values above the fourth quartile can be treated more conservatively, although those in the next third quartile probably should be reviewed within 1–2 years.

CLINICAL PROTOCOL

Prevention of bone loss in asymptomatic women is generally achieved using two complementary approaches, behavior modification and pharmacologic intervention. Again this is similar to the management of hypertension and hypercholesterolemia.

The initial approach to the patient is based on modification of the risk factor profile. However, its effectiveness in patients with low bone mass is not established. Therefore, early pharmacologic intervention has become more widely used in this population. At the time of menopause, we evaluate each patient for the presence of risk factors, ascertained as part of a complete medical history. We assist in the modification of the patient's behavior to reduce the impact of the factors that are amenable to intervention. Elimination of secondary causes of osteoporosis is a mandatory part of this initial evaluation (see Chapters 56, 61 and 63).

For prevention of primary (postmenopausal) osteoporosis, alterations in nutrition and lifestyle form the preliminary approach, on the assumption that a reduction in risk factor profile will be beneficial. Reductions in alcohol consumption and elimination of cigarette use are amenable to intervention and are particularly detrimental to the patient's general health.

Physical Activity

Changing the pattern of physical activity may be difficult, especially for patients who are less positively motivated. This is especially true when discussing prevention with patients, who are, by definition, asymptomatic. Most of the patients seen in our clinic are at a relatively low level of fitness and require formal cardiovascular evaluation before beginning an exercise program. We suggest that the exercise activity chosen be fun to improve compliance. In the absence of proven benefit for any exercise for prevention of osteoporosis, any weight-bearing activity suffices (5). Recreational therapy, which has a social component, may serve to improve patient compliance. However, even simple activities such as walking are useful and can be added to the daily routine with minimal difficulty. Back-strengthening exercise is probably also of value, and patients may be referred to a trainer for specific instructions, because there may be limitations of exercises that force spinal flexion. In addition to any potential beneficial effects on the skeleton, continued activity in their daily lives reduces the risk of falls, trauma from falls, and fracture.

Calcium Supplementation

Although calcium is a nutrient and adequate intake should be obtained from nutritional sources (6), in practice it is difficult for many people to achieve a dietary intake >800 mg/day (the current recommended daily allowance). Self-imposed calorie restrictions and the avoidance of cholesterol results in limitation of dairy produce, the major source of dietary calcium in the Western world. Other sources of calcium include green vegetables, nuts, and certain fish. Bioavailability of calcium from foods is ~30%, with only calcium in spinach being unavailable for absorption.

In providing advice about calcium intake the intent is to ensure that the majority of the population obtain sufficient calcium to maintain calcium balance. Recommendations include an intake of 800 mg until age 10; 1,500 mg during adolescence; and 1,200 mg thereafter, increasing to 1,500 mg during pregnancy, lactation, and if at increased risk of osteoporosis (6). To achieve such intakes, it is commonly necessary to resort to calcium supplementation, and most individuals require only 500–1,000 mg/day as a supplement to dietary sources to achieve these intakes.

There are many forms of calcium available as supplement, and the advice to the patient should be a simple as possible. First, it is important that the calcium be bioavailable. Studies suggest that name brands are in general more soluble than generic varieties, and although some of the latter are clearly adequate, in general the former are preferred. Because calcium absorption is better in an acid environment for the carbonate, we recommend the supplement be taken with food. The addition of a modest calcium supplement to each meal is a regimen to which the patient can easily adhere. Both calcium carbonate and citrate offer the highest calcium content per unit tablet weight (40% and 30% respectively). Absorption of calcium as the citrate is slightly more efficient and not dependent on gastric acidity. However, this may not be biologically important for most patients, and citrate is generally more expensive.

At the recommended dietary intakes, calcium supplementation is virtually free of side effects. If eructation, intestinal colic, and constipation occur with the carbonate, then citrate is a useful alternative. Care should be taken in prescribing calcium supplements to patients with a history of renal stones. If urine calcium excretion is not increased, the citrate salt may be used.

Pharmacologic Therapy to Prevent Bone Loss

A considerable body of data supports the concept that estrogen administration to postmenopausal women reduces skeletal turnover and reduces the rate of bone loss (7). Epidemiological data indicate that estrogen use is associated with a reduction in the risk of fracture, especially fractures of the hip and wrist (Colles' fracture). Risk reduction averaged over several studies appears to be in the order of 50%. For vertebral fractures the interpretation of the few prospective data available suggest that estrogens also reduce the risk of vertebral fracture by as much as 75%.

Several general guidelines can be given for the use of estrogen for this indication. Because estrogens primarily reduce the rate of bone loss, the earlier therapy is begun, the more likely the bone mass and structure will be preserved. However, recent data suggest that estrogen therapy reduces the rate of bone loss in estrogen-deficient women independent of age, with reduction in bone loss among older individuals, at least up to the eighth decade (8). The minimum effective dose of estrogen for most individuals is 0.625 mg conjugated equine estrogen or its equivalent (9). Efficacy has been demonstrated for several other estrogens, including estradiol and estrone sulfate. It is also apparent that the route of administration is not important, and several studies have demonstrated that transdermal estrogen is effective (10).

The effects of estrogen continue for as long as treatment is provided, whereas bone loss ensues when treatment is discontinued at a rate comparable to the rate of bone loss that occurs immediately after ovariectomy. Prospective studies have confirmed the long-term efficacy of estrogen for at least 10 years.

Practical Aspects of Estrogen Administration

Although menopausal symptoms remain the most frequent indication for estrogen therapy, prevention of osteoporosis is becoming a more widely recognized indication for therapy for postmenopausal women. Treatment of menopausal symptoms are accompanied by an excellent response to therapy. For control of bone loss, however, the majority of patients are in the asymptomatic phase of bone loss. The physician always faces the problems in providing therapy for an asymptomatic phase of a disease whether it is hypertension, hypercholesterolemia, or osteoporosis. The epidemiological data that estrogens may reduce the risk of ischemic heart disease may be an added potential benefit for estrogen prescription. The potential complications of endometrial and breast malignancies must also be discussed with each patient.

When the patient presents for an assessment of the risk

of osteoporosis we begin with evaluation of the risk factors. It must be remembered that these factors do not allow clinically meaningful stratification of patients, and specifically do not identify individuals with low bone mass. Rather the assessment of these risk factors allows discussion of behaviors that should be changed to lower the risk of osteoporosis. When therapy is being considered specifically for osteoporosis prevention, a bone mass measurement allows determination of the future risk of fracture for the individual patient. The lower the bone mineral density, the greater the likelihood that therapy is required. As yet there are no specific guidelines on the level of bone mass that requires intervention, but certainly a value toward the lower quartile of the young normal range should prompt strong consideration of intervention. When bone mass is in average range ±1 SD for young adults, a wait-and-see approach can be proposed, with follow-up bone mass measurement at 1- or 2-year intervals. Those individuals at the upper end (first and second quartiles) of the young normal range are at low risk of osteoporotic fracture, and general health guidelines for nutrition and lifestyle may be is required.

In our clinic we include a discussion about the other effects of estrogen. Estrogens, given unopposed by progestins, increase the risk of endometrial hyperplasia and carcinoma. There is more doubt about the effect of estrogen on breast cancer, but long-term therapy (>15 years) may increase the risk slightly (10–30%) (11). On the other hand, estrogens alleviate menopausal symptoms, improve urogenital atrophy, and appear to reduce the risk of ischemic heart disease by as much as 50% (12). Estrogens have been associated with improved overall mortality, including reduction in mortality from breast cancer. Thus, estrogen use is considerably more complex than simply its effects on the skeleton.

The specific protocol for estrogen use remains a subject of considerable discussion and controversy. Some general recommendations can be made. All patients should have a mammography and be taught breast self-examination before therapy is initiated. The schedule for mammography in this age range should be based on the National Cancer Institute's guidelines and be independent of the decision to treat, but treatment certainly mandates it. If the patient has gone through a natural menopause and still has her uterus, combination or sequential therapy with a progestin is used to protect the endometrium (13). There is no rationale at present for progestin in patients who have undergone hysterectomy. There is no evidence that addition of a progestin will negatively impact on the estrogen effect on the skeleton. One study using norethindrone acetate, a 19-nortestosterone derivative suggested that there may be an additive effect when given along with estrogens (14). For younger women approaching menopause, we favor a sequential regimen. Estrogen is given every day, with rest periods at the end of each month for those who have significant mastalgia with therapy, whereas the progestin is given from the first of each calendar month for at least 12 days (2 weeks is often simpler). Most patients will have some endometrial shedding, often fairly light, between the 11th and 21st of each month (15). Recurrent bleeding not on that schedule requires investigation. The progestin dose should be the minimum required for endometrial protection. For medroxyprogesterone acetate, the most commonly used progestin in the United States, 5 mg/day is the minimum, but must be increased to 10 mg if bleeding is out of schedule. Norethindrone is available in 5 mg tablets in the United States, but this is an excessive dose. If there are symptoms with medroxyprogesterone acetate, norethindrone [one-half tablet/day (2.5 mg)] may be tried, or two tablets/day of the progestin, the only oral contraceptive that contains 0.35 mg/norgestrel tablet. The latter is an expensive regimen even when used for only 2 weeks each month. The estrogen dose required to reduce bone loss in most individuals is 0.625 mg conjugated equine estrogen or its equivalent (9). The 0.05 mg estradiol patch also appears to be sufficient (10). Because some patients will continue to lose bone on these doses (perhaps as many as 5–15%) measurement of bone mass after 1 year with the highly precise DXA technique may be advantageous. It is not clear if those individuals who lose bone on estrogen therapy are nonresponders or partial responders who will subsequently respond to an increase in the daily dose.

Older women and those who wish to avoid monthly vaginal bleeding may consider a combined continuous regimen. In this regimen the estrogen and progestin are both given each day of the month. The estrogen dose is similar to that recommended above, but the progestin dose may be reduced by one-half. This regimen is associated with some irregular, unheralded bleeding in the first 2–3 months of treatment in ~50% of patients, but close to 80% will become amenorrheic thereafter. Because the early bleeding is often light and may just be spotting, many patients will suffer this temporary inconvenience in return for the promise of no further bleeding. Long-term endometrial safety using the combined regimen are not available.

Side effects of therapy include occasional weight gain and rarely an idiosyncratic increase in blood pressure. Therefore, blood pressure should be measured in all patients after 3 months of therapy. Progestin side effects include irritability and mood swings, often described as being premenstrual, which may become sufficiently troublesome to require the progestin dose to be reduced to the minimum.

For prevention of osteoporosis, treatment should be continued for as long as feasible, at least 5–10 years. As a practical issue we review each patient on an annual basis and evaluate with her the benefits and her concerns regarding treatment. Modifications can be made at this time. We now use repeat measurements of bone mass by DXA to monitor patients to ensure that bone loss is not progressing. This can also be used as an aid to compliance, which is notably poor with estrogens, primarily because of bleeding and the perceived risk of cancer. An alternative to bone mass measurement is to measure the biochemical indices of bone remodeling before and at some time, often 3 months, after the institution of treatment. Estrogens are associated with a reduction in β-glycerophosphatase, alkaline, and acid phosphatase, and urinary hydroxyproline and deoxypyridinoline and pyridinoline cross-links (16). A biochemical response usually indicates a skeletal response, but may not be absolutely predictive. The high rate appears most often associated with failure to educate the patient adequately about the expected results of therapy and the potential problems. In practice once patients are established on therapy for 6 months to 1 year, they usually are comfortable remaining on treatment for many years thereafter.

The main contraindication to estrogen therapy is the presence or history of an estrogen-dependent tumor, especially breast malignancy. Other relative contraindications include undiagnosed vaginal bleeding, a prior history of endometrial malignancy (>3 years posthysterectomy), active thromboembolic disease, and grossly abnormal liver or renal function. Hypertension and diabetes are not contraindications, but must be controlled before therapy is begun.

Alternatives to Estrogen

In the United States, salmon calcitonin is a Food and Drug Administration (FDA)-approved alternative to estrogen for the treatment of osteoporosis, but not as yet been proven effective for prevention (17). The major disadvantages to salmon calcitonin are that it must be given by subcutaneous or intramuscular injection, and it is expensive. Preparations of salmon calcitonin, which can be given by intranasal spray, are effective in both prevention and treatment of osteoporosis through stabilization of bone mass. When the data from recent controlled studies conducted in the Untied States are evaluated by the FDA, it is possible that intranasal calcitonin will become an acceptable alternative to estrogen for prevention of the disease, especially for postmenopausal women who cannot or should not take estrogen. Calcitonin will also be a useful drug for prevention of steroid osteoporosis and for treatment of osteoporosis in men. The absence of significant side effects is a major advantage to calcitonin's use in primary prevention.

Another significant development likely to improve treatment for prevention of osteoporosis in the near future is the development of the class of drugs known as bisphosphonates (18). These agents are derivatives of pyrophosphate, but are not metabolized by the body. The bisphosphonates are potent inhibitors of bone remodeling; however, the mode of action of these drugs is still not entirely clear, and each of the bisphosphonates may affect remodeling with subtle but important differences. The agents appear to be well tolerated and to date are without significant side effects. The major advantages of bisphosphonates include the oral route of administration, and their dose may be titratable for individual patients. As yet no significant antifracture efficacy has been demonstrated, and none of these drugs are presently approved by the FDA for either treatment or prevention. Because of their low level of side effects, they may become important therapies in the prevention of osteoporosis of all types.

Certain progestins by themselves appear to have bone-sparing effects but are unlikely to be used in prevention. The addition of a progestin to estrogen, as previously noted, does not negatively impact on the skeletal effect of the estrogen, and certain progestins may enhance the bone-sparing effects of estrogens (14). For postmenopausal patients with a history of breast cancer, there is some evidence that the so-called antiestrogen, tamoxifen, in doses usually used to prevent cancer recurrence (20–30 mg/day) (19,20) may reduce the rate of bone loss and prevent osteoporosis, a potentially serious problem for this group of patients. Tamoxifen is not FDA-approved for osteoporosis prevention, and patients who are at high risk for breast cancer and who are on tamoxifen should have bone mass carefully monitored so that a bone-specific agent can be added early in the course of bone loss.

CONCLUSIONS

The initial approach to osteoporosis prevention consists of identification of those subjects likely to be at risk; behavior modification to eliminate risk factors and improve nutrition and lifestyle; and estrogen intervention, which remains the cornerstone of prevention for the postmenopausal patient. Calcitonin (injectable and nasal spray) and oral bisphosphonates may be alternatives available in the near future.

REFERENCES

1. Riggs BL, Melton LJ III: Involutional osteoporosis. *N Engl J Med* 314:1676–1686, 1986
2. Consensus Development Conference: Prophylaxis and treatment of osteoporosis. *Osteo Int* 1:114–126, 1991
3. Hui SL, Slemenda CW, Johnston CC Jr: Baseline measurement of bone mass predicts fracture in white women. *Ann Intern Med* 111:355–361, 1989
4. Johnston CC Jr, Melton LJ III, Lindsay R, et al.: Clinical indications for bone mass measurement. *J Bone Miner Res* 4:1–28, 1989
5. Dalsky GP, Stocke KS, Ehsani AA, et al.: Weight-bearing exercise training and lumbar bone mineral content in postmenopausal women. *Ann Intern Med* 108:824–828, 1988
6. Heaney RP: Effect of calcium on skeletal development, bone loss, and risk of fractures. *Am J Med* 91:23S–28S, 1991
7. Lindsay R: Sex steroids in the pathogenesis and prevention of osteoporosis. In: Riggs BL (ed) *Osteoporosis: Etiology, Diagnosis and Management*. Raven Press, New York, pp 333–358, 1988
8. Lindsay R, Tohme J: Estrogen treatment of patients with established postmenopausal osteoporosis. *Obstet Gynecol* 76:290–295, 1990
9. Lindsay R, Hart DM, Clark DM: The minimum effective dose of estrogen for prevention of postmenopausal bone loss. *Obstet Gynecol* 63:759–763, 1984
10. Stevenson JC, Cust MP, Gangar KF, et al.: Effects of transdermal versus oral hormone replacement therapy on bone density in spine and proximal femur in postmenopausal women. *Lancet* 336:265–269, 1990
11. Hulka BS: Hormone-replacement therapy and the risk of breast cancer. *Cancer* 40:289–296, 1990
12. Barrett-Connor E, Bush TL: Estrogen and coronary heart disease in women. *JAMA* 265:1861–1967, 1991
13. Voight LF, Weiss NS, Chu J, et al.: Progestogen supplementation of exogenous estrogens and the risk of endometrial cancer. *Lancet* 338:274–277, 1991
14. Christiansen C, Riis BJ: 17β-Estradiol and continuous norethistrone: A unique treatment for established osteoporosis in elderly women. *J Clin Endocrinol Metab* 71:836–841, 1990
15. Padwick ML, Pryse-Davies J, Whitehead MI: A simple method

for determining the optimal dosage of progestin in postmenopausal women receiving estrogen. *N Engl J Med* 315:930–934, 1986

16. Uebelhart D, Schlemmer A, Johansen JS, Gineyts E, Christiansen C, Delmas PD: Effect of menopause and hormone replacement therapy on the urinary excretion of pyridinoline crosslinks. *J Clin Endocrinol Metab* 72:367–373, 1991

17. Avioli LV, Gennari C: Calcitonin therapy in osteoporotic syndromes. In Avioli LV (ed). *The Osteoporotic Syndrome, 3rd ed.* Wiley Liss, New York, pp 137–154, 1992

18. Fleisch H: The possible use of bisphosphonates in osteoporosis. In DeLuca HF, Mazess R (eds) *Osteoporosis: Physiological Basis, Assessment and Treatment.* Elsevier, New York, pp 323–330, 1990

19. Turken S, Siris E, Seldin D, Lindsay R: Effects of tamoxifen on spinal bone density. *J Natl Cancer Inst* 81:1086–1088, 1989

20. Love RR, Mazess RB, Barden HS, et al.: Effects of tamoxifen on bone mineral density in postmenopausal women with breast cancer. *N Engl J Med* 326:852–856, 1992

59. Juvenile Osteoporosis

Michael E. Norman, M.D.

Department of Pediatrics, Alfred I. duPont Institute, Wilmington, Delaware, and Jefferson Medical College, Philadelphia, Pennsylvania

Diagnosis of osteoporosis in children is usually made when skeletal radiographs reveal a generalized decrease in mineralized bone (e.g., osteopenia) in the absence of rickets or excessive bone resorption (e.g., osteitis fibrosa). Juvenile osteoporosis occurs typically before the onset of puberty, but it may also be seen in younger children, especially when they are growing rapidly. It may be due to an inherited condition that is clinically evident from birth or early infancy, or it may be acquired during childhood. There is a primary or idiopathic form and a number of secondary forms of juvenile osteoporosis. The condition is uncommon; between 1939 and 1991 ~60 cases of idiopathic juvenile osteoporosis were reported in the literature. However, the onset of osteoporosis just before or after the onset of puberty can have far-reaching effects, because one-half of skeletal mass is acquired during the adolescent years.

PATHOPHYSIOLOGY

True osteoporosis is defined histomorphometrically by a decreased total amount of normally formed bone. During bone formation (modeling) and bone remodeling, two fundamental defects may occur, singly or in combination, including 1) a defect in bone-forming cells leading to decreased or defective matrix formation; and 2) abnormalities in the coupling of bone formation and resorption, in which an imbalance develops between matrix formation (mineralization) and bone resorption. An inherited group of disorders known as osteogenesis imperfecta represent a defect of bone-forming cells in which abnormal types of collagen produce defective matrix (see Chapter 77). Idiopathic juvenile osteoporosis (IJO) and the secondary causes of osteoporosis represent various expressions of the latter type of defect. Idiopathic juvenile osteoporosis and chronic corticosteroid therapy are the most important forms of acquired juvenile osteoporosis. Early reports of calcium balance suggested that IJO changes, with negative or inappropriately neutral balances initially (1,2), progressing to positive balance during the healing phase (2,3), and in response to vitamin D administration. Jowsey and

Johnson (4) and Hoekman et al. (5) presented histologic evidence for increased bone resorption, whereas Smith (6) and Evans et al. (7) found decreased bone formation as the major pathophysiologic event in IJO. Marder et al. (8) and Saggese et al. (9) suggested a role for 1,25-dihydroxyvitamin D deficiency in the pathogenesis of IJO. Several reports have also suggested a role for calcitonin deficiency in some patients (10). The bone loss noted in astronauts undergoing prolonged periods of weightlessness in space may be analogous to IJO with rapid resorption of weight-bearing bones and suppressed bone formation. Both weightlessness and IJO appear to be reversible (6). Some have speculated that IJO, like weightlessness, consists of some fundamental disturbance in the mechanical forces that stimulate new bone formation in the growing and young adult skeleton.

CLINICAL FEATURES

The typical child presenting with IJO is immediately prepubertal and healthy. Symptoms begin with an insidious onset of pain in the lower back, hips, and feet and difficulty walking. Knee and ankle pain and fractures of the lower extremities may be present. IJO affects both sexes equally; family and dietary histories are negative. Physical examination may be entirely normal, or reveal thoracolumbar kyphosis, or kyphoscoliosis, pigeon chest deformity, crown:pubis to pubis:heel ratio of less than 1.0, loss of height, deformities of the long bones, and limp. Generally, these physical abnormalities are reversible, although several of Dent's original patients subsequently developed crippling deformities that left them wheelchair-bound with cardiorespiratory abnormalities (1).

The history and physical examination of children with secondary forms of osteoporosis reflect the primary disease more than the osteoporosis (Table 1). There is usually a family history of osteoporosis or the primary disease, evidence of failure to thrive, immobilization, or administration of corticosteroid or anticonvulsant drugs.

TABLE 1. *Differential diagnosis of juvenile osteoporosis*

I. Primary
   A. Calcium Deficiency
   B. Idiopathic Juvenile Osteoporosis
   C. Osteogenesis Imperfecta
      1. Multiple subtypes
II. Secondary
   A. Endocrine
      1. Cushing's syndrome
      2. Diabetes mellitus
      3. Glucocorticoid therapy
      4. Thyrotoxicosis
   B. Gastrointestinal
      1. Biliary atresia
      2. Glycogen storage disease, type I
      3. Hepatitis
      4. Malabsorption
   C. Inborn Errors of Metabolism
      1. Homocystinuria
      2. Lysinuric protein intolerance
   D. Miscellaneous
      1. Acute lymphoblastic leukemia
      2. Anticonvulsant therapy
      3. Cyanotic congenital heart disease
      4. Immobilization

BIOCHEMICAL FEATURES

There are no known biochemical abnormalities characteristic of IJO, and no known endocrine disorder has been identified. In some children (1,2,5) calcium balance is markedly negative or inappropriately neutral, and serum calcium levels are normal. Urine calcium excretion may be normal or elevated. Serum phosphorus, bicarbonate, magnesium, and alkaline phosphatase levels are also normal. The disease eventually resolves with time and onset of puberty and can be detected by improvement in calcium balance. Increased urinary hydroxyproline excretion, an indirect indicator of increased bone resorption, hypercalcemia, and suppressed parathyroid hormone secretion have been observed in some patients. Suppression of parathyroid hormone secretion reduces 1,25-dihydroxyvitamin D synthesis and decreases intestinal calcium absorption contributing to the negative calcium balance (5).

In secondary forms of osteoporosis, biochemical and clinical clues to diagnosis depend on the underlying primary disease (2,7).

RADIOLOGIC FEATURES

Conventional radiography is a relatively insensitive method for detecting bone loss; ~30% of skeletal mineral must be lost before osteopenia can be appreciated. In the absence of fractures or rickets, osteomalacia may be difficult to distinguish from osteoporosis as the cause of osteopenia. Looser's lines or changes of secondary hyperparathyroidism favors rickets or osteomalacia, whereas biconcave vertebral deformities favor osteoporosis (see Chapter 24). Children with fully expressed IJO present with generalized osteopenia, fractures of the weight-bearing bones, and collapsed or misshapen vertebrae. Disc spaces may be widened asymmetrically due to wedging of the vertebral bodies (Fig. 1A,B). Sclerosis may be noted. Long bones are usually normal in length and cortical width, unlike the thin gracile bones of children with osteogenesis imperfecta (see Chapter 76). The pathognomonic x-ray finding of IJO is neoosseous osteoporosis, an impaction-type fracture occurring at sites of newly formed weight-bearing metaphyseal bone. Typically, such fractures are seen at the distal tibiae, adjacent to the ankle joint and adjacent to the knee and hip joints (2,6). Using photon absorptiometry and computerized axial tomography for detection of decreased bone mineral density, childhood osteoporosis may be diagnosed much earlier.

BONE BIOPSY

Few qualitative or quantitative studies of bone tissue have been performed in childhood osteoporosis. From microradiographs of bone, Cloutier et al. (3) and Jowsey and Johnson (4) reported increased bone resorption in IJO. They speculated that excessive dietary phosphorus intake may have stimulated parathyroid-mediated bone resorption. In contrast, Smith (6), using quantitative static histology of iliac bone, found indirect evidence for decreased bone formation. Evans et al. (7) found no abnormalities of endosteal bone formation by histomorphometry (using double tetracycline labeling) in a 12-year-old boy with severe IJO. They suggested that the major evidence for impaired periosteal new bone formation in IJO would come from careful study of skeletal radiographs and not from bone biopsy material.

DIFFERENTIAL DIAGNOSIS

Osteogenesis imperfecta is the most important entity to consider in the differential diagnosis of IJO (11). Comparisons with IJO are listed in Table 2 (see Chapter 76). Osteogenesis imperfecta can usually be differentiated from IJO by clinical characteristics, radiologic findings, and a positive family history. Diseases resulting in osteoporosis in childhood that must be differentiated from IJO are outlined in Table 1. Secondary causes of osteoporosis must be excluded in those children who present without the typical features of IJO. As a result, the diagnosis of IJO is reached by excluding secondary causes of osteoporosis and osteogenesis imperfecta.

THERAPY

Prompt and definitive diagnosis early in the course of the disease is important, although there is no specific medical or surgical therapy. Supportive care is instituted promptly (nonweight-bearing, crutch walking, and physical therapy) in anticipation of spontaneous recovery with onset of puberty. There may be a role for supplemental calcitriol therapy in selected patients (8,9). Sodium fluo-

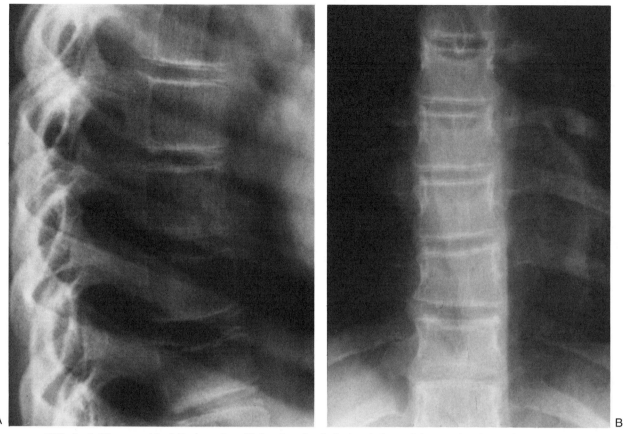

FIG. 1. A 10-year-old white female with back pain. **A:** Lateral view of thoracolumbar spine reveals wedge compression fracture of T8 and T9 with patchy sclerosis of T7. There was generalized osteopenia of the skeleton, confirmed by computerized axial tomography. **B:** Anterior view of the same patient reveals loss of height of T8 on the right side. The vertebral bodies are osteopenic.

ride increases bone mass and has been reported to reduce fracture rates in primary vertebral osteoporosis (12). Fluoride treatment has been associated with a number of toxicity symptoms and musculoskeletal complaints in adults, and it remains unclear if the hyperosteoidosis associated with this therapy produces increased bone strength. The author has used long-term fluoride therapy with a positive clinical response in one patient with IJO (unpublished observations). Based on findings of increased bone resorption on bone biopsy of one child, Hoekman et al. (5) re-

TABLE 2. *Differential diagnosis: osteogenesis imperfecta (OI) vs. idiopathic juvenile osteoporosis (IJO)*

Characteristic	OI	IJO
Family history	Often positive	Negative
Age of onset	Birth	2–3 yr before puberty
Duration of signs/symptoms	Lifelong	1–4 yr
Physical findings	Thin gracile bones	Upper:lower segment ratio <1.0
	Multiple deformities and contractures	Dorsal kyphoscoliosis
		Pectus carinatum
	Blue sclerae[a]	Abnormal gait
	Lax joints	
	Abnormal dentition	
Calcium balance	Positive	Negative in acute phase
Radiologic findings	Long narrow bones	Long bones with thin cortices
	Thin ribs	Wedge compression fractures of spine
	Pathologic fractures, rarely metaphyseal in location	Metaphyseal fractures common, with neoosseous osteoporosis
	Wormian skull bones	
Molecular studies (dermal fibroblasts)	Abnormal collagen	Normal collagen

[a] Classic dominant inherited form, with associated nerve deafness.

ported dramatic clinical, biochemical, and radiologic response with bisphosphonate, which inhibits bone resorption. Osteoporosis in most patients is reversible. Treatment of secondary causes of osteoporosis requires careful management of the underlying disease to minimize bone loss.

PROGNOSIS

With the exception of a few patients who develop progressive lower extremity, spine, and chest wall deformities and confinement to wheelchairs or bed, the prognosis of IJO is generally excellent. Distinguishing features have been recognized that identify the subgroup of children with poor prognosis. The prognosis of osteogenesis imperfecta is dependent on the inherited subtype and is discussed in Chapter 77. The most effective treatment of secondary osteoporosis is successful therapy of the underlying disease. Failing this, supportive care should be provided as with IJO.

REFERENCES

1. Dent CE, Friedman M: Idiopathic juvenile osteoporosis. *Q J Med* 34:177–210, 1965

2. Brenton DP, Dent CE: Idiopathic juvenile osteoporosis. In: Bickel JH, Stern J (eds) *Inborn Errors of Calcium and Bone Metabolism.* University Park Press, Baltimore, pp 223–238, 1976
3. Cloutier MD, Hayles AB, Riggs BL, Jowsey J, Bickel WH: Juvenile osteoporosis: Report of a case including a description of some metabolic and microradiographic studies. *Pediatrics* 40: 649–655, 1967
4. Jowsey J, Johnson KA: Juvenile osteoporosis: Bone findings in seven patients. *J Pediatr* 81:511–517, 1972
5. Hoekman K, Papapoulos SE, Peters ACB, Bijvoet OL: Characteristics and bisphosphonate treatment of a patient with juvenile osteoporosis. *J Clin Endocrinol Metab* 61:952–955, 1985
6. Smith R: Idiopathic osteoporosis in the young. *J Bone Joint Surg* 62-B:417–427, 1980
7. Evans RA, Dunstan CR, Hills E: Bone metabolism in idiopathic juvenile osteoporosis: A case report. *Calcif Tissue Int* 35:5–8, 1983
8. Marder HK, Tsang RC, Hug G, Crawford AC: Calcitriol deficiency in idiopathic juvenile osteoporosis. *Am J Dis Child* 136: 914–917, 1982
9. Saggese G, Bertelloni S, Baroncelli GI, Perri G, Calderazzi A: Mineral metabolism and calcitriol therapy in idiopathic juvenile osteoporosis. *Am J Dis Child* 145:457–461, 1991
10. Jackson EC, Strife CF, Tsang RC, Marder HK: Effect of calcitonin replacement therapy in idiopathic juvenile osteoporosis. *Am J Dis Child* 142:1237–1239, 1988
11. Teotia M, Teotia SPS, Singh RK: Idiopathic juvenile osteoporosis. *Am J Dis Child* 133:894–900, 1979
12. Harrison JE: Fluoride treatment for osteoporosis. *Calcif Tissue Int* 46:287–288, 1990

60. Regional Osteoporosis

Howard Duncan, M.D.

Rheumatology Division, Henry Ford Hospital, Detroit, Michigan

Localized osteoporosis is most often seen radiographically as an incidental finding in limbs that have been immobilized more than 4 weeks. Severe regional osteoporosis may occur with the reflex sympathetic dystrophy syndrome, a symptom complex characterized by severe pain, swelling, autonomic dysfunction, and impaired mobility of an extremity, which may occur without a precipitating cause.

The development of an acute, painful, swollen extremity following trauma, infection, or burn has been recognized for many centuries. Weir Mitchell in 1864 gave the classical description of the syndrome he called causalgia, which followed gunshot injury to a major nerve of the limb. Reflex sympathetic dystrophy syndrome is the term applied to a similar set of symptoms and signs when the peripheral nerve has not been injured. Precipitating events that have been associated with the reflex sympathetic dystrophy include trauma, surgical operation, acute cerebrovascular injuries, stroke, myocardial infarction, intrathoracic disease, primary diseases of the joints, drug therapy (barbiturates, antiepileptic agents, and antituberculous agents), malignancy, and pregnancy. Many cases of reflex sympathetic dystrophy syndrome have no precipitating event. Although typical forms involving a single

site may be readily diagnosed, many partial forms are overlooked. The variable presentations of the syndrome have resulted in several names for the syndrome, including algodystrophy, the preferred European term (1); Sudeck's atrophy; reflex neurovascular dystrophy; shoulder-hand syndrome; traumatic angiospasm; migratory osteoporosis; and transient osteoporosis.

CLINICAL FEATURES

Typical signs and symptoms include pain and swelling of an extremity, usually unilateral, that may become bilateral in 30% of patients. The pain is usually burning, aching, or even "bursting" and can be sufficiently intense to prevent movement of an affected digit or joint. Blowing on the skin may produce discomfort. Affected lower limbs may become more painful during weight-bearing. Signs of autonomic instability are usually present, including tight, shining, warm, and ruddy skin. Pallor, cyanosis, coldness, nonpitting edema, and hyperhidrosis may also be present.

The involved area is not limited to a dermatome, myotome, or peripheral nerve distribution, but may involve a foot, hand, knee, or shoulder. Partial or incomplete forms may exist involving a portion of the hand or foot, or one only of the femoral condyles at the knee may be involved with symptoms and signs localized to that side of the joint (2). Localized areas of involvement along with a preexisting illness, such as rheumatoid arthritis, may account for the rapid changes that are sometimes attributed to the underlying disease. Steinbrocker et al. (3) have described three distinct clinical stages of the syndrome. Although most patients pass through these distinct phases in a predictable pattern, overlap may be noted, or one stage may be completely bypassed.

Stage I may have a dramatic onset and last from 1–6 months. The main symptom is persistent deep burning pain aggravated by movement, contact, or emotional disturbance. The skin is warm, dry, or moist; hyperesthetic; tender to minor pressure; and accompanied by nonpitting edema. Usually, all digits are painful in the interarticular as well as the articular sites and are sensitive to palpation. Roentgenographic changes may show rapid demineralization in a patchy or diffuse distribution. The trabeculae in the immediate subchondral area undergo the most severe change, leaving the subchondral plate more clearly delineated than normal. A positive bone scan with technetium pertechnitate may develop before x-ray changes are evident and may identify early involvement of the opposite limb (4).

Stage II may last 3–6 months with partial resolution of some of the symptoms of stage I followed by a tendency for atrophy of the subcutaneous tissue, wasting of the interstitial muscles, thickening of joint capsules, stiffness with flexion deformity of the fingers, induration of the skin, and features reminiscent of scleroderma. At this juncture there is usually a marked degree of osteopenia.

Stage III is characterized by trophic changes and contracture of the skin and joints with x-ray evidence of severe demineralization.

Although single episodes are most common, symptoms may follow a migratory pattern. Individual episodes may last 6–9 months followed by spontaneous or assisted resolutions (5). A patient may experience six or more episodes.

PATHOGENESIS

The pathogenesis of these syndromes is not clear. The injured axons have increased sensitivity to norepinephrine and other substances released by local sympathetic nerves. The sensitivity is blocked by intravenous sympatholytic agents such as propanalol and auanethidine. New growth sprouts from injured nerves are known to be very sensitive to pressure and sympathetic amines. Increased orthodromic impulses on both A- and C-fibers and pressure on new free nerve endings may provide constant bursts of activity, particularly in response to touch. It is possible that injury to the smaller nerves and nerve terminals produces reflex sympathetic dystrophy (algodystrophy), whereas injury to the larger nerves produces causalgia.

LABORATORY FEATURES

There are usually no characteristic biochemical abnormalities. The sedimentation rate may be elevated, depending on the presence of a primary, precipitating process.

RADIOGRAPHY

Radiological changes may occur rapidly during the first 3 or 4 weeks. The majority of patients have patchy demineralization in the affected area, either involving a whole region (hand or foot) or a portion of the limb. Bilateral x-rays are suggested because the earliest changes may be subtle. The most marked changes occur in the articular surfaces of subchondral bone where the support trabeculae may rapidly diminish in size and number. Trabecular bone loss exaggerates the definition of the subchondral plate, which appears as a pencil line between the joint space cavity and remaining trabeculae. The pattern of bone loss is often patchy in the earlier phases of hip and knee involvement, with only a segment of the end of the bone affected (6,7). Occasionally, a band of demineralization up to 1-cm wide may occur in children and young adults, particularly in the old epiphyseal growth plate. The cause is not clear, but may accompany other demineralizing disorders. Cortical streaking or lacunae representing the "remodeling space" in high-turnover bone is a feature of the radiography. Short-term illness of 3 months or less may have no detectable loss of trabeculae. Chronic involvement, 6–9 months, is usually associated with loss of some trabeculae, whereas the remaining trabeculae may become thickened and more prominent with reactivation of the limb. Cortical bone width may remain diminished.

SCINTIGRAPHY

Affected joints occasionally develop small non-inflammatory effusions and small justaarticular joint erosions in the early phase of the disease (4). Technetium-99 bone scans are more sensitive and can demonstrate affected areas, both symptomatic and asymptomatic.

THERAPY

Early therapeutic intervention is important. Pain control with nonsteroidal and antiinflammatory agents is the initial choice, but stronger analgesics may be necessary. Protective and assisted mobilization of the affected limb is essential to prevent disuse and to control peripheral edema. Vigorous physical therapy is essential, and treatment of any underlying condition imperative.

Oral glucocorticoids (30–40 mg of prednisone) (4,5) in the first 4–6 weeks for 2 weeks may be useful to reduce the high-turnover metabolic state. Sympathetic blockade with local anesthetic (lidocaine or bupevocaine) have been useful. β-Blocking agents such as propanalol have been used and require monitoring of the peripheral pulse. Guanethidine can be injected into vessels proximal to the occlusion. None of these therapeutic programs have been tested by double-blind trials; however, in a modified trial, calcitonin has been very effective (1). The use of antidepressants, splints, psychotherapy, acupuncture, and electric stimulation (TENS-transcutaneous nerve stimulating unit) have all been used with other therapeutic regimens, with inconclusive results.

REFERENCES

1. Doury P, Dirheimer Y, Pattin S: *Algodystrophy: Diagnosis and Therapy of a Frequent Disease of the Locomotor Apparatus.* Springer Verlag, New York, 1981
2. Lagier R: Partial algodystrophy of the knee. *J Rheum* 10:255–260, 1983
3. Steinbrocker O, Spitzer N, Friedman H: The shoulder-hand syndrome in reflex dystrophy of the upper extremity. *Ann Intern Med* 29:22–52, 1948
4. Kozin F, McCarty DJ, Sims J, Genant H: The reflex sympathetic dystrophy syndrome. *Am J Med* 60:321–337, 1976
5. Duncan H, Frame B, Frost HM, Arnstein R: Regional migrating osteoporosis. *South Med J* 62:41–44, 1969
6. Lequesne M: Transient osteoporosis of the hip: A non-traumatic variety of Sudek atrophy. *Ann Rheum Dis* 27:463, 1968
7. Lakharpal S, Ginsburg WW, Luthra HS, Hunder GC: Transient osteoporosis: A study of 56 cases and a review of the literature. *Ann Intern Med* 106:444–450, 1987

61. Steroid and Drug-Induced Osteopenia

Theodore J. Hahn, M.D.

*Division of Geriatrics and GRECC, West Los Angeles Veterans
Administration Medical Center, Los Angeles, California*

GLUCOCORTICOID-INDUCED OSTEOPENIA

Clinical Features

Cushing's disease or chronic treatment with pharmacologic doses of glucocorticoids frequently produces a severe osteopenia that clinically resembles age-related osteoporosis. On occasion, typical Cushingoid features may not be apparent, and the osteopenia can be the major presenting problem. The disorder appears to be the result of 1) direct glucocorticoid suppression of osteoblastic bone-forming activity and 2) increased bone resorption caused by parathyroid hormone (PTH) stimulation of osteoclastic activity. Bone loss is more severe in those regions of the skeleton with a high content of trabecular bone. Thus, fractures are especially common in the ribs, vertebrae, and ends of long bones. Chronic glucocorticoid therapy is by far the most common iatrogenic cause of osteopenia and is a major risk factor for bone loss. The reported incidence of bone fractures in steroid-treated patients ranges from 8–18% and is 2- to 3-fold greater than in similar patients treated with other agents (1).

There are a number of *risk factors* (Table 1) for the development of glucocorticoid-induced osteopenia (1–3). A direct relationship has been demonstrated between the cumulative dose of glucocorticoids and both the degree of bone loss and the incidence of bone fractures. Moreover, patients with inflammatory arthritis exhibit a greater degree of bone loss, presumably due to the additive effects of relative immobilization, although the systemic effects of increased interleukin-1, interleukin-6, and tumor necrosis factor production may also play a role. Age, meno-

pausal status and activity level are important determinants of fracture risk. The incidence of clinically significant osteopenia is highest in children, postmenopausal women, patients of both sexes over the age of 50, and relatively immobilized individuals. In older, immobilized, and postmenopausal patients, a preexisting low level of bone mass predisposes to the rapid development of clinically significant osteopenia. In younger individuals, the high rate of bone turnover predisposes to more rapid bone loss. Current data indicates that a rapid loss of bone occurs immediately after the initiation of glucocorticoid therapy, with 12–15% or more loss of trabecular mass occurring over the first 12–18 months followed by a less marked acceleration in the rate of bone loss thereafter (4,5).

The *biochemical changes* in patients with glucocorticoid-induced osteopenia are generally not striking (6). Fasting serum calcium, phosphate, and vitamin D metabolite levels are usually within normal limits. The serum immunoreactive PTH (iPTH) concentration may be normal or mildly elevated. Serum alkaline phosphatase and osteocalcin levels decline progressively after the initiation of glucocorticoid therapy, reflecting the decline in osteoblastic bone forming activity (7,8). However, alkaline phosphatase values usually remain within the normal range, and increase transiently following bone fractures. Urinary calcium excretion is frequently increased during the first several years of steroid therapy, despite the fact that intestinal calcium absorption is reduced. This calciuric effect apparently reflects both a "spillover" of calcium not assimilated into bone due to suppressed osteoblastic activity, combined with a direct calciuric effect

TABLE 1. *Risk factors for glucocorticoid-induced osteopenia*

Major
  High total cumulative dose of glucocorticoids
  Age <15 or >50 years
  Postmenopausal status
Secondary
  Long duration of glucocorticoid therapy
  Disorders associated with increased interleukin-1, interleukin-6, or tumor necrosis factor production (e.g., rheumatoid arthritis)
  General osteoporosis risk factors
    Female sex
    Caucasian or Asian ancestry
    Relative immobilization
    Small body build

of glucocorticoids at the renal level. However, after several years of glucocorticoid therapy, urinary calcium excretion usually declines to within the normal range.

Pathogenesis

Glucocorticoid excess produces bone loss primarily by suppressing osteoblast function. An additional contributing factor is the inhibition of intestinal calcium absorption leading to mild secondary hyperparathyroidism and increased osteoclastic bone resorption (Fig. 1). In addition, glucocorticoids also promote bone loss by directly stimulating renal calcium excretion, and may possibly directly stimulate PTH secretion and enhance osteoclastic responsiveness to PTH (1). The suppression of osteoblastic bone-forming activity is apparently a direct effect of glucocorticoids (9). Inhibition of osteoblast precursor maturation, suppression of the stimulatory autocrine effects of prostaglandins and growth factors, and enhancement of the inhibitory effects of PTH on mature osteoblast function may all contribute to reduced osteoblast activity (10).

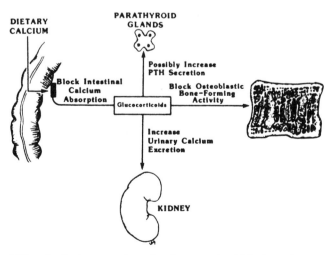

FIG. 1. Pathogenesis of glucocorticoid-induced osteopenia.

The decrease in intestinal calcium absorption produced by glucocorticoids appears to be caused by a direct inhibitory effect on intestinal mucosal cell function, because there are no significant alterations in serum vitamin D metabolite levels (6,8). Bone histology demonstrates reduced osteoblast number and function, and increased osteoclastic bone resorption (6).

Diagnosis and Management

The diagnosis of steroid-induced osteopenia is made on the basis of the clinical situation and the exclusion of other causes of osteopenia. Occasionally, bone biopsy may be helpful in this regard. Following adrenalectomy in patients with Cushing's disease, there is histologic evidence of increased bone mass. A similar rebound increase in bone-forming activity also occurs following the discontinuation of chronic glucocorticoid therapy (11). This presumably reflects a normal osteoblastic response to weight-bearing stress on reduced bone mass following removal of the inhibitory effects of glucocorticoids. However, bone mass is not restored to previous levels and usually remains markedly subnormal. In patients maintained on chronic steroid therapy, reducing the *glucocorticoid dose* to the lowest possible level should be of benefit in reducing deleterious effects on bone mass, (Table 2)

TABLE 2. *Management of glucocorticoid-induced osteopenia*

Prophylaxis
  1. Maintain glucocorticoid dose at lowest possible level.
  2. General measures
    a. Maintain regular program of weight-bearing physical activity.
    b. Maintain adequate intake of calcium (800–1,200 mg/day premenopausal and 1,500–2,000 mg/day postmenopausal) and vitamin D (400–800 U/day).
    c. Eliminate adverse health habits—smoking and alcohol excess.
  3. Reduce urinary calcium loss with hydrochlorothiazide.
  4. Start estrogen replacement therapy in postmenopausal women unless contraindicated.
  5. Consider prophylactic calcitonin or diphosphonate therapy in high-risk patients.
  6. Follow serum testosterone levels in men and start testosterone replacement therapy when indicated.
Established Osteopenia
  1. Rule out endocrine disorders, osteomalacia, and multiple myeloma.
  2. Maintain glucocorticoid dose at lowest possible level.
  3. Use general measures as for prophylaxis.
  4. Reduce urinary calcium loss with hydrochlorothiazide.
  5. Maintain normal gonadal hormone status—estrogen replacement therapy in postmenopausal or amenorrheic women and testosterone replacement where indicated in men.
  6. Start calcitonin or diphosphonate therapy.

although significant osteopenia has been observed in patients treated chronically with doses as low as 7.5–10 mg prednisone/day (1). Also, although animal studies have suggested that alternate-day glucocorticoid regimens may reduce the severity of bone loss, clinical studies have failed to demonstrate any significant advantage of such regimens with regard to bone loss and fracture incidence in man (12). The use of short-acting glucocorticoids where possible should theoretically be of benefit. Deflazacort, a recently developed oxazoline derivative of prednisolone, has been reported to have reduced deleterious effects on bone mass relative to its antiinflammatory actions (5). However, long-term controlled studies will be required to confirm that this property results in decreased fracture incidence.

It would be highly desirable to have an effective means of directly *stimulating bone formation*. Weight-bearing exercise can be helpful, but there are obvious limits to this approach. Sodium fluoride administration has been suggested to be of possible potential benefit on the basis of its ability to stimulate increased bone density and increased trabecular bone volume in steroid-treated patients (13). Also, short-term studies have shown a stimulatory effect of nandrolone deconate on bone density in postmenopausal women on glucocorticoids (14). However, these regimens remain unproven in glucocorticoid osteopenia. In contrast, reduced serum testosterone levels occur frequently in steroid-treated males due to the suppression of adrenal androgen production and such individuals should be treated with appropriate testosterone supplementation (e.g., 50–200 mg testosterone ethantate intramuscularly every 3 weeks) to help maintain bone and muscle mass.

On the other hand, *inhibiting bone resorption* is more readily accomplished and appears to be of benefit. Earlier studies demonstrated that the reduced intestinal calcium absorption in patients on glucocorticoids could be reversed by administering *vitamin D* (50,000 U) 2–3 times weekly, or 25-hydroxyvitamin D [25OHD (40–50 μg/day)], in combination with calcium (500 mg/day) (6). This produced a suppression of PTH levels, an increase in bone mass relative to controls, and improved bone histology. However, bone mass values remained below normal levels. Moreover, vitamin D metabolite therapy carries with it a significant risk of hypercalciuria and hypercalcemia, and requires biochemical monitoring at monthly intervals. On the other hand, supplementation with *calcium* (1,000 mg/day) can somewhat reduce bone resorption and decrease the loss of bone mass (15), and is a relatively safe regimen. A complementary approach is to reduce urinary calcium loss with *hydrochlorothiazide* (25 mg twice daily). Thiazide therapy has been shown to reduce serum PTH levels in glucocorticoid-treated patients (16) and will also reduce the risk of hypercalciuria. In peri- or postmenopausal women, estrogen replacement therapy should be instituted where possible to reduce bone loss (17).

Short-term studies of parenteral *calcitonin* administration in steroid-treated patients have shown a significant reduction of bone loss. In one recent study, patients treated prophylactically with calcitonin intramuscularly (100 U daily for 1 month, then every other day) experienced no significant loss of vertebral bone mass for 2 years after the initiation of moderate-dose prednisone therapy, in contrast to a 15% loss in the control group (18). *Diphosphonates* may prove to have a major role in the treatment of glucocorticoid osteopenia. In patients treated chronically with glucocorticoids, oral pamidronate (APD) administration produced an initial increase in appendicular and vertebral bone density followed by stabilization of bone mass over the subsequent 18 months, in association with biochemical evidence of reduced bone resorption (19). Sodium etidronate, the only diphosphonate currently available in the United States, has not been examined for its efficacy in steroid osteomalacia.

In summary, the first approach to minimizing glucocorticoid-induced bone loss is to maintain an intake of 400–800 U vitamin D and 1,500–2,000 mg calcium/day. Hydrochlorothiazide is a useful adjuvant to reduce urinary calcium losses. Weight-bearing exercise, especially walking, should be encouraged to stimulate bone-forming activity, and gonadal hormone deficiencies should be promptly corrected. Calcitonin and the diphosphonates appear to be potentially useful agents for preventing or partially reversing bone loss. However, the efficacy of all of these regimens in reducing fractures remains to be demonstrated.

ANTICONVULSANT DRUG-INDUCED MINERAL DISORDERS

Clinical Features

Chronic treatment with anticonvulsant drugs can produce a variety of disorders of vitamin D, mineral, and bone metabolism. Among the most common abnormalities are hypocalcemia, increased serum alkaline phosphatase, reduced serum 25OHD levels, mildly increased serum PTH concentration, decreased bone mass, increased fracture incidence, and histologic evidence of osteomalacia (1). Most of these clinical manifestations appear to be the result of two processes: drug-induced alterations in the hepatic metabolism of vitamin D and direct inhibitory effects of certain drugs on cellular function. This group of drug-induced mineral disorders is commonly referred to as "anticonvulsant osteomalacia."

The reported *incidence* of this disorder varies from 4–70%, depending on the population studied and the sensitivity of the techniques used. Anticonvulsant osteomalacia presents a rather broad clinical spectrum. Rarely, a patient may present with a full-blown clinical picture of repeated bone fractures, marked hypocalcemia and hypophosphatemia, proximal myopathy, severe osteopenia with radiographic signs of rickets (in children) or pseudofractures (in adults), and florid osteomalacia on bone biopsy. However, the usual patient has a much more subtle presentation. Bone symptoms are often minimal or absent, serum calcium, phosphate, and alkaline phosphatase concentrations may lie within, or close to, the normal range, and routine x-rays may not reveal clear-cut osteopenia. In most large series, the average reduction in serum calcium concentration is on the order of 0.3–0.8

mg/dL, whereas the incidence of frank hypocalcemia varies from 4 to 30%, and alkaline phosphatase levels are elevated in 24–40% of patients (1).

The use of sensitive techniques permits demonstration of significant abnormalities in a large proportion of patients (20–22). For example, serum 25OHD concentrations in anticonvulsant-treated patients are reduced by 40–70% relative to matched controls. In addition, mild elevations of serum iPTH occur in a significant number of patients, correlating inversely with serum calcium and 25OHD levels. Using photon-absorption techniques, it has been demonstrated that mean bone mass in anticonvulsant-treated patients is reduced by 10–30% relative to age-normal values.

Within any group of anticonvulsant-treated patients there is a wide range in the severity of clinical manifestations, and a number of specific *risk factors* (1) affect the presentation of the disorder (Table 3). Drug dose and duration of therapy are extremely important factors in determining the incidence of clinical abnormalities. Multiple-drug regimens produce more severe reductions in serum calcium, 25OHD, and bone mass than do single-drug regimens. Moreover, the larger the total daily drug dose, the more severe are the derangements in mineral metabolism. In addition, the incidence of abnormalities increases with the duration of therapy, although significant changes in mineral parameters have been observed after as little as 6 months of treatment. Among the most commonly implicated drugs are phenobarbital, diphenylhydantoin, and mesantoin. Other drugs capable of inducing increased hepatic oxidase enzyme activity, such as gluthetimide and rifampin (1,23), can produce similar disorders.

In both normal individuals and in patients on anticonvulsant therapy, *serum 25OHD levels* correlate with vitamin D intake (20,21). However, at any given level of intake, mean 25OHD levels in anticonvulsant-treated patients are lower than those in control subjects, and the degree of reduction in 25OHD correlates directly with the total daily drug dose. On average, anticonvulsant drug therapy increases the average vitamin D intake required to maintain normal serum 25OHD levels by 400–1,000 U/day. Hence, suboptimal vitamin D intake is associated with an increased incidence of mineral disorders in patients on anticonvulsant drugs. Sunlight exposure, which increases cutaneous production of vitamin D_3, is another major source of vitamin D in man. In situations where sunlight exposure is reduced, the incidence of vitamin D deficiency is increased. Thus, the incidence of biochemical and radiologic abnormalities is much higher in institu-

tionalized or elderly patients who are largely confined indoors. However, even among outpatients, serum 25OHD and calcium levels are lower in individuals with limited sunlight exposure. Seasonal changes in sunlight exposure may also play a role, because the period of lowest 25OHD concentration and greatest risk of disordered mineral metabolism is during the winter months.

In severe or atypical cases of epilepsy, various forms of *adjuvant therapy* may be used that can aggravate the disordered state of mineral metabolism. Acetazolamide, often used in poorly controlled patients, accelerates the course of drug-induced osteomalacia, probably due both to its phosphaturic effect and to the production of a systemic acidosis that may both directly accelerate bone loss and also impair renal 1,25-dihydroxyvitamin D production (1). Similarly, the deleterious effects of ketogenic diet therapy may also be attributable to the production of a systemic acidosis (24). Reduced physical activity, due either to the sedative effects of the anticonvulsant drugs or to the effects of associated neurologic disorders, appears to contribute to the severity of the osteopenia by reducing the weight-bearing stimulus for bone formation. Radiologic evidence of osteopenia in anticonvulsant-treated patients occurs most commonly in nonambulatory individuals. Indeed, a significant portion of the osteopenia seen in many patients on anticonvulsant drugs may be the result of chronic physical inactivity.

Pathogenesis

Many drugs, including virtually all of the common anticonvulsants, stimulate increased *hepatic microsomal mixed function oxidase* activity. One major consequence of this action is that degradative metabolism of steroid hormones such as estrogens, androgen, and cortisol is increased 2- to 4-fold in individuals treated with high doses of these drugs. However, hypothalamic-pituitary axis feedback regulation maintains normal levels of these steroid hormones in most cases. The vitamin D sterols share this hepatic microsomal degradative pathway, and thus chronic anticonvulsant drug administration results in a marked acceleration of the serum disappearance of vitamin D and 25OHD, with an associated increase in the rate of appearance of polar, biologically inactive products that are excreted in the bile and urine (25). However, feedback regulation of serum 25OHD levels is limited, because vitamin D input is dependent on intake and sunlight exposure, and the hepatic production of 25OHD is subject to only modest feedback control. Hence, drug-induced acceleration of hepatic inactivation of the vitamin D sterols can readily reduce serum 25OHD levels. In situations where vitamin D input is limited, reduction of serum 25OHD to levels of 2–10 ng/mL, a range corresponding to vitamin D deficiency, is often achieved. Serum 24,25-dihydroxyvitamin D levels are reduced in parallel with 25OHD. However, early in the course of the disorder serum 1,25-dihydroxyvitamin D is usually normal, or even mildly elevated in response to the secondary hyperparathyroidism resulting from decreased intestinal calcium ab-

TABLE 3. *Risk factors for anticonvulsant osteomalacia*

1. High-dose, multiple drug regimens
2. Long duration of therapy
3. Low vitamin D intake and limited sunlight exposure
4. Reduced level of physical activity
5. Use of adjuvant regimens such as acetazolamide or ketogenic diet
6. Use of other hepatic enzyme-inducing drugs such as gluthetimide or rifampin

sorption, and then subsequently declines with increasing vitamin D deficiency.

In addition, anticonvulsant drugs have direct *effects on cellular metabolism* independent of their effects on vitamin D. This is particularly true for diphenylhydantoin (DPH), which inhibits cation transport in a variety of tissues (1). For example, DPH causes a direct inhibition of intestinal calcium transport, and supranormal levels of vitamin D metabolites are required to maintain normal intestinal calcium transport in patients on DPH therapy. Moreover, both phenobarbital and DPH directly inhibit the bone resorptive response to PTH and vitamin D metabolites, although DPH is far more potent in this regard (26). In addition, DPH has been shown to suppress collagen formation directly by bone explants *in vitro* (27). Thus, DPH directly suppresses both osteoblastic and osteoclastic activity *in vitro,* a pattern that contrasts with the increased osteoclastic activity seen in patients with severe vitamin D deficiency. Clearly, the net effect of anticonvulsant drugs on bone cell metabolism *in vivo* represents a summation of the effects of decreased vitamin D metabolite levels, increased PTH secretion, and the direct effects of anticonvulsant drugs on cellular function. In general, when vitamin D levels are low, bone histology demonstrates osteomalacia and increased osteoclastic activity, whereas anticonvulsant-treated patients with relatively normal vitamin D metabolite levels often exhibit reduced osteoblastic and osteoclastic activities.

Diagnosis and Treatment

The diagnosis of anticonvulsant osteomalacia should be suspected on the basis of a history of chronic anticonvulsant drug treatment and the presence of one or more of the risk factors discussed previously. Reduced fasting serum calcium and phosphate levels, and an elevated alkaline phosphatase, are often but not invariably present. Twenty-four-hour urinary calcium excretion is usually reduced below 1 mg/kg body weight. The diagnosis is established by the above criteria in combination with a reduced serum 25OHD level, mildly increased serum iPTH, and osteopenia documented by dual-beam absorptiometry or quantitated computed tomography measurement of lumbar spine bone density. When the diagnosis is uncertain, bone biopsy may be helpful.

In patients with established disease characterized by osteopenia and reduced serum 25OHD and calcium levels, appropriate initial treatment consists of ~100,000 U vitamin D/1.7 m² body area/week in divided doses, plus 1,000 mg calcium/day (1,22). Alternately, 25OHD₃ (50 μg three times weekly) plus calcium supplementation are also effective (Table 4). This regimen is continued with appropriate adjustments in dose for a period of 6–24 months until the biochemical parameters (serum and urine calcium and serum 25OHD) are normalized, and the lumbar spine bone mass, measured at 6-month intervals, has reached normal levels or has stabilized. At that point, chronic maintenance therapy with 800 U vitamin D plus 1,000 mg calcium/day is begun. This dose of vitamin D is conveniently given as two standard multivitamin tablets

TABLE 4. *Management of anticonvulsant-induced osteomalacia*

Prophylaxis
1. Maintain 800 U vitamin D plus 800 mg calcium/day.
2. Maintain physical activity as possible.
3. Avoid adjuvant regimens and hepatic enzyme-inducing drugs where possible.

Established Osteopenia
1. Rule out other osteopenic disorders.
2. Vitamin D [50,000 U (or 25-hydroxyvitamin D)] 1–3 times/week plus calcium (1,000 mg/day) for 6–24 months until biochemical parameters are normalized and bone mass is stabilized.
3. Maintain physical activity as possible.

daily. It is extremely important to carefully monitor 24-hr urine calcium excretion and serum calcium levels during high-dose vitamin D treatment to reduce the risk of inadvertent overdosage. If 24-hr urine calcium excretion exceeds 4 mg/kg body weight, vitamin D should be discontinued. Patients being started on long-term anticonvulsant therapy should be placed on a prophylactic regimen of 800 U vitamin D/day plus calcium supplementation to reduce the risk of clinically significant mineral disorders.

REFERENCES

1. Hahn TJ: Drug-induced disorders of vitamin D and mineral metabolism. *Clin Endocrinol Metab* 9:107–129, 1980
2. Dykman TR, Gluck OS, Murphy WA, Hahn TJ, Hahn BH: Evaluation of factors associated with glucocorticoid-induced osteopenia in patients with rheumatic diseases. *Arthr Rheum* 28: 361–368, 1985
3. Als OS, Gotfredsen A, Christiansen C: The effect of glucocorticoids on bone mass in rheumatoid arthritis patients. Influence of menopausal state. *Arthr Rheum* 28:369–375, 1985
4. LoCascio V, Bonucci E, Imbimbo B, Ballanti P, Tartarotti D, Galvanni G, Fucella L, Adami S: Bone loss after glucocorticoid therapy. *Calcif Tiss Int* 36:435–438, 1984
5. Olgaard K, Storm T, van Wooeren N, Daugaard H, Egfjord M, Lewin E, Brabdi L: Glucocorticoid-induced osteoporosis in the lumbar spine, forearm, and mandible of nephrotic patients: A double-blind study on the high-dose, long-term effects of prednisone versus deflazacort. *Calcif Tiss Int* 50:490–497, 1992
6. Hahn TJ, Halstead SL, Hahn BH: Altered mineral metabolism in glucocorticoid-induced osteopenia: Effect of 25-hydroxyvitamin D administration. *J Clin Invest* 64:655–665, 1979
7. Reid IR, Chapman GE, Fraser TRC, Davies AD, Surus AS, Meyer J, Huq NL, Ibbertson HK: Low serum osteocalcin levels in glucocorticoid-treated asthmatics. *J Clin Endocrinol Metab* 62:378–388, 1986
8. Hahn TJ, Halstead LR, Baran DT: Effects of short-term glucocorticoid administration on intestinal calcium absorption and circulating vitamin D metabolite concentration in man. *J Clin Endocrinol Metab* 52:111–115, 1981
9. Canalis E: Effects of glucocorticoids on type I collagen synthesis, alkaline phosphatase activity, and deoxyribonucleic acid content in cultured rat calvariae. *Endocrinology* 112:931–939, 1983
10. Raisz LG, Kream BE: Regulation of bone formation. *N Engl J Med* 309:29–36, 83–89, 1983
11. Pocock NA, Eisman JA, Dunstan CR, Evans RA, Thomas DH, Huq NL: Recovery from steroid-induced osteoporosis. *Ann Intern Med* 107:319–323, 1987

12. Gluck OS, Murphy WA, Hahn TJ, Hahn B: Bone loss in adults receiving alternate day glucocorticoid therapy. A comparison with daily therapy. *Arthr Rheum* 24:892–898, 1981

13. Spector S, Greenwald M, Silverman SA: Successful treatment of osteoporosis due to steroid-dependent COPD and asthma. *Am Rev Respir Dis* 139:A16, 1989

14. Need AG: Corticosteroids and osteoporosis. *Aus NZ J Med* 17: 267–272, 1987

15. Reid IR, Ibbertson HK: Calcium supplements in the prevention of steroid-induced osteoporosis. *Am J Clin Nutr* 44:287–290, 1986.

16. Suzuki Y, Ichikawa Y, Homma M: Importance of increased urinary calcium excretion in the development of secondary hyperparathyroidism patients under glucocorticoid therapy. *Metabolism* 32:151–157, 1983

17. Lukert BP, Johnson BE, Robinson RG: Estrogen and progesterone replacement therapy reduces glucocorticoid-induced bone loss, *J Bone Miner Res* 7:1063–1069, 1992

18. Montemurro L, Schiraldi G, Fraioli P, Tosi G, Riboldi A, Rizzato G: Prevention of corticosteroid-induced osteoporosis with salmon calcitonin. *Calcif Tiss Int* 49:71–76, 1991

19. Reid IR, Schooler BA, Steward AW: Prevention of glucocorticoid-induced osteoporosis. *J Bone Miner Res* 5:619–623, 1990

20. Hahn TJ, Hendin BA, Scharp CR, Haddad JG: Effect of chronic anticonvulsant therapy on serum 25-hydroxycholecalciferol levels in adults. *N Engl J Med* 287:900–904, 1972

21. Hahn TJ, Hendin BA, Scharp CR, Boisseau VC, Haddad JG: Serum 25-hydroxycalciferol levels and bone mass in children on chronic anticonvulsant therapy. *N Engl J Med* 292:550–554, 1975

22. Hahn TJ, Halstead LR: Anticonvulsant drug-induced osteomalacia: Alterations in mineral metabolism and response to vitamin D_3 administration. *Calcif Tiss Int* 27:13–18, 1979

23. Brodie MJ, Boobis AR, Dollery CT, Hillyard CJ, Brown DJ, MacIntyre I, Park BK: Rifampin and vitamin D metabolism. *Clin Pharmacol Ther* 27:801–914, 1980

24. Hahn TJ, Halstead LR, DeVivo DC: Disordered mineral metabolism produced by ketogenic diet therapy. *Calcif Tiss Int* 28: 17–22, 1979

25. Hahn TJ, Birge SJ, Scharp CR, Avioli LV: Phenobarbital-induced alteration in vitamin D metabolism. *J Clin Invest* 51: 741–748, 1972

26. Hahn TJ, Scharp CR, Richardson CA, Halstead LR, Kahn AJ, Teitelbaum SL: Interaction of diphenylhydantoin and phenobarbital with hormonal mediation of fetal rat bone resorption in vitro. *J Clin Invest* 62:406–414, 1978

27. Dietrich JW, Duffield R: Effects of diphenylhydantoin on synthesis of collagen and noncollagen protein in tissue culture. *Endocrinology* 106:606–610, 1980

62. Osteoporosis in Men

Jeffrey A. Jackson, M.D.

Division of Endocrinology, Scott & White Clinic and Memorial Hospital,
Texas A&M University Health Science Center, College of Medicine,
Temple, Texas

Osteoporosis in men has received much less attention than its counterpart in women. One-seventh of all osteoporotic vertebral compression fractures occur in men. The greatest morbidity, mortality, and societal expense, however, is caused by hip fractures in men that account for one-fourth to one-fifth of all hip fractures. The lower incidence of osteoporosis in men is due to higher peak bone mass, shorter life expectancy, and the absence of a distinct menopause-equivalent with associated marked acceleration of bone loss.

The differential diagnosis of osteopenia (i.e., reduced bone mass without fractures) and osteoporosis in men is shown in Table 1. This list also applies to other groups of patients such as black and premenopausal women.

HYPOGONADISM

Long-standing testosterone deficiency is typical of ~30% of men presenting with spinal osteoporosis (1). These men most commonly present in the sixth decade and in retrospect, most have had hypogonadal symptoms of impotence and decreased libido in excess of 20–30 years. Virtually any cause of hypogonadism (primary or secondary) may be associated with osteoporosis in men, including Klinefelter syndrome, hypogonadotropic hypogonadism, hyperprolactinemia, hemochromatosis,

mumps orchitis, and castration (2). Testosterone deficiency may be a significant risk factor for hip fracture in elderly men (3) and may contribute to bone loss associated with aging in general, malignancy, and other systemic diseases (see Chapter 63), malnutrition, ethanol abuse, and glucocorticoid excess (see Chapter 61).

Detection of hypogonadism in osteoporotic men may be quite challenging. Pitfalls include lack of palpably abnormal testes (not uncommon in secondary hypogonadism occurring after puberty), denial of hypogonadal symptoms (testosterone-deficient men may be capable of adequate sexual function), and presence of "normal" serum total testosterone levels despite clear elevations in serum luteinizing hormone (sometimes due to associated increases in sex steroid-binding globulin). Every osteopenic or osteoporotic man should have routine measurement of serum testosterone and luteinizing hormone.

Histomorphometric heterogeneity in hypogonadal osteoporotic men [similar to that of postmenopausal osteoporosis except for lack of subnormal bone formation rates (1)] may reflect a gradual transition from osteoclast- to osteoblast-dependent bone loss over time. The increased remodeling activation and bone turnover in such men appears to be correctable by testosterone replacement (1) or calcitonin (2). Testosterone deficiency may reduce calcitonin secretion and synthesis of 1,25-dihydroxyvitamin D may be impaired, particularly when substrate (25-hy-

TABLE 1. *Differential diagnosis of osteopenia and osteoporosis in men*[a]

Endocrinopathies: hypogonadism, Cushing's syndrome, hyperthyroidism, primary hyperparathyroidism, hyperprolactinemia, acromegaly, and hypercalciuria.

Osteomalacia: vitamin D deficiency, phosphate wasting syndromes, metabolic acidosis, and inhibitors of mineralization.

Neoplastic disease: multiple myeloma, systemic mastocytosis, diffuse bony metastases, vertebral metastases, myelo- and lymphoproliferative disorders.

Drug-induced: glucocorticoids, ethanol, excessive thyroid hormone, heparin, anticonvulsants, and tobacco smoking.

Hereditary disorders: osteogenesis imperfecta, Ehlers–Danlos and Marfan syndromes, and homocystinuria.

Other disorders: immobilization, chronic disease (rheumatoid arthritis, liver/kidney failure), malnutrition, skeletal sarcoidosis, Gaucher's disease, hypophosphatasia, and hemoglobinopathies.

Idiopathic: juvenile and adult.

[a] Adapted from Jackson JA, Kleerekoper M: Osteoporosis in men: Diagnosis, pathophysiology, and prevention. *Medicine* 69:139–152, 1990.

droxyvitamin D) is deficient (1,4). Parallels between the bone effects of gonadal hormone deficiency in men and women may be due to similar direct effects on bone; both estrogen and androgen receptors have now been demonstrated in human osteoblast-like cells *in vitro*.

Study of the effects of testosterone replacement therapy on bone mineral density has been quite limited. Significant increases in radial and spinal bone mineral densities have been reported in patients with hypogonadotropic hypogonadism and initially open epiphyses with testosterone treatment for ~2 years but those with initially closed epiphyses showed minimal improvement (5). Restoration of gonadal function after successful treatment of hyperprolactinemic hypogonadal men resulted in significant increases in only cortical bone density (6). Spine and forearm bone mineral densities increase in hypogonadal men with hemochromatosis treated by testosterone replacement and venesection (7).

OTHER ENDOCRINOPATHIES

Cushing's syndrome may present with osteoporosis and no other typical stigmata of hypercortisolism. Accelerated bone loss may also occur in hyperthyroidism, primary hyperparathyroidism, and idiopathic renal hypercalciuria, all of which are characterized histologically by increased bone turnover.

OSTEOMALACIA

Osteomalacia may coexist with osteoporosis and remain undetected in a patient presenting with a fracture, particularly of the hip or pelvis. Typical features of hypophosphatemia, hypocalcemia, and elevation of serum alkaline phosphatase may be absent, and bone histomorphometry may be necessary for definitive diagnosis. Measurement of 25-hydroxyvitamin D levels is indicated in any osteoporotic man with prior gastric surgery or history suggesting intestinal malabsorption of vitamin D (see Chapters 65 and 66).

NEOPLASTIC DISEASE

Diffuse osteopenia may be caused by multiple myeloma, systemic mastocytosis, diffuse bony metastases, and myelo- and lymphoproliferative disorders (see Chapter 63). Serum immunoelectrophoresis, radionuclide bone scans, vertebral computed tomography/magnetic resonance imaging or biopsy, and bone marrow aspiration/biopsy may be useful to exclude these diseases.

DRUG-INDUCED BONE LOSS

Glucocorticoid therapy causes both suppression of bone formation and increased bone resorption due to secondary hyperparathyroidism (related to direct inhibition of gastrointestinal calcium absorption). Chronic alcoholics frequently manifest osteoporosis due to impaired osteoblast function; nutritional deficiency of calcium, vitamin D, and protein; decreased sunlight exposure; and an increased tendency to fall. Excessive thyroid replacement and chronic heparin or anticonvulsant therapy may cause accelerated bone loss. Cigarette smoking is a major risk factor for osteoporosis in men (8), possibly due to impaired gastrointestinal calcium absorption.

OTHER DISORDERS

Hereditary disorders in collagen metabolism represent a spectrum, including osteogenesis imperfecta, Ehlers–Danlos and Marfan syndromes, and homocystinuria. These may be recognized by suggestive family history (including hearing loss and dentinogenesis), blue sclerae, joint hyperextensibility, and/or typical habitus. Chronic diseases such as hepatic/renal failure and rheumatoid arthritis, prolonged immobilization, and malnutrition may cause abnormal bone loss.

IDIOPATHIC

The diagnosis of idiopathic osteoporosis should be made only after all other causes have been excluded. Idiopathic juvenile osteoporosis is discussed in Chapter 59. In adults, men predominate by a 10:1 ratio, presenting with vertebral compressions in the third to sixth decades. Bone histomorphometry has revealed defective osteoblastic function with low bone formation rates (1,9), although there appears to be a subgroup with hypercalciuria and increased bone turnover (10) perhaps related to excessive interleukin-1 or other humoral growth factors. Alterations in 1,25-dihydroxyvitamin D synthesis may also contribute to bone loss in some of these patients.

INVOLUTIONAL BONE LOSS IN MEN

Most studies of bone mass and density in aging men have shown gradual decline in bone mineral content at cortical sites (3–4% loss per decade after age 40) and greater rate of fall at cancellous sites (7–12% loss per decade after ages 30–35). These changes are similar but occur at a slower rate than those in women (see Chapter 56). Cancellous bone with its greater surface area and metabolic activity appears more susceptible to structural loss than is compact bone. Recent evidence suggests that, in addition to the amount of bone present, the three-dimensional trabecular microstructure makes a major contribution to bone strength (11). Slow bone loss as characterizes that of aging may preferentially involve insufficient osteoblast deposition of new bone in resorptive cavities of normal or decreased depth. Increased depth of cavities may occur in involutional osteopenia, particularly in women, but is typical of rapid bone turnover of any cause (i.e., glucocorticoids, hyperthyroidism, or sudden development of gonadal deficiency). If rapid bone turnover is interposed on the aging skeleton, perforation of trabecular plates may result in loss (presently irreversible) of entire structural elements that in turn causes discontinuity of the trabecular skeleton and disproportionate reduction in biomechanical strength.

Figure 1 summarizes the current understanding of the multifactorial pathophysiology of involutional bone loss in men (12). A major factor appears to be reduction in osteoblast function with age, possibly due to decreased osteoblast longevity or impaired regulation of osteoblast activity and recruitment or formation-resorption coupling by systemic or local skeletal growth factors. Decreased mechanical loading, exercise, and muscle mass in the elderly may impair remodeling activity. Negative calcium balance in aging men is due to insufficient oral calcium intake and decreased gastrointestinal calcium absorptive efficiency, which appears to be caused primarily by reduction in synthesis of 1,25-dihydroxyvitamin D. Age-related increase in bone resorption may be related to several hormonal factors. Increases in serum parathyroid hormone with age have been reported by most investigators. Although calcitonin levels (measured by monomeric assays) do not fall with age in either sex, the higher calcitonin levels in men than in women may contribute to their greater bone mass. A fall in gonadal function with age (13) may contribute significantly to involutional bone loss in men. Increased propensity to fall also plays a major role in involutional fractures; women over age 50 fall four times more often than men.

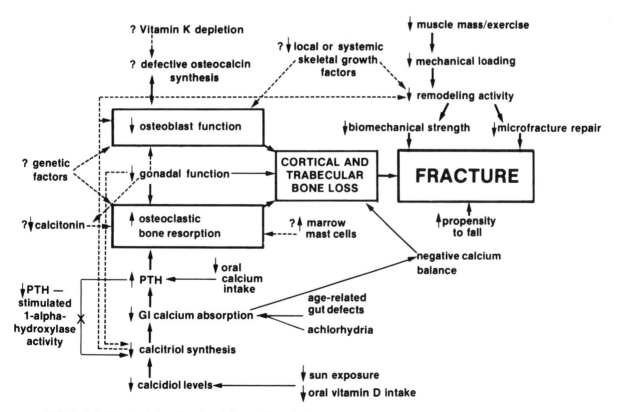

FIG. 1. Multifactorial pathophysiology of involutional bone loss in men. (From Jackson JA, Kleerekoper M: Osteoporosis in men: Diagnosis, pathophysiology, and prevention. *Medicine* 69: 139–152, 1990.)

TABLE 2. *Prevention of osteoporosis in men: general measures*[a]

Routine maintenance of adequate calcium intake throughout life: 1,000 mg/day elemental calcium in young men and boys; 1,500 mg/day (or more) in men > ages 55–60.

Routine maintenance of adequate vitamin D intake throughout life: low-dose vitamin D supplementation to push total intake to 600–800 IU/day in men > ages 55–60.

Lifelong regular physical exercise.

Recognize and treat testosterone deficiency early; consider screening testicular function every decade in men > ages 55–60 (earlier in men with prior unilateral orchiectomy/orchitis/testicular atrophy).

Limit ethanol use and avoid tobacco smoking.

Recognize other high-risk men (Table 3); consider specific prophylactic treatment regimens:
  Postgastric surgery (oral calcium ± vitamin D)
  Chronic glucocorticoid therapy (oral calcium ± vitamin D and thiazides).

Avoidance of falls.

[a] See Table 1 footnote.

PREVENTION

Because current therapy of established osteoporosis is inadequate and no therapeutic agent has yet convincingly proven efficacious in preventing osteoporotic fractures, emphasis must be placed on prevention of bone loss (Table 2). Specific measures may include routine calcium

TABLE 3. *Risk factors for osteoporosis in men*[a]

Caucasion (?Asiatic) ancestry
Low dietary calcium intake
Lean body build
Inactive lifestyle
Impaired gonadal function
Significant ethanol use
Drugs, particularly glucocorticoids
Chronic illness/immobilization
Cigarette smoking
Postgastric surgery or intestinal resection
?Family history of osteoporotic fractures
?Chronic excess sodium, caffeine, protein, and phosphorus intake

[a] See Table 1 footnote.

and vitamin D supplementation in men after ages 55–60, lifelong regular exercise, prompt recognition and treatment of testosterone deficiency, moderation of ethanol intake, and avoidance of tobacco smoking. Recognition of risk factors for osteoporosis in men [(8) listed roughly in order of importance in Table 3] is also important. In the future, specific programs for prevention of falls will likely yield beneficial results for the elderly.

REFERENCES

1. Jackson JA, Kleerekoper M, Parfitt AM, Rao DS, Villanueva AR, Frame B: Bone histomorphometry in hypogonadal and eugonadal men with spinal osteoporosis. *J Clin Endocrinol Metab* 65:53–58, 1987
2. Stepan JJ, Lachman M, Zverina J, Pacovsky V, Baylink DJ: Castrated men exhibit bone loss: Effect of calcitonin treatment on biochemical indices of bone remodeling. *J Clin Endocrinol Metab* 69:523–527, 1989
3. Jackson JA, Riggs MW, Spiekerman AM: Testosterone deficiency as a risk factor for hip fractures in men: a case-control study. *Am J Med Sci* 304:4–8, 1992
4. Francis RM, Peacock M, Aaron JE, et al.: Osteoporosis in hypogonadal men: Role of decreased plasma, 1,25-dihydroxyvitamin D, calcium malabsorption and low bone formation. *Bone* 7: 261–268, 1986
5. Finkelstein JS, Klibanski A, Neer RM, Doppelt SH, Rosenthal DI, Segre GV, Crowley WF Jr: Increases in bone density during treatment of men with idiopathic hypogonadotropic hypogonadism. *J Clin Endocrinol Metab* 69:776–783, 1989
6. Greenspan SL, Oppenheim DS, Klibanski A: Importance of gonadal steroids to bone mass in men with hyperprolactinemic hypogonadism. *Ann Intern Med* 110:526–531, 1989
7. Diamond T, Stiel D, Posen S: Effects of testosterone and venesection on spinal and peripheral bone mineral in six hypogonadal men with hemochromatosis. *J Bone Miner Res* 6:39–43, 1991
8. Seeman E, Melton LJ III, O'Fallon WM, Riggs BL: Risk factors for spinal osteoporosis in men. *Am J Med* 75:977–983, 1983
9. Zerwekh JE, Sakhaee K, Breslau NA, Gottschalk F, Pak CY: Impaired bone formation in male idiopathic osteoporosis: Further reduction in the presence of concomitant hypercalciuria. *Osteoporosis Int* 2:128–134, 1992
10. Perry HM, Fallon MD, Bergfield M, Teitelbaum SL, Avioli LV: Osteoporosis in young men: A syndrome of hypercalciuria and accelerated bone turnover. *Arch Intern Med* 142:1295–1298, 1982
11. Parfitt AM: Age-related structural changes in trabecular and cortical bone: Cellular mechanisms and biomechanical consequences. *Calcif Tissue Int* 36:S123–128, 1984
12. Jackson JA, Kleerekoper M: Osteoporosis in men: Diagnosis, pathophysiology, and prevention. *Medicine* 69:139–152, 1990
13. Vermeulen A: Androgens in the aging male. *J Clin Endocrinol Metab* 73:221–224, 1991

63. Miscellaneous Causes of Osteoporosis

Malachi J. McKenna, M.D., F.A.C.P.

Department of Medicine, St. Michael's Hospital and St. Vincent's Hospital, Dublin, Ireland

Generalized osteoporosis has been reported in a variety of uncommon circumstances (Table 1). Because some are associated with other bone lesions (including focal osteolysis, hyperostosis, focal and generalized osteosclerosis, osteomalacia, and abnormalities at ossification centers), they are also discussed in other sections.

TABLE 1. *Miscellaneous causes of osteoporosis*

Marrow Disorders
    Plasma cell dyscrasias
    Leukemia
    Lymphomas
    Systemic mastocytosis
    Anemias
    Lipidoses
    Mucopolysaccharidoses
Connective Tissue Disorders
    Osteogenesis imperfecta
    Ehlers–Danlos
    Marfans syndrome
    Cutis laxa
    Homocystinuria
    Menkes's syndrome
    Scurvy
Drug-Related
    Corticosteroid
    Heparin
    Oral anticoagulants
    Anticonvulsants
    Methotrexate
    Thyroid hormone
    Lithium
    Gonadotrophin-releasing analogs
Miscellaneous
    Pregnancy/lactation
    Chronic hypophosphatemia
    Hyperphosphatasia
    Insulin-dependent diabetes mellitus
    Anorexia nervosa
    Cadmium poisoning

MARROW-RELATED DISORDERS

Cancellous and endocortical bone surfaces are in close apposition to bone marrow. Any marrow process can modify remodeling activity and thus exacerbate the proclivity to loss of cancellous and endocortical bone leading to cortical thinning, expansion of the marrow cavity, and reduction in cancellous bone volume (1).

Plasma Cell Dyscrasias

Plasma cell dyscrasias, namely multiple myeloma and macroglobulinemia, are known to be associated with several bone disorders (see Chapters 34 and 79 and ref. 2). Typically, multiple myeloma is manifest by numerous osteolytic lesions at multiple sites where red marrow prevails. Bone-seeking tracers do not concentrate amid the bone lesions, serum alkaline phosphatase is not elevated, and urine hydroxyproline excretion is high; this suggests an uncoupling of bone resorption and bone formation. The identification of osteoclast-activating factor in the 1970s (3) gave biochemical support to this hypothesis. Since then a number of bone resorbing cytokines (interleukin 1, tumor necrosis factor, and lymphotoxin) have been identified and implicated in the process of bone destruction (4,5). Furthermore, parathyroid hormone-related peptide released by myeloma cells may add to an enhanced resorptive state (6). Focal areas of sclerosis may occur and very rarely generalized osteosclerosis has been documented, indicating other as yet unidentified and unexplained local influences on bone remodeling.

Systemic Mastocytosis

Mast cells are connective tissue elements. Although primarily located at cutaneous and mucosal surfaces, they also inhabit the bone marrow of normal individuals. They process cytoplasmic granules that exhibit a quality of metachromasia, staining pink or red when exposed to a basic blue dye (8). The mast cell is a storehouse for many potent chemical mediators, including biogenic amines (i.e., histamine), enzymes, chemotactic peptides, structural proteoglycans (i.e., heparin), and cytokines, and is the source of arachidonic acid metabolites after degranulation (9). It is known that heparin can result in osteoporosis, and it is likely that other cell products can contribute to this process (10).

Systemic mastocytosis (Fig. 1), an abnormal proliferation of mast cells, usually results in mixed sclerotic-porotic lesions that present in a diffuse or circumscribed manner (see ref. 5 and Chapter 81). Rarely, generalized osteoporosis may be the only radiologic manifestation (9,11–14). Dynamic histomorphometric analysis of bone in subjects with generalized osteoporosis and systemic mastocytosis has reported both a high-turnover state (11,14) and an imbalance of remodeling activity where formation is less than resorption, the latter appearing to be nonosteoclastic-mediated (Fig. 1) (9). An analogous excess of marrow mast cells is seen in postmenopausal osteoporosis (15–17). Whether they are two distinct conditions or similar disorders differing only in severity is not known, but does support the opinion that systemic mastocytosis can lead to osteoporosis. It would appear that the milder form of systemic mastocytosis (urticaria pigmentosa being a pathognomic feature) is apt to result in osteoporosis alone (17).

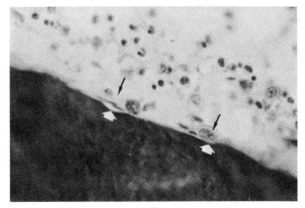

FIG. 1. Photomicrograph of bone section stained with toluidine blue picturing mast cell (*black arrows*) adjacent to resorption cavities (*white arrows*) (original magnification, 250 ×). (From McKenna MJ, Frame B: The mast cell and bone. *Clin Orthop* 200:226–233, 1985.)

Leukemias

Leukemia, a malignant disorder originating and dispersed throughout the marrow, can result in osteoporosis. This occurs more commonly in adolescents than in adults (18). In children, diffuse osteoporosis, particularly involving the spine, is observed. Other features include transverse radiolucent bands at the metaphyseal ends of long bones and focal osteolytic lesions; less commonly a moth-eaten appearance permeating bones is seen (2). The tendency to osteoporosis can be aggravated by the use of methotrexate, which is known to induce bone pain and fractures (19). In chronic leukemia, osteoporosis is mainly seen in flat bones where active marrow persists in adulthood. It is possible that cytokines directly influencing bone remodeling activity are involved in the pathogenesis.

Lymphomas

Lymphomatous involvement of the skeleton, although not rare, is usually focal in nature (2). Hypercalcemia of lymphoma is the result of unregulated extrarenal generation of calcitriol in malignant tissue. Generalized osteoporosis with hypercalcemia as a presenting feature of lymphoma has been documented (20). Whether intramarrow 1,25-dihydroxyvitamin D [1,25(OH)$_2$D] production had role in the genesis of osteoporosis is unknown.

Anemias

Chronic anemias that predispose to marrow hyperplasia such as sickle cell disease and β-thalassemia can result in osteoporosis (2). In sickle cell disease there is widening of the medullary cavity and the intertrabecular spaces with thinning of the remaining trabeculae. Radiographic evidence of osteoporosis is found in the axial skeleton, skull, and mandible. The diploic spaces are widened, and there is a coarse granular appearance to all of the vault except the occipital bone. There are step-like indentations in the central portion of the vertebral endplates—the "H" vertebrae. Other features include focal osteonecrosis, a propensity to osteomyelitis, and deformities due to growth disturbances. In homozygous β-thalassemia major the whole skull tends to be osteoporotic (2). There is diffuse expansion of the facial bones leading to deformity. Vertebrae rarely show the squared-off indentations of sickle cell disease. There is osteoporosis of the ribs and clavicle. Unlike sickle cell disease, there is underconstriction and flaring of the distal femoral metaphysis, the Erlenmeyer flask deformity of altered bone modeling during growth (2). It is now apparent that even β-thalassemia minor can result in severe osteopenia of the axial skeleton with relative sparing of the appendicular skeleton (21).

Lipidoses

Bone disease is a common feature of Gaucher's disease (22,23), whereas it is much less common in the related Niemann–Pick disease. The Gaucher cell, a peculiar lipid-laden cell, is found throughout the reticuloendothelial system, most notably in the spleen, liver, and bone marrow. It is an altered macrophage; cells of monocyte-macrophage lineage include the osteoclast. A deficiency in a lysosomal enzyme, β-glucosidase, leads to an accumulation of glucosylceramide in phagocytic cells of the reticuloendothelial system.

Skeletal abnormalities are a customary feature but do not correlate with the extent of visceral involvement, bone marrow depression, degree of enzyme deficiency, or concentration of circulating glucosylceramide (23). In the growing skeleton, a failure of modeling results in an Erlenmeyer deformity, most notably at the distal femora and proximal tibiae. Osteoporosis may be generalized (typically seen in the femur and characterized by cortical thinning) or focal with a propensity to pathological fracture. Vertebral compression deformities occur and there is a predilection to fractures of the femur and rib. Other radiological findings include osteosclerotic lesions (thought to be a manifestation of cancellous osteonecrosis), corticomedullary osteonecrosis (that may be silent if occurring in a bone shaft or symptomatic if appearing in the femoral head), Gaucher crisis (bone pain of abrupt onset with normal radiology of affected bone that probably is due to infarction and is likely to be the precursor state of osteosclerosis), and rarely osteomyelitis (23).

It is likely the Gaucher cell alters bone modeling and remodeling activity at contiguous sites accounting for skeletal abnormalities but the mechanisms are unknown (23). In addition, compromise of blood flow with resultant hypoxia and cell death must be a direct consequence of either the space-occupying infiltrative process or sudden release of lysosomal contents (23).

CONNECTIVE TISSUE DISORDERS

Scurvy

Vitamin C, a potent reducing agent, is essential for the proper synthesis of collagen. Scurvy in the infant may be manifest by generalized osteoporosis; the bone radiographs have a ground-glass appearance (24). Severe cortical thinning is evident, and there is blurring or almost complete disappearance of the trabecular striations. Certain specific features are seen, including transverse metaphyseal lines of increased and decreased density, metaphyseal excrescences, subperiosteal hemorrhages, and an epiphyseal shell of increased calcification encompassing central lucency.

UNCLASSIFIED CONDITIONS

Pregnancy/Lactation

Osteoporosis of pregnancy is a rare and poorly studied entity, although the association has been known for over

40 years. Within the short period of gestation, severe osteoporosis may manifest with multiple vertebral compression deformities as well as bone pain in the appendicular skeleton and a propensity to hip fracture. The disease is limited to the period of pregnancy or lactation, and does not necessarily recur during future gestations (25). There is an increased need for calcium during pregnancy primarily for the calcification of fetal bones but also probably in preparation for lactation. Homeostatic mechanisms necessary to meet this requirement include an increase in $1,25(OH)_2D$ production and possibly an increase in calcitonin secretion. It has been suggested that failure or inefficiency of these mechanisms is the pathogenetic mechanism. Because it may not recur, this suggests either a serendipitous occurrence or that additional factors are associated with a particular pregnancy (25). Accurate studies of bone turnover, both histomorphometric and radiotracer, are obviously prohibited and dynamic histomorphometric studies post hoc have in general excluded any persistent abnormality in bone remodeling activity (26). Modest calcium supplementation during pregnancy may not be preventative.

Hypophosphatemia

Typically, one associates prolonged hypophosphatemia with a mineralization defect resulting in osteomalacia as personified by the syndromes of vitamin D-resistant rickets and oncogenous osteomalacia (see Chapters 55 and 67–69). Minor degrees of hypophosphatemia with reduction in the renal phosphate threshold are observed in a subset of patients with idiopathic hypercalciuria, apparently without any deleterious skeletal effect. Histomorphometric studies in a group of hypophosphatemic subjects with osteopenia and vertebral compression excluded osteomalacia, but demonstrated a tendency to a low bone turnover state (27). It is hypothesized that chronic low-grade hypophosphatemia impairs osteoblastic bone formation.

Insulin-Dependent Diabetes Mellitus

Bone disease as a complication of diabetes mellitus has drawn limited attention (28–30). Recent studies have disclosed three phenomena related to bone disease in diabetes mellitus: frequent occurrence of low bone mineral density (BMD) in insulin-dependent diabetes mellitus (IDDM); low, normal, and even high BMD in noninsulin-dependent diabetes mellitus (NIDDM); but no increase in fracture risk compared with the nondiabetic population. Add to these observations the problem of stress fractures in the foot bones, then bone disease in diabetes mellitus acquires a relevant clinical dimension. To date, this conflicting information on BMD in IDDM and NIDDM has not been explained. In the 1960s dynamic bone histomorphometry on cortical bone from the rib demonstrated that the bone formation rate was low in diabetes mellitus (31). More recent studies have confirmed low bone formation in cortical and cancellous bone from the ilium (32). In

clinical surveys low levels of osteocalcin are reported in support of the histological finding of low bone formation rate (33,34). It is possible that a low bone turnover state results in low BMD during periods of net bone gain such as longitudinal growth of the skeleton or age up to attainment of peak adult bone mass (32). During periods of net bone loss at older ages, a protective effect of low bone turnover on BMD would be expected (32). However a reduction in bone turnover rate, a process of bone renewal that replaces old bone with new bone, could increases bone fragility and the tendency to stress fractures in the foot bones (32).

REFERENCES

1. Frost HM: The upper IO (L3). In: *Intermediary Organization of the Skeleton*, vol 1. CRC Press, Boca Raton, FL, pp 147–197, 1986
2. Resnick D: Disorders of the hemopoietic system. In: Resnick D, Niwayama G (eds) *The Metabolic Basis of Inherited Disease*. McGraw-Hill, New York, pp 1884–2040, 1981
3. Mundy GR, Raisz LG, Cooper RA, Schechter GP, Salmon SE: Evidence for the secretion of an osteoclast stimulating factor in myeloma. *N Engl J Med* 291:1041–1046, 1974
4. Garret IR, Durie BGM, Nedwin GE, Gillespie A, Bringman T, Sabatini M, Bertolini DR, Mundy GR: Production of lymphotoxin, a bone-resorbing cytokine, by cultured human myeloma cells. *N Engl J Med* 317:526–532, 1987
5. Lowik CWGM, van der Pluijm G, Bloys H, et al.: Parathyroid hormone (PTH) and PTH-like protein (PLP) stimulate interleukin-6 production by osteogenic cells: A possible role of interleukin-6 in osteoclastogenesis. *Biochem Biophys Res Commun* 162:1546–1552, 1989
6. Budayr AA, Nussebsib RA, Klein RF, et al.: Increased serum levels of a parathyroid hormone-like protein in malignancy-associated hypercalcaemia. *Ann Intern Med* 111:1106–1112, 1989
7. McKenna MJ, Sarvaria S, Brunner J, Rosenbaum R, Kleerekoper M, Goldberg M: Osteosclerotic metastases with severe hypocalcemia, parathyroid resistance, anemia and cardiac failure. *Am J Med* 84:175–176, 1988
8. McKenna MJ, Lundin D, Villaneuva AR, Parfitt AM: Staining for mast cells in undecalcified bone sections. *J Histotechnol* 13:49–51, 1990
9. McKenna MJ, Frame B: The mast cell and bone. *Clin Orthop* 200:226–233, 1985
10. Raisz LG: Local and systemic factors in the pathogenesis of osteoporosis. *N Engl J Med* 318:818–828, 1988
11. Fallon MD, Whyte MP, Teitlebaum SL: Systemic mastocytosis associated with generalized osteoporosis. *Hum Pathol* 12:813–820, 1981
12. Harvey JA, Anderson HC, Borek D, Morris D, Lukert BP: Osteoporosis associated with mastocytosis confined to bone: Report of two cases. *Bone* 10:237–241, 1989
13. Lidor C, Frisch B, Gazit D, Gepstein R, Hallel T, Mekori YA: Osteoporosis as the sole presentation of bone marrow mastocytosis. *J Bone Miner Res* 5:871–876, 1990
14. Chines A, Pacifici R, Avioli LV, Teitlebaum SL, Korenblat PE: Systemic mastocytosis presenting as osteoporosis: a clinical and histomorphometric study. *J Clin Endocrinol Metab* 72:140–144, 1991
15. Frame B, Nixon RK: Bone marrow mast cells in osteoporosis and aging. *N Engl J Med* 279:626–630, 1968
16. Fallon MD, Whyte MP, Craig B Jr, Teitlebaum SL: Mast-cell proliferation in postmenopausal osteoporosis. *Calcif Tissue Int* 35:29–31, 1983
17. McKenna MJ: New indices for quantifying mast cells in bone: Comparison of normal bone, osteoporosis, and mastocytosis. *Bone Miner* 17(suppl 1):178, 1992
18. Newman AJ, Melhorn DK: Vertebral compression in childhood leukaemia. *Am J Dis Child* 125:863–865, 1973

19. Regab AH, Frech RS, Vietti TJ: Osteoporotic fractures secondary to methotrexate therapy of acute leukaemia in remission. *Cancer* 25:580–585, 1969

20. Child JA, Smith IE: Lymphoma presenting as "idiopathic" juvenile osteoporosis. *Br Med J* 1:720–721, 1975

21. Greep N, Andersen A-LJ, Gallagher JC: Thalassemia minor: A risk factor for osteoporosis. *Bone Miner* 16:63–72, 1992

22. Brady RO, Barranger JA: Glucosylceramide lipidosis: Gaucher's disease. In: Stanbury JB, Wyngaarden JB, Fredrickson DS, Goldstein JL, Brown MS (eds) *The Metabolic Basis of Inherited of Disease, 5th ed.* McGraw-Hill, New York, pp 842–856, 1983

23. Mankin HJ, Doppelt SH, Rosenberg AE, Barranger JA: Metabolic bone disease in patients with Gaucher's disease. In: Avioli LV, Krane SM (eds) *Metabolic Bone Disease and Clinically Related Disorders, 2nd ed.* W.B. Saunders Company, Philadelphia, pp 730–752, 1990

24. Resnick D: Hypervitaminoses and hypovitaminoses. In: Resnick D, Niwayama G (eds) *Diagnosis of Bone and Joint Disorders, vol 3.* McGraw Hill, New York, pp 2385–2395, 1983

25. Smith R, Stevenson JC, Winearls CG, Woods CG, Woodsworth BP: Osteoporosis in pregnancy. *Lancet* 1:1178–1180, 1985

26. Gruber HE, Gutteridge DH, Baylink DJ: Osteoporosis associated pregnancy and lactation: Bone biopsy and skeletal features in three patients. *Bone* 5:159–165, 1984

27. de Vernejoul MC, Marie PJ, Miravet L, Ryckewaert A: Chronic hypophosphataemia without osteomalacia. In: Frame B, Potts JT Jr (eds) *Clinical Disorders of Bone and Mineral Metabolism.* Exerpta Medica, Amsterdam, pp 232–236, 1983

28. McNair P: Bone mineral metabolism in human type I (insulin dependent) diabetes mellitus. *Danish Med Bull* 35:109–121, 1988

29. Selby PL: Osteopenia and diabetes. *Diabetic Med* 5:423–428, 1988

30. Melchior TM, Sorensen OH, Thamsborg G, Sykuluski R, Storm T: Bone tissue alterations in diabetes. In: Belfiore F, Molinatti GM, Reaven GM (eds) *Tissue-Specific Metabolic Alterations in Diabetes.* Front Diabetes, vol 10. Karger, Basel, pp 40–53, 1990

31. Klein M, Wu K, Frost HM: The numbers of bone resorption and formation foci in rib in diabetes mellitus. *Henry Ford Hosp Med Bull* 12:527–536, 1964

32. Krakauer J, McKenna MJ, Rao DS, Whitehouse FW, Parfitt AM: Low bone turnover in diabetes mellitus accounts for preservation of bone mineral density. *Diabetologia* 35(suppl 1):A192, 1992

33. Pietschmann P, Schernthaner G, Woloszczuk W: Serum osteocalcin levels in diabetes mellitus: Analysis of the type of diabetes and microvascular complications. *Diabetologia* 31:891–895, 1988

34. Rico H, Hernandez ER, Cabranes JA, Gomes-Castresana F: Suggestion of a deficient osteoblastic function in diabetes mellitus: The possible cause of osteopenia in diabetics. *Calcif Tissue Int* 45:71–73, 1989

64. Serum Fluoride Levels

David J. Baylink, M.D.

Mineral Metabolism Unit, Jerry Pettis Veterans Administration and Department of Medicine, Loma Linda University, Loma Linda, California

Man is exposed to fluoride, the thirteenth most abundant element on the earth's crust, in a wide range of concentrations from multiple sources, including water, soil, atmosphere, vegetation, livestock, the food chain (from the use of fluoridated water in commercial food processing), dental products, anesthetics, and as a drug for prevention of dental caries and for treatment of osteoporosis. Indications for measurement of serum fluoride include: 1) an evaluation of possible intoxication, which might result either from an industrial exposure (fluoride in the atmosphere) or from living in a community where large amounts of fluoride are present in water and soil, or from a fluoride medication overdose (1); or 2) an evaluation of the use of fluoride in the treatment of bone-wasting diseases, particularly osteoporosis (2). In the United States, the primary use of serum fluoride measurement is for the evaluation of the use of this drug in the treatment of osteoporosis, and this will be the focus of this chapter.

Serum levels of fluoride in patients receiving fluoride for the treatment for osteoporosis are obtained for two reasons: 1) to detect abnormally high levels or 2) to detect levels below those considered to be therapeutic. The usual dose of fluoride is 20–30 mg of elemental fluoride daily. This dose is used in an attempt to achieve a serum level of ~10 μM. By comparison, normal adult serum fluoride ranges from 0.5 to 2.3 μM in males and females from 18–80 years of age; lowest values are seen in young adults and levels progressively increase with age to reach peak values of ~2 μM in the six to eight decades (3).

The rationale for designating 10 μM serum fluoride as a safe and effective level is as follows: patients who are good responders to fluoride may show a response in terms of increased bone density with levels of only 5 μM; however, more consistently positive responses are seen at a serum level of 10 μM. There is a dose range of action of fluoride to increase bone cell proliferation *in vitro* that extends over an order of magnitude. However, it is not yet clear whether levels higher than 10 μM will result in superior results in patients. That level of serum fluoride that results in the first evident toxic symptoms or changes is not known. We know that serum levels of ~50 μM will result in a decreased concentrating ability by the kidneys (4). Peak serum fluoride levels after a 10 mg dose do not reach such high levels. Accordingly, the peak level usually does not exceed three times the morning predose level (i.e., the level just before the morning fluoride dose) under such conditions. Until more information becomes available in terms of the efficacy and toxicity of fluoride, we feel that the morning predose level of 10 μM should be the goal for adult patients being treated for osteoporosis and other bone-wasting diseases.

There are basically two means by which patients can develop levels above what we consider the safe level: 1) excessive doses of fluoride and 2) normal doses in the presence of impaired renal function. There is a strong correlation between fluoride and creatinine clearances ($r = 0.90, p < 0.001$) (5). Thus, as renal function declines, fluoride renal clearance also declines and as a result serum fluoride levels rise. Many patients being treated with fluoride are in their seventh and eighth decades, an age when renal function has declined. It is therefore not surprising that the most common cause of high serum fluoride levels in patients being treated with this drug is impaired renal function.

Our protocol for serum fluoride measurements includes a serum fluoride 2 months after starting the drug. High values at this time require a reduction in the dose of the medication. If the values are less at this point in time than 10 μM, we do not adjust the dose upward, because there is some evidence that the morning predose serum level of fluoride does not reach a maximum level until after several months of therapy. If after 6–9 months of therapy the morning predose serum fluoride is less than 10 μM, we increase the daily dose by 10 mg of elemental fluoride. In summary, we measure the blood level early on to detect toxicity and after several months in order to determine whether the patient is receiving an adequate dose of fluoride. It should be remembered that patients with only one kidney will require a lower dose of fluoride as will patients who have renal tubular acidosis, inasmuch as acidosis tends to reduce fluoride excretion in the urine. One will seldom see a fluoride level much above 10 μM at a dose of fluoride of 20–30 mg/day unless the patient has impaired renal function.

If fluoride is to be used in children, with osteogenesis imperfecta tarda or other diseases of reduced bone density, one will not see morning predose serum fluoride levels of more than ~5 μM with doses of fluoride at 1 mg/kg body weight even though a similar dose in an adult would produce a serum fluoride of >10 μM. It is possible that the bone clearance of fluoride is so avid in children that we do not see a morning predose level that reaches up to 10 μM although the cause for this apparent discrepancy is not yet settled.

When the serum fluoride level is low and the dose is appropriate, one should consider that the patient: 1) has impaired absorption due to achlorhydria or other gastrointestinal disturbances: 2) is ingesting drugs that might interfere with fluoride absorption such as H_2-receptor blockers or calcium salts that will cause a precipitation of insoluble calcium fluoride in the gut; or 3) is drinking enormous amounts of liquid inasmuch as the urine excretion of fluoride is proportional to the free water clearance. Although fluoride is alleged to be 90–100% bioavailable, we doubt that this is the case in some of our elderly osteoporotic patients.

Some investigators have advocated the measurement of urine fluoride or bone fluoride in addition to, or instead of, serum fluoride. Indeed in one investigation there was a finding of an increase in urine excretion of fluoride in patients who were good responders as opposed to those who were poor responders (6). When renal function is normal, urine fluoride excretion and serum level tend to be related, in which case one could get similar information from measuring either serum or urine. On the other hand, in a patient with a reduced renal function, the urine level will not necessarily reflect the serum level. Moreover, we feel that it is the serum level, rather than the urine or bone level, that is important in terms of therapeutic assessment of fluoride dosage, largely because fluoride has been shown to act directly on bone cells *in vitro* (7). Similarly, we do not feel that bone fluoride measurements are helpful in terms of assessing adequate fluoride dosage, because the bone fluoride deposition rate is related not only to the serum fluoride level, but also to the bone formation rate, such that the bone level is not a good index of serum fluoride. Some investigators suggest that when the bone fluoride level reaches a certain level, fluoride therapy should be stopped in order to avoid adverse effects on bone mechanical performance. We feel that there is insufficient information at this time to recommend bone fluoride measurements for general use. Until evidence arrives to the contrary, we feel that the most appropriate way to assess fluoride efficacy and safety is through measurement of the morning predose serum levels.

In osteoporotic patients, serum fluoride should be measured in the morning in a fasting state, 12 hr after the last oral fluoride preparation. If the blood sample is obtained shortly after the patient consumes fluoride orally, the serum levels obtained will be two- or more-fold higher than those 12 hr after the medication.

The method for measuring fluoride in biological fluids, including serum, utilizes an Orion Fluoride Ion-Specific Electrode that measures ionic fluoride, a relevant parameter because fluoride circulates in a nonprotein-bound form (8). The analytical procedure to measure fluoride in biological fluids has been published in detail (3).

REFERENCES

1. Van Kesteren RG, Duursma SA, Van Der Sluys Veer J: A subacute fluoride intoxication during treatment of osteoporosis with sodium fluoride (NaF). *Neth J Med* 24:14–16, 1981
2. Farley SMG, Wergedal JE, Smith LC, Lundy MW, Farley JR, Baylink DJ: Fluoride therapy for osteoporosis: Characterization of the skeletal response by serial measurements of serum alkaline phosphatase activity. *Metabolism* 36:211–218, 1987
3. Husdan H, Vogl R, Oreopoulos D, Gryfe C, Rapoport A: Serum ionic fluoride: Normal range and relationship to age and sex. *Clin Chem* 22(11):1884–1888, 1976
4. van Dyke R: Fluoride from anesthetics and its consequences. In: Johansen E, Taves DR, Olsen TO (eds) Continuing Evaluation of the Use of Fluorides. *A.A.A.S. Selected Symposium no II, vol 10.* Westview Press, Boulder, Colorado, pp 241–249, 1979
5. Kraenzlin ME, Kraenzlin C, Farley SMG, Fitzsimmons RJ, Baylink DJ: Fluoride pharmacokinetics in good and poor responders to fluoride therapy. *J Bone Miner Res* 5(1):S49–S52, 1990
6. Duursma SA, Glerum JH, Van Dijk A, Bosch R, Kerkhoff H, Van Putten J, Raymakers JA: Responders and non-responders after fluoride therapy in osteoporosis. *Bone* 8:131–136, 1987
7. Farley JE, Wergedal JE, Baylink DJ: Fluoride directly stimulates proliferation and alkaline phosphatase activity of bone-forming cells. *Science* 222:330–332, 1983
8. Ekstand J, Ericsson Y, Rosell: Absence of protein-bound fluoride from human blood plasma. *Arch Oral Biol* 22:299–232, 1977

65. Nutritional Rickets and Osteomalacia

Gordon L. Klein, M.D., M.P.H.

Department of Pediatrics and Nutrition, University of Texas Medical Branch, Galveston, Texas

Recommended dietary intakes of vitamin D and minerals for infants, children, and adults are listed elsewhere (see Appendix IV). Intakes of vitamin D, calcium, or phosphorus substantially below these recommendations may result in rickets or osteomalacia. Rickets is a disorder of mineralization of the bone matrix, or osteoid, in growing bone; it involves both the growth plate (epiphysis) and newly formed trabecular and cortical bone. Osteomalacia is also a defect in bone matrix mineralization, but it occurs after the cessation of growth and involves only the bone and not the growth plate. The mineralization defects in rickets, resulting from inadequate calcium and/or phosphate deposition in the matrix, has an uncertain etiology. However, experimental evidence suggests that matrix of both cartilage and bone may be abnormal and thus less able to be mineralized. Deficiencies of vitamin D, calcium, or phosphorus due to inadequate nutritional intake (Table 1), can result in defective bone mineralization. We will consider each separately.

VITAMIN D DEFICIENCY

The main natural sources of vitamin D in foods are the fish liver foods. Otherwise, fortification of foods such as milk and eggs have been necessary to prevent vitamin D deficiency from occurring in the United States (1,2). However, consumption of unfortified foods in an environment with reduced exposure to sunlight can lead to vitamin D deficiency in many developing countries (1,2). This is especially true of Asian women who wear veils, consume unfortified foods when they become pregnant, and nurse their infants.

Another group at risk for vitamin D deficiency is that of breast-fed infants who do not receive vitamin D supplementation. Breast milk has been shown to be low in vitamin D, and cases of rickets in breast-fed infants have been reported (2).

Rickets can also develop in infants receiving total parenteral nutrition (TPN) solution exclusively from which vitamin D and calcium were inadvertently omitted (3). However, it is unclear whether absence of vitamin D alone would have been sufficient to produce bone disease. Adults who received TPN devoid of vitamin D for up to 1 year, did not develop osteomalacia although their serum levels of 25-hydroxyvitamin D (25OHD) were very low (3).

Pathogenesis

A diagram illustrating the steps in the pathogenesis of vitamin D-deficient rickets is shown in Fig. 1. The most biologically active vitamin D metabolite, 1,25-dihydroxy-vitamin D [1,25(OH)$_2$D], is made in the kidney by hydroxylation of 25OHD that comes from the liver (see Chapter 13). 1,25-Dihydroxyvitamin D enhances calcium and phosphate absorption from the small intestine. During vitamin D deficiency, intestinal calcium and phosphate absorption are reduced, causing hypocalcemia. The hypocalcemia in turn stimulates the parathyroid glands to secrete increased quantities of parathyroid hormone (PTH). Parathyroid hormone acts indirectly on osteoclasts to promote bone resorption and increase calcium and phosphorus available to the blood. In addition, PTH acts on the kidney to promote tubular calcium reabsorption and increase phosphate excretion. Parathyroid hormone also stimulates the renal conversion of 25OHD to 1,25(OH)$_2$D. 1,25-Dihydroxyvitamin D stimulates the small intestine to absorb more calcium and phosphorus (2).

Clinical and Laboratory Manifestations

Clinical manifestations of rickets include hypotonia, muscle weakness, and, in severe cases, tetany. Weight-bearing produces a bowing deformity of the long bones. Prominence of the costochondral junction, the so-called rachitic rosary, can also be seen (Fig. 2). as can an indentation of the lower ribs, Harrison's groove, due to softening. Occasionally there is indentation of the sternum in response to the force exerted by the diaphragm and intercostal muscles. Deformities of the back, including kyphosis and lordosis, along with limb bowing, can contribute to a waddling gait. There is also an increased frequency of fractures.

Abnormalities of the skull, especially in younger infants, include a softened calvarium (craniotabes), parietal flattening, and frontal bossing. There is delayed eruption of permanent dentition and enamel defects can occur (2).

Diffuse bone pain is the most common manifestation of osteomalacia, although there is some tendency for localization of pain in the hip area. Pelvic deformities and a waddling gait may also be present.

Roentgenographically the long bones are the earliest and most common sites of change. Typically there is thinning of the cortex and rarefaction of the shaft with widening, fraying, and cupping of the distal ends of the shaft and disappearance of the zone of provisional cartilaginous calcification (Fig. 3). Thin cortical radiolucent lines (stress fractures) at right angles to the bone shaft may be seen in osteomalacia as well as other metabolic bone disorders. These are most often symmetrical and bilateral. Decreased bone density is also seen. The pelvis and ribs are the most frequently affected areas (2).

Biochemical findings, as expected, include low or normal serum levels of calcium, low serum levels of phospho-

TABLE 1. *Causes and recommended management of nutritional rickets and ostomalacia*

Condition	Causes	Recommended management (ref.)
Vitamin D deficiency	Lack of adequate sunlight	Ultraviolet lamp or increased sunlight exposure (1)
	Consumption of diet low in fortified foods	*Vitamin D₂ Treatment* Variable: usually 1,500–5,000 IU/day orally (2) 10,000–50,000 IU/month intramuscularly (2)
	Unsupplemented breast-fed infant	*Prevention* Vitamin D₂ 400 IU/day orally (2) *For Premature Infants*
	Total parenteral nutrition	400–800 IU/day orally (6,10) 20–25 IU/kg/day in total parenteral nutrition (5)
Calcium deficiency	Lack of dietary calcium —infants and children	*Treatment* 700 mg/day orally (7) 1–2 g/day orally (9)
	High phytate diet Inadequate calcium in total parenteral nutrition —Breast-fed infants	30 mg/kg/day orally in breast-fed infant (13) *Prevention* In premature infants 200 mg/kg/day orally (10) 20–60 mg/dL (5–15 mM) in parenteral nutrition (5)
Phosphate deficiency	Breast-fed infants Inadequate phosphate in total parenteral nutrition—premature infants Chronic antacid therapy renal failure, and dialysis therapy	*Treatment* 25 mg/kg/day in breast-fed infants (13) Withdrawal of aluminum-containing antacids (14) *Prevention* 115–120 mg/kg/day orally in premature infants (10) 15–47 mg/dL (5–15 mM) in parenteral nutrition (5)

rus, and markedly elevated serum alkaline phosphatase levels. This enzyme elevation probably reflects increased bone turnover. Serum PTH levels are elevated when hypocalcemia is present. Serum levels of 25OHD are low in vitamin D deficiency; secondary hyperparathyroidism and low serum phosphorus stimulate renal production of 1,25(OH)₂D so that levels of this hormone are either normal or high if adequate vitamin D is present (2). Serum osteocalcin concentrations are within the normal range, although insufficient data are available to be definitive.

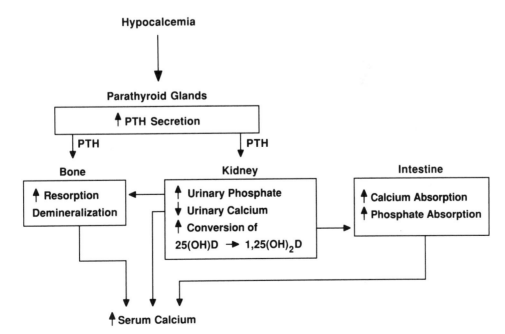

FIG. 1. Body's reaction to hypocalcemia with the consequent resorption of bone.

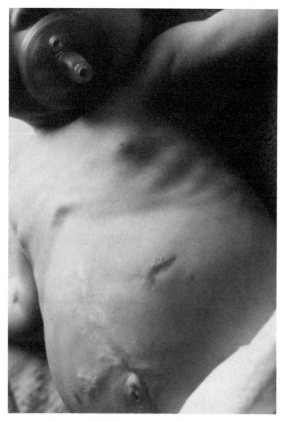

FIG. 2. An infant with nutritional rickets displaying a rachitic rosary at the costochondral junction.

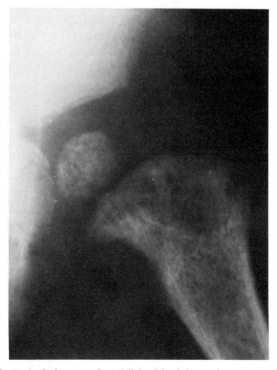

FIG. 3. Left femur of a child with rickets demonstrating gross demineralization, a coarse trabecular pattern, loss of epiphyseal definition, and a cupping deformity of the epiphysis.

Treatment and Prevention

Recommended doses of vitamin D for treatment and prevention of vitamin D deficiency rickets are given in Table 1. In vitamin D-deficiency due to fat malabsorption, use of a more polar compound, such as 25OHD, 20–30 μg/day, or 1,25(OH)$_2$D, 0.15–0.5 μg/day, may be more efficacious. Alternatively, ergocalciferol (vitamin D$_2$ in oil) given intramuscularly may be effective (3). The dose and frequency of administration must be adjusted depending on the serum levels of calcium, phosphorus, alkaline phosphatase, and 25OHD. In infants doses have ranged from 10,000 to 50,000 IU (250–1250 μg/month. Complications of vitamin D$_2$ therapy include hypercalcemia and hypercalciuria (2). Alternatively, for patients whose rickets or osteomalacia results from lack of exposure to sunlight either increased exposure to sunlight, or ultraviolet lamp treatment may prove beneficial (1).

Rickets of prematurity is generally considered a disease of calcium and/or phosphate deficiency rather than vitamin D-deficiency. When long-term TPN therapy is involved, aluminum accumulation may also be a contributing factor (4). Currently, doses of vitamin D$_2$ for parenteral use in TPN-fed infants are 20–25 IU (0.5 μg/kg/day) (5). The oral dose of vitamin D$_2$ is between 400 and 800 IU (10 and 20 μg) daily (6,10).

For prevention of vitamin D deficiency not due to malabsorption or prematurity, daily exposure to adequate sunlight, consumption of fortified milk, or dietary supplementation of 400 IU (10 μg) is recommended.

CALCIUM DEFICIENCY

Decreased calcium intake or intestinal absorption has been associated with rickets. Kooh and colleagues (7) described rickets in an infant receiving prolonged nutrition with lamb-base formula, which provided adequate phosphorus, but only 180 mg/day of calcium. Vitamin D supplements were provided to give this child up to 800 IU (20 μg) per day. With the provision of 700 mg calcium/day there was marked biochemical and roentgenographic improvement after 1 month (7).

Similarly Pettifor and coworkers identified a population of children in South Africa who consumed no milk or dairy products and whose daily calcium intake was estimated to be only 125 mg, whereas phosphate intake was adequate. Biochemical and roentgenographic evidence of rickets were present. Moreover, bone histology in three children revealed increased unmineralized osteoid (matrix) and decreased bone turnover, diagnostic of osteomalacia (8,9). Calcium supplementation led to both biochemical and histologic improvement (9).

Reduction in calcium absorption may contribute to calcium-deficiency rickets. Consumption of cereals and other grain products high in phytate could lead to intraluminal calcium phytate complexation and consequent calcium malabsorption. This has been postulated by Stamp (1) and colleagues in Asian populations living in London. However, they subsequently demonstrated in two children that despite continued consumption of a high phytate diet, rickets improved with ultraviolet light therapy (1). Thus, it is possible that lack of sunlight rather than phytate-induced calcium malabsorption was responsible for the rickets in these children.

Another source of calcium deficiency-induced bone disease is total parenteral nutrition. Early in the development of TPN therapy, inadvertent omission of calcium led to rickets that was reversed by addition of calcium (3). Today, relative lack of calcium in the TPN solutions may be in part responsible for the osteopenia and rickets of prematurity.

Pathogenesis

The pathogenesis of calcium deficiency rickets is similar to that of vitamin D deficiency rickets in that hypocalcemia causes secondary hyperparathyroidism. Parathyroid hormone increases bone resorption and enhances the renal conversion of 25OHD to 1,25(OH)$_2$D to increase intestinal calcium and phosphorus absorption. Alkaline phosphatase also reflects elevated osteoblastic bone cell activity. Both the patients of Kooh et al. (7), and those of Pettifor and colleagues (8,9) had normal serum 25OHD levels, demonstrating that they were not vitamin D-deficient. The patient of Kooh et al. was hypophosphatemic, whereas those from South Africa were not.

Clinical manifestations of calcium deficiency rickets are similar to those described for vitamin D deficiency.

Treatment and Prevention

In the cases described from Canada and South Africa, oral calcium treatment was given (7–9) as shown in Table 1. Response to treatment was assessed by reduction in serum alkaline phosphatase levels and improvement in roentgenographic and histologic abnormalities. Special premature formulas now contain 75–150 mg calcium/dL. Currently, ~200 mg/kg/day is the goal for daily oral calcium intake (10). Parenteral solutions contain from 20 to 60 mg calcium/dL (5). Use of solutions containing 20 mg/dL of calcium resulted in a 20% incidence of rickets and osteopenia among premature infants in an intensive care nursery (11). Experience with 60 mg calcium/dL has been too limited to determine whether it reduces the incidence of rickets.

PHOSPHATE DEFICIENCY

Phosphate deficiency has been reported to cause rickets and osteomalacia. During the early development of TPN, omission of phosphate resulted in rickets that resolved with appropriate phosphate supplementation (3). However, premature infants may still receive inadequate phosphate relative to their needs (5). The calcium and phosphate added to parenteral nutrition solutions are limited by the possibility of calcium phosphate precipitation. According to Mierzwa (12), the following equation may serve

as a guide to determining whether calcium and phosphate will precipitate in solutions:

$$\frac{\text{Phosphate (mmol)} \times 1.8}{\text{Volume (L)}} = A$$

$$\frac{\dfrac{\text{Calcium gluconate (mg)} \times 4.6}{1,000}}{\text{Volume (L)}} = B$$

If $A \times B$ is less than 300 the parenteral nutrition solution is not likely to precipitate. Preliminary reports indicate that newer amino acid formulations supplemented with the sulfur-containing amino acids taurine and cysteine allow greater quantities of calcium and phosphate to remain in solution in TPN formulations (5).

Nutritional hypophosphatemic rickets has also been reported in a premature infant who was breast-fed without calcium or phosphate supplements (13).

Others at risk for hyphophosphatemic osteomalacia include those who have been taking antacids for long periods of time (14) and those on dialysis with osteomalacia (see Chapter 74). Antacid-induced osteomalacia results from aluminum complexation with dietary phosphate in the intestinal lumen that prevents phosphate absorption. Aluminum itself does not become deposited in bone in significant quantities (14).

Pathogenesis

The pathogenesis of phosphate deficiency rickets differs from that of vitamin D and calcium deficiency in that neither hyperparathyroidism nor vitamin D deficiency are present. Patients become phosphate-deficient, causing a reduction in serum phosphorus. Phosphate deficiency and hypophosphatemia increase renal production of 1,25(OH)$_2$D. 1,25-Dihydroxyvitamin D increases bone resorption *in vitro,* and it is possible but not proven that elevated serum levels of 1,25(OH)$_2$D cause bone resorption in these patients (13), although there is evidence that it may do so in adults (15).

Treatment and Prevention

Recommended parenteral phosphate intake for premature infants and phosphate and calcium supplementation for breast-fed prematures are given in Table 1. Roentgenographic changes of rickets resolved in one-breast-fed infant after 3 months of calcium and phosphate supplements (13). However, these recommendations may not be sufficient to ensure optimal bone mineral content (10). The phosphate available in specialized premature infant formulas is ~75 mg/dL (10). Long-term evaluation must be completed before one can conclude that this supplementation is effective in reducing the incidence of osteopenia and rickets in prematures.

For patients requiring long-term antiulcer therapy, use of nonaluminum-containing medications such as cimetidine or ranitidine should be considered.

REFERENCES

1. Stamp TCB: Factors in human vitamin D nutrition and in the production and cure of classical rickets. *Proc Nutr Soc* 34: 119–130, 1975
2. Sandstead HH: Clinical manifestations of certain classical deficiency diseases. In: Goodhart RS, Shils ME (eds) *Modern Nutrition in Health and Disease 6th ed*. Lea and Febiger, Philadelphia, pp 693–696, 1980
3. Klein GL, Chesney RW: Metabolic bone disease associated with total parenteral nutrition. In: Lebenthal E (ed) *Total Parenteral Nutrition: Indication, Utilization, Complications, and Pathophysiological Considerations*, 1st ed. Raven Press, New York, pp 431–443, 1986
4. Sedman AB, Klein GL, Merritt RJ, Miller NL, Weber KO, Gill WL, Anand H, Alfrey AC: Evidence of aluminum loading in infants receiving intravenous therapy. *N Engl J Med* 312: 1337–1343, 1985
5. Koo WWK, Kaplan LA, Bendon R, Succop P, Tsang RC, Horn J, Steichen D: Response to aluminum in parenteral nutrition during infancy. *J Pediatr* 109:877–883, 1986
6. Hillman LS; Neonatal osteopenia-diagnosis and management. In: Frame B, Potts JT Jr (eds) *Clinical Disorders of Bone and Mineral Metabolism*. Excerpta Medica, Amsterdam, pp 427–430, 1983
7. Kooh SW, Fraser D, Reilly BJ, Hamilton JR, Gall DG, Bell L: Rickets due to calcium deficiency. *N Engl J Med* 297:1264–1266, 1977
8. Pettifor JM, Ross FP, Travers R, Glorieux FH, DeLuca HF: Dietary calcium deficiency: A syndrome associated with bone deformities and elevated serum 1,25-dihydroxyvitamin D concentrations. *Metab Bone Dis Rel Res* 2:301–306, 1981
9. Marie PJ, Pettifor JM, Ross FP, Glorieux FH: Histological osteomalacia due to dietary calcium deficiency in children. *N Engl J Med* 307:584–588, 1982
10. Greer FR, Steichen JJ, Tsang RC: Effects of increased calcium, phosphorus and vitamin D intake on bone mineralization in very low birth weight infants fed formulas with polycose and medium chain triglycerides. *J Pediatr* 100:951–955, 1982
11. Koo WWK, Oestreich A, Tsang RC, Sherman R, Steichen J: Natural history of rickets and fractures in very low birth weight (VLBW) infants during infancy. *J Bone Miner Res* 1:123(abstract 255), 1986
12. Mierzwa MW: Stability and compatibility in preparing TPN solution. In: Lebenthal E (ed) *Total Parenteral Nutrition: Indications, Utilization, Complications, and Pathophysiological Considerations*. 1st ed. Raven Press, New York, pp 219–230, 1986
13. Rowe JC, Wood DH, Rowe DW, Raisz LG: Nutritional hypophosphatemia rickets in a premature infant fed breast milk. *N Engl J Med* 300:293–296, 1979
14. Carmichael KA, Fallon MD, Dalinka M, Kaplan FS, Axel L, Haddad JG: Osteomalacia and osteitis fibrosa in a man ingesting aluminum hydroxide antacid. *Am J Med* 76:1137–1143, 1984
15. Maierhofer WJ, Gray RW, Cheung H, Lemann J Jr: Bone resorption stimulated by elevated serum 1,25(OH)$_2$-vitamin D concentrations in healthy men. *Kidney Int* 24:555–560, 1983

66. Metabolic Bone Disease in Gastrointestinal and Biliary Disorders

D. Sudhaker Rao, M.B.B.S.

Bone and Mineral Division, Henry Ford Hospital, Detroit, Michigan

Because gastrointestinal tract is the major route of nutrient absorption, it is therefore, not surprising to find significant abnormalities in bone and mineral metabolism in patients with various gastrointestinal disorders. In a number of gastrointestinal, hepatobiliary, and pancreatic diseases, there is impaired absorption and/or catabolism of vitamin D and its metabolites (1–3) and malabsorption of calcium (4,5). In a few patients there may even be an increased urinary and fecal loss of calcium and calcidiol (25-hydroxyvitamin D). Symptoms related to the underlying malabsorption syndrome may not always be obvious and in some patients metabolic bone disease (MBD) may be the only presenting manifestation of an occult malabsorption syndrome (6,7). Careful and systematic evaluation is therefore needed to uncover such abnormalities.

The prevalence an the type of MBD in gastrointestinal diseases varies with the duration, type, and severity of malabsorption. MBD is uncommon, for instance, in patients with pancreatic insufficiency, but may approach 50–70% in those with gluten enteropathy. Conversely, prior gastrectomy is a strong risk factor for postmenopausal osteoporosis (8). Because of the varied response of the skeleton to alterations in mineral homeostasis, the spectrum of bone disease in gastrointestinal disorders may range from subjective impression of "decreased bone density" seen on routine skeletal roentgenograms, to severe osteomalacia with its classic clinical, biochemical, and radiologic findings; all gradations between these two extremes may be encountered.

MORPHOLOGIC AND KINETIC CHARACTERISTICS OF METABOLIC BONE DISEASE AND DEFINITION OF OSTEOMALACIA (9,10)

Both in normal subjects and in patients with osteoporosis, there is no relationship between mean osteoid seam thickness (O.Th; measured directly in μm, see Chapter 27) and osteoid surface (OS; measured directly as percentage of total bone surface). By contrast, in patients with vitamin D depletion there is a hyperbolic relationship between these two variables (Fig. 1A). This indicates that OS increases first and that O.Th increases only slightly until OS exceeds 70%, beyond which any further rise in OS is accompanied by a substantial increase in O.Th. The relationship between O.Th and adjusted apposition rate [(AjAR) as determined by tetracycline labeling, see Chapter 27] is more complex. When AjAR is above 0.1 $\mu g/day$,

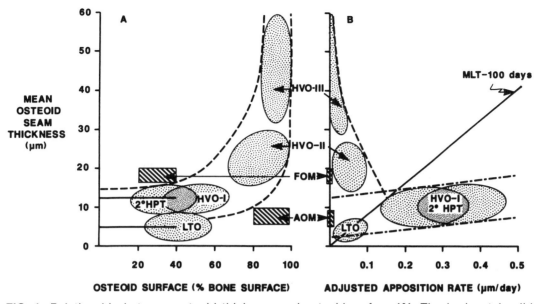

FIG. 1. Relationship between osteoid thickness and osteoid surface **(A).** The *horizontal solid lines* indicate the range for these variables in normal subjects. The *interrupted curvilinear lines* depict the hyperbolic relationship between these two variables in various metabolic bone diseases and in different stages of osteomalacia. On the *right* **(B),** the *straight interrupted lines* show the positive relationship between osteoid thickness and adjusted mineral apposition rate. The *oblique interrupted line* indicates the reversal of this relationship in patients with osteomalacia, a cardinal feature of this condition unlike all other conditions. The *solid straight line* represents a mineralization lag time of 100 days and separates patients with and without osteomalacia. Location of each category of MBD is diagrammatically shown for the sake of clarity. Note that there is significant overlap between patients with secondary hyperparathyroidism with (HVO-I) and without (secondary hyperparathyroidism alone) vitamin D depletion; the latter group represents patients with intestinal malabsorption of calcium alone. *HVO,* hypovitaminosis D osteopathy; *FOM,* focal osteomalacia; *AOM,* atypical osteomalacia; *LTO,* low-turnover osteoporosis. (From Parfitt AM: Osteomalacia and related disorders. In: Krane SM (ed) *Metabolic Bone Diseases, 2nd ed.* Grune and Stratton, New York, pp 329–396, 1990.)

there is a positive relationship between O.Th and AjAR, but below this value any reduction in AjAR is accompanied by a *rise* in O.Th in patients with vitamin D deficiency and by a *fall* in O.Th in all other conditions (Fig. 1B). This reversal of relationship between O.Th and AjAR is *the cardinal kinetic feature* of osteomalacia. A mineralization lag time (Mlt = O.Th ÷ AjAR, expressed in days) of 100 days separates patients with and without osteomalacia. Accordingly, osteomalacia is defined by a combination of O.Th >15 μm and an Mlt of >100 days (8,9). Patients with vitamin D deficiency who do not meet the above criteria are considered as having preosteomalacia or hypovitaminosis D osteopathy-stage I (HVO-I). Based on these morphologic and kinetic characteristics, it is possible to identify three distinct types of bone lesions in patients with various gastrointestinal disorders.

Secondary Hyperparathyroidism With or Without Vitamin D Deficiency

It is characterized by increased surface and volume, *but not the thickness* of osteoid (Table 1). In patients with

vitamin D deficiency additional features of reduced AjAR and prolongation of Mlt (usually <100 days) will be present. In both types there is accelerated loss of mainly cortical bone. Serum calcium (Ca), phosphate (P), and Ca × P product are normal but serum alkaline phosphatase (SAP) may be elevated in up to 80% of the patients. There is biochemical evidence of secondary hyperparathyroidism with increased nephrogenous cAMP (NcAMP) and parathyroid hormone (PTH), and decreased tubular maximum for phosphate reabsorption. Although 24-hr urine calcium is frequently <100 mg/day, it varies with dietary intake. Clinically, most patients are asymptomatic and present mainly with a history of skeletal fracture. Bone pain and muscle weakness are uncommon.

Osteomalacia

As defined previously, it is characterized by O.Th of >15 μm and an Mlt of >100 days. Both the surface and volume, as well as the thickness, of osteoid are increased (Table 1). Within this group two further stages are identified: HVO-II, in which some mineralization of osteoid

TABLE 1. *Morphologic and kinetic characteristics of bone diseases*

Measurement	Secondary HPT		Osteomalacia		
	D+	D− (HVO-I)	HVO-II	HVO-III	LTO
Osteoid surface (% BS)	↑	↑	↑ ↑	↑ ↑	N
Osteoid volume (% BV)	N	N/	↑ ↑	↑ ↑	N
Osteoid thickness (μm)	N	N/	↑ ↑	↑ ↑	N/ ↓
Mlt (days)	N	<100	>100	>100	<100
Osteoclast surface (% MdS)	↑	↑	↑ ↑	↑ ↑	N/ ↓
BFR (μm³/μm²/yr)	↑	↑	↓	0	N/ ↓

HPT, hyperparathyroidism; D, vitamin D; LTO, low-turnover osteoporosis; HVO, hypervitaminosis D osteopathy (stages I, II, and III); BS, bone surface; BV, bone volume; Mlt, mineralization lag time; MdS, mineralized surface; BFR, bone formation rate; N, normal; ↑, increased; ↓, decreased.

still occurs with preservation of double tetracycline labels; and HVO-III, where mineralization ceases to occur. Biochemical abnormalities are common in osteomalacia with reductions in Ca, P, and Ca × P product and elevations in SAP, NcAMP, and PTH. Classic radiologic features of osteomalacia such as pseudofractures, biconcave vertebrae, triradiate pelvis, and protrusio acetabuli are seen only in this group. Patients are symptomatic with diffuse bone pain and muscle weakness and may present with waddling gait that is typical of osteomalacia.

Two additional types of osteomalacia (focal and atypical) that are not related to vitamin D deficiency are recognized on careful analysis of bone histomorphometry. These are discussed in more detail in Chapter 72.

Low-Turnover Osteoporosis

This is probably the most common and the least understood form of MBD in patients with gastrointestinal disorders. Protein and other micronutrient deficiencies might contribute to the development of this bone disease. It is characterized by normal or reduced O.Th, decreased bone formation rate (Table 1), and slight reduction in AjAR resembling in some ways postmenopausal osteoporosis (8). Vertebral compression fractures are more common than in the other two types of bone lesions. Biochemical abnormalities are less frequent and secondary hyperparathyroidism is absent. Symptoms are usually related to the attendant skeletal fractures.

All seven types of bone lesions (secondary hyperparathyroidism, HVO-I, HVO-II, HVO-III, low-turnover osteoporosis; and focal and atypical osteomalacia) are diagrammatically shown in Fig. 1A, B, and the salient histomorphometric features are summarized in Table 1.

Two comments deserve emphasis: 1) secondary hyperparathyroidism is a consistent feature in all patients with vitamin D deficiency leading to an accelerated loss of mainly cortical bone; and 2) involutional or postmenopausal osteoporosis frequently accompanies the vitamin D-related bone disease and does not respond to therapy with vitamin D or its metabolites. Currently, transiliac bone biopsy after tetracycline labeling is the only definitive way of determining the exact nature of the underlying bone disease.

SPECIFIC ASPECTS OF METABOLIC BONE DISEASE IN GASTROINTESTINAL DISORDERS

Postgastrectomy Bone Disease (11–16)

Metabolic bone disease following gastrectomy or the more recent gastric stapling procedure is much more common than is generally appreciated. This is partly due to the incorrect notion that bone disease after gastric exclusion surgery is infrequent because of the routine fortification of milk and other dairy products with vitamin D in this country. However, because of the rarity of dietary vitamin D deficiency, gastrectomy alone accounts for half of all cases of osteomalacia seen in this country followed by, in the order of frequency, intestinal malabsorption, primary biliary cirrhosis, and pancreatic insufficiency. Several factors contribute to the development of bone disease following gastrectomy. These include poor dietary intake or self-imposed restrictions of dairy products to avoid diarrhea and dumping syndrome; rapid transit of food; the anatomic changes in gastrointestinal tract resulting in impaired absorption of vitamin D and its metabolites (Fig. 2) and of calcium; increased catabolism of vitamin D and its metabolites; and phosphate depletion due to excessive use of phosphate binding antacids. Patients with Billroth-II or total gastrectomy appear to be more at risk of developing MBD than those who have had Billroth-I operation. Bone disease is seldom detected early, and most patients present five or more years after gastrectomy. The onset is insidious, and there is frequent association of osteoporosis. Many patients are asymptomatic in the early postoperative period, and the bone loss can be detected only by sensitive techniques (see Chapter 26). Routine skeletal surveys are neither sensitive nor specific to be useful for screening purposes.

Hypocalcemia and hypophosphatemia are uncommon early in the course and tend to occur when the bone disease has advanced to HVO stage II or III. Elevated SAP level may indicate an underlying bone disease in the absence of hepatobiliary or Paget's disease, and thus serves as a useful screening test. Measurement of serum calcidiol concentration is another useful screening test to detect early vitamin D depletion and is available through commercial laboratories. When there is decreased bone min-

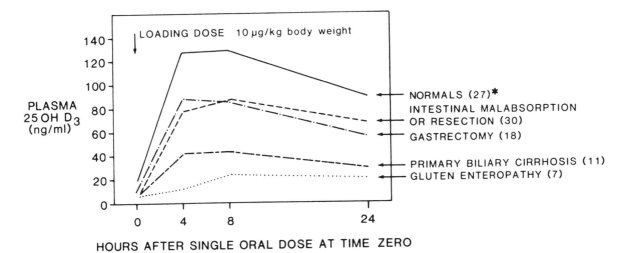

FIG. 2. Calcidiol absorption tests in normal subjects and in patients with various gastrointestinal disorders. Only the mean values were used to construct the curves for the sake of clarity. There is wide variation both in normal subjects and in patients. The scatter is much wider at 4 hr than at 8 hr, but the mean level at 4 and 8 hr for each group is significantly lower than in normal persons. Data were compiled from published reports as well as from personal experience. *Numbers in parenthesis represent the total number of normal patients studied. [From Rao DS: Bone and mineral metabolism. In: Berk JE (ed) *Bockus Gastroenterology, 5th ed.* W. B. Saunders, Philadelphia, 1993 (in press).]

eral content or low serum calcidiol level or both, bone histology is almost always abnormal. Approximately 20% of such patients will have osteomalacia as defined previously, and the remainder show evidence of secondary hyperparathyroidism.

As vitamin D depletion becomes more severe, which is usually a function of time since gastrectomy, patients develop diffuse bone pain, muscle weakness, and typical waddling gait. Classic radiologic signs of osteomalacia will be present, and the bone disease is far advanced with significant irreversible bone loss. Bone histology shows either HVO-II or HVO-III, and the clinical syndrome resembles more closely the traditional descriptions of osteomalacia. Hypocalcemia, hypophosphatemia, and elevated SAP are uniform findings at this stage of the disease. Although treatment greatly improves the clinical status of the patient, recovery of bone mineral deficit is negligible, and patients are at risk of fractures for the rest of their lives. It is, therefore, important to diagnose the bone disease at the earliest possible time and prevent long-term morbidity. This policy is no different from that of iron, folate, or vitamin B_{12} deficiencies.

Lifelong therapy with vitamin D or its metabolites and calcium is needed, with close monitoring of serum Ca, SAP, and renal function during the years of treatment. Despite similar risk factor(s) it is unclear why some patients develop HVO after gastrectomy, whereas others manifest only low turnover osteoporosis. General malnutrition, protein, and other micronutrient deficiencies may contribute to the pathogenesis of the latter. As might be expected, low turnover osteoporosis does not respond to vitamin D therapy, and therapeutic strategies similar to that used in the treatment of postmenopausal osteoporosis (see Chapter 56) might offer promise.

Malabsorption Syndromes (17,18)

In patients with intestinal disease, resection, or bypass, there is impaired absorption of both vitamin D and calcium; in some patients there may even be an increased endogenous fecal loss of calcium and vitamin D. The degree of malabsorption of vitamin D and calcium depletion is quite variable and, in general, depends on the severity of intestinal malabsorption. In Crohn's disease, for instance, vitamin D depletion is uncommon in the absence of intestinal resection or concomitant cholestyramine therapy. In gluten enteropathy, on the other hand, vitamin D depletion is common because of more severe malabsorption (Fig. 2). The prevalence of osteomalacia may approach 50–70% in such patients and, occasionally, osteomalacia may be the only presenting manifestation of gluten enteropathy (6,7). In patients with intestinal bypass surgery for morbid obesity, bone disease may develop even when prophylactic vitamin D therapy is instituted soon after surgery. Both osteopenia and osteoporosis are more frequent and severe than in patients with gastrectomy. Detection, surveillance, and treatment of metabolic bone disease is similar to that detailed for postgastrectomy patients.

Hepatobiliary Diseases (19–22)

Because of a large functional reserve, abnormalities in bone and mineral metabolism are relatively rare in the usual types of parenchymal liver diseases. Bone disease in chronic alcoholism is probably related to the direct effect of alcohol on bone (see Chapters 61 and 62) rather than to the associated liver disease. In severe hepatic impairment, such as primary biliary cirrhosis or biliary atresia in children, abnormalities of bone and mineral metabolism are commonplace. Factors that contribute to MBD include inadequate intake of dairy products because of anorexia; impaired absorption of dietary vitamin D and calcidiol (Fig. 2); urinary and fecal loss of vitamin D and its metabolites; binding of vitamin D or its metabolites by bile acid sequestering agents; and impaired 25-hydroxylation of vitamin D in the liver.

Biochemical abnormalities are more pronounced than in patients with gastrectomy or malabsorption syndrome. Hypocalcemia is frequent and is due to associated hypoalbuminemia or hypoproteinemia. Because elevated SAP is a uniform finding in various liver diseases, its significance in detecting an underlying bone disease is negated unless liver and bone isoenzymes are measured. Secondary hyperparathyroidism is less common than in patients with gastrectomy or intestinal malabsorption.

Osteopenia and low turnover osteoporosis are far more common than osteomalacia. Indeed, osteomalacia as defined by rigorous criteria has occurred only in two cases (10). Both the lack of clinically significant bone disease and the infrequency of osteomalacia are probably related to the serious nature of the liver disease so that skeletal manifestations become less clinically relevant. In a small number of patients, bone disease, especially osteomalacia, may contribute to the morbidity of already ill patients. With improvement in long-term survival, metabolic bone disease may dominate the clinical course of their illness, just as renal osteodystrophy has become a major problem in patients receiving maintenance hemodialysis.

Bone pain, when present, is often related to multiple long bone and rib fractures as a result of severe cortical bone loss rather than to osteomalacia. Even in asymptomatic patients vertebral compression fractures may occur. Muscle weakness is also unrelated to vitamin D deficiency in the majority of patients.

Treatment of hepatic osteodystrophy is unsatisfactory at present, except in those with unequivocal osteomalacia. Bone histology after tetracycline labeling is essential in planning therapeutic options in these patients. Either calcidiol or calcitriol (1,25-dihydroxyvitamin D) is better suited than vitamin D because of severe impairment of liver function.

Pancreatic Insufficiency (23)

Even in the presence of significant fat malabsorption and steatorrhea, metabolic bone disease is infrequent in patients with pancreatic insufficiency. Normal mucosal integrity may partly explain this infrequency. Nevertheless, patients are at risk of developing malabsorption of vitamin D and calcium. Ethanol abuse, a common feature among such patients, may also contribute to bone loss independently (see Chapters 61 and 62). Hypocalcemia is more common in acute pancreatitis than in chronic pancreatic disease. Other biochemical abnormalities are uncommon, and low calcidiol levels, when present, are related to poor dietary intake. Osteopenia may be more prevalent and osteomalacia is distinctly rare. Systematic studies of bone disease in patients with pancreatic insufficiency are not available and therefore the spectrum of bone disease in such patients remains unknown.

CALCIDIOL ABSORPTION TEST (1–3,24)

Availability of sensitive assays for measurement of serum calcidiol concentration made it possible to test for the presence of calcidiol malabsorption directly in various gastrointestinal disorders (Fig. 2). The test also provides an additional advantage of rapid repletion of body stores in patients with significant vitamin D depletion. The test is performed by administering 10 μg/kg of body weight of calcidiol in a single oral dose in the fasting state. Serum levels of calcidiol are measured at 4-hr intervals for 24 hr. A modified short test measuring only preabsorptive and 4- and 8-hr postabsorptive levels also provides useful information, because peak levels occur at either of these two times. Although the test does not replace other specific tests for malabsorption syndrome, it has a reasonable diagnostic and therapeutic utility. The known minor differences in absorption of vitamin D and calcidiol do not diminish its usefulness. Figure 2 shows typical absorption curves of calcidiol in various gastrointestinal diseases (24).

THERAPEUTIC PLAN AND CHOICE OF VITAMIN D OR ITS METABOLITES IN THE MANAGEMENT OF HVO

Prevention of HVO depends on the awareness of its existence in an appropriate clinical setting and the ability to screen the population at risk. To be effective the prevention program must begin before significant cortical bone loss has occurred. Yearly screening of patients at risk with SAP and serum calcidiol appears reasonable. Whether this is cost-effective is unknown, but considering the morbidity that an undiagnosed HVO confers, it is probably justifiable. Some have recommended yearly injections of 2.5 mg vitamin D_3 for all patients with gastrectomy, but its effectiveness in the prevention of HVO is unsubstantiated. Furthermore, absorption of such parenteral preparations is unpredictable, and suitable intravenous preparations are not available. With the availability of calcidiol for therapeutic use and the ability to monitor its serum concentrations, it is prudent to use this preparation. Doses should be adjusted to maintain a serum calcidiol level of 30–50 ng/mL. Although oral vitamin D is effective in many patients, variable bioavailability, chemical deterioration, and problems in monitoring the dose make these preparations unsuitable for long-term management. Calcidiol, on the other hand, is available in gelatin-coated capsules, less likely subject to chemical deterioration, has shorter half-life that reduces the potential for toxicity, is easily monitored by serum levels, and its conversion to calcitriol remains under homeostatic control. In conditions such as primary biliary cirrhosis, calcidiol may be the drug of choice because of defective 25-hydroxylation of vitamin D. *In most patients with HVO as a result of gastrointestinal disorders, renal function is normal and there is very little justification for the use of calcitriol.*

Treatment of established HVO is best achieved by performing calcidiol absorption test, which rapidly restores body stores, followed by continuation of therapy with calcidiol. Further dosage adjustments must be guided by the serum levels of calcidiol as described previously for prevention.

Because many patients require life-long therapy, periodic monitoring of serum Ca, SAP, and renal function is necessary. Hypercalcemia may occur at any time and should be treated promptly, as discussed in Chapter 28. Education of patients about the nature of their bone disease, necessity for life-long therapy, and the potential for future fracture risk even after resolution of HVO is essential both for compliance and to avoid complications related to calcidiol toxicity. It is worth reemphasizing that HVO in its early stages is asymptomatic but has already caused significant irreversible cortical bone loss and increased fracture risk. Therapy only repletes body stores and alleviates symptoms but rarely reverses bone loss. It is, therefore, important to keep all patients with gastrointestinal disorders under lifelong surveillance to avoid preventable morbidity.

REFERENCES

1. Gertner JM, Lilburn M, Domenech M: 25-Hydroxycholecalciferol absorption in steatorrhea and post-gastrectomy osteomalacia. *Br Med J* 1:1310–1312, 1977
2. Compston JE, Creamer B: Plasma levels and intestinal absorption of 25-hydroxy vitamin D in patients with small bowel resection. *Gut* 18:171–175, 1977
3. Compston JE, Thompson RPH: Intestinal absorption of 25-hydroxyvitamin D and osteomalacia in primary biliary cirrhosis. *Lancet* 1:721–724, 1977
4. Sjoberg HE, Nilsson LH: Retention of oral [47]Ca in patients with intestinal malabsorption: Regional enteritis and pancreatic insufficiency. *Scand J Gastroenterol* 5:265–273, 1970
5. Harris OD, Philips HM, Cooke WT: [47]Ca studies in adult coeliac disease and other gastrointestinal conditions with particular reference to osteomalacia. *Scand J Gastroenterol* 5:169–175, 1970
6. Hajjar ET, Vincenti F, Salti CS: Gluten-induced enteropathy; osteomalacia as a principal manifestation. *Arch Intern Med* 134:565–566, 1974
7. De-Boer WA, Tytgat GN: A patient with osteomalacia as single presenting symptom of gluten-sensitive enteropathy. *J Intern Med* 232:81–85, 1992
8. Rao DS, Kleerekoper M, Rogers M, et al.: Is gastrectomy a risk factor for osteoporosis? In: Christiansen C, et al. (eds) *Osteoporosis, vol 2.* Copenhagen Internal Symposium on Osteoporosis, Denmark, pp 775–777, 1984
9. Rao DS, Villanueva AR, Mathews M, et al.: Histologic evolution of vitamin-D depletion in patients with intestinal malabsorption or dietary deficiency. In: Frame B, Potts JT (eds) *Clinical Disorders of Bone and Mineral Metabolism.* Excerpta Medica, Amsterdam, pp 224–226, 1983
10. Parfitt AM: Osteomalacia and related disorders. In: Krane SM (ed) *Metabolic Bone Disease,* 2nd ed. Grune and Stratton, New York, pp 329–396, 1990
11. Bordier PH, Matrait H, Hiolo D, Hepner GW, Thompson GR, Booth CC: Subclinical vitamin-D deficiency following gastric surgery: Histologic evidence of bone. *Lancet* 1:437–440, 1968
12. Morgan DB, Hunt G, Paterson CR: The osteomalacia syndrome after stomach operations. *Q J Med* 39:395–410, 1970
13. Garrick R, Ireland AW, Posen S: Bone abnormalities after gastric surgery, a prospective histological study. *Ann Intern Med* 75:221–225, 1971
14. Imawari M, Kozawa K, Akanuma Y, Koizumi S, Itakura H, Kosaka K: Serum 25-hydroxyvitamin D and vitamin D-binding protein levels and mineral metabolism after partial and total gastrectomy. *Gastroenterology* 79:255–258, 1980
15. Nilas L, Christiansen C, Christiansen J: Regulation of vitamin D and calcium metabolism after gastrectomy. *Gut* 26:252–257, 1985
16. Klein KB, Orwoll ES, Lieberman DA, Meier DE, McLung MR, Parfitt AM: Metabolic bone disease in asymptomatic men after partial gastrectomy with Billroth-II anastomosis. *Gastroenterology* 92:608–612, 1987
17. Compston JE, Horton LWL, Creamer B: Osteomalacia after small intestine resection. *Lancet* 1:9–12, 1978
18. Parfitt AM, Miller MJ, Frame B, Villanueva AR, Rao DS, Oliver I, Thompson DL: Metabolic bone disease after intestinal bypass for treatment of obesity. *Ann Intern Med* 89:193, 1978
19. Dibble JB, Sheridan P, Hampshire R, Hardy GJ, Losowsky MS: Evidence for secondary hyperparathyroidism in the osteomalacia associated with chronic liver disease. *Clin Endocrinol* 15:373–383, 1981
20. Reed JS, Meredith SC, Nemchansky BA, Rosenberg IH, Bover JL: Bone disease in primary biliary cirrhosis: Reversal of osteomalacia with oral 25-hydroxyvitamin D. *Gastroenterology* 79:512–517, 1980
21. Matloff DS, Kaplan MM, Neer RM, Goldberg MJ, Bitman W, Wolfe HI: Osteoporosis in primary biliary cirrhosis: Effects of 25-hydroxy vitamin D treatment. *Gastroenterology* 83:97–102, 1982
22. Herlong FH, Recker RR, Maddrey WC: Bone disease in primary biliary cirrhosis: Histologic features and response to 25-hydroxy vitamin D. *Gastroenterology* 83:103–108, 1982
23. Hahn TJ, Squires AE, Halstead LR, Stronninger DB: Reduced serum 25-hydroxy vitamin D concentration and disordered mineral metabolism in patients with cystic fibrosis. *J Pediatr* 94:38–42, 1979
24. Rao DS: Bone and mineral metabolism. In: Berk JE (ed) *Bockus Gastroenterology,* 5th ed. W. B. Saunders, Philadelphia, 1993 (in press)

67. Vitamin D Dependent Rickets

*Uri A. Liberman, M.D., Ph.D. and †Stephen J. Marx, M.D.

*Division of Metabolic Diseases, Beilinson Medical Center, Petah-Tiqva,
and Department of Physiology and Pharmacology, Sackler School of
Medicine, Tel Aviv University, Tel Aviv, Israel and †Mineral Metabolism
Section, Metabolic Disease Branch, National Institutes of Health,
Bethesda, Maryland*

Pseudovitamin D deficiency or vitamin D dependent rickets (VDDR) type I and II are rare inborn errors of vitamin D metabolism, characterized by all the classical clinical, radiological, biochemical, and histological features of vitamin D deficiency (Chapter 65) despite adequate vitamin D intake and without a therapeutic response to an accepted vitamin D replacement therapy. The two syndromes differ (Table 1) in the circulating concentration of 1,25-dihydroxyvitamin D [$1,25(OH)_2D$], the therapeutic response to 1-α-hydroxylated active vitamin D metabolites, and obviously in the primary defect in vitamin D metabolism.

VITAMIN D DEPENDENT RICKETS TYPE I (VDDR-I)

Prader et al. (1) in 1961 were the first to report two young children with VDDR-I and to coin the phrase *pseudovitamin D deficiency* to describe this syndrome. The disease manifest itself before 2 years of age and often during the first 6 months of life. Complete remission could be obtained but was dependent on continuous therapy with high doses of vitamin D. Family studies revealed this to be a genetic disorder with a pattern suggestive of autosomal recessive inheritance (2). Although there are no direct enzymatic measurements in humans to prove defective activity of the renal 25-hydroxyvitamin D-1-α-hydroxylase [25(OH)D-1-hydroxylase], there are several indirect measurements to support this etiology. First, serum concentrations of 25-hydroxyvitamin D (25OHD) were normal or markedly elevated in patients treated with high doses of vitamin D or $25OHD_3$. Second, blood levels of $1,25(OH)_2D$ were very low in several studies of children with VDDR-I. Finally, while massive doses of vitamin D and $25OHD_3$ (1000 to 3000 μg/day and 200 to 900 μg/day, respectively, 100 to 300 times the recommended daily dose) are required to maintain remission of rickets in VDDR-I, 0.25 to 1.0 μg/day of $1,25(OH)_2D_3$ (a normal physiological dose) are sufficient to achieve the same effect. Taken together, these observations support the thesis that many if not all patients with VDDR-I have a hereditary defect in the renal tubular 25OHD-1-hydroxylase. The beneficial therapeutic effect of high circulating levels of 25OHD in patients with VDDR-I treated with vitamin D or $25OHD_3$ where $1,25(OH)_2D$ concentrations remain low has several possible explanations. First, 25OHD at high concentrations may activate the specific intracellular receptor for $1,25(OH)_2D$ whose affinity of 25OHD is about two orders of magnitude lower than for the active hor-

mone (Chapter 13). Second, high concentration of the substrate 25OHD may drive the local production of $1,25(OH)_2D$ in some tissue in a paracrine or autocrine manner. Finally, a metabolite of 25OHD may act directly on target tissues.

A similar syndrome has been studied in a mutant strain of pigs (3) in which the mode of inheritance as well as the clinical, radiological, and biochemical pictures are similar to the human disease. In a recent study (4) of piglets affected by this disease, circulating levels of 25OHD were elevated, $1,25(OH)_2D$ were low or undetectable, concentrations of specific [^3H]$1,25(OH)_2D_3$ binding sites were normal, and no 25OHD-1-hydroxylase activity could be measured in renal cortical homogenates. Thus, there is strong evidence that the disease state in the pig is caused solely by an inherited defect in the renal 25OHD-1-hydroxylase system. It is likely that a similar defect occurs in human VDDR-I.

VITAMIN D DEPENDENT RICKETS TYPE II (VDDR-II)

In 1978, Brooks et al. (5) described a patient with hypocalcemia, osteomalacia, and elevated circulating levels of $1,25(OH)_2D$. Treatment with vitamin D_3 resulted in a further increase in serum $1,25(OH)_2D$ levels and corrected the hypocalcemia of the patient. The term *vitamin D dependent rickets type II* was suggested to describe this disorder. Based on additional case reports, in which about half of the patients with this disorder did not respond to any form of vitamin D therapy and therefore were not dependent on the vitamin, and some *in vivo* and *in vitro* studies to be discussed, the term VDDR-II seems to be a misnomer. We therefore suggest the term **hereditary resistance to $1,25(OH)_2D$** as more appropriate to describe this syndrome. However, due to convention and convenience the term VDDR-II will be retained in this chapter.

Clinical Manifestations

The clinical, radiological, histological, and biochemical characteristics common to all patients with VDDR-II are rickets and/or osteomalacia of varying severity; no history or biochemical evidence of vitamin D or calcium deficiency; hypocalcemia and/or secondary hyperparathyroidism; no remission with physiological doses of vitamin D or its active metabolites; and increased serum levels

TABLE 1. *Vitamin D dependent rickets (VDDR)*

| | Serum concentrations | | | | |
	Calcium	25(OH)D	1,25(OH)$_2$D	iPTH	Presumed defect
VDDR-I	↓	N– ↑	↓ ↓	↑	renal 25OHD 1-hydroxylase
VDDR-II	↓	N– ↑	N– ↑	↑	intracellular 1,25(OH)$_2$D receptor

of 1,25(OH)$_2$D before or during treatment with calciferol preparations (6). There are less than 50 known patients with this syndrome (a partial list in references 6–21 and personal communications). Contrary to the homogeneity of the clinical and biochemical presentation of VDDR-I, a marked heterogeneity exists in VDDR-II.

Affected children appear normal at birth, and the metabolic bone disease presents early, usually before 2 years of age. However, late onset of the disease was reported in several sporadic cases, presenting in some patients in their teens (5); in one patient the onset of osteomalacia was at 45 years of age (10). All cases with late presentation have been normocalcemic, and they represent the mildest form of the disease.

A peculiar feature of the syndrome that appears in about two thirds of the kindreds is alopecia that varies from sparse hair to total alopecia without eye lashes (Fig. 1). In some patients additional ectodermal anomalies as multiple milia, epidermal cysts (Fig. 1), and oligodontia appear as well (9). The alopecia may be obvious at birth but usually develops during the first months of life. Alopecia seems to be a marker of a more severe form of the disease as judged by the earlier age of the presentation of the disease, the marked clinical aberrations, the number of patients that did not respond to treatment with high

doses of vitamin D and metabolites, and the high levels of serum 1,25(OH)$_2$D recorded during successful and unsuccessful therapy (6,23). Though some patients with alopecia have a satisfactory calcemic response to high doses of vitamin D and metabolites, none have shown improvement of hair growth.

Parental consanguinity and multiple siblings with the same defect occur in about half of the reported kindreds with VDDR-II, suggesting an autosomal recessive mode of inheritance in these and perhaps all kindreds. Parents of patients appear phenotypically normal. However, *in vitro* studies of cultured cells (see the following discussion) from parents of two kindreds with VDDR-II revealed heterogeneity of their 1,25(OH)$_2$D$_3$ receptor (VDR), i.e., expression of both a normal and an abnormal VDR allele. The affected children expressed only the abnormal allele (24,25). There is a striking clustering of patients close to the Mediterranean, and most of the patients reported from Europe and North American are descendants of families originating from around the Mediterranean as well. Notable exceptions are several kindreds reported from Japan (10,11,22).

Pathogenesis

Patients with VDDR-II show the highest serum levels of 1,25(OH)$_2$D found in any living system. These levels could represent the end result of synergistic action of three potential stimulators of the 25OHD-1-hydroxylase, namely hypocalcemia, secondary hyperparathyroidism, and hypophosphatemia; or they might also reflect an additional defect in regulation of the renal hydroxylase. This problem was investigated by Marx et al. and Balsan et al. (6,14) in a patient whose disease was in therapeutic remission. At this time the serum concentrations of calcium, PTH, and phosphorus were all normal. A brief change of medication from 1-α-(OH)D$_3$ to 25OHD$_3$ resulted in extremely high levels of 1,25(OH)$_2$D in serum derived from endogenous production, while serum calcium, PTH, and phosphorus remained in the normal range. It seems possible that under these conditions, the patient exhibited the consequences of defective feedback inhibition normally exerted by 1,25(OH)$_2$D on the renal 25OHD-1-hydroxylase. Such "aberrant" regulation of the enzyme might in fact be beneficial to some patients by maintaining high enough levels of 1,25(OH)$_2$D to sustain remission of the disease. 1,25(OH)$_2$D is a potent inducer of the 25-hydroxyvitamin D-24-hydroxylase [25OHD-24-hydroxylase] *in vivo* and *in vitro*. In patients with VDDR-II, serum levels of 24,25-(OH)$_2$D have been low or inappropriately low in face of the high levels of 1,25(OH)$_2$D

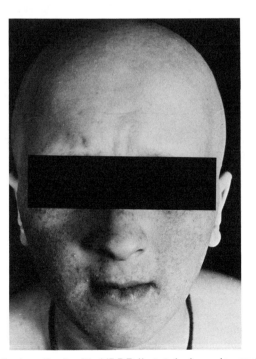

FIG. 1. A patient with VDDR-II: total alopecia, multiple milia, and epidermal cysts.

(6,9,21). This probably reflects decreased synthesis due to defective induction of the renal 25OHD-24-hydroxylase by 1,25(OH)$_2$D and indicates the importance of the 1,25(OH)$_2$D vitamin D receptor in the regulation of vitamin D metabolism. Complete remission of hypocalcemia, secondary hyperparathyroidism, and metabolic bone disease was achieved with moderate to extraordinarily high doses of bioactive vitamin D analogs in all kindred with normal hair [with a questionable one exception (20)], but only in some of the kindreds with total alopecia.

The notion that total alopecia is probably a direct consequence of resistance to 1,25(OH)$_2$D is supported by the following observations: (A) Alopecia is present in kindreds with different biochemical and molecular defects in the 1,25(OH)$_2$D receptor-effector system; (B) high-affinity uptake of [^{3}H]1,25(OH)$_2$D$_3$ occurred in the nucleus of the outer root sheath cells of the hair follicle of rodents; and (C) the epidermis and hair follicles contain a calcium-binding protein that is at least partially vitamin D dependent. Alopecia has been observed only with end-organ resistance to 1,25(OH)$_2$D and has not been noted with hereditary or acquired states associated with low circulating levels of 1,25(OH)$_2$D. Thus, either the deficiency in vitamin D action is more severe in VDDR-II or, alternatively, 1,25(OH)$_2$D may have an effect on differentiation of the hair follicle in the fetus that is unrelated to mineral homeostatis.

Classification by Cellular Defect

Studies on the nature of the intracellular defect in the 1,25(OH)$_2$D receptor-effector system of patients with VDDR-II became possible with demonstration that cells originating from tissues easily accessible for biopsy contain receptors for the hormone that are similar if not identical to those of classical target tissues. The cells used are mainly dermal fibroblasts, but keratinocytes, cells derived from bone, and recently peripheral blood mononuclear (PBM) cells (mitogen-stimulated T-lymphocytes and Epstein-Barr (EB) virus–transformed lymphocytes) have been used as well (6,12–16,25–28). These cells are used to assess most of the steps in 1,25(OH)$_2$D action from cellular uptake to bioresponse and to elucidate the molecular aberrations in the hormone receptor-protein and the nuclear DNA that encodes for it (24,25).

Several methods have been used to characterize the hormone-receptor interaction, including binding capacity and affinity of [^{3}H]1,25(OH)$_2$D$_3$ to intact cells, nuclei, or high salt soluble extract (cytosol) (6,12,13,16); measurements of receptor content by monoclonal antibodies (24,29); and characterization of the hormone-receptor complex on continuous sucrose gradient and heterologous DNA-cellulose columns (6,13,19,30). *In vitro* bioeffects of 1,25(OH)$_2$D on the various cells have been assayed by induction of the 25OHD-24-hydroxylase in skin- and bone-derived cells (17,31–33), osteocalcin (BGP) synthesis in cells derived from bone (33), inhibition of cell proliferation in PBM cells (27,28) and dermal fibroblasts (15,34), a mitogenic effect on dermal fibroblasts (34), and

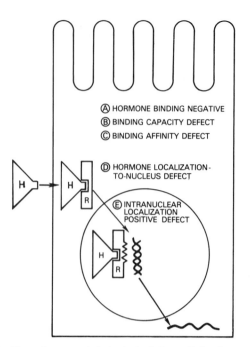

FIG. 2. Five classes of defects in intracellular interaction with 1,25(OH)$_2$D$_3$ associated with VDDR-II. This is a pictorial formulation not intended to prejudge the issue of the normal location of unoccupied receptors and the question of whether some or all of the mutations affect the structure of the receptor.

stimulation of cyclic cGMP production in cultured skin fibroblasts (35).

With these methods at least five phenotypically different intracellular defects have been identified (Fig. 2).

1. Hormone binding negative. Unmeasurable specific binding of [^{3}H]1,25(OH)$_2$D$_3$ to either high salt soluble cell extract and/or intact cells or nuclei. This is the most common abnormality observed. In the majority of these patients, high concentrations of 1,25(OH)$_2$D in serum or culture medium did not evoke a biological or biochemical response *in vivo* or *in vitro*. In four patients from different kindreds, normal amounts of receptor were found in soluble dermal fibroblast extract with a monoclonal antibody against the chick receptor that cross-reacts with the human receptor (29). This suggests that at least in these kindreds, there is a focal abnormality in the hormone-binding domain and not receptor deletion. Recently, however, a point mutation causing truncation of the vitamin D receptor protein was described (29A). In four affected children from three related families, genomic DNA from EB virus–transformed lymphocytes was isolated and amplified by PCR technique. DNA from all affected subjects exhibited a single C to A base substitution within exon 7 at nucleotide 970. This mutation resulted in the conversion of the normal codon for thyrosine into a premature termination codon at amino acid 292 of the vitamin D receptor protein, thus causing a deletion of a large portion of the 1,25(OH)$_2$D binding domain.

2. Defect in Hormone-binding capacity. The number of binding sites is about 10% of control with an apparent normal affinity. A patient with this defect showed no calcemic response to prolonged treatment with high doses of active calciferol metabolites (14).
3. Defect in hormone-binding affinity. $[^3H]1,25(OH)_2D_3$ binding affinity is reduced 20- to 30-fold with normal binding capacity of soluble (cytosolic) dermal fibroblasts extract. A complete remission of the disease in these patients could be achieved by high doses of vitamin D or its active metabolites (21).
4. Deficient nuclear localization. Normal or near normal binding affinity and capacity of $[^3H]1,25(OH)_2D_3$ binding to soluble cell extract. Normal binding to heterologous DNA but unmeasurable localization of $[^3H]1,25(OH)_2D_3$ to nuclei in intact cells. An identical defect was demonstrated with cells cultured from a bone biopsy of one patient (12) and in mitogen-stimulated PBM cells from several kindreds (22). These patients were treated successfully with high doses of vitamin D and its active metabolites (7,12,22).
5. Normal or near normal $[^3H]1,25(OH)_2D_3$ binding to soluble cell extract and to nuclei of intact cells, but decreased affinity of the hormone-receptor complex to heterologous DNA (19,25,30). No biological response to high doses of vitamin D or its active metabolites either in vivo or in vitro was documented in almost all patients with this type of defect (9,19,30). Recently a single nucleotide mutation in the exons encoding the DNA binding domain of the VDR was demonstrated in genomic DNA isolated from fibroblasts and/or EB virus–transformed lymphocytes from members from five kindreds with type 5 defect (25,25A). Four different single nucleotide mutations were found in the five kindreds. All mutations caused a single amino acid substitution localized to the region of the two zinc fingers of the vitamin D receptor protein. This region is essential for DNA binding of the hormone-receptor complex. It is worthwhile to mention that the DNA-binding domain of VDR is evolutionarily highly conserved throughout all members of the v-ERB-A related proteins that include the receptors for steroid hormone, thyroid hormones, and retinoic acid.

Though the number of patients with VDDR-II is small in each subgroup (categorized by type of receptor defect), it seems that patients with type 3 (deficient affinity) and type 4 (deficient nuclear localization) defects will respond to high doses of vitamin D with complete clinical and biochemical remission; patients with type 2 (low capacity) and most patients with type 1 (receptor negative) and 5 (receptor positive) defects could not be cured with high doses of vitamin D or metabolites. However, it should be emphasized that not all of these patients received the treatment long enough and with sufficiently high doses (see the following section). Measurements of an in vitro bioresponse of cells to $1,25(OH)_2D_3$ were carried out in less than half of the kindreds with VDDR-II. Induction of 25OHD-24-hydroxylase by $1,25(OH)_2D_3$ in cultured dermal fibroblasts showed an invariable correlation to the therapeutic response to vitamin D and metabolites in vivo (17,31,32).

Treatment

If the predictive therapeutic value of the in vitro bioresponse to $1,25(OH)_2D_3$ could be substantiated, it may eliminate the need for expensive and time-consuming therapy trials with vitamin D and metabolites. In the meantime it is mandatory to treat every patient with VDDR-II, regardless of the type of receptor defect. An adequate therapeutic trail must include (A) vitamin D_2 alone for the mildest cases, though in more severe typical cases therapy should be initiated with high doses of vitamin D analogs that will ensure maintenance of high serum concentrations of $1,25(OH)_2D$ (this can be accomplished by treatment with $1,25(OH)_2D_3$ or $1-\alpha(OH)D_3$ at daily doses in the range of up to 6 μg per kilogram body weight or a total of 30 to 60 μg); (B) supplemental calcium of up to 3 g elementary calcium per day; and (C) a duration of therapy (about 3–5 mo) sufficient to mineralize depleted bones and thus allow recovery from the hypocalcemia of "hungry bones." A close follow-up is essential and consists of clinical signs and symptoms; bone x-rays; serum levels of calcium, phosphorus, alkaline phosphatase, and creatinine; urinary excretion of calcium, phosphorus, and creatinine; parameters of parathyroid function; and serum $1,25(OH)_2D$ levels. Failure of therapy may be considered if no change in any of these parameters occurs during the treatment period while $1,25(OH)_2D$ serum levels are maintained above 100 times the mean normal range. It was reported recently that remarkable clinical and biochemical remission including catch-up growth and histological healing of defective osteoid mineralization was achieved by long-term therapy with high-dose oral calcium in one patient (36) or long-term intracaval infusion of calcium in several unusual patients with VDDR-II who did not respond to adequate trial with active vitamin D metabolites (33,37,38). These important studies imply that clinical remission could be achieved by calcium administration even in the most resistant patients with VDDR-II.

CONCLUSION

In summary, two inborn errors in vitamin D metabolism are presented and discussed. The important message is not just the description of a rare curiosity of nature, but rather the finding that rare aberrations of natural metabolic processes are important to unveil basic physiological, biochemical, and molecular mechanisms in general and in human beings in particular.

REFERENCES

1. Prader A, Illig R, Heierli E: Eline besondere Form der primaren vitamin D-resistenten Rachitis mit Hypocalcemie und autoso-

mal-dominanten Erbgang: Die hereditare Psuedo-Mangelrachitis. *Helv Paediatr Acta* 16:452–468, 1961

2. Scriver CR, Fraser D, Kooh SW: Hereditary rickets. In: Heath D, Marx SJ (eds), *Calcium Disorders,* Butterworth, London, 1982

3. Harmeyer JV, Grabe C, Winkley I: Pseudovitamin D deficiency rickets in pigs. An animal model for the study of familial vitamin D dependency. *Experimental Biol Med* 7:117–125, 1982

4. Fox J, Maunder EMW, Ranall VA, Care AD: Vitamin D dependent rickets type I in pigs. *Clin Sci* 69:541–548, 1985

5. Brooks MH, Bell NH, Love L, Stern PH, Ordei E, Queener SJ, Hamstra AJ, DeLuca HF: Vitamin D dependent rickets type II, resistance of target organs to 1,25-dihydroxyvitamin D. *N Engl J Med* 293:996–999, 1978

6. Marx SJ, Liberman UA, Eil C, Gamblin GT, DeGrange DA, Balsan S: Hereditary resistance to 1,25-dihydroxyvitamin D. *Recent Prog Hormone Res* 40:589–620, 1984

7. Marx SJ, Spiegel AM, Brown EM, Gardner DG, Downs RW Jr, Attie M, Hamstra AJ, DeLuca HF: A familial syndrome of decrease in sensitivity to 1,25-dihydroxyvitamin D. *J Clin Endocrinol Metab* 47:1303–1310, 1978

8. Rosen JF, Fleischman AR, Finberg L, Hamstra A, DeLuca HF: Rickets with alopecia: an inborn error of vitamin D metabolism. *J Pediatr* 94:729–735, 1979

9. Liberman UA, Samuel R, Halabe A, Kauli R, Edelstein S, Weisman Y, Papapoulos SE, Clemens TL, Fraher LJ, O'Riordan JLH: Eng-organ resistance to 1,25-dihydroxy cholecalciferol. *Lancet* 1:504–506, 1980

10. Fujita T, Nomura M, Okajima S, Suzuya H: Adult-onset vitamin D-resistant osteomalacia with unresponsiveness to parathyroid hormone. *J Clin Endocrinol Metab* 50:927–931, 1980

11. Tsuchiya Y, Matsuo N, Cho H, Kumagai M, Yasaka A, Suda T, Orimo H, Shiraki M: An unusual form of vitamin D-dependent rickets in a child: alopecia and marked end-organ hyposensitivity to biological active vitamin D. *J Clin Endocrinol Metab* 51:685–690, 1980

12. Eil C, Liberman UA, Rosen JF, Marx SJ; A cellular defect in hereditary vitamin D-dependent rickets type II: defective nuclear uptake of 1,25-dihydroxyvitamin D in cultured skin fibroblasts. *N Engl J Med* 304:1588–1591, 1981

13. Feldman D, Chen T, Cone C, Hirst M, Shari S, Benderli A, Hochberg Z: Vitamin D resistant rickets with alopecia: cultured skin fibroblasts exhibit defective cytoplasmic receptors and unresponsiveness to 1,25(OH)$_2$D$_3$. *J Clin Endocrinol Metab* 55:1020–1025, 1982

14. Balsan A, Garabedian M, Liberman UA, Eil C, Bourdeau A, Guillozo H, Grimberg R, DeDeunff MJ, Lieberherr M, Guimbaud P, Broyer M, Marx SJ: Rickets and alopecia with resistance to 1,25-dihydroxyvitamin D: two different clinical courses with two different cellular defects. *J Clin Endocrinol Metab* 57:803–811, 1983

15. Clemems TL, Adams JC, Horiuchi N, Gilchrist BA, Cho H, Ysuchiya Y, Matsuo N, Suda T, Holick MF: Interaction of 1,25-dihydroxyvitamin D$_3$ with keratinocytes and fibroblasts from skin of a subject with vitamin D-dependent rickets type II: a model for the study of action of 1,25-dihydroxyvitamin D$_3$. *J Clin Endocrinol Metab* 56:824–830, 1983

16. Liberman UA, Eil C, Marx SJ: Resistance of 1,25-dihydroxyvitamin D: association with heterogeneous defects in cultured skin fibroblasts. *J Clin Invest* 71:192–200, 1983

17. Chen TL, Hirst MA, Cone CM, Hochberg Z, Tietze HU, Feldman D: 1,25-dihydroxyvitamin D resistance, rickets and alopecia: analysis of receptors and bioresponse in cultured skin fibroblasts from patients and parents. *J Clin Endocrinol Metab* 59:383–388, 1984

18. Hochberg Z, Benderli Z, Levy J, Weisman Y, Chen T, Feldman D: 1,25-dihydroxyvitamin D resistance, rickets, and alopecia. *Am J Med* 77:805–811, 1984

19. Hirst MA, Hochman HI, Feldman D: Vitamin D resistance and alopecia: a kindred with normal 1,25-dihydroxyvitamin D$_3$ binding, but decreased receptor affinity for deoxyribonucleic acid. *J Clin Endocrinol Metab* 60:490–495, 1985

20. Fraher LJ, Karmali R, Hinde FRJ, Hendy GN, Jani H, Nicholson L, Grant D, O'Riordan JLH: Vitamin D-dependent rickets

type II: extreme end organ resistance to 1,25-dihydroxyvitamin D$_3$ in a patient without alopecia. *Eur J Pediatr* 145:389–395, 1986.

21. Castells S, Greig F, Fusi MA, Finberg L, Yasumura S, Liberman UA, Eil C, Marx SJ: Severely deficient binding of 1,25-dihydroxyvitamin D to its receptor in a patient responsive to high doses of this hormone. *J Clin Endocrinol Metab* 63:252–256, 1986

22. Tajkeda E, Kuroda Y, Saijo T, Naito E, Kobashi H, Yokota I, Miyao M; 1-α-hydroxyvitamin D$_3$ treatment of three patients with 1,25-dihydroxyvitamin D-receptor-defect rickets and alopecia. *Pediatrics* 80:97–101, 1987

23. Marx SJ, Bliziotes MM, Nanes M: Analysis of the relation between alopecia and resistance to 1,25-dihydroxyvitamin D. *Clin Endocrinol* 25:373–381, 1986

24. Malloy PJ, Hochberg Z, Pike JW, Feldman D: Abnormal binding of vitamin D receptors to deoxyribonucleic acid in a kindred with vitamin D dependent rickets, type II. *J Clin Endocrinol Metab* 68:263–269, 1989

25. Hughes MR, Malloy PJ, Kieback DG, Kesterson RA, Pike JW, Feldman D, O'Malley BW: Point mutations in the human vitamin D receptor gene associated with hypocalcemia rickets. *Science* 242:1702–1705, 1988

25A. Sone T, Marx SJ, Liberman UA, Pike JW: A unique point mutation in the human vitamin D receptor chromosomal gene confers hereditary resistance to 1,25-dihydroxyvitamin D$_3$. *Mol Endocrinol* 4:623–631, 1990

26. Liberman UA, Eil C, Holst P, Rosen JF, Marx JS: Hereditary resistance to 1,25-dihydroxyvitamin D: defective function of receptors for 1,25-dihydroxyvitamin D in cells cultured from bone. *J Clin Endocrinol Metab* 57:958–962, 1983

27. Koren R, Ravid A, Liberman UA, Hochberg Z, Weisman J, Novogrodsky A: Defective binding and function of 1,25-dihydroxyvitamin D$_3$ receptors in peripheral mononuclear cells of patients with end-organ resistance to 1,25-dihydroxyvitamin D. *J Clin Invest* 76:2012–2015, 1985

28. Takeda E, Kuzoda Y, Saijo T, Toshima K, Naito E, Kobashi H, Iwakuni Y, Miyao M: Rapid diagnosis of vitamin d-dependent rickets type II by use of phytohemagglutinin-stimulated lymphocytes. *Clin Chim Acta* 155:245–250, 1986

29. Pike JW, Dokoh S, Haussler MR, Liberman UA, Marx SJ, Eil C: Vitamin D-resistant fibroblasts have immunoassayable 1,25-dihydroxyvitamin D$_3$ receptors. *Science* 224:879–881, 1984

29A. Ritchie HH, Hughes MR, Thompson ET, Hochberg Z, Feldman D, Pike JW, O'Mally BW: An ochre mutation in the vitamin D receptor gene causes hereditary 1,25-dihydroxyvitamin-D$_3$ resistant rickets in three families. *Proc Natl Acad Sci USA* 86:9783–9787, 1989

30. Liberman UA, Eil C, Marx SJ: Receptor positive hereditary resistance to 1,25-dihydroxyvitamin D: chromatography of hormone-receptor complexes on DNA-cellulose shows two classes of mutation. *J Clin Endocrinol Metab* 62:122–126, 1986

31. Griffin JE, Zerwekh JE: Impaired stimulation of 25-hydroxyvitamin D-24-hydroxylase in fibroblasts from a patient with vitamin D-dependent rickets, type II. *J Clin Invest* 72:1190–1199, 1983

32. Gamblin GT, Liberman UA, Eil C, Downs RW Jr, DeGrange DA, Marx SJ: Vitamin D-dependent rickets type II, defective induction of 25-hydroxyvitamin D$_3$-24-hydroxylase by 1,25-dihydroxyvitamin D$_3$ in cultured skin fibroblasts. *J Clin Invest* 75:954–960, 1985

33. Balsan S, Garabedian M, Larchet M, Gorski AM, Cournot G, Tau C, Bourdeau A, Silve C, Ricour C: Long-term nocturnal calcium infusions can cure rickets and promote normal mineralization in hereditary resistance to 1,25-dihydroxyvitamin D. *J Clin Invest* 77:1661–1667, 1986

34. Barsony J, McKoy W, DeGrange DA, Liberman UA, Marx SJ: Selective expression of a normal action of 1,25-dihydroxyvitamin D$_3$ receptor in human skin fibroblasts with hereditary severe defects in multiple action of this receptor. *J Clin Invest* 83:2093–2101, 1989

35. Barsony J, Marx SJ: Receptor-mediated rapid action of 1-α-25-dihydroxy-cholecalciferol: increase of intracellular cGMP in human skin fibroblasts. *Proc Natl Acad Sci USA* 85:1223–1226, 1988

36. Sakati N, Woodhouse NTY, Niles N, Harji H, DeGrange DA, Marx SJ: Hereditary resistance to 1,25-dihydroxyvitamin D:

clinical and radiological improvement during high-dose oral calcium therapy. *Hormone Res* 24:280–287, 1986

37. Weisman Y, Bab I, Gazit D, Spirer Z, Jaffe M, Hochberg Z: Long-term intracaval calcium infusion therapy in end-organ resistance to 1,25-dihydroxyvitamin D. *Am J Med* 83:984–990, 1987

38. Bliziotes M, Yergey AL, Nanes MS, Muenzer J, Begley MG, Vieira NE, Kher KK, Brandi ML, Marx SJ: Absent intestinal response to calciferols in hereditary resistance to 1,25-dihydroxyvitamin D: documentation and effective therapy with high dose intravenous calcium infusions. *J Clin Endocrinol Metab* 66: 294–300, 1988

68. Hypophosphatemic Vitamin D Resistant Rickets

Francis H. Glorieux, M.D., Ph.D.

Departments of Surgery, Pediatrics, and Human Genetics, McGill University, and Genetics Unit, Shriners Hospital, Montréal, Québec, Canada

Bone growth and mineralization require adequate availability of calcium and phosphate, the two major constituents of hydroxyapatite, the crystalline part of bone tissue. Defective supply of either calcium or phosphate will result in impaired mineralization, which will cause rickets at the growth plate level and osteomalacia at the cortico-endosteal level. Thus, in growing individuals, both lesions will be present, although by definition only osteomalacia can possibly develop in adults.

Deficiency in calcium, as a consequence of either insufficient intake (1), or vitamin D deficiency or abnormal metabolism (2) will induce hypocalcemia, rickets, and osteomalacia. The latter will be characterized by osteopenia, as a consequence of the increased resorption induced by hyperparathyroidism secondary to hypocalcemia.

In chronic hypophosphatemia, although clinical and radiologic manifestations of rickets are similar to those seen in calcium deficiency, osteomalacia is characterized by an accumulation of unmineralized osteoid along the trabeculae. Because calcemia is normal, there is no secondary hyperparathyroidism and thus neither increased osteoclast activity nor excessive resorption. Consequently, bone mass is not decreased. It is, in fact, often measured above normal values for age.

CLASSIFICATION OF HYPOPHOSPHATEMIC SYNDROMES

Both acquired and congenital forms occur. In most instances, the acquired forms can be controlled by acting on the underlying causes (insufficient phosphate intake, increased renal loss secondary to a mesenchymal tumor or an altered tubular function). The inherited syndromes, however, present a challenge—sometimes for diagnosis and always for management. The most frequent of the hypophosphatemic syndromes was described more than 50 years ago by Albright et al. (3), who coined the term *hypophosphatemic vitamin D resistant rickets*. It is inherited as an X-linked dominant trait (4) with the mutant gene located in the distal part of the short arm of the X chromo-

some (5); hence, it is now referred to as X-linked hypophosphatemia (XLH). In 1976 a homologous mutation was discovered in the mouse (Hyp) (6). The high degree of conservatism of the mammalian X chromosome and comparative mapping of the human and mouse gonosomes (7) support the contention of a close analogy between the XLH and Hyp mutations. Active studies have thus been pursued in parallel in the two species to better understand the phenotypic expression of the abnormal genes.

CLINICAL EXPRESSION

The classic triad, fully expressed in hemizygous male patients, consists of (a) hypophosphatemia, (b) lower limb deformities, and (c) stunted growth rate. Although low serum phosphate (P) is evident early after birth, it is only at time of weight bearing that leg deformities and progressive departure from normal growth rate become sufficiently striking to attract attention and make parents seek medical opinion. An often overlooked clinical sign is the appearance of the teeth. There is no enamel hypoplasia in XLH, as opposed to what is seen in hypocalcemic rickets. Hypophosphatemic rickets presents with dentine defects that are not apparent on examination but which may cause dental abscesses and early decay in the young adult. In several families, isolated hypophosphatemia can be found in some heterozygous females; thus, this trait is considered the marker for the mutation. These healthy trait carriers provide evidence that hypophosphatemia and renal P waste alone cannot explain the abnormal phenotype.

RENAL DEFECT

It is generally accepted that hypophosphatemia is the consequence of a primary inborn error of phosphate transport probably located in the proximal nephron (8). It is noteworthy that the defect is less severe in heterozygotes than it is in hemizygotes. This gene dose effect indicates that the abnormality is close to the abnormal gene product. The abnormality in the Hyp mouse has been localized in the brush border of the proximal tubular cells (9). The possibility that it would be secondary to the presence of a humoral "hypophosphatemic factor" (10) has received experimental support in the mouse model (11). Whether these findings can be directly extrapolated to human subjects is not established. In particular, they would not explain the gene dose effect that is present in humans but not readily evident in the murine model.

Because of the close link between the phosphate repletion status and 1,25-dihydroxyvitamin D (1,25D) synthesis, the metabolism of this hormone has been extensively studied in mutant individuals. It is important to point out that there is no simple 1,25D deficiency (as seen in vitamin D pseudodeficiency) and that no close correlation exists between extracellular P concentration and 1,25D synthesis. Rather, the reported inappropriate response of 1,25D synthesis to a low phosphate challenge (12), although there is no abnormality in the response to a low calcium challenge (13), points toward the vitamin D metabolism abnormality as secondary to the primary P transport defect and its consequences on intracellular P economy.

RESPONSE TO TREATMENT

Based on the established renal P waste, therapy has centered on often aggressive P replacement (1–3 g elemental P/d in 4–5 doses). To offset the hypocalcemic effect of P supplementation, which has caused sometimes severe secondary hyperparathyroidism, large (20–75,000 IU/d) amounts of vitamin D were added to the regimen. With adequate compliance to such a combined treatment, growth rate was markedly improved and radiologic evidence of healed rickets was noted (14,15). The early observation that heterozygous girls responded better to treatment than hemizygous boys (14) has recently been substantiated, supporting the concept of a gene dose effect in this X-linked dominant disorder (16). However, histologic studies of iliac crest bone biopsies showed that the osteomalacic component of the bone disease was hardly improved (17). Only with the substitution of 1,25D for vitamin D at the dose of 30–70 ng/kg/d was improvement and sometimes healing of the mineralization defect observed on the trabecular surfaces (18–21). Interestingly, the hypomineralized periosteocytic lesions (HPL), which are a hallmark of XLH, never completely disappear even after active mineralization has been restored at the endosteal surfaces. After more than 2 yr of efficient therapy, HPL are still present around 20% of the osteocytes in the newly formed osteons (22). Because HPL are never present in other chronic hypophosphatemic states, this observation gives substance to the early proposal that there may be an osteoblast primary metabolic defect in XLH (23). The lesions are also present in the Hyp mouse (24), where an abnormal osteoblast response to 1,25D has been demonstrated (25). Studies recently conducted with osteoblasts isolated from mouse calvaria have provided morphologic evidence that Hyp osteoblasts, even when transplanted in a normal environment, are unable to produce adequate amounts of mineralized matrix (26). Al-

though more work will be needed to characterize the osteoblast defect precisely, it is tempting to speculate that the osteoblast shares, with the renal tubular cell, a gene product that would specifically affect phosphate transport and, in an ancillary fashion, 1,25D synthesis.

LONG-TERM EFFECTS OF TREATMENT

Except for occasional osmotic diarrhea, P supplementation has not caused any harmful effects. Coated tablets are preferable to liquid forms because tablets provide a slower rate of absorption. Tablets are also made of a mixture of sodium and potassium salts, avoiding the high sodium load so frequent with the solutions.

Before 1978 large amounts of vitamin D were administered to offset the hypocalcemic effect of P supplementation and the ensuing iatrogenic hyperparathyroidism. This was often difficult to control, and several cases of autonomous hyperparathyroidism were encountered that could be treated only surgically (14). The substitution of 1,25D for vitamin D has now allowed a more precise control of PTH secretion throughout the treatment period. It thus appears that 1,25D, through its direct effect on PTH release, is able to maintain euparathyroidism together with adequate bone modeling and remodeling (20,27).

One major concern with long-term administration of 1,25D is a possible deterioration of renal function through interstitial nephrocalcinosis. Indeed, frequent ultrasound observations of echodense renal pyramids have been reported (28). Recent histologic studies have confirmed that they correspond to mineral deposits made exclusively of calcium phosphate (29). Whether the induction of such deposits is related primarily to the phosphate load or to the long-term use of 1,25D is unclear at present. Such findings, however, are not directly related to evidence of decreased renal function. In our experience, in 18 patients treated for an average of 8 yr, two-thirds of patients present with profiles of increased echogenecity of the renal pyramids (too quickly labeled nephrocalcinosis) but no alteration of renal function (unpublished). Thus, long-term use of 1,25D associated with supplemental P and with frequent monitoring of urinary calcium excretion to avoid episodes of hypercalciuria should be considered a safe and efficient way to control the clinical expression of the XLH mutation. When hypercalciuria develops, adjustment of the 1,25D dosage is necessary.

Because stunted growth is a major consequence of the XLH phenotype, the use of biosynthetic growth hormone, as a third therapeutic component, was recently advocated (30). The hormone increased serum P levels, and over a 24-wk period, appeared to affect growth rate positively in 11 XLH children. Other such studies will be needed before concluding that the basic treatment protocol should be uniformly modified.

TREATMENT OF GROWN-UP PATIENTS

With early initiation of therapy and good compliance throughout the growing period, clinical results are usually satisfactory in terms of stature achieved and prevention of lower limb deformities. An important question is whether one should maintain the demanding treatment schedule combining 1,25D and phosphate after fusion of the epiphyseal plates. Because growth has ceased and bone turnover is reduced, the appropriateness of maintaining a high phosphate intake can rightly be questioned. The demonstration that the treatment resulted in significant clinical and histomorphometric improvement in 18 symptomatic XLH adult patients who received P + 1,25D for 4 years (31) suggests that such an approach is worthwhile. Its optimal duration, however, remains unresolved. Because strict compliance to P supplements on a 5 dose/day schedule is difficult, one may envisage that continuing 1,25D alone, through its stimulation of bone turnover and intestinal phosphate absorption, would maintain the good results obtained with the combined therapy. Preliminary observations in 6 XLH patients indicate that 1,25D alone (at a dose of 1–2 µg/d) has positively influenced the parameters of bone mineralization over a 11–17 mo period (unpublished). This study, still in progress, should allow us to better define our long-term strategy of metabolic and clinical control of XLH patients.

CONCLUSION

Despite the persistent questions about the pathogenesis of XLH, medical control of its clinical expression has greatly improved over the past 15 yr. The combination of large amounts of phosphate salts and supraphysiologic doses of 1,25D has allowed normal growth and adequate bone matrix mineralization. With close and careful follow-up the regimen is safe, and no deleterious effects on renal function should be expected. Uncertainty continues with regard to the treatment of asymptomatic adult XLH subjects.

REFERENCES

1. Marie PJ, Pettifor JM, Ross FP, Glorieux FH: Histologic osteomalacia due to dietary calcium deficiency in children. *N Engl J Med* 307:584, 1982
2. Glorieux FH, Pettifor JM: Metabolic bone disease. In: Kelley VC (ed), *Practice of Pediatrics*, Harper & Row, Philadelphia 7:34, 1984
3. Albright F, Butler AM, Bloomberg E. Rickets resistant to vitamin D therapy. *Am J Dis Child* 54:529, 1937
4. Winters RW, Graham JB, Williams TF, McFalls VW, Burnett CH: A genetic study of familial hypophosphatemia and vitamin-D resistant rickets with a review of the literature. *Medicine* 37:97, 1958
5. Thakker RV, Read AP, Davies KE, Whyte WP, Weksberg R, Glorieux FH, Davies M, Mountford RC, King A, Kim GS, Harris R, and O'Riordan JLH: Bridging markers defining the map position of X-linked hypophosphatemic rickets. *J Med Genet* 24:756, 1987
6. Eicher EM, Southard JL, Scriver CR, Glorieux FH: Hypophosphatemia: mouse model for human familial hypophosphatemic (vitamin-D resistant) rickets. *Proc Natl Acad Sci (USA)* 73:4667, 1976
7. Davisson MT: X-linked genetic homologies between mouse and man. *Genomics* 1:213, 1987
8. Glorieux F, Scriver CR: Loss of a PTH sensitive component of phosphate transport in X-linked hypophosphatemia. *Science* 175:997, 1972
9. Tenenhouse HS, Scriver CR, McInnes RR, Glorieux FH: Renal handling of phosphate in vivo and in vitro by the X-linked hypophosphatemic male mouse (Hyp/Y). Evidence for a defect in the brush border membrane. *Kidney Int* 14:236, 1978
10. Bonjour J-P, Caverzasio J, Muhlbauer R, Trechsel U, Troechler U: Are 1,25(OH)$_2$D$_3$ production and tubular phosphate transport regulated by one common mechanism which would be defective in X-linked hypophosphatemic rickets? In: Norman AW, Schaefer K, Herrath DV, Grigoleit H-G (eds), *Vitamin D, Chemical Biochemical and Clinical Endocrinology of Calcium Metabolism,* Walter de Gruyter, Berlin, New York, 427–433, 1982
11. Nesbitt T, Coffman TM, Griffiths R, Drezner MK: Crosstransplantation of kidneys in normal and Hyp mice. Evidence that the Hyp mouse phenotype is unrelated to an intrinsic renal defect. *J Clin Invest* 89:1453, 1992
12. Lobaugh B, Drezner MK: Abnormal regulation of renal 25-dihydroxyvitamin D-1α-hydroxylase activity in the X-linked hypophosphatemic mouse. *J Clin Invest* 71:400, 1983
13. Meyer RA Jr, Gray RW, Roos BA, Kiebzak GM: Increased plasma 1,25-dihydroxyvitamin D after low calcium challenge in X-linked hypophosphatemic mice. *Endocrinology* 11:174, 1982
14. Glorieux FH, Scriver CR, Reade TM, Goldman H, Roseborough A: The use of phosphate and vitamin D to prevent dwarfism and rickets in X-linked hypophosphatemia. *N Engl J Med* 281:481, 1972
15. Verge CF, Lam A, Simpson JM, Cowell CR, Howard NJ, Silink M: Effects of therapy in X-linked hypophosphatemic rickets. *N Engl J Med* 325:1843, 1991
16. Petersen DJ, Boniface AM, Schranck FW, Rupich RC, Whyte MP: X-linked hypophosphatemic rickets: a study (with literature review) of linear growth response to calcitriol and phosphate therapy. *J Bone Miner Res* 7:583, 1992
17. Glorieux FH, Bordier PJ, Marie P, Delvin EE, Travers R: Inadequate bone response to phosphate and vitamin D in familial hypophosphatemic rickets. In: Massry S, Ritz E, Rapado A (eds), *Homeostasis of Phosphate and Other Minerals,* Plenum, New York, 227–232, 1980
18. Glorieux FH, Marie PJ, Pettifor JM, Delvin EE: Bone response to phosphate salts, ergocalciferol and calcitriol in hypophosphatemic vitamin-D resistant rickets. *N Engl J Med* 303:1023, 1980
19. Costa T, Marie PJ, Scriver CR, Cole DEC, Reade TM, Nogrady B, Glorieux FH, Delvin EE: XO-linked hypophosphatemia. Effect of calcitriol on renal handling of phosphate, serum phosphate, and bone mineralization. *J Clin Endocrinol Metab* 52:463, 1981
20. Drezner MK, Lyles KW, Haussler MR, Harrelson JM: Evaluation of a role for 1,25-dihydroxyvitamin D in the pathogenesis and treatment of X-linked hypophosphatemic rickets and osteomalacia. *J Clin Invest* 66:1020, 1980
21. Harrell RM, Lyles KW, Harrelson JM, Friedman NE, Drezner MK: Healing of bone disease in X-linked hypophosphatemic rickets/osteomalacia. Induction and maintenance with phosphorous and calcitriol. *J Clin Invest* 75:1858, 1985
22. Marie PJ, Glorieux FH: Relation between hypomineralized periosteocytic lesions and bone mineralization in vitamin D resistant rickets. *Calif Tissue Int* 35:443, 1983
23. Frost HM: Some observations on bone mineral in a case of vitamin D resistant rickets. *Henry Ford Hosp Med Bull* 6:300, 1958
24. Glorieux FH, Ecarot-Charrier B: X-linked vitamin-D resistant rickets: is osteoblast activity defective? In: Cohn DV, Martin TJ, Meunier PJ (eds), *Calcium Regulation and Bone Metabolism,* Excerpta Medica, Amsterdam, New York, Oxford, 9:227–231, 1987
25. Yamamoto T, Ecarot B, Glorieux FH: Abnormal response of osteoblasts from Hyp mice to 1,25-dihydroxyvitamin D$_3$. *Bone* 13:209, 1992
26. Ecarot-Charrier E, Glorieux FH, Travers R, Desbarats M, Bouchard F, Hinek A: Defective bone formation by transplanted Hyp mouse bone cells into normal mice. *Endocrinology* 123:768, 1988
27. Bettinelli A, Bianchi ML, Mazazucchi E, Gandolini G, Appliani AC: Acute effects of calcitriol and phosphate salts on mineral metabolism in children with hypophosphatemic rickets. *J Pediatr* 118:373, 1991

28. Goodyer PR, Kronick JB, Jequier S, Reade TM, Scriver CR: Nephrocalcinosis and its relationship to treatment of hereditary rickets. *J Pediatr* 111:700, 1987
29. Alon U, Donaldson DL, Hellerstein S, Warady BA, Harris DJ: Metabolic and histologic investigation of the nature of nephrocalcinosis in children with hypophosphatemic rickets and in the Hyp mouse. *J Pediatr* 120:899, 1992
30. Wilson DM, Lee PDK, Morris AH, Reiter EO, Gertner JM, Marcus R, Quarmby VE, Rosenfeld RG: Growth hormone therapy in hypophosphatemic rickets. *Am J Dis Child* 145:1165, 1991
31. Sullivan W, Carpenter T, Glorieux FH, Travers R, Insogna K: A prospective trial of phosphate and 1,25-dihydroxyvitamin D$_3$ therapy in symptomatic adults with X-linked hypophosphatemic rickets. *J Clin Endocrinol Metab* 75:879, 1992

69. Tumor-Associated Rickets and Osteomalacia

Marc K. Drezner, M.D.

Department of Medicine, Duke University Medical Center,
Durham, North Carolina

TUMOR-ASSOCIATED RICKETS AND OSTEOMALACIA

Since 1959 there have been reports of approximately 79 patients (1–61) in whom rickets and/or osteomalacia has been associated with various types of tumors (Table 1). Indeed, with greater awareness of the disease, physician-scientists have recognized >40% of known affected subjects within the past decade. The syndrome is characterized, in general, by remission of the unexplained bone disease after resection of the coexisting tumor. Patients usually present with bone and muscle pain, muscle weakness, and occasionally recurrent fractures of long bones. Additional symptoms common to younger patients are fatigue, gait disturbances, slow growth, and skeletal abnormalities, including bowing of the lower extremities. The duration of symptoms before diagnosis ranges from 5 mo to 17 yr with an average of more than 4 yr. The age at diagnosis is generally the fourth decade, with a range of 9 to 73 years of age. Approximately 10% of patients are younger than 18 years at presentation.

The biochemical findings characterizing this disorder prior to tumor removal include hypophosphatemia and an abnormally low renal tubular maximum for the reabsorption of phosphorus per liter of glomerular filtrate (TmP/GFR), indicative of renal phosphate wasting. The serum phosphorus values average 1.4 mg/dl with a range of 0.7–2.2 mg/dl. After removal of the tumor the level returns to normal, averaging 3.6 mg/dl. Additional abnormalities include gastrointestinal malabsorption of phosphorus, which, coupled with renal phosphorus wasting, results in a negative phosphorus balance. Serum 25(OH)D is normal (in 13 of 16 patients) and serum 1,25(OH)$_2$D overtly low (in 12 of 14 patients) or inappropriately normal relative to the hypophosphatemia. Aminoaciduria, most frequently glycinuria, and glucosuria are occasionally present. Radiographic abnormalities include generalized osteopenia, pseudofractures, and coarsened trabeculae as well as widened epiphyseal plates in children.

TUMORS

The tumors present in patients with tumor-associated osteomalacia have been of mesenchymal origin in the large majority of patients (Table 1). However, the frequent occurrence of Looser zones in the radiographs of moribund patients with carcinomas of epidermal and endodermal derivation (62) indicates that the disease may be secondary to a variety of tumor types. Indeed, the recent observation of tumor-associated osteomalacia concurrent with breast carcinoma (63), prostate carcinoma (30,44), oat cell carcinoma (41), multiple myeloma, and chronic lymphocytic leukemia (53) supports this conclusion. The occurrence of osteomalacia in patients with widespread fibrous dysplasia of bone (64), neurofibromatosis (55,65), and linear nevus sebaceous syndrome (47) could also be tumor associated. Proof of a causal relationship has been precluded by the multiplicity of lesions and the consequent inability to effect surgical cure. However, in one case of fibrous dysplasia, removal of virtually all of the abnormal bone did result in appropriate biochemical and radiographic improvement (64).

The mesenchymal tumors associated with this osteomalacia syndrome have been variably described as sclerosing angioma, benign angiofibroma, hemangiopericytoma, chondrosarcoma, primitive mesenchymal tumor, soft-parts chondromalike tumor, and giant cell tumor of bone. The diversity of these diagnostic labels underscores the morphologic complexity of these tumors. However, Weidner and Cruz (65) have recently established that the histologically polymorphous mesenchymal tumors can be subdivided into four distinct morphologic patterns: (A) primitive-appearing, mixed connective tissue tumors; (B) osteoblastomalike tumors; (C) nonossifying fibromalike tumors; and (D) ossifying fibromalike tumors. The most common of these, the mixed connective tissue variant, is characterized by variable numbers of primitive-appearing stromal cells growing in poorly defined sheets and punctuated by clusters of osteoclastlike giant cells. Vascularity is also often prominent, but in less vascular areas poorly developed cartilage or foci of osteoid or bone are commonly present. The primitive stromal cells are likely the

TABLE 1. *Tumor-associated osteomalacia*[a]

Reference	Age/sex	Symptom duration (yrs)	Serum phosphorus pre-op (mg/dl)	Serum phosphorus post-op (mg/dl)	Tumor type/site	Symptoms
McCance (1)	15/F	9.0	2.1	4.7	Degenerated osteoid/femur	Muscle weakness
Hauge (2)	55/M				Malignant neuroma/axilla	
Prader et al. (3)	11/F	1.0	1.9	4.1	Giant cell granuloma/rib	Lower limb pain/fatigue
Yoshikawa et al. (4)	54/F	6.0	0.9	5.4	Cavernous hemangioma/popliteal region	Lower limb pain
Krane (5)	56/M	3.0	1.4	3.2	Giant cell tumor/hip	Bone pain
Salassa et al. (6)	38/M	4.0	1.4	4.6	Sclerosing hemangioma/groin	Bone pain/weakness
	30/M	3.0	1.2	3.3	Sclerosing hemangioma/popliteal area	Bone pain
Evans and Azzopardi (7)	47/F	1.5	1.7	3.6	Primary bone tumor (type?)/femur	Bone pain/femur fracture weakness
Olefsky et al. (8)	40/M	10.0	1.1	3.5	Ossifying mesenchymal tumor/pharynx	Bone pain/weakness
Pollack et al. (9)	9/F	1.5	1.7	4.8	Non-ossifying fibroma/radius	Gait disturbance/weakness
Moser and Fessel (10)	54/M	1.0	1.7		Ossifying mesenchymal tumor/toe	Joint pain
Willhoite (11)	11/F	3.5	1.7	4.4	Ossifying mesenchymal tumor/ulna	Genu valgum/delayed growth
Linovitz et al. (12)	36/M	9.0	1.4	4	Hemangiopericytoma/medial malleolus	Back pain
	51/M	4.0	0.9	1.6	Hemangioma/knee	Back pain
Renton and Shaw (13)	53/F	5.0	1.2		Hemangiopericytoma/ethnoid	Leg pain
	58/M	14.0	1.6		Hemangiopericytoma/abdominal wall	Bone pain
	43/F	2.0	1.5	1.8	Hemangiopericytoma/femur	Bone and joint pain
Morita (14)	30/M	5.0	0.7	3.5	Fibrous xanthoma/thigh	Bone pain/muscle weakness
Aschinberg et al. (15)	12/M	7.0	1	3.9	Fibroangioma/skin (face/lower limb)	Bone pain/muscle weakness
Drezner and Feinglos (16)	42/F	8.0	1.3	3.2	Giant cell tumor of bone/ileum	Fatigue/muscle weakness/bone pain
Yoshikawa et al. (17)	18/M	5.0	1.5	4	Benign osteoblastoma/metacarpal	Profound weakness
	18/F	5.0	1.2	5	Benign osteoblastoma/humerus	Profound weakness
Wyman et al. (18)	44/M	5.0	1.2	3.5	Sarcoma/tibia	Muscle, joint and bone pain
Leite et al. (19)	50/M				Hemangiofibroma	
Lau et al. (20)			2	4.1	Sclerosing hemangioma/unknown	
Werner et al. (21)			1.9		Atypical chondroma/hand	Back pain/myopathy
Turner and Dalinka (22)	56/F	8.0			Cavernous hemangioma/foot	Bone pain
Nortman et al. (23)	49/F	4.0	1.5	1.5	Mesenchymoma/nose	Bone pain/muscle weakness
Daniels and Weisenfeld (24)	34/M	0.8	1.8		Hemangioma/skull, pelvis, ribs	Back pain/muscle weakness
Fukumoto et al. (25)	27/F		1.5	3.1	Osteoblastoma/tibia	Proximal muscle weakness
Lejeune et al. (26)	62/F	2.5	1.75	3.6	Benign connective tissue/radius	Lumbar pain
Crouzet et al. (27)	37/M	6.0	1.7	3.4	Hemangiopericytoma/frontal bone	Vertebral compression fracture/ankle pain
Camus et al. (28)	37/F	1.0	2.2	3.2	Hemangioma/rectum	Bone pain
	37/M	9.0	1.6	3.4	Hemangiopericytoma/frontal bone	Bone pain/femoral fracture
	72/M	0.5	1.8	3.4	Neuroma/nerve root	Lumbar pain/sciatica
Sweet et al. (29)	25/F	1.0	1.5	2.7	Hemangiopericytoma/middle turbinate	Painful feet/muscle weakness
Lyles et al. (30)	61/M	0.5	1.4		Prostatic carcinoma	Bone pain
	74/M	4.0	1.7		Prostatic carcinoma	Bone pain
Nitzan et al. (31)	26/M	2.0	1.5	3.1	Brown tumor/jaw	Bone pain/muscle weakness
Asnes et al. (32)	14/F	1.0	1.7	3.8	Non-ossifying fibroma/femur	Joint pain
Parker et al. (33)	15/M	1.0	2.1	4.2	Non-ossifying fibroma/radius	Bone pain/muscle weakness
Chacko and Joseph (34)	56/F	5.0	1.7	1.2	Hemangiopericytoma/nostril	Back pain
Hioco et al. (35)	65/F				Cavernous hemangioma/quadriceps	
Barcelo et al. (36)	44/F	3.0	1.3		Fibroangioma/foot	Bone pain/muscle weakness
Nomura et al. (37)	29/M	2.0	1.3	3.6	Osteosarcoma/mandible	Lumbar pain/muscle weakness

TABLE 1. *Continued.*

Reference	Age/sex	Symptom duration (yrs)	Serum phosphorus		Tumor type/site	Symptoms
			pre-op (mg/dl)	post-op (mg/dl)		
Ryan and Reiss (38)	64/M	4.0	1.8	2.1	Primary bone tumor (type?)/ femur	Bone pain/muscle weakness
	66/F	2.5	1.3		Type?/frontal bone	Bone pain
Firth et al. (39)	44/M	1.0	1.2	2.4	Malignant chondroblastoma/ femur	Bone pain
Taylor et al. (40)	57/M	0.3	1.5		Oat cell carcinoma/pulmonary (metastases: liver; spine)	Cervical pain/weakness
Leehey et al. (41)	20/M	1.0	1.6	3.5	Non-ossifying fibroma/tibia	Bone pain and fractures
Seshadri et al. (42)	73/M		1.7		Giant cell tumor/tendon sheath (thigh)	
	40/F		1.1		Hemangiopericytoma/ethnoid sinus	
	14/M		2.2		Odontogenic fibroma/ mandible	
Cotton and Van Puffelen (43)	44/M	1.0	1.2	2.4	Malignant chondroblastoma/ femur	Bone pain
Murphy et al. (44)	4 Patients		2		Prostatic carcinoma	Bone pain/muscle weakness
Gitelis et al. (45)	44/F	0.3	1.4	2.6	Hemangiopericytoma/forearm (soft tissue)	Bone and joint pain/bone fractures
	48/F	3.0	1.15	3.8	Mesenchymal tumor (type?)/	Bone pain/muscle weakness
Rico et al. (46)	31/M	9.0	0.9	4.7	Giant cell fibrous malignant histiocytoma/thigh	Bone pain/muscle weakness/ fractures/osteopenia
Carey et al. (47)	7/M	5.0	2.6		Epidermal nevi (linear nevus sebaceous syndrome)	Bone pain/muscle weakness/ genu valgum/osteopenia
	23/F	14.0	1.2		Epidermal nevi (linear nevus sebaceous syndrome)	Bone pain/recurrent fractures
Siris et al. (48)	44/M	2.0	2.1	3.5	Vascular mesenchymoma (type?)/sole of foot	Bone pain/weakness/ osteopenia fractures
Reid et al. (49)	57/F	16.0	1.1	2.7	Mixed mesenchymal tumor/ extensor hallucis tendon	Diffuse pain and immobilization
Prowse and Brooks (50)	73/M	1.0	1.6	3.4	Diffuse giant cell tumor/ tendon sheath	Diffuse bone pain/osteopenia/ fracture
Sparagana (51)	19/M	0.5	1.6	3.9	Ossifying fibroma/tibia	Bone pain/fractures
	50/M	3.0	1.8	3.7	Low-grade fibrosarcoma/skull	Bone and muscle pain/ fractures/weakness and immobilization
Rao et al. (52)	69/F		2.4	3.1	Myelomatosis	Back pain/muscle weakness/ generalized osteopenia
	70/F		2.4	3	Chronic lymphocytic leukemia	Severe proximal muscle weakness
McClure and Smith (53)	60/F	2.0	1.2		Hemangiopericytoma/femur	Bone pain/weakness/ immobilization
Miyauchi et al. (54)	54/M	7.0	1	3.9	Hemangiopericytoma/thigh	Muscle weakness/bone pain/ waddling gait
Konishi et al. (55)	40/F	10.0	1.02		Neurofibromatosis	Muscle weakness/bone pain/ loss of height
Nitzan et al. (56)	53/M	19.0	2	6	Fibrosarcoma/maxilla	Muscle weakness/bone pain
McGuire et al. (57)	34/F	1.0	1.3	4.1	Benign undifferentiated tumor of mesenchymal origin	Back and thigh pain/muscle weakness
Schultze et al. (58)	51/M	6.0	2.1	3.8	Hemangiopericytoma/condylar aspect, r. femur	Pain/multiple rib fractures
Leicht et al. (59)	34/F	2.0	1.2	4	Synovial sarcoma/first metatarsal space	Progressive bone pain
Uchida et al. (60)	53/F	17.0	1.5	6	Benign ossifying mesenchymal tumor of bone	Polyarthralgia/bone pain
Papotti et al. (61)	62/M	2.0	1.6		Hemangiopericytoma/ subcutaneous nodule knee	Muscle weakness/bone pain
	24/W	1.8	1.6		Chondroid, giant cell tumor/ left thigh	Muscle weakness/pain
	38/W	2.0	1.2		Hemangiopericytoma/l. maxillary sinus	Weakness/gait disturbance/ exophthalmos/nasal bleeding

[a] Modified from Cotton GE and Van Puffelen P: Hypophosphatemic osteomalacia secondary to neoplasia. *J Bone Joint Surg* 68A:129–133, 1986.

source of the hormonal factor(s) that causes the syndrome. Whether similar mesenchymal elements exist in the epidermal and endodermal tumors associated with the syndrome remains unknown. However, fibrous mesenchymal components are present in many neural tumors, and metastatic carcinoma of the prostate is frequently an osteoblastic lesion associated with varying degrees of fibrous tissue proliferation. Thus, it is possible that the expression of tumor-associated osteomalacia, concurrent with the presence of epidermal or endodermal tumors, depends upon the presence and activity of such mesenchymal elements in many cases.

Regardless of the cell type responsible for the syndrome, the tumors at fault are often small, difficult to locate, and present in obscure areas. In this regard, many of the reported lesions have been located in a relatively inaccessible area within bone, such as within the femur or tibia, the nasopharynx, or a sinus. Alternatively, small lesions have been found in the popliteal region, the groin, and the suprapatellar area. In any case, a careful and thorough examination is necessary to document or exclude the presence of such a tumor.

PATHOPHYSIOLOGY

The pathophysiological basis underlying tumor-associated osteomalacia remains unknown. Such incomplete understanding of the disorder undoubtedly relates to its infrequent occurrence and, consequently, the few physiologic studies of the disease. Nevertheless, most investigators agree that the probable pathogenesis of the syndrome is tumor production of a humoral factor(s) that may affect multiple functions of the proximal renal tubule—particularly phosphate reabsorption—and which may result in hypophosphatemia. This possibility has been supported by (A) the presence of phosphaturic activity in tumor extracts from 2 of 3 patients with tumor-associated osteomalacia (15), (B) the occurrence of hypophosphatemia and increased urinary phosphate excretion in heterotransplanted tumor-bearing athymic nude mice (54), and (C) the coincidence of aminoaciduria and glycosuria with renal phosphate wasting in some affected subjects, indicative of complex alterations in proximal renal tubular function (16). However, the recent observation that mesenchymal tumors from affected subjects do not secrete phosphaturic factors into culture medium indicates that the pathogenesis of the disorder may be more complicated than currently appreciated (56).

In this regard, abnormal vitamin D metabolism has been identified as an additional factor that may contribute to the pathogenesis of the tumor-associated osteomalacia. Several observations support this possibility, including (A) the decreased circulating $1,25(OH)_2D$ level observed in virtually all patients who manifest the characteristic syndrome; (B) normalization of the serum $1,25(OH)_2D$ concentration rapidly after surgical removal of the coincident tumor, and in association with resolution of the biochemical abnormalities of the syndrome; and (C) diminished renal $25(OH)D-1\alpha$-hydroxylase activity in het-

erotransplanted tumor-bearing athymic nude mice (66) and in kidney cell cultures exposed to tumor extracts (54).

In any case, the interrelationship between the abnormal renal phosphate transport and the defect in vitamin D metabolism evident in affected subjects remains unknown. An innate heterogeneity in the pathogenesis of the syndrome cannot be excluded. However, an interplay between these abnormalities likely contributes to the phenotypic expression of the disorder in the majority of patients.

In contrast to these observations, patients with tumor-associated osteomalacia secondary to hematogenous malignancy manifest abnormalities of the syndrome owing to a distinctly different mechanism. In these subjects the nephropathy associated with light chain proteinuria results in the decreased renal tubular reabsorption of phosphate characteristic of the disease. To date at least 15 patients have been reported who potentially manifest this form of the disorder (53). In many instances, however, the diagnosis of tumor-associated osteomalacia was not considered. Nevertheless, at least in some cases of this syndrome, renal tubular damage may be mediated by tissue deposition of light chains or of some other immunoglobulin derivative with similar toxic effects on the kidney. Thus, light-chain nephropathy must be considered one possible mechanism for the tumor-associated osteomalacic syndrome.

DIFFERENTIAL DIAGNOSIS

The tumor-associated osteomalacia syndrome has all the classic biochemical and radiologic criteria of the hypophosphatemic osteomalacias. Diagnosis, therefore, depends upon a diligent search for tumors in all patients with hypophosphatemic vitamin D resistant rachitic/osteomalacic disease. Tumors may range from small to large and benign to malignant. Moreover, the tumor may be present for many years before the clinical appearance of bone disease. Thus, regardless of the temporal association between the onset of the osteomalacia and the clinical awareness of tumor, tumor-associated osteomalacia should be considered. Indeed, where possible, resection of any associated tumor should be attempted both to confirm the diagnosis and possibly to induce resolution of the syndrome.

When the tumor cannot be totally resected, diagnosis remains inferential. However, several observations can support the diagnosis: (A) a normal serum $25(OH)D$ level; (B) a selective deficiency of $1,25(OH)_2D$, manifest by a decreased serum concentration; (C) presence of light-chain proteinuria; (D) demonstration of phosphaturic activity in tumor extracts; and/or (E) induction of the tumor-associated osteomalacia syndrome in athymic nude mice upon heterotransplantation of tumor tissue from affected subjects.

In the absence of tumor and/or family history of disease, and after exclusion of common causes of osteomalacia, the possibility of adult onset hypophosphatemic osteomalacia with or without Fanconi's syndrome must be considered. This syndrome may result from acquired or genetic causes, and age of onset is extremely variable. Biochemical abnormalities are indistinguishable from those in patients with tumor-associated osteomalacia. Thus, in the absence of genetic transmission of the disorder, careful long-term follow-up for tumor occurrence must be maintained in all patients with hypophosphatemic osteomalacia.

TREATMENT

The first and foremost treatment of tumor-associated osteomalacia is complete resection of the associated tumor. However, recurrence of mesenchymal tumors, such as giant cell tumors of bone, or inability to resect completely certain malignancies, such as prostatic carcinoma, has resulted in the need for developing effective therapeutic intervention for the tumor-associated osteomalacia syndrome. Historically, pharmacologic doses of vitamin D have been used in an effort to heal the bone disease. For the most part, the trials have been short and the results have not been assessed in detail. Nevertheless, it appears certain that this treatment does not cure the rachitic or osteomalacic components of the syndrome. Moreover, no resolution of the abnormal biochemistries ensues.

More recently, administration of 1,25(OH)$_2$D alone or in combination with phosphorus supplementation has served as effective therapy for the tumor-associated osteomalacia. In this regard, Drezner and Feingios (16) and Lobaugh et al. (66) have noted striking improvement of the biochemical and bone abnormalities of the syndrome in response to calcitriol (2.0–3.0 mg/d). In two such patients the serum phosphorus level increased from pretreatment levels of 1.5 ± 0.7 and 2.2 ± 0.1 mg/dl to normal values of 3.7 ± 0.03 and 2.8 ± 0.08 mg/dl, respectively. Similarly, the renal TmP/GFR rose from an abnormally low level, 0.8 ± 0.03 and 1.9 ± 0.03 mg/dl, to normal 3.0 ± 0.01 and 2.8 ± 0.09 mg/dl. Commensurately, evidence of bone healing was present in bone biopsies from these subjects.

In contrast, several investigators have observed only modest symptomatic, biochemical, and histologic improvement in response to calcitriol. However, such patients generally responded well to combination therapy with pharmacologic amounts of 1,25(OH)$_2$D and phosphorus (59). In this regard, phosphorus supplementation (2–4 g/d) directly replaces the ongoing renal loss of inorganic phosphorus, whereas calcitriol (1.5–3 μg/d) serves to replace insufficient renal production of the sterol and to enhance renal phosphate reabsorption. Such therapy normalizes the biochemical abnormalities of the syndrome and results in healing of the osteomalacia. These data indicate that patients with tumor-associated osteomalacia may benefit from a combination drug regimen.

COMPLICATIONS OF THERAPY

Little information is available regarding the long-term consequences of therapy in patients with tumor-associ-

ated osteomalacia. The doses of medicines used, however, raise the possibility that nephrolithiasis, nephrocalcinosis, and hypercalcemia may frequently complicate the therapeutic course. Indeed, hypercalcemia secondary to parathyroid hyperfunction has been documented in five affected subjects, representing approximately 6% of the reported cases. All of these patients had received phosphorus (as part of a combination regimen with vitamin D$_2$ or 1,25(OH)$_2$D), which may have stimulated parathyroid hormone secretion and ultimately led to parathyroid autonomy. Thus, careful assessment of parathyroid function, serum, and urinary calcium and renal function is essential to ensure safe and efficacious therapy.

REFERENCES

1. McCance RA: Osteomalacia with Looser's nodes (milkman's syndrome) due to a raised resistance to vitamin D acquired about the age of 15 years. *Q J Med* 16:33–46, 1947
2. Hauge BM: Vitamin D resistant osteomalacia. *Acta Med Scand* 153:271–282, 1956
3. Prader AV, Illig R, Uehlilinger E, Stalder G: Rachitis infolge knochentumors. *Helv Paediatr Acta* 14:554–565, 1959
4. Yoshikawa S, Kawabata M, Hatsuyama Y, Hosokawa O, Fujita T: Atypical vitamin-D resistant osteomalacia. Report of a Case. *J Bone Joint Surg* 45A:998–1007, 1964
5. Krane SM: Case records of the Massachusetts General Hospital. *N Engl J Med* 273:1330, 1965
6. Salassa RM, Jowsey J, Arnaud CD: Hypophosphatemic osteomalacia associated with "nonendocrine" tumors. *N Engl J Med* 283:65–70, 1970
7. Evans DJ, Azzopardi JG: Distinctive tumours of bone and soft tissue causing acquired vitamin-D-resistant osteomalacia. *Lancet* 1:353–354, 1972
8. Olefsky J, Kempson R, Jones H, Reaven G: "Tertiary" hyperparathyroidism and apparent "cure" of vitamin-D-resistant rickets after removal of an ossifying mesenchymal tumor of the pharynx. *N Engl J Med* 286:740–745, 1972
9. Pollack JA, Schiller AL, Crawford JD: Rickets and myopathy cured by removal of a nonossifying fibroma of bone. *Pediatrics* 52:364–371, 1973
10. Moser CR, Fessel WJ: Rheumatic manifestations of hypophosphatemia. *Arch Intern Med* 134:674–678, 1974
11. Willhoite DR: Acquired rickets and solitary bone tumor. The question of a causal relationship [abstract]. *Clin Orthop* 109:210–211, 1975
12. Linovitz RJ, Resnick D, Keissling P, Kondon JJ, Sehler B, Nejdi RJ, Rowe JH, Deftos LJ: Tumor-induced osteomalacia and rickets: a surgically curable syndrome. Report of two cases. *J Bone Joint Surg* 58A:419–423, 1976
13. Renton P, Shaw DG: Hypophosphatemic osteomalacia secondary to vascular tumors of bone and soft tissue. *Skeletal Radiol* 1:21–24, 1975
14. Morita M: [A case of adult onset vitamin D–resistant osteomalacia associated with soft tissue tumor.] *Kotsu Taisha* [Bone Metabolism] 9:286–291, 1976
15. Aschinberg LC, Soloman LM, Zeis PM, Justice P, Rosenthal IM: Vitamin D–resistant rickets associated with epidermal nevus syndrome: demonstration of a phosphaturic substance in the dermal lesions. *J Pediatr* 91:56–60, 1977
16. Drezner MK, Feingios MN: Osteomalacia due to 1,25-dihydroxy-cholecalciferol deficiency. Association with a giant cell tumor of bone. *J Clin Invest* 60:1046–1053, 1977
17. Yoshikawa S, Nakamura T, Takagi M, Imamura T, Okano K, Sasaki S: Benign osteoblastoma as a cause of osteomalacia. A report of two cases. *J Bone Joint Surg* 59B(3):279–289, 1977
18. Wyman AL, Paradinas FJ, Daly JR: Hypophosphataemic osteomalacia associated with a malignant tumour of the tibia: report of a case. *J Clin Pathol* 30:328–335, 1977

19. Leite MOR, Borelli A, de Ulhoa Cintra AB: Osteomalacia hipofosfatemica asociada a hemangio-fibroma. Consideracoes etiopaogenicas. *Rev Hosp Clin Fac Med Sao Paulo* 33:65–67, 1978

20. Lau K, Strom MC, Goldberg M, Goldfarb S, Gray RW, Lemann R Jr, Agus ZS: Evidence for a humoral phosphaturic factor in oncogenic hypophosphatemic osteomalacia [abstract]. *Clin Res* 27:421A, 1979

21. Wener M, Cohen L, Bar RS, Strottmann MP, DeLuca H: Regulation of phosphate and calcium metabolism by vitamin D metabolites: studies in a patient with oncogenic osteomalacia [abstract]. *Arthritis Rheum* 22:672–673, 1979

22. Turner ML, Dalinka MK: Osteomalacia: uncommon causes. *Am J Roentgenol* 133:539–540, 1979

23. Nortman DF, Coburn JW, Brautbar N, Sherrard DJ, Haussler MR, Singer FR, Brickman AS, Barton RT: Treatment of mesenchymal tumor associated osteomalacia (MTAO) with 1,24(OH)$_2$D$_3$. Report of a case. In: Norman AW (ed), *Vitamin D, Basic Research and Its Clinical Application. Proceedings of the Fourth Workshop on Vitamin D,* De Gruyter, Berlin: 1167–1168, 1979

24. Daniels RA, Weisenfeld I: Tumorous phosphaturic osteomalacia. Report of a case associated with multiple hemangiomas of bone. *Am J Med* 67:155–159, 1979

25. Fukumoto Y, Tarui S, Tsuklyama K, Ichihara K, Moriwaki K, Nonaka K, Mizushima T, Kobayashi Y, Dokoh S, Fukunaga M, Morita R: Tumor-induced vitamin D–resistant hypophosphatemic osteomalacia associated with proximal renal tubular dysfunction and 1,25-dihydroxyvitamin D deficiency. *J Clin Endocrinol Metab* 49:873–878, 1979

26. Lejeune E, Bouvier M, Meunier P, Vauzelle JL, Deplante JP, David L, Liorca G, Andre-Fouet E: L'osteomalacle des tumeurs mesenchymateuses. A propos d'une noouvelle observation. *Rev Rhumat* 46:187–193, 1979

27. Crouzet J, Camus JP, Gatti JM, Descamps H, Beraneck L: Osteomalacie hypophosphoremique et hemangiopericytome de la voute du crane. *Rev Rheumat* 47:523–528, 1980

28. Camus JP, Courzet J, Prier A, Guillemant S, Ulmann A, Koeger AC: Osteomalacies hypophosphoremiques gueries par l'ablation de tumeurs benignes du tissu conjonctif: etude de trois observations avec dosages pre- et post-operatoires des metabolites de la vitamine D. *Ann Med Interne* (Paris) 131:422–426, 1980

29. Sweet RA, Males JL, Hamstra AJ, Deluca HF: Vitamin D metabolite levels in oncogenic osteomalacia. *Ann Intern Med* 93:279–280, 1980

30. Lyles KW, Berry WR, Haussler M, Harrelson JM, Drezner MK: Hypophosphatemic osteomalacia: Association with prostatic carcinoma. *Ann Intern Med* 93:275–278, 1980

31. Nitzan DW, Marmary Y, Azaz B: Mandibular tumor-induced muscular weakness and osteomalacia. *Oral Surg Oral Med Oral Pathol* 52:253–256, 1981

32. Asnes RS, Berdon WE, Bassett CA: Hypophosphatemic rickets in an adolescent cured by excision of a nonossifying fibroma. *Clin Pediatr* (Phila) 20:646–648, 1981

33. Parker MS, Klein I, Haussler MR, Mintz DH: Tumor-induced osteomalacia. Evidence of a surgically correctable alteration in vitamin D metabolism. *JAMA* 245:492–493, 1990

34. Chacko V, Joseph B: Osteomalacia associated with hemiangiopericytoma. *J Indian Med Assoc* 76:173–175, 1981

35. Hioco J, Chanzy MO, Hioco F, Voisin MC, Villiaumey J: Osteomalacia with mesenchymal tumors—two new cases [abstract]. *Rev Rhum Spec* 890, 1981

36. Barcelo P Jr, Asensi E, Paso M, Obach J, Barcelo P Sr: Osteomalacia hipofosforemica secundaria as histiocitoma fibroso vascular [abstract]. *Rev Rhum Spec* 1352, 1981

37. Nomura G, Koshino Y, Morimoto H, Kida H, Noura S, Tamai K: Vitamin D resistant hypophosphatemic osteomalacia associated with osteosarcoma of the mandible. Report of a case. *Jpn J Med* 21:35–39, 1982

38. Ryan EA, Reiss E: Oncogenous osteomalacia. Review of the world literature and report of two new cases. *Am J Med* 77: 501–512, 1984

39. Firth RG, Grant CS, Riggs BL: Development of hypercalcemic hyperparathyroidism after long-term phosphate supplementation in hypophosphatemic osteomalacia. Report of two cases. *Am J Med* 78:669–673, 1985

40. Taylor HC, Fallon MD, Velasco ME: Oncogenic osteomalacia and inappropriate antidiuretic hormone secretion due to oat-cell carcinoma. *Ann Intern Med* 101:786–788, 1984

41. Leehey DJ, Ing TS, Daugirdas JT: Fanconi syndrome associated with a non-ossifying fibroma of bone. *Am J Med* 78:708–710, 1985

42. Seshadri MS, Cornish CJ, Mason RS, Posen S: Parathyroid hormone-like bioactivity in tumours from patients with oncogenic osteomalacia. *Clin Endocrinol* (Oxf) 23:689–697, 1985

43. Cotton GE, Van Puffelen P: Hypophosphatemic osteomalacia secondary to neoplasia. *J Bone Joint Surg* 68A:129–133, 1986

44. Murphy P, Wright G, Rai GS: Hypophosphatemic osteomalacia associated with prostatic carcinoma. *Br Med J* 290:1945, 1985

45. Gitelis S, Ryan WG, Rosenberg AG, Templeton AC: Adult-onset hypophosphatemic osteomalacia secondary to neoplasm: a case report and review of the pathophysiology. *J Bone Joint Surg* 68A:134–138, 1986

46. Rico H, Fernandez-Miranda E, Sanz J, Gomez-Castresana F, Escriba A, Hernandez ER, Krsnik I: Oncogenous osteomalacia: a new case secondary to a malignant tumor. *Bone* 7:325–329, 1986

47. Carey DE, Drezner MK, Hamdan JA, Mange M, Ashmad MS, Mubarak S, Nyhan WL: Hypophosphatemic rickets/osteomalacia in linear sebaceous nevus syndrome: a variant of tumor-induced osteomalacia. *J Pediatr* 109:994–1000, 1986

48. Siris ES, Clemens TL, Dempster DW, Shane E, Segre GV, Lindsay R, Bilezekian JP: Tumor-induced osteomalacia: kinetics of calcium phosphorus and vitamin D metabolism and characteristics of bone histomorphometry. *Am J Med* 82:307–312, 1987

49. Reid IR, Teitelbaum SL, Dusso A, Whyte MP: Hypercalcemic hyperparathyroidism complicating oncogenic osteomalacia: effect of successful tumor resection on mineral homeostasis. *Am J Med* 83:350–354, 1987

50. Prowse M, Brooks PM: Oncogenic hypophosphatemic osteomalacia associated with a giant cell tumour of a tendon sheath. *Aust NZ J Med* 17:330–332, 1987

51. Sparagana M: Tumor-induced osteomalacia: long-term follow-up of two patients cured by removal of their tumors. *J Surg Oncol* 36:198–205, 1987

52. Rao DS, Parfitt AM, Villanueva AR, Dorman PJ, Kleerekoper M: Hypophosphatemic osteomalacia and adult Fanconi syndrome due to light-chain nephropathy: another form of oncogenous osteomalacia. *Am J Med* 82:333–338, 1987

53. McClure J, Smith PS: Oncogenic osteomalacia. *J Clin Pathol* 40:446–453, 1987

54. Miyauchi A, Fukase M, Tsutsumi M, Fujita T: Hemangiopericytoma-induced osteomalacia: tumor transplantation in nude mice causes hypophosphatemia and tumor extracts inhibit renal 25-hydroxyvitamin D-1-hydroxylase activity. *J Clin Endocrinol Metab* 67:46–53, 1988

55. Konishi K, Nakamura M, Yamakawa H, Suzuki H, Saruta T, Hanaoka H, Davatchi T: Case report: hypophosphatemic osteomalacia in von Recklinghausen neurofibromatosis. *Am J Med Sci* 301:322–328, 1991

56. Nitzan DW, Horowitz AT, Darmon D, Friedlaender MM, Rubinger D, Stein P, Bab I, Popovtzer MM, Silver J: Oncogenous osteomalacia: a case study. *Bone Miner* 6:191–197, 1989

57. McGuire MH, Merenda JT, Etzkorn JR, Sundaram M: Oncogenic osteomalacia: a case report. *Clin Orthop* 244:305–308, 1989

58. Schultze D, Deiling G, Faensen M, Haubold R, Loy V, Molzahn M, Pommer W, Semier J, Trempenau B: Onkogene hypophosphatamische Osteomalazie. *Kurze Originalien Falberichte* 114: 1073–1078, 1989

59. Leicht E, Biro G, Langer H-J: Tumor-induced osteomalacia: pre- and postoperative biochemical findings. *Horm Metab Res* 22:640–643, 1990

60. Uchida H, Yokoyama S, Kashima K, Nakayama I, Shimizu, Masumi S: Oncogenic vitamin D resistant hypophosphatemic osteomalacia (benign ossifying mesenchymal tumor of bone): case report. *Jpn J Clin Oncol* 21:218–226, 1991

61. Papotti M, Foschini MP, Isia G, Rizzi G, Betts C, Eusebl V: Hypophosphatemic oncogenic osteomalacia: report of three new cases. *Tumori* 74:599–607, 1988
62. Dent CE, Stamp TCB: Vitamin D rickets and osteomalacia. In: Avioli LV, Krane S (eds), *Metabolic Bone Disease*, Academic Press, New York, 1:237, 1978
63. Dent CE, Gertner JM: Hypophosphatemic osteomalacia in fibrous dysplasia. *Q J Med* 45:411–420, 1975
64. Saville PD, Nassim JR, Stevenson FH: Osteomalacia in von Recklinghausen's neurofibromatosis: metabolic study of a case. *Br Med J* 1:1311–1313, 1955
65. Weidner N, Cruz DS: Phosphaturic mesenchymal tumors: a polymorphous group causing osteomalacia or rickets. *Cancer* 59:1442–1454, 1987
66. Lobaugh B, Burch WM Jr, Drezner MK: Abnormalities of vitamin D metabolism and action in the vitamin D resistant rachitic and osteomalacic diseases. In: Rumar R (ed), *Vitamin D*, Martinus Nijhoff, Boston, 665–720, 1984

70. Hypophosphatasia

Michael P. Whyte, M.D.

Metabolic Research Unit, Shriners Hospital for Crippled Children, St. Louis, Missouri, and Division of Bone and Mineral Diseases, The Jewish Hospital of St. Louis, Washington University School of Medicine, St. Louis, Missouri

Hypophosphatasia is a rare heritable type of rickets or osteomalacia (1,2). About 300 cases have been reported. It occurs in all races with an incidence of about 1/100,000 live births for the severe forms. This inborn error of metabolism is characterized by a generalized reduction of activity of the tissue-nonspecific (liver/bone/kidney) isoenzyme of alkaline phosphatase (ALP). Activity of the tissue-specific intestinal, placental, and germ cell ALP isoenzymes is normal (3).

Although distinct separation of the various clinical forms of hypophosphatasia is impossible, four principal types are reported depending upon the age at which skeletal lesions are first noted: perinatal, infantile, childhood, and adult. Premature loss of deciduous teeth is a clinical hallmark in affected children. When dental manifestations alone are present, the disorder is regarded as "odontohypophosphatasia." In general, the earlier the presentation of skeletal problems, the more severe the disease (1,2).

CLINICAL PRESENTATION

Although at least some tissue-nonspecific ALP appears to be present in all tissues, hypophosphatasia affects predominantly the skeleton and dentition. The severity of clinical expression, however, is remarkably variable. Death may occur *in utero,* or symptoms may never appear (1,2).

Perinatal hypophosphatasia manifests during gestation. The pregnancy may be complicated by polyhydramnios. Typically, extreme skeletal hypomineralization causing short and deformed limbs and caput membraneceum is present at birth. Rarely, unusual bony spurs occur at the ends of long bones. There may be a high-pitched cry. Some newborns survive several days but suffer increasing respiratory compromise, unexplained fever, anemia (perhaps from encroachment on the marrow space by excessive osteoid), failure to gain weight, irritability, periodic apnea with cyanosis and bradycardia, intracranial hemorrhage, and idiopathic seizures. This is a lethal condition (1,2).

Infantile hypophosphatasia becomes clinically apparent before age 6 mo. Development often seems normal until poor feeding, inadequate weight gain, hypotonia, and wide fontanels are noted. Progressive rachitic deformities are typical. Hypercalcemia and hypercalciuria can cause recurrent vomiting, nephrocalcinosis, and ultimately renal compromise. Despite widely "open" fontanels (actually hypomineralized areas of calvarium), functional craniosynostosis is common. Mild hypertelorism and brachycephaly can be present. Raised intracranial pressure causes bulging of the anterior fontanel, proptosis, and papilledema. A flail chest predisposes to pneumonia. Infantile hypophosphatasia may show progressive deterioration during the months after diagnosis and is fatal in about 50% of affected subjects. The prognosis improves with survival beyond infancy (1,2).

Childhood hypophosphatasia varies greatly in clinical severity. Premature loss of deciduous teeth (earlier than 5 yr of age) from hypoplasia or aplasia of dental cementum may be the only clinical abnormality. Odontohypophosphatasia is present when radiographs show no evidence of skeletal disease. The incisors are typically lost first, but in severe cases the entire dentition can be affected. There is only minimal tooth root resorption. Dental radiographs often show enlarged pulp chambers and root canals that characterize "shell teeth." When rickets occurs, delayed walking with a waddling gait, short stature, a dolichocephalic skull with frontal bossing, and other consistent physical changes are often present. Childhood hypophosphatasia may improve spontaneously, but recurrence of skeletal disease during adulthood is likely (1,2).

Adult hypophosphatasia usually presents during middle age, often with painful and poorly healing recurrent metatarsal stress fractures. Pain in the thighs or hips may be due to femoral pseudofractures. About 50% of affected adults will have a history of rickets and/or premature loss of deciduous teeth during childhood. Loss or extraction of adult teeth is also common. Chondrocalcinosis occurs frequently and calcium pyrophosphate dihydrate crystal deposition disease and calcific periarthritis affect some patients (see the following section) (4). Recurrent stress fractures heal slowly; persistent femoral pseudofractures will mend following orthopedic rodding (5).

LABORATORY FINDINGS

Hypophosphatasia is diagnosed from a consistent clinical history and physical findings, radiologic evidence of rickets or osteomalacia, and the presence of low serum ALP activity (hypophosphatasemia) (1). It is important to recognize that there are age-related changes in the normal range for serum ALP activity and that several disorders and treatments can cause hypophosphatasemia (6).

The rickets/osteomalacia of hypophosphatasia is unusual in that it occurs although neither serum levels of calcium nor inorganic phosphate (Pi) is reduced. Indeed, hypercalciuria and hypercalcemia occur frequently in perinatal and infantile hypophosphatasia, apparently from dyssynergy between gut absorption of calcium and defective bone mineralization. Furthermore, children and adults with hypophosphatasia typically have serum Pi levels that are above the control mean level, and about 50% of these subjects are frankly hyperphosphatemic. Enhanced renal reclamation of Pi (increased TmP/GFR) accounts for this finding. In serum, 25-hydroxyvitamin D, 1,25-dihydroxyvitamin D, and immunoreactive parathyroid hormone levels are usually normal (1). Other routine biochemical measurements are generally unremarkable.

Endogenous levels of three phosphocompounds are increased in hypophosphatasia (1): phosphoethanolamine (PEA); inorganic pyrophosphate (PPi); and pyridoxal 5'-phosphate (PLP). Demonstration of phosphoethanolaminuria supports the diagnosis but is not diagnostic. Urinary PEA levels can be modestly increased in a variety of other disorders, and normal levels can occur in mild cases of hypophosphatasia. Assay of PPi in plasma and urine remains a research technique. An elevated plasma level of PLP is a sensitive and specific marker for hypophosphatasia (subjects should not be taking vitamin B$_6$ supplements when tested). In general, the greater the plasma PLP level, the more severe the clinical expression (1,3).

RADIOLOGIC FINDINGS

In perinatal hypophosphatasia, skeletal radiographs show diagnostic abnormalities (7). Marked bony undermineralization occurs with severe rachitic changes. In extreme cases, the skeleton may be so poorly mineralized that only the base of the skull is apparent. In less remarkable cases, the cranial bones may be ossified at their central portions and thereby give the illusion that the sutures are open and widely separated. Fracture is common.

Infantile hypophosphatasia causes characteristic, but less severe, changes. Abrupt transition from a relatively normal diaphyses to a hypomineralized metaphysis may

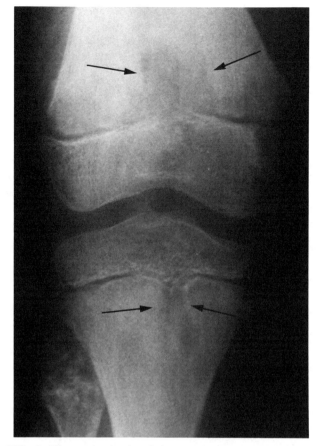

FIG. 1. The metaphysis of the proximal tibia of this 10-year-old boy with mild childhood hypophosphatasia shows a subtle but characteristic "tongue" of radiolucency (*arrows*). Note, however, that the growth plate is not widened.

suggest a sudden metabolic deterioration. Progressive skeletal demineralization can occur. Skeletal scintigraphy may help to show premature closure of cranial sutures that appear "widened" on conventional radiographs.

Childhood hypophosphatasia characteristically causes "tongues" of radiolucency to project from rachitic growth plates into metaphyses (Fig. 1). True premature fusion of cranial sutures occurs whereby radiographs of the skull typically show a "beaten-copper" appearance.

In adult hypophosphatasia, there may be osteopenia, recurrent poorly healing stress fractures of the metatarsals, chondrocalcinosis, and femoral pseudofractures.

HISTOPATHOLOGIC FINDINGS

Nondecalcified sections of bone reveal typical histologic features of rickets or osteomalacia in all clinical forms of hypophosphatasia except odontohypophosphatasia, in which the skeleton may be unremarkable. However, biochemical or histochemical studies of bone ALP activity can distinguish hypophosphatasia from other forms of rickets/osteomalacia.

Open cranial "sutures" are not typical fibrous tissue

but are uncalcified osteoid. Dental histopathology shows aplasia or hypoplasia of cementum. Enlarged pulp chambers ("shell teeth") indicate retarded dentinogenesis. These changes generally reflect the severity of the skeletal disease but do vary from tooth to tooth.

INHERITANCE

Perinatal and infantile hypophosphatasia are inherited as autosomal recessive disorders. Parents of severely affected subjects may have low or low-normal serum ALP activity, mildly elevated plasma PLP levels, and modest phosphoethanolaminuria. Challenge with a course of pyridoxine orally is followed by a distinctly abnormal increase in plasma PLP levels in carriers and especially in patients (3).

The mode of inheritance for the milder forms of hypophosphatasia is less clear. Some cases of odontohypophosphatasia and adult-onset disease may reflect clinical expression in heterozygous subjects where the disorder is transmitted as an autosomal dominant trait (see the following section) (1,2).

BIOCHEMICAL/GENETIC DEFECT

In keeping with an inborn error of metabolism that affects the tissue-nonspecific ALP isoenzyme, autopsy studies of subjects with the perinatal and infantile forms of hypophosphatasia have demonstrated a profound deficiency of ALP activity in liver, bone, and kidney, but not in the intestine or placenta. A variety of missense mutations in the coding sequence of the tissue-nonspecific ALP gene have been shown to cause severe forms of hypophosphatasia (8). Some patients, however, may have a regulatory defect (1). Some cases of childhood and adult hypophosphatasia are due to compound heterozygosity for missense mutations (8). Studies of vitamin B6 metabolism in hypophosphatasia indicate that tissue-nonspecific ALP acts to regulate the extracellular concentration of a variety of phosphocompounds (3). Accumulation of PPi may account for the impaired skeletal mineralization (3).

TREATMENT

There is no established medical therapy. Traditional treatments for rickets or osteomalacia (e.g., vitamin D and mineral supplementation) are important to avoid, because serum levels of calcium, Pi, and $1,25(OH)_2D$ are not re-duced (1). Furthermore, vitamin D may exacerbate any predisposition to hypercalcemia and hypercalciuria.

The hypercalcemia of perinatal or infantile hypophosphatasia will respond to restriction of dietary calcium and/or to glucocorticoid therapy. Fractures in children and adults do mend; however, this process may be slow, and delayed healing after osteotomy with casting has been observed. Placement of intramedullary rods, rather than load-sparing plates, is best for the acute or prophylactic treatment of fractures and pseudofractures in adults (5). Dentures may be necessary for some affected children.

PRENATAL DIAGNOSIS

Perinatal hypophosphatasia can be detected prenatally. Combined use of serial ultrasonography (with attention to the limbs as well as skull), assay of ALP activity in amniotic fluid cells by an experienced laboratory, and radiologic study of the fetus enable reliable early prenatal diagnosis of severe cases in the second trimester (9). First trimester diagnosis using chorionic villus samples has also been described (10).

REFERENCES

1. Whyte MP: Hypophosphatasia. In: Scriver CR, Beaudet AL, Sly WS, Valle D (eds), *The Metabolic Basis of Inherited Disease, 6th ed.* McGraw-Hill, New York, 2843–2856, 1989
2. Caswell AM, Whyte MP, Russell RGG: Hypophosphatasia and the extracellular metabolism of inorganic pyrophosphate: clinical and laboratory aspects. *Crit Rev Clin Lab Sci* 28:175–232, 1992
3. Whyte MP: Alkaline phosphatase: physiologic role explored in hypophosphatasia. In: Peck WA (ed), *Bone and Mineral Research, 6th ed.* Elsevier Science Publishers, Amsterdam, 175–218, 1989
4. Chuck AJ, Pattrick MG, Hamilton E, Wilson R, Doherty M: Crystal deposition in hypophosphatasia: a reappraisal. *Ann Rheum Dis* 48:571–576, 1989
5. Coe JD, Murphy WA, Whyte MP: Management of femoral fractures and pseudofractures in adult hypophosphatasia. *J Bone Joint Surg* 68A:981–990, 1986
6. Weinstein RS, Whyte MP: Heterogeneity of adult hypophosphatasia: report of severe and mild cases. *Arch Intern Med* 141:727–731, 1981
7. Shohat M, Rimoin DL, Gerber HE, Lachman RS: Perinatal hypophosphatasia: clinical, radiologic, and morphologic findings. *Pediatr Radiol* 21:421, 1991
8. Henthorn PS, Raducha M, Fedde KN, Lafferty MA, Whyte MP: Different missense mutations at the tissue-nonspecific alkaline phosphatase gene locus in autosomal recessively inherited forms of mild and severe hypophosphatasia. *Proc Natl Acad Sci USA* 89:9924–9928, 1992
9. Kousseff BG, Mulivor RA: Prenatal diagnosis of hypophosphatasia. *Obstet Gynecol* 57:6(suppl):9S, 1981
10. Brock DJH, Barron L: First-trimester prenatal diagnosis of hypophosphatasia: experience with 16 cases. *Prenat Diagn* 11:387, 1991

71. Fanconi Syndrome and Renal Tubular Acidosis

Russell W. Chesney, M.D.

Department of Pediatrics, LeBonheur Children's Medical Center,
Memphis, Tennessee

Osteomalacia with or without rickets is a common feature of Fanconi syndrome and certain forms of renal tubular acidosis (RTA). The renal Fanconi syndrome is characterized by a generalized defect in renal proximal tubule transport capacity including impaired reabsorption of glucose, phosphate, amino acids, bicarbonate, uric acid, citrate and other organic acids, and low molecular weight proteins (<50,000 D). Calcium, magnesium, sodium, potassium, and water are also excreted in excess (1). This syndrome is often the ultimate expression of toxic and/or metabolic injury to the proximal tubule; hence, the syndrome has many associated disorders that play a role in its pathogenesis (Tables 1 and 2). Familial and hereditary disorders associated with the syndrome are listed in Table 1, and acquired conditions in Table 2. Because the syndrome represents a global tubulopathy and has a large number of associated disorders, the most likely pathogenic sequence involves deranged intracellular metabolic regulation rather than a defect in individual solute or ion transport sites. Abnormal intracellular metabolism could result either in a reduction in high-energy phosphate compounds necessary for active transport processes or in defective membrane biosynthesis (2). The syndrome has also been seen in association with vitamin D deficiency (3), although autosomal recessive cystine storage disease (cystinosis) and light-chain myeloma are the most common causes in children and adults, respectively (4). Some cases of the Fanconi syndrome are not linked to any of the known associations, and these idiopathic cases can be seen in both children and adults by a sporadic, recessive, dominant or sex-linked hereditary pattern (4).

Renal tubular acidosis (RTA) is a disorder in which the kidney is incapable of conserving bicarbonate; thus, patients develop a decline in plasma bicarbonate concentrations and systemic metabolic acidosis (5). The underlying renal defect consists of a reduction in tubular bicarbonate reabsorption, the inability to secrete protons (H+) so that a pH gradient between blood and the lumen cannot be formed, or the back-diffusion of previously secreted hydrogen ions across a cell membrane that cannot sustain a pH gradient (5). The causes and associations with RTA are given in Table 3. A current classification of the types of RTA considers a distal tubular hydrogen ion gradient limited form (type I), a proximal tubular bicarbonate wasting form (type II), and a hyperkalemic form (type IV). The term *type III* is no longer used and is thought to have represented a hybrid of types I and II. The magnitude of bicarbonate wasting into the urine is greatest in type II and least in type IV (2). Some patients with RTA will have a limited gradient defect and demonstrate renal bicarbonate wasting and a low plasma bicarbonate concentration but no systemic metabolic acidosis; this type is difficult to classify.

McSherry (6) has divided type IV RTA into several subtypes: Subtype 1 is related to aldosterone deficiency in the absence of overt intrinsic renal insufficiency, and subtype 2 arises from hyporeninemic hypoaldosteronism. Another subtype is associated with partial or total end-organ resistance to aldosterone. If these patients have total lack of responsiveness to the hormone, with high circulating values of aldosterone, this disorder is termed *pseudohypoaldosteronism.*

Metabolic bone disease is a feature of both the Fanconi syndrome and RTA (1–6); each will be discussed individually.

Both rickets and osteomalacia are common in many forms of the Fanconi syndrome (Table 4). Ascribed mechanisms for this metabolic bone disorder include hypophosphatemia due to phosphaturia, increased urinary calcium excretion, abnormal vitamin D metabolism, and renal insufficiency (7). Since 85% to 90% of filtered phosphate is reabsorbed by the S_1 and S_2 segments of the proximal tubule, the global defect in proximal tubule transport capacity limits phosphate reclamation. Despite any other alterations in mineral or hormone regulation in the Fanconi syndrome, this persistent phosphaturia is a major factor in the development and maintenance of rickets and/or osteomalacia, since phosphate levels in the extracellular fluid are diminished. This hypophosphatemic osteomalacia can result in osteonecrosis as a result of microfractures (8) and may be a late feature of lifelong Fanconi syndrome (9).

Hypercalciuria and nephrocalcinosis are especially common in Wilson's disease, in which both a proximal and a distal RTA are present—hence the finding of calcium deposition in the renal interstitium. Nevertheless, the serum calcium concentration is not reduced, and hypocalcemia probably does not cause metabolic bone disease.

Abnormalities of vitamin D metabolism have been described in the Fanconi syndrome. As indicated, vitamin D deficiency can result in a proximal tubulopathy resembling the Fanconi syndrome that is reversed by vitamin D treatment (3). Galactosemia, Wilson's disease, tyrosinemia, the Fanconi Bickel syndrome, and fructose intolerance could result in sufficient hepatic damage and cirrhosis to impair the 25-hydroxylation of vitamin D (10). The circulating values of 1,25(OH)$_2$D are either low or normal but are not elevated, as would be anticipated in the face of hypophosphatemia and secondary hyperparathyroidism (11). Whenever 1,25(OH)$_2$D values are reduced, bone demineralization appears to be greater (12). This reduction in 1,25(OH)$_2$D circulating values may be related to impaired proximal tubule cell metabolism or to structural changes in this tissue, since the 25(OH)D-1-α-

TABLE 1. *Familial and hereditary disorders associated with the Fanconi syndrome*

Primary or idiopathic disorders (no identifiable associated disorder)
1. Familial
2. Sporadic

Hereditary disorders
1. Cystinosis (Lignac-Fanconi disease)
2. Lowe's syndrome
3. Hereditary fructose intolerance
4. Tyrosinemia, type I (tyrosinosis)
5. Galactosemia
6. Glycogen storage disease
7. Wilson's disease
8. Others
  A. Hereditary mitochrondial myopathy with lactic acidemia
  B. Metachromatic leukodystrophy
  C. Subacute necrotizing encephalomyelopathy (Leigh's syndrome)
  D. Hereditary nephritis (Alport's syndrome)
  E. Medullary cystic disease

hydroxylase is localized to proximal tubule cell mitochondria (2). Other researchers, however, have shown reduced production of $1,25(OH)_2D$ only when renal insufficiency is demonstrable (13), especially in cystinosis, a disorder associated with progressive renal insufficiency (7).

Light-chain nephropathy may result in bone disease due to defective vitamin D metabolism (reflected in low serum $1,25(OH_2D$ values) and hypophosphatemic osteomalacia (14).

Osteomalacia has also been reported as being related to the presence of a tumor that possibly elaborated a tubulopathic substance resulting in the features of the Fanconi syndrome (15). As in oncogenous rickets, removal of the bone tumor reverses all signs of the Fanconi syndrome, including metabolic bone disease.

Wilson's disease has been associated with hypoparathyroidism, which could also contribute to the development of osteomalacia. This association is presumably related to copper deposition in the parathyroid glands (16).

Bone disease may occur in association with the Fanconi syndrome found in patients with chronic rejection of a renal transplant (17). Presumably the bone disease is due to phosphaturic hypophosphatemia and steroid-induced osteopenia related to the use of glucocorticoids as part of antirejection therapy.

Many patients with cystinosis have been stated to demonstrate osteoporosis (4). These patients have not undergone bone biopsies using modern histomorphometric analysis and double tetracycline labeling. Many of these patients are malnourished and have bone roentgenograms that display a severe degree of osteopenia that has been termed osteomalacia and/or osteoporosis.

The therapy of osteomalacia/rickets in the Fanconi syndrome is predicated on the cause of the bone disease. In general, oral phosphate supplements, either in the form of neutral phosphate or Joulie's solution, are provided at doses between 1 g to 4 g daily given in 4 to 6 daily divided doses (4). In patients with vitamin D deficiency, treatment with appropriate doses may reverse the bone disease

(3,7). Many patients with the Fanconi syndrome and osteomalacia will benefit from therapy with the 1a-hydroxylated vitamin D analogs or dihydrotachysterol (DHT) in appropriate doses (4,9–13). In patients with myeloma, therapy of the underlying monoclonal gammopathy is often curative, but oral phosphate and vitamin D may also be required. Finally, in patients with the unexpected occurrence of osteomalacia and the Fanconi syndrome, a bone scan may be indicated to seek a nonossifying fibroma that hopefully can then be fully extirpated.

Osteomalacia and/or rickets in RTA also has several causes (Table 5). Rickets is rare in children with RTA type I, as is osteomalacia in adults with the same condition (2,18). Nevertheless, these patients have erosion of bone as a result of systemic metabolic acidosis and release of calcium from bone as calcium carbonate is used as a buffer (2). This additional calcium is excreted into the urine, and many of these patients are hypercalciuric by any criteria used, with a urine calcium level greater than 4 mg/kg/day or a urine calcium/creatinine ratio greater than 0.2

TABLE 2. *Acquired disorders associated with the Fanconi syndrome*

1. Disorders of protein metabolism/excretion
  a. Multiple myeloma
  b. Benign monoclonal gammopathy
  c. Light-chain nephropathy
  d. Amyloidosis
  e. Sjogren's syndrome
  f. Nephrotic syndrome
2. Immunologic disorders
  a. Interstitial nephritis with anti-TBM antibody
  b. Renal transplantation
  c. Malignancy
3. Other renal disorders
  a. Balkan nephropathy
  b. Paroxysmal nocturnal hemoglobinuria
  c. Renal vein thrombosis in newborn infant
4. Vitamin D disorders with secondary hyperparathyroidism
  a. Vitamin D deficiency
  b. Vitamin D dependent rickets
5. Disorders linked with drug, heavy metal, or other toxin exposure
  A. Drug-related courses
    a. Outdated, degraded tetracycline
    b. Methyl-3 chromone
    c. 6-Mercaptopurine
    d. Gentamicin and aminoglycoside antibiotics
    e. Valproic acid
    f. Streptozotocin
    g. Isophthalanilide
    h. Ifosfamide
  B. Heavy metal exposure
    a. Cadmium
    b. Lead
    c. Mercury
    d. Uranium
    e. *Cis*-platinum
  C. Other toxin exposure
    a. Paraquat poisoning
    b. Lysol burn
    c. Toluene inhalation (glue sniffing)

TABLE 3. *Classification of RTA*

Site	Hereditary	Acquired

Proximal tubule	**RTA type II**
	Familial
	Transient (infants)
		RTA type II
		Drugs
		  Acetazolamide
		  Mafenide acetate
		  Sulfanilamide
		Chronic active hepatitis
		Associated with tetralogy of Fallot

	Fanconi's syndrome
	Familial
	Sporadic
	Cystinosis
	Wilson's disease
	Galactosemia
	Hereditary fructose intolerance
	Lowe's syndrome
	Tyrosinemia
	Pyruvate carboxylase deficiency
		Fanconi's Syndrome
		Drugs
		  Outdated tetracycline
		  Methyl-5-chrome
		  6-mercaptopurine
		  Cephalothin
		  Gentamicin
		Heavy metals: Pb, Cd, Hg, U
		Secondary hyperparathyroidism
		Immunologic disorders
		Multiple myeloma
		Monoclonal gammopathy
		Systemic lupus
		Sjogren's syndrome
		Renal transplantation
		Amyloidosis
		Burkitt's lymphoma
		Interstitial nephritis
		Balkan nephropathy
		Nephrotic syndrome
		Osteopetrosis
		Paroxysmal nocturnal hemoglobinuria

Distal tubule	**RTA type I**
	Primary
	Secondary
	Hereditary fructose intolerance
	Ehlers-Danlos syndrome
	Fabry's disease
	Hereditary eliptocytosis
	Medullary sponge kidney
	Hypercalciuria
	Polycystic kidney disease
	Associated with nerve deafness
		RTA type I
		Sporadic
		Metabolic disorders
		Hyperthyroidism with nephrocalcinosis
		Hypothyroidism
		Primary hyperparathyroidism with nephrocalcinosis
		Galactorrhea with hyperprolactinemia
		Idiopathic hypercalciuria
		Hypomagnesemia
		Hypergammaglobulinemic states
		Idiopathic
		Hyperglobulinemic purpura
		Cryoglobulinemia
		Sjogren's syndrome
		SLE
		Sarcoidosis
		Hodgkin's disease
		Tuberculosis
		Takayusu's arteritis
		Chronic active hepatitis
		Thyroiditis
		Starvation and malnutrition
		Hepatic cirrhosis
		Primary biliary cirrhosis
		Acute tubular necrosis
		Pyelonephritis
		Renal transplantation
		Obstructive uropathy
		Drugs
		  Lithium
		  Amphotericin B
		  Toluene
		  Analgesic nephropathy

TABLE 3. *Continued.*

Site	Hereditary	Acquired
	RTA type IV	**RTA type IV**
	Combined aldosterone, glucocorticoid deficiency	Combined aldosterone, glucocorticoid deficiency
	21-hydroxylase deficiency	Addison's disease
	Aldosterone deficiency (isolated)	Bilateral adrenalectomy
	Corticosterone methyl oxidase deficiency	Aldosterone deficiency (isolated)
		Primary, idiopathic
		Secondary, deficient renin secretion
		Chronic renal parenchymal disease
		Diabetic nephropathy
		Interstitial nephritis
		Obstructive uropathy
		Renal transplantation
		Drugs
		Nonsteroidal anti-inflammatory
		Secondary (without hyporeninemia)
		Drugs
		Heparin
		Converting enzyme inhibitors
		Adrenal insensitivity to AII
	Pseudohypoaldosteronism of infancy, type 1	Pseudohypoaldosteronism
	21-hydroxylase deficiency	Secondary
		Interstitial nephritis
		Drugs
		Spironolactone
		Amiloride
		Triamterene
	Aldosterone deficiency plus resistance	Aldosterone deficiency plus resistance
		Secondary
	21-hydroxylase deficiency	Chronic renal parenchymal disease
	Pseudohypoaldosteronism, type II	Obstructive uropathy
		Renal transplantation
		Lupus nephritis
	RTA combined types I and IV	**RTA combined types I and IV**
	SS hemoglobinopathy	Secondary
	SC hemoglobinopathy	Chronic renal parenchymal disease
		Obstructive uropathy
		Drugs
		Amiloride
		Triamterene

Calcium excretion decreases with correction of metabolic acidosis (19). Hence, oral $NaHCO_3$ or Shohl's solution will reverse this bone demineralization. As noted by numerous groups, nephrocalcinosis may persist long after correction of systemic metabolic acidosis (2).

Rickets and osteomalacia are common features of RTA type II, particularly if the proximal tubular bicarbonaturia is a component of a more global tubulopathy. The mechanisms and therapy for metabolic bone disease in RTA type II are covered in the previous section on the Fanconi syndrome. Nephrocalcinosis and hypercalciuria are not as common, since the final urine pH in proximal RTA is often acidic and thus the deposition of calcium phosphate complexes is not favored (5).

In type II RTA, which is isolated, systemic metabolic acidosis presumably results in demineralization; however, this has not been systematically evaluated.

Certain patients with vitamin D deficiency on a nutritional basis show evidence of bicarbonate wasting, although this is not usually an isolated event (2). In view of experimental studies in animals, an impaired conversion of 25(OH)D to 1,25(OH)$_2$D may be a consequence of systemic metabolic acidosis (20). A somewhat similar study in normal men who were made acidotic by an ammonium chloride challenge indicated impaired conversion of vitamin D to its active metabolite (21). However, this effect was seen only acutely. Chronic acidosis did not impair conversion of 25(OH)D to 1,25(OH)$_2$D in a study in children with RTA types I and II. Several had never been treated with bicarbonate therapy and had normal values of 1,25(OH)$_2$D in serum (22). Hence, there is little evidence for the role of impaired metabolic conversion in bone demineralization.

Whenever type IV RTA is associated with renal insufficiency, renal osteodystrophy may be expected to occur as renal failure progresses (2).

TABLE 4. *Factors contributing to osteomalacia and rickets in the Fanconi syndrome*

1. Hypophosphatemia due to a renal tubular phosphate hyperexcretion
2. Hypercalciuria—probably a minor component
3. Vitamin D deficiency
   A. Malabsorption
   B. Failure of 25-hydroxylation in disorders associated with the Fanconi syndrome and cirrhosis
4. Reduced 1a-hydroxylation of 25(OH)D
   A. Not responsive to hypophosphatemic stimulus
   B. Result of proximal tubule damage, which also leads to global proximal tubulopathy
   C. Renal insufficiency, especially in nephropathic cystinosis and chronic idiopathic Fanconi syndrome with renal insufficiency
   D. Kappa light-chain deposition in the proximal tubule in myeloma or leukemia
5. Mesenchymal tumor–elaborating substance, which results in the complex tubulopathy and osteomalacia
6. Hypoparathyroidism in Wilson's disease, presumably due to copper deposition in the parathyroid glands
7. Chronic renal transplant rejection resulting in a global tubulopathy with phosphaturia and steroid-induced osteopenia

A rare form of RTA is associated with osteopetrosis (2). This is discussed elsewhere but clearly does not result in bone demineralization.

The therapy of RTA includes correction of systemic metabolic acidemia by oral $NaHCO_3$ therapy; the doses vary according to the nephron segment affected. Type I RTA is generally treated with 1–2 mEq/kg/24 hr of oral $NaHCO_3$, but higher doses may be needed in young children (19). Type II RTA requires 10–15 mEq/kg/24 hr or slightly lower doses if thiazides are used in addition (2). Thiazides reduce plasma volume and thereby enhance tubule bicarbonate reabsorption. Patients with type IV disease may also require fluorinated glucocorticoids in supraphysiologic doses that augment potassium secretion (2). Hypercalciuria and bone resorption are reversed by $NaHCO_3$ therapy.

TABLE 5. *Causes of osteomalacia/rickets in renal tubular acidosis*

1. Bone resorption and hypercalciuria in association with type I RTA
2. Osteomalacia and/or rickets with type II RTA as part of Fanconi syndrome (See Table 4); predominately related to hypophosphatemia
3. Vitamin D deficiency
4. Defect in the conversion of 25(OH)D to 1,25(OH)$_2$D
   A) Animal model
   B) Possible presence in humans
5. Type IV RTA associated with renal insufficiency and renal osteodystrophy
6. Association between osteopetrosis and RTA with carbonic anhydrase

REFERENCES

1. Roth KS, Foreman JW, Segal S: The Fanconi syndrome and mechanisms of tubular transport dysfunction. *Kidney Int* 20: 705–716, 1981
2. Roth KS, Buckalew VM Jr, Chan JCM: Renal tubular disorders. In: Gonick H (ed) *Current Nephrology* Yearbook, Chicago, 87–117, 1985
3. Chesney RW, Harrison HE: Fanconi syndrome following bowel surgery and hepatitis reversed by 25-hydroxycholecalciferol. *J Pediatr* 86:857–861, 1975
4. Brewer ED: The Fanconi syndrome: clinical disorders. In: Gonick HC, Buckalew VM (eds), *Renal Tubular Disorders,* Marcel Dekker, New York, 475–544, 1985
5. Battle DC, Kurtzman NA: The defect in distal tubular acidosis. In: Gonick HC, Buckalew VM (eds), *Renal Tubular Disorders,* Marcel Dekker, New York, 281–306, 1985
6. McSherry E: Renal tubular acidosis in childhood. *Kidney Int* 20:799–809, 1982
7. Friedman AL, Chesney RW: Isolated renal tubular defects. In: Schrier R, Gottschalk C (eds), *Diseases of the Kidney, 5th ed.,* Little Brown, Boston, 663–690, 1988
8. Gaucher A, Thomas JL, Netter P, Faure G: Osteomalacia, pseudosacroiliitis and necrosis of the femoral heads in Fanconi syndrome in an adult. *J Rheumatol* 8:512–515, 1981
9. Brenton DP, Isenberg DA, Ainsworth DC, Garrod P, Krywawych S, Stamp TC: The adult presenting idiopathic Fanconi syndrome. *J Inherit Metab Dis* 4:211–215, 1981
10. Kitagawa T, Akatsuka A, Owada M, Mano T: Biologic and therapeutic effects of 1 alpha-hydroxycholecalciferol in different types of Fanconi syndrome. *Contrib Nephrol* 22:107–119, 1980
11. Baran DT, March TW: Evidence for a defect in vitamin D metabolism in a patient with incomplete Fanconi syndrome. *J Clin Endocrinol Metab* 59:998–1001, 1984
12. Colussi G, DeFerrari ME, Surean M, Malberti F, Rombola G, Ponlomero G, Galvanini G, Minetti L: Vitamin D metabolites and osteomalacia in the human Fanconi syndrome. *Proc Eur Dial Transplant Assoc* 21:756–760, 1985
13. Steinberg R, Chesney RW, Schulman J, DeLuca HF, Phelps M: Circulating vitamin D metabolites in nephropathic cystinosis. *J Pediatr* 120:592–594, 1983
14. Rao DS, Parfitt AM, Villanueva AR, Dorman PJ, Kleerekoper M: Hypophosphatemic osteomalacia and adult Fanconi syndrome due to light chain nephropathy. Another form of oncogenous osteomalacia. *Am J Med* 82:333–338, 1987
15. Leehey DJ, Ing TS, Daugirdas JT: Fanconi syndrome associated with a non-ossifying fibroma of bone. *Am J Med* 78:708–710, 1985
16. Carpenter TO, Carnes DL, Anast CS: Hypoparathyroidism in Wilson's disease. *N Engl J Med* 309:873–877, 1983
17. Friedman AL, Chesney RW: Fanconi's syndrome in renal transplation. *Am J Nephrol* 1:45–47, 1981
18. Brenner RJ, Spring DB, Sebastian A: Incidence of radiographically evident bone disease, nephrocalcinosis and nephrolithiasis in various types of renal tubular acidosis. *N Engl J Med* 307: 217–221, 1982
19. Rodriguez-Soriano J, Vallo A, Vastillo G: Natural history of primary distal renal tubular acidosis treated since infancy. *J Pediatr* 101:669–676, 1982
20. Lee SW, Russell J, Avioli LV: 25-hydroxycholecalciferol to 1,25-dihydroxycholecalciferol: conversion impaired by sysemic metabolic acidosis. *Science* 195:994, 1977
21. Kraut JF, Gordon EM, Ranson JC: Effect of chronic metabolic acidosis on vitamin D metabolism in humans. *Kidney Int* 24: 644–648, 1983
22. Chesney RW, Kaplan BS, Phelps M, De Luca HG: Renal tubular acidosis does not alter circulating values of calcitriol. *J Pediatr* 104:51–55, 1984

72. Drug-Induced Osteomalacia

A. Michael Parfitt, M.D.

Bone and Mineral Research Laboratory, Henry Ford Hospital,
Detroit, Michigan

Osteomalacia is usually due to a defect either in vitamin D metabolism or in phosphate metabolism (1). Drugs can cause osteomalacia indirectly by one of these well-established mechanisms or directly by some more specific but less well understood effect on mineralization (Table 1). Osteomalacia has been attributed to malabsorption of vitamin D secondary to laxative-induced diarrhea (2), but the histologic diagnosis of osteomalacia did not conform to current criteria. Cholestyramine given for bile salt diarrhea impairs vitamin D absorption and contributes to osteomalacia in patients with intestinal resection for Crohn's disease (3), but it does not cause osteomalacia by itself. A common complication of many drugs is renal tubular dysfunction, including both impaired reabsorption of bicarbonate alone and the complete Fanconi syndrome (Chapter 71), but histologically verified osteomalacia has not been reported. Either the drug-induced defects are reversible, or the disease for which the drug was given does not allow long enough survival for osteomalacia to develop.

MORPHOLOGIC AND KINETIC CHARACTERISTICS OF DRUG-INDUCED OSTEOMALACIA

The cardinal kinetic characteristic of impaired mineralization is reversal of the usual positive relationship between osteoid thickness and adjusted apposition rate, so osteoid thickness increases instead of decreases as adjusted apposition rate declines (Chapter 27). As the mineralization defect becomes more severe, the mineralized bone formation rate declines and eventually becomes zero. Rigorous diagnostic criteria have been formulated based on these kinetic characteristics (Table 2). In addition, two variant forms of osteomalacia can be identified. In focal osteomalacia, contrary to the general rule, osteoid thickness increases earlier or to a relatively greater extent than osteoid surface, and osteoid volume increases only moderately (4). Focal osteomalacia occurs when the initial increase in remodeling activation that characterizes hypovitaminosis D osteopathy (HVO) (Table 2) is absent. In atypical osteomalacia, substantial osteoid accumulation occurs in the absence of increased osteoid thickness because of a more severe than usual impairment of osteoblast matrix synthesis. Atypical osteomalacia is rare in vitamin D-related forms but is a stage in the evolution of hypophosphatemic osteomalacia (1). When induced by drugs, osteomalacia is very commonly either focal or atypical in its morphologic and kinetic features.

INCREASED VITAMIN D CATABOLISM AND ANTICONVULSANT BONE DISEASE

Some patients on long-term anticonvulsant therapy develop a syndrome of low plasma 25-hydroxyvitamin D (25OHD) intestinal malabsorption of calcium, slight fall in plasma calcium, secondary hyperparathyroidism, and cortical osteopenia (1,5, and Chapters 51 and 61). Although commonly referred to as anticonvulsant osteomalacia, this term is misleading on several counts. Radiographic evidence of mild rickets has been found in 8% of children, but systematic surveys of bone histology in adults have invariably failed to disclose osteomalacia, except where privational vitamin D depletion is common. With double tetracycline labeling, the bone formation rate is increased without defective mineralization (6), and in this and every other respect the syndrome conforms exactly to the description of HVOi (1, Table 2). Osteomalacia is largely confined to patients with only marginally adequate vitamin D supply, prolonged treatment with multiple drugs, or other risk factors.

The term *anticonvulsant osteomalacia* (see Chapter 69) is also misleading because the implication of uniform pathogenesis takes no account of significant differences between drugs (1,7). Phenobarbital is a more potent inducer of hepatic microsomal enzymes than phenytoin and enhances the catabolism of vitamin D and 25OHD in the liver, but it does not usually by itself reduce plasma 25OHD levels or cause rickets, probably because the formation of 25OHD is increased as well as its destruction. Phenytoin has not been shown to have any direct effect of vitamin D catabolism but is more commonly associated with abnormal bone mineral metabolism than phenobarbital because it can lead to hypocalcemia and secondary hyperparathyroidism by mechanisms unrelated to vitamin D, such as impaired calcium release from bone and reduced intestinal calcium absorption. Paradoxically, the best evidence for the clinical importance of enzyme induction and enhanced vitamin D catabolism comes from studies not with anticonvulsants but with rifampicin and isoniazid (8).

Whatever the mechanism, anticonvulsant administration appears to increase vitamin D requirement by 10–15 µg/day in children and possibly more in adults (9), the extent depending on the dose and especially the number of drugs used but also reflecting individual susceptibility to enzyme induction. Whether the increased requirement is clinically significant depends on the total dermal and dietary supply of vitamin D. In some institutions fractures due in part to anticonvulsant-induced osteopenia are a major health problem and overt rickets is common (9), but in other institutions prolonged immobility appears a

TABLE 1. *Classification of drug-induced osteomalacia*

Indirect:	Vitamin D mediated—Anticonvulsants
	Phosphate mediated—Antacids
Direct:	Sodium etidronate
	Sodium fluoride
	Aluminum salts

more important determinant of bone density than anticonvulsant therapy (1). Symptomatic bone disease is rare in noninstitutional settings, but the long-term effects of asymptomatic osteopenia are unknown.

Although the clinical biochemical, and histological abnormalities respond well to treatment, cortical bone loss is largely irreversible (5). There is currently no consensus on whether all or only some anticonvulsant-treated patients should be given prophylactic vitamin D, if the latter, how they should be selected, and in either case whether ergo(vitamin D_2)- or cholecalciferol (vitamin D_3) is more effective (10).

ANTACID-INDUCED PHOSPHORUS DEPLETION

Osteomalacia, according to reasonable criteria, has resulted from chronic phosphorus depletion in 12 cases (1). Patients had taken phosphate-binding antacids in large quantities, usually for at least 2 yr. The clinical and radiographic features do not differ from osteomalacia in general, although symptoms of general debility may be more frequent and severe (11). The plasma alkaline phosphatase is usually raised, but the abnormalities of bone mineral metabolism are unique. Plasma calcium is always normal and plasma phosphate usually but not invariably very low (0.9–3.2 mg/dl). The most consistent and diagnostically reliable abnormality is that urine phosphorus excretion is always less than 50 mg/24h and often much lower (1). By contrast, urinary calcium excretion is increased, sometimes to very high levels; in one case nephrolithiasis resulted, leading to unnecessary parathyroid surgery (12). The clinical and biochemical syndrome of phosphorus depletion (Chapter 55), except for osteomalacia, can be induced experimentally within a few weeks in normal subjects by high-dose antacid administration (13).

The osteomalacia is histologically typical, without evidence of aluminum deposition, and with increased osteoclast extent, less than in HVO but more than in other forms of primary hypophosphatemia. Consequently, the hypercalciuria probably results from increased net bone resorption as well as from increased intestinal calcium absorption (14). Since plasma 25OHD and PTH levels are normal, both sources of urinary calcium probably depend on an increased plasma 1,25-dihydroxyvitamin D [1,25 $(OH)_2D$] concentration, known to be induced by phosphate depletion and demonstrated in the two most recent cases (1). In retrospect, this abnormality was first observed more than 20 years ago in a patient with an increased plasma level of vitamin D activity, measurable at that time by bioassay (11). All manifestations are quickly reversed with cessation of antacid administration, combined if necessary with supplemental phosphate. Looser's zones have been observed to heal, but there is no histologic verification that osteomalacia can be completely cured.

DRUG-INDUCED INHIBITION OF MINERALIZATION

Sodium Etidronate

This agent blocks mineralization *in vitro* and probably binds to the crystal surface of newly deposited mineral *in vivo*. Osteoid accumulation and reduced tetracycline uptake are regularly seen in the treatment of Paget's disease with a dose of 10 mg/kg/day or more and are associated with increasing bone pain and increased fracture risk (1,15). The mineralization defect is focal or atypical in about half the cases (16, Fig. 1) and develops earlier and is more severe in pagetic than in normal bone, presumably because of the difference in turnover. Although a dose of 5 mg/kg/day is generally considered to be safe, focal osteomalacia is quite common after treatment with this dose for 6 mo or longer (4, Fig. 2); in one case there was generalized osteomalacia presenting with a pathologic fracture (17). The high frequency of focal osteomalacia probably results from the depression of remodeling activation by etidronate, leading to reduced bone turnover before the emergence of a significant mineralization defect. Etidronate-induced osteomalacia is reversible, but the excess osteoid may not begin to mineralize for 3–6 mo after the drug is discontinued (18).

Sodium Fluoride

In patients with osteoporosis treated with sodium fluoride significant increases in the surface extent, thickness, and volume of unmineralized osteoid have usually been observed. In most cases these changes result from stimu-

TABLE 2. *Diagnostic criteria for morphologic forms of osteomalacia*

Form	Osteoid thickness	Mineralization lag time	Osteoid surface	Bone formation rate
Pre[a]	N	N	↑↑	↑
Generalized	↑	↑	↑↑	↓
Focal	↑	↑	N	↓
Atypical	N	↑	↑	↓

[a] Pre, Stage I of hypovitaminosis D osteopathy (HVO), due to secondary hyperparathyroidism (see Chapter 65).

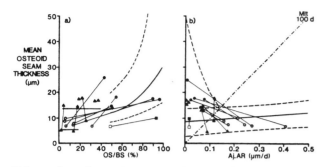

FIG. 1. Osteoid thickness relationships in drug-induced osteomalacia. Solid and interrupted lines are regressions and confidence intervals in normal subjects and patients with various stages of HVO. Static measurements on left and kinetic measurements on right. OS/BS—osteoid surface/bone surface. Aj.AR is adjusted apposition rate. Data are from three patients with Paget's disease treated with EHDP 5 mg/kg bw for 12–20 mo giving rise to focal osteomalacia (single closed triangles) and from 10 patients with osteoporosis treated with sodium fluoride in various regimens, with pretreatment values (open symbols) and posttreatment values (closed symbols) joined. Osteomalacia was focal in three cases (triangles), atypical in one case (squares), and generalized in six cases (circles). Note that complete arrest of mineralization was observed in all three EHDP treated patients but in only one of ten fluoride treated patients. (Reprinted with permission from Parfitt AM: Osteomalacia and related disorders. In: Avioli LV, Krane SM (eds), *Metabolic Bone Disease and Clinically Related Disorders, 2nd ed.* WB Saunders, Philadelphia, 329–396, 1990.)

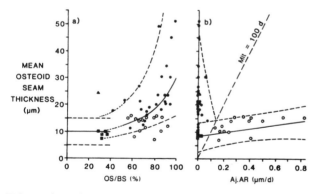

FIG. 2. Osteoid thickness relationships in aluminum-related osteomalacia occurring during maintenance hemodialysis. Layout and abbreviations as in Fig. 1, with static measurements on left and kinetic measurements on right. Data are from 46 patients, 15 with osteitis fibrosa (open circles), 25 with generalized osteomalacia (closed circles), 1 with focal osteomalacia (closed triangle), and 5 with aplastic bone disease (closed squares); these represent an early stage of atypical osteomalacia with osteoid volume/bone volume between 5% and 10%. Note that there is considerable overlap in patients with and without osteomalacia by the static measurements, but clear demarcation by the kinetic measurements (Reprinted with permission from Parfitt AM: Osteomalacia and related disorders. In: Avioli LV, Krane SM (eds), *Metabolic Bone Disease and Clinically Related Disorders, 2nd ed.* WB Saunders, Philadelphia, 329–396, 1990.)

lation of matrix synthesis rather than from impaired mineralization (1,19). Histologic evidence of osteomalacia was found in 8 of 14 patients after 2 yr of treatment but was clinically manifest only in one patient (19). Symptomatic osteomalacia attributed to fluoride treatment has been reported in only a few individual cases (1), probably because osteoid is usually added to mineralized bone rather than replacing it, so that structural failure is less likely (18). We have observed osteomalacia in 10 cases, of which 6 were generalized, 3 focal, and 1 atypical (Fig. 1). Symptoms were present only in one patient with focal osteomalacia who had a painful stress fracture of a pubic ramus resembling a Looser's zone.

The available data suggest that sodium fluoride in high doses significantly impairs mineralization in some patients, but the defect is not prevented by physiologic level of vitamin D or related to abnormal vitamin D metabolism, is not caused by lack of substrate for mineralization, is not associated with secondary hyperparathyroidism, and probably reflects a direct toxic effect on osteoblasts. Osteomalacia is also found in some patients after prolonged treatment with niflumic acid, a fluorine containing antiinflammatory agent (20). Osteomalacia could be a stage in the evolution of a successful therapeutic response rather than a harmful side effect, but it may contribute to the increased fracture rate in the first year of fluoride treatment, especially if the dose is too high.

Aluminum

Disabling osteomalacia with multiple spontaneous fractures, sometimes including the sternum, was frequently found during the early years of maintenance hemodialysis, especially after parathyroidectomy (1,21, Chapter 74). The severe epidemic form due to high dialysate aluminum level is now giving way to a more subtle sporadic disorder that results from widespread use of aluminum-containing antacids to control hyperphosphatemia (22). Proximal muscle weakness can occur in either form, probably reflecting the neurotoxicity of aluminum (23). Bisphosphonate uptake by bone is reduced, and biochemical markers of bone formation are relatively low despite abundant osteoid (1). Such findings, combined with relatively low serum PTH levels, osteopenia rather than osteosclerosis (24), more than three fractures, and high basal and postdeferoxamine serum aluminum levels (25), are highly suggestive of aluminum-induced bone disease (Chapters 23 and 74). Bone biopsy is necessary not only for diagnosis but for proper management (21), particularly the avoidance of injudicious parathyroid surgery (26).

Both atypical osteomalacia (referred to in this context as aplastic or type II) and focal osteomalacia are common, and some patients have low turnover nonosteomalacic osteopenia (Table 3), similar to that occuring in gastrointestinal and hepatobiliary disease (1, Chapter 66). The different histologic patterns reflect varying severity of prior hyperparathyroid bone disease and of independent effects of aluminum to preferentially inhibit either bone matrix synthesis or mineralization (Table 3). In patients with generalized osteomalacia the bone formation rate is no lower

TABLE 3. *Morphologic patterns of aluminum-related bone disease*[a]

	Osteomalacia			Osteopenia[b]	
	Generalized	Focal	Atypical	LT	HT
Prior hyperparathyroidism	+ +	0– +	+ +	+	+ + +
Impaired mineralization	+ + +	+ + +	+ +	+	+
Impaired matrix production	+	+	+ +	+ + +	+
Osteoid surface	↑	N	↑	N or ↑	↑
Osteoid thickness	↑	↑	N	N or ↓	N[c]
Bone formation rate	↓	↓	↓	↓	↑

[a] Relationship to severity of three functional abnormalities (0, +, + +, + + +) and to directional change of three histologic features (↑, N, ↓).

[b] LT, low turnover; HT, high turnover. Atypical osteomalacia and low turnover osteopenia (and some cases of focal osteomalacia) together comprise aplastic bone disease. In comparison with the absence of aluminum; absolute value for amount of bone may be normal.

[c] In relation to adjusted apposition rate; absolute value may be high. (Reprinted with permission from Parfitt AM: The localization of aluminum in bone: implications for the mechanism of fixation and for the pathogenesis of aluminum-related bone disease. *Int J Artif Organs* 11:79–90, 1988.

than that in the osteomalacia of vitamin D depletion, but there is a closer resemblance to hypophosphatemic osteomalacia (1,21, Fig. 2). In contrast to HVO, the morphologic expression of hyperparathyroidism is less apparent and the mineralization defect is more severe, and these abnormalities are inversely rather than directly related (1,21).

Aluminum inhibits mineralization both *in vitro* and *in vivo*, and dialysis osteomalacia is undoubtedly associated with aluminum deposition at the osteoid-bone interface (1,21). But aluminum in the cement line, which is the initial location of the bone interface, frequently does not block mineralization in patients with osteitis fibrosa, and mineralization resumes after renal transplantation despite persistence of stainable aluminum (21). Furthermore, nonuremic vitamin D–deficient animals given aluminum accumulate it in bone without impairing the healing response to vitamin D (21). Clearly, other factors must be involved in the pathogenesis of the different forms of aluminum related bone disease, such as the plasma level of citrate, which complexes aluminum to form a more potent inhibitor of mineralization than any other aluminum salt (27), and relative hypophosphatemia and possible phosphate depletion as an independent effect of antacid administration (1). Finally, aluminum accumulation can both inhibit and stimulate osteoblasts in different circumstances (21).

The management of aluminum-related bone disease is based on minimizing dialysate aluminum levels, use of nonaluminum-containing phosphate binders such as calcium carbonate, and removal of aluminum by chelation or by renal transplantation, either alone or in combination (28) (Chapter 74).

REFERENCES

1. Parfitt AM: Osteomalacia and related disorders. In: Avioli LV, Krane SM (eds), *Metabolic Bone Disease and Clinically Related Disorders,* 2nd ed. WB Saunders, Philadelphia, 329–396, 1990
2. Frame B, Guiang HL, Frost HM, Reynolds WA: Osteomalacia induced by laxative (phenolphthalein) ingestion. *Arch Intern Med* 128:794–796, 1971
3. Compston JE, Horton LWL: Oral 25-hydroxyvitamin D₃ in treatment of osteomalacia associated with ileal resection and cholestyramine therapy. *Gastroenterology* 74:900–902, 1978
4. Boyce BF, Smith L, Fogelman I, Johnston E, Ralston S, Boyle IT: focal osteomalacia due to low-dose diphosphonate therapy in Paget's disease. *Lancet* 1:821–824, 1984
5. Hahn TJ: Drug-induced disorders of vitamin D and mineral metabolism. *Clin Endocrinol Metab* 9:107–129, 1980
6. Weinstein RS, Bryce GF, Sappington LJ, King DW, Gallagher BB: Decreased serum ionized calcium and normal vitamin D metabolite levels with anti-convulsant drug treatment. *J Clin Endocrinol Metab* 58:1003–1009, 1984
7. Mimaki T, Waison PD, Haussler MR: Anticonvulsant therapy and vitamin D metabolism: evidence for different mechanisms for phenytoin and phenobarbital. *Pediatr Pharmacol* 1:105–112, 1980
8. Brodie MJ, Boobis AR, Hillyard CJ, Abeyasekera G, Stevenson JC, McIntyre I, Park BK: Effect of rifampicin and isoniazid on vitamin D metabolism. *Clin Pharmacol Ther* 32:525–530, 1982
9. Davie MWJ, Emberson CE, Lawson DEM, Roberts GE, Barnes JLC, Barnes ND, Heeley AF: Low plasma 25-hydroxyvitamin D and serum calcium levels in institutionalized epileptic subjects: associated risk factors, consequences and response to treatment with vitamin D. *Q J Med* 52:79–91, 1983
10. Tjellesen L, Gotfredsen A, Christiansen C: Different actions of vitamin D₂ and D₃ on bone metabolism in patients treated with pheonbarbitone/phenytoin. *Calcif Tissue Int* 37:218–222, 1985
11. Lotz M, Zisman E, Bartter FC: Evidence for a phosphorus-depletion syndrome in man. *N Engl J Med* 278:409–452, 1968
12. Cooke N, Teitelbaum S, Avioli LV: Antacid-induced osteomalacia and nephrolithiasis. *Arch Intern Med* 138:1007–1009, 1978
13. Dominguez JH, Gray RW, Lemann J Jr: Dietary phosphate deprivation in women and men. Effects on mineral and acid balances, parathyroid hormone and metabolism of 25-OH-vitamin D. *J Clin Endocrinol Metab* 43:1056–1068, 1976
14. Parfitt AM: Bone as a source of urinary calcium-osseous hypercalciuria. In: Coe F (ed), *Hypercalciuric States—Pathogenesis, Consequences and Treatment.* New York, Grune & Stratton, 313–378, 1984
15. Krane SM: Etidronate disodium in the treatment of Paget's disease of bone. *Ann Intern Med* 96:619–625, 1982
16. Khairi MRA, Altman RD, DeRosa GP, Zimmerman J, Schenk RK, Johnston CC: Sodium etidronate in the treatment of Paget's disease of bone. A study of long-term results. *Ann Intern Med* 87:656–663, 1977
17. Evans RA, Dunstan CR, Hills E, Wong SYP: Pathologic fracture due to severe osteomalacia following low-dose diphosphonate

treatment of Paget's disease of bone. *Aust NZ J Med* 13: 277–279, 1983

18. Schenk RK, Olah AJ: What is osteomalacia? *Adv Exp Biol Med* 128:549–562, 1980

19. Briancon D, Meunier PJ: Treatment of osteoporosis with fluoride, calcium, and vitamin D. *Orthop Clin North Am* 12:629–648, 1981

20. Bonvoisin B, Bouvier M, Meunier PJ, Lejeune E: Osteomalacie histologique induit par l'administration prolongee d'acide nifumique. *La Nouvelle Presse Medicale* 11:1636, 1982

21. Parfitt AM: The localization of aluminum in bone: implications for the mechanism of fixation and for the pathogenesis of aluminum-related bone disease. *Int J Artif Organs* 11:79–90, 1988

22. Norris KC, Crooks PW, Nebeker HG, et al.: Clinical and laboratory features of aluminum-related bone disease: differences between sporadic and "epidemic" forms of the syndrome. *Am J Kidney Dis* 6:342–347, 1985

23. Wills MR, Savory J: Aluminum poisoning: dialysis encephalopathy, osteomalacia, and anaemia. *Lancet* 2:29–34, 1983

24. Kriegschauser JS, Swee RG, McCarthy JT, Hauser MF: Aluminum toxicity in patients undergoing dialysis: radiographic findings and prediction of bone biopsy results. *Radiology* 164: 399–403, 1987

25. Hodsman AB, Hood SA, Brown P, Cordy PE: Do serum aluminum levels reflect underlying skeletal aluminum accumulation and bone histology before or after chelation by deferoxamine? *J Lab Clin Med* 106:674–681, 1985

26. Sherrard DJ, Ott SM, Andress DL: Pseudohyperparathyroidism. Syndrome associated with aluminum intoxication in patients with renal failure. *Am J Med* 79:127–130, 1985

27. Thomas WC, Meyer JL: Aluminum-induced osteomalacia: an explanation *Am J Nephrol* 4:201–203, 1984

28. Parfitt AM: Are bone problems of dialysis patients always solved by renal transplantation? A CPC Series: *Cases in Metabolic Bone Disease 1, No. 4.* Medical Projects, New York, 1986

73. Metabolic Bone Disease of Total Parenteral Nutrition

Gordon L. Klein, M.D., M.P.H.

Department of Pediatrics and Nutrition, University of Texas Medical Branch, Galveston, Texas

Total parenteral nutrition (TPN) is a therapeutic regimen designed to provide for the administration of all nutritional requirements in a concentrated solution infused either into a central or a peripheral vein. This method of treatment is generally used in patients with gastrointestinal disease severe enough to prevent adequate oral or enteral nutrition. Because parenteral requirements for various nutrients are unknown and because the purity of individual intravenous solutions is variable, TPN therapy may be subject to the inadequate provision of certain nutrients as well as to the inadvertent contamination of solutions with toxic substances. Bone disease may be a manifestation of the various deficiencies or toxicities.

Bone disease resulting from inadequate provision of calcium or phosphate in the TPN solution has been discussed in Chapter 65.

This chapter deals with bone disease brought about by aluminum toxicity in adults. It also covers the role of aluminum in the metabolic bone disease in a group of infants and children receiving long-term TPN therapy.

BONE DISEASE IN ADULTS

Clinical Presentation

The initial and, in many cases, only clinical presentation of bone disease in a group of patients studied in Los Angeles and Seattle was periarticular bone pain, especially in weight-bearing bones, lower back, or ribs. The pain presented from 2 to 36 mo after initiation of TPN therapy, increased in intensity, and did not respond to narcotic analgesics. In some instances movement was so painful that patients confined themselves to bed. Improvement occurred only when TPN treatment was discontinued (1, Fig. 1). However, only about 20% of the patients evaluated prospectively were symptomatic.

Roentgenographic Findings

Approximately 80% of patients evaluated had diffuse osteopenia (1). Photon absorptiometry of the radius in one patient revealed decreased bone mineral content. Neutron activation studies in a similar series of patients in Toronto revealed that bone mass decreased to the level seen in osteoporosis in 60% of the subjects, whereas 40% had intermediate values between normal and osteoporotic (2).

Histologic Evaluation

Within 4 mo of initiating TPN treatment, hyperkinetic, rapidly turning-over bone (increased formation and resorption) was described, which changed to low-turnover osteomalacia after at least 1 yr of therapy (3). Patchy osteomalacia was found in patients from Los Angeles and Seattle who had bone biopsies performed after at least 1 yr of TPN. Increased unmineralized osteoid and decreased bone formation were seen (Fig. 2).

Biochemical Features

In both the Canadian and American reports, serum calcium and phosphorus levels were normal or mildly ele-

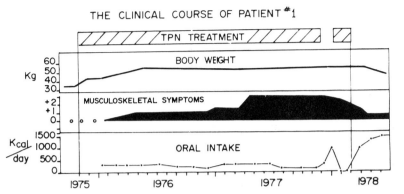

THE CLINICAL COURSE OF PATIENT #1

FIG. 1. Changes in bone pain in relation to TPN therapy in the index case with TPN bone disease, modified from Klein et al. *Lancet* 2: 1041–1044, 1980 (1).

vated. Serum levels of alkaline phosphatase were often elevated, but the cholestatic complications of TPN treatment interfered with interpretation. A striking hypercalciuria, often with negative calcium balance, was found in most TPN patients. Because the hypercalciuria resolved when TPN was stopped, and because the urinary calcium excretion was not related to serum levels of immunoreactive parathyroid hormone (iPTH), the hypercalciuria was thought to be due to increased filtered load of calcium from and possibly the protein load in the TPN solutions (1,4).

Serum levels of immunoreactive PTH were in the low-normal range, whereas serum levels of 1,25-dihydroxyvitamin D [1,25(OH)$_2$D] were very low, giving rise to the possibility of TPN-induced hypoparathyroidism. However, when calcium was removed from the TPN solution in two patients, serum PTH levels rose without any de-

tectable rise in serum levels of 1,25(OH)$_2$D. Serum levels of 25-hydroxyvitamin D (25OHD) and 24,25-dihydroxyvitamin D were normal (5). Cessation of TPN treatment in one patient with low serum levels of 1,25(OH)$_2$D resulted in a rise in serum levels to normal within 6 wk after discontinuing TPN treatment (5). The possibility has been raised that a component of the TPN solution was acting as a toxin.

Aluminum

Because osteomalacia with decreased bone formation had been observed in patients with renal failure undergoing hemodialysis and because aluminum accumulation in bone had been previously observed (6), bone biopsies were obtained from TPN patients (7). Aluminum content

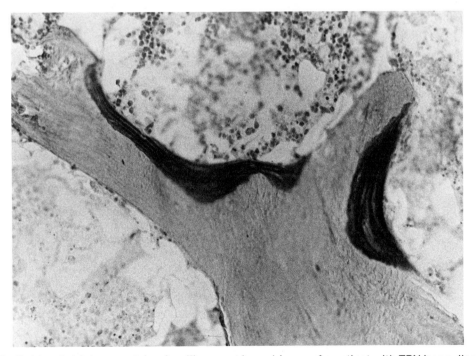

FIG. 2. Goldner's trichrome stain of an iliac crest bone biopsy of a patient with TPN bone disease, magnification × 160. Mineralized bone is shown in gray; unmineralized osteoid is shown in black. This patient has patchy areas of excessive unmineralized osteoid, one of the diagnostic features of osteomalacia. Photo courtesy of Dr. DJ Sherrard, VA Medical Center, Seattle, WA.

in biopsy specimens was elevated, up to 30 times normal, and elevated aluminum levels were also found in plasma and urine (7). Analysis of the TPN solutions revealed that casein hydrolysate was found to contain large quantities of aluminum, up to 1 mg/L, which provided a parenteral aluminum intake of 2000–3000 µg/day (7). Substitution for casein hydrolysate of a synthetic amino acid mixture containing only about 2% of the aluminum in casein resulted in an acute decline in plasma aluminum concentration and urinary aluminum excretion. However, aluminum retention by tissues such as bone persisted for up to 3 yr after discontinuing casein (4,8).

The primary route of aluminum disposal is urinary excretion; however, patients receiving TPN have relatively normal renal function (7). One possibility for the accumulation of aluminum in patients with normal renal function is the fact that plasma ultrafilterable aluminum is only about 5% of total plasma aluminum (8). Therefore, most circulating aluminum is protein-bound and not filtered. We have suggested that there are at least two pools of aluminum in the body: a rapidly exchangeable pool that is quickly depleted on reduction or cessation of aluminum loading and a slowly exchangeable pool, which may represent a tissue pool in equilibrium with plasma.

Proposed Pathogenesis of the Adult Form of TPN Bone Disease

Aluminum has been localized by aurin tricarboxylic acid stain to the mineralization front of bone, both in patients with TPN bone disease and in those with dialysis osteomalacia (Chapters 23, 71, 73). Under conditions of chronic aluminum loading, the extent of surface stainable aluminum in bone correlates very closely with quantitative bone aluminum determined by flameless atomic absorption spectroscopy. However, surface stainable bone aluminum was inversely correlated with rate of bone formation (6, Fig. 3). It remains unknown whether aluminum

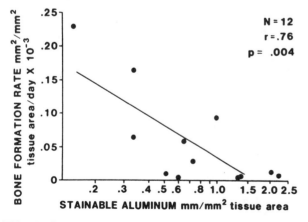

FIG. 3. Correlation between bone formation rate and stainable aluminum in patients receiving total parenteral nutrition who had received casein hydrolysate. The values for bone aluminum are plotted on a logarithmic scale. From Ott et al. *Ann Intern Med* 98:910–914, 1983 (6). Reprinted by permission from *Ann Intern Med*.

impairs bone formation directly by affecting bone, indirectly by accumulating in the parathyroid glands and interfering with PTH secretion (6), or by altering vitamin D metabolism (6).

The Role of Vitamin D

Removal of vitamin D from the TPN solutions resulted in low serum levels of 25OHD but no clinical or histologic manifestations of bone disease (3). In another study patients receiving chronic parenteral nutrition failed to develop osteomalacia even though they received amounts of vitamin D comparable to the quantities postulated to provoke osteomalacia in aluminum-loaded patients (9). Although vitamin D is in standard multivitamin mixes for parenteral use, the role of vitamin D in the pathogenesis of TPN bone disease remains open to question.

Treatment and Prevention

Replacement of casein hydrolysate, the chief source of aluminum from the TPN solutions, with a synthetic amino acid solution resulted in reduction of bone pain and hypercalciuria, improvement in bone formation rate, and return of serum levels of 1,25(HO)$_2$D to normal (4). Whether aluminum reduction was the only factor resulting in improvement is not certain because the amounts of protein and vitamin D$_2$ in the TPN solution were also reduced (4). The reduction in protein content may have corrected the hypercalciuria, though it was probably not responsible for the increase in bone formation rate (4). It is also unlikely that the reduction in vitamin D content played a major role in the increased bone formation rate.

A recent report showed that bone histology in TPN patients is heterogeneous in the absence of stainable bone aluminum (10). Bone formation rate was not lower than normal subjects but was higher than that in aluminum-toxic TPN patients (10). Another study describes low-turnover TPN bone disease in the absence of stainable bone aluminum but with elevated serum aluminum levels (11).

Bone biopsies in aluminum-loaded patients who had casein hydrolysate removed from their TPN solutions showed inverse relationships between bone formation rate and surface stainable aluminum and between bone formation rate and plasma aluminum (4). This latter relationship suggests that plasma aluminum, even before it accumulates in bone, reduces bone formation. It would appear that TPN bone disease can be reduced or eliminated if care is taken to avoid contamination of the solution with calcium-containing additives. Because the current aluminum content of TPN solutions is highly variable, measurements of aluminum in blood, urine, and TPN solution is advisable in patients who develop bone disease while receiving TPN therapy.

One caveat remains. The attribution of metabolic bone disease is to TPN therapy may be mistaken if preexisting bone disease is not excluded. Malabsorption of vitamin D, calcium, or phosphorus, for example, could result in

TABLE 1. *Sources of aluminum in common intravenously administered products*[a]

Solution	Number of lots tested	Aluminum content, μg/L	Reference
Potassium phosphate	3	16,598 ± 1801	12
Sodium phosphate	1	5977	12
10% Calcium gluconate	5	5056 ± 335	12
Heparin (1,000 μ/ml)	3	684 ± 761	12
25% Normal serum albumin	4	1822 ± 2503	12
Trace metal solution	7	972 ± 108	11

[a] Values are given as mean ± SD.

osteomalacia secondary to gastrointestinal disease. Elderly women requiring TPN treatment may have postmenopausal osteoporosis. Therefore, evaluation of bone density, histology, and biochemistry early in the course of TPN therapy can help to determine the presence of preexisting metabolic bone disease.

BONE DISEASE IN INFANTS

Long-term treatment with TPN has been associated with rickets or osteopenia in premature infants (12). Although insufficient provision of calcium or phosphate may be primarily responsible for the rickets, aluminum loading may be a complicating factor. Evidence supporting this is as follows.

Significant quantities of aluminum may still be found in TPN solutions, mainly in calcium and phosphate salts, heparin, and albumin (12). These sources can result in aluminum concentrations of some TPN solutions form 30–306 μg/L (13,14) (see Table 1).

This concentration of aluminum can result in aluminum administration to premature infants of from 15–30 μg/kg/day (14). Adult patients receiving TPN with normal renal function who were loaded with aluminum to the point of bone toxicity received 60 μg/kg/day, while others receiving long-term TPN therapy with crystalline amino acids instead of casein hydrolysate received only 1 μg/kg/day. The latter groups had no evidence of elevated serum, urine, or bone content of aluminum (14). Thus, premature infants receive aluminum in TPN solutions intermediate between known safe and known toxic amounts.

Because renal function in premature infants is developmentally reduced, the risk of aluminum retention is increased. Older term infants receiving chronic TPN treatment retain approximately 75% of the intravenous aluminum load (12).

In premature infants aluminum has been observed to accumulate in bone, blood and urine, occasionally to high levels (12,13). Autopsy specimens of vertebrae from two infants who died while receiving TPN revealed a positive aurin tricarboxylic acid stain for aluminum at the level of the mineralization front (13). Thus, premature infants receiving TPN therapy may accumulate aluminum in bone at the mineralization front in a manner similar to adults.

Although accumulation of aluminum at the mineralization front in premature infants is not by itself evidence of aluminum toxicity, aluminum accumulation in bone has been associated with decreased bone formation and probably osteomalacia in adults (6).

In addition, long-term TPN therapy in three infants led to rickets despite the provision of 1,000 IU (25 μg) daily vitamin D_2 in the TPN solution. The rickets finally resolved after high-dose vitamin D_2 (ergocalciferol in oil) was given (12). The reason for vitamin D dependent rickets with long-term TPN therapy is unclear. However, all three patients were subsequently found to have accumulated large quantities of aluminum.

Treatment and Prevention

Every attempt should be made to provide, especially to premature infants, as much calcium and phosphate as permitted by the TPN solution.

Until manufacturers reduce the aluminum content of these products, periodic monitoring of infants receiving TPN for roentgenographic evidence of bone disease is recommended. Periodic determinations of serum levels of calcium, phosphorus, PTH, 25OHD, and $1,25(OH)_2D$ can identify associated hyperparathyroidism and vitamin D deficiency (low 25OHD). If bone disease persists despite maximal calcium and phosphate supplementation, and if 24-hour urine excretion of calcium and phosphorus does not exceed intake, then aluminum in plasma, urine, and the TPN solution should be obtained. Specimens must be collected in plastic containers and sent to a specialized laboratory for analysis.

Plasma aluminum concentration exceeding 100 μg/L and/or urine aluminum/creatinine (μg/mg) greater than 0.3 (normal <0.05) require analysis of the components of the TPN solution for aluminum content: Inform the hospital pharmacists of the source(s) of the high levels of aluminum so that they may inform the manufacturer, and if possible stop or reduce TPN. Although deferoxamine therapy has been useful in chelating aluminum from the bones of adults with dialysis osteomalacia, there has been insufficient experience with this drug in infants to recommend its general use.

REFERENCES

1. Klein GL, Targoff CM, Ament ME, Sherrard DJ, Bluestone R, Young JH, Norman AW, Coburn JW: Bone disease associated with total parenteral nutrition *Lancet* 2:1041–1044, 1980
2. Harrison JE, Jeejeebhoy KN, Track NS: The effect of total par-

enteral nutrition (TPN) on bone mass. In: Coburn JW, Klein GL (eds), *Metabolic Bone Disease in Total Parenteral Nutrition.* Urban and Schwarzenberg, Baltimore/Munich, 53–61, 1985

3. Jeejeebhoy KN, Shike M, Sturtridge WC, Tam CS, Jones G, Murray TM, Harrison JE: TPN bone disease at Toronto. In: Coburn JW, Klein GL (eds), *Metabolic Bone Disease in Total Parenteral Nutrition.* Urban and Schwarzenberg, Baltimore/Munich, 17–29, 1985

4. Vargas JH, Klein GL, Ament ME, Ott SM, Sherrard DJ, Horst RL, Berquist WE, Alfrey AC, Slatopolsky E, Coburn JW: Metabolic bone disease of total parenteral nutrition: course after changing from casein to amino acids in parenteral solutions with reduced aluminum content. *Am J Clin Nutr* 48:1070–1078,1988

5. Klein GL, Horst RL, Norman AW, Ament ME, Slatopolsky E, Coburn JW: Reduced serum levels of 1α,25-dihydroxyvitamin D during long term parenteral nutrition. *Ann Intern Med* 94: 638–643, 1981

6. Ott SM, Maloney NA, Klein GL, Alfrey AC, Ament ME, Coburn JW, Sherrard DJ: Aluminum is associated with low bone formation in patients receiving chronic parenteral nutrition. *Ann Intern Med* 98:910–914, 1983

7. Klein GL, Alfrey AC, Miller NL, Sherrard DJ, Hazlet TK, Ament ME, Coburn JW: Aluminum loading during total parenteral nutrition. *Am J Clin Nutr* 35:1425–1429, 1982

8. Klein GL, Ott SM, Alfrey AC, Sherrard DJ, Hazlet TK, Miller NL, Maloney NA, Berquist WE, Ament ME, Coburn JW: Aluminum as a factor in the bone disease of long-term parenteral nutrition. *Trans Assoc Am Phys* 95:155–164, 1982

9. Shike M, Shils ME, Heller A, Alcock N, Vigorita V, Brockman R, Holick MF, Lane J, Flombaum C: Bone disease in prolonged parenteral nutrition: osteopenia without mineralization defect. *Am J Clin Nutr* 44:89–98, 1986

10. Lipkin EW, Ott SM, Klein GL: Heterogeneity of bone histology in parenteral nutrition patients. *Am J Clin Nutr* 46:673–680, 1987

11. DeVernejoul MC, Messing B, Modrowski D, Bielakoff J, Buisine A, Miravet L: Multifactorial low remodeling bone disease during cyclic total parenteral nutrition. *J Clin Endocrinol Metab* 60:109–113, 1985

12. Sedman AB, Klein GL, Merritt RJ, Miller NL, Weber KO, Gill WL, Anand H, Alfrey AC: Evidence of aluminum loading in infants receiving intravenous therapy. *N Engl J Med* 312: 1337–1343, 1985

13. Koo WWK, Kaplan LA, Bendon R, Succop P, Tsang RC, Horn J, Steicha JJ: Response to aluminum in parenteral nutrition during infancy. *J Pediatr* 109:877–883, 1986

14. Klein GL: Unusual sources of aluminum. In: DeBroe ME, Coburn JW (eds), *Aluminum and Renal Failure.* Kluwes, Dorsdrecht/Boston/Lancaster, pp. 203–211, 1990

74. Renal Osteodystrophy in Adults and Children

William G. Goodman, M.D., Jack W. Coburn, M.D., Jorge A. Ramirez, M.D., Eduardo Slatopolsky, M.D., and Isidro B. Salusky, M.D.

Departments of Radiological Sciences, Medicine and Pediatrics, UCLA School of Medicine, and Veterans Administration Medical Center, West Los Angeles, Wadsworth Division, Los Angeles, California and the Renal Division, Washington University, St. Louis, Missouri

The physiologic control of mineral metabolism is a closely integrated process that involves the kidneys, intestine, parathyroid glands, and bone. Because the kidney plays a critical role in the overall regulation of mineral homeostasis, the development of renal disease has widespread consequences for the skeleton and for a variety of soft tissues. In its broadest sense, the term *renal osteodystrophy* encompasses the full spectrum of bone and soft tissue disorders associated with renal failure.

The kidney serves to regulate the external balances of calcium, phosphorus, and magnesium by modulating the excretion of these minerals in the urine. Other exogenous and endogenous substances, such as aluminum and beta-2-microglobulin, are also removed from the body by renal excretion, and their retention in patients undergoing long-term dialysis can lead to specific disorders of the joints and bone (1,2). In addition, the cells of the proximal nephron are the primary site for the synthesis of 1,25-dihydroxyvitamin D, or calcitriol; this vitamin D sterol is a major determinant of intestinal calcium absorption and an important regulator of parathyroid hormone (PTH) secretion. The kidney also serves both as a target organ for the actions of PTH and as a site for the degradation of PTH. Since each of these metabolic and excretory functions is disturbed to some degree in patients with chronic renal failure, even moderate reductions in nephron mass can result in substantial alterations in bone and mineral metabolism (3).

This chapter provides an overview of the pathogenesis, signs and symptoms, histologic features, and roentgenographic characteristics of renal osteodystrophy. Differences between adult and pediatric patients in the manifestations of renal osteodystrophy are discussed, and bone disease in renal transplant recipients is reviewed. Current approaches to the prevention and treatment of renal osteodystrophy are summarized, and the features of amyloidosis in patients with chronic renal failure are briefly described.

PATHOGENESIS OF RENAL OSTEODYSTROPHY

PTH and calcitriol, or $1,25(OH)_2D_3$, are two of the most important hormonal regulators of calcium and bone metabolism, and their physiologic regulation is closely integrated. Overall, both hormones act to raise serum calcium levels. PTH decreases calcium excretion in the urine and enhances the mobilization of calcium from bone in addition to increasing renal phosphorus excretion; if sustained, high serum PTH levels result in increased rates of bone remodeling and turnover (3). PTH also promotes the renal synthesis of calcitriol, the most potent metabolite of vitamin D. Calcitriol separately enhances the release of calcium from bone, represents the primary determinant of active intestinal calcium absorption, and participates in the inhibitory feedback control of PTH secretion (4). Although PTH and calcitriol production normally increase during hypocalcemia and decrease during hypercalcemia, the regulation of the parathyroid–vitamin D axis is disturbed in renal failure; thus, serum calcitriol levels are characteristically reduced, whereas serum PTH levels are usually elevated. In addition, aluminum can independently inhibit the release of PTH by the parathyroid glands, whereas its accumulation in bone can directly impair bone formation and mineralization (5–7).

Interactions among these and other factors ultimately determine the type of bone disease that develops in patients with renal failure (8). Generally, the renal bone diseases are classified as either high-turnover lesions, which are due to persistently high serum PTH levels, or low-turnover lesions, which are related either to excess bone aluminum deposition or to normal or reduced serum PTH levels. Each group of disorders is considered separately here, but it should be noted that the skeletal manifestations in an individual patient can represent the combined response to more than one pathogenic process (9,10). The histopathologic manifestations of renal bone disease probably represent portions of a continuum that encompasses both the low-turnover and high-turnover skeletal disorders.

High-Turnover Bone Disease (Secondary Hyperparathyroidism)

Several factors contribute to sustained increases in PTH secretion and, ultimately, to parathyroid gland hyperplasia and high-turnover lesions of bone in patients with chronic renal failure. Among these are hyperphosphatemia due to diminished renal phosphorus excretion, hypocalcemia, impaired renal calcitriol production, disturbances in the control of PTH secretion, and skeletal resistance to the calcemic actions of PTH (3).

Phosphorus retention and hyperphosphatemia have been recognized for many years as important factors in the pathogenesis of secondary hyperparathyroidism (11). The development of secondary hyperparathyroidism can be prevented in experimental animals with chronic renal failure when dietary phosphorus intake is lowered in proportion to reductions in glomerular filtration rate (12); dietary phosphate restriction can also reduce the serum levels of PTH in patients with moderate renal failure (13,14). Available information suggests that phosphate retention promotes the secretion of PTH in several ways. First, hyperphosphatemia can lower serum ionized calcium levels directly, thereby stimulating the release of PTH by the parathyroid glands (15). Second, excess phosphorus reduces renal 1α-hydroxylase activity, which is responsible for the conversion of 25-hydroxyvitamin D to $1,25(OH)_2D_3$ (16); a high rate of transepithelial phosphate transport in the proximal tubule may be partly responsible for this change when glomerular filtration is reduced (14). Third, phosphorus retention may enhance the synthesis

and/or release of PTH directly without associated changes in serum ionized calcium or calcitriol levels (17,18). Regardless of the precise mechanism responsible, increased serum PTH levels and low serum calcitriol levels are commonly found in patients with mild to moderate renal failure.

In addition to disturbances in phosphorus metabolism, the regulation of PTH secretion appears to be altered in patients with chronic renal failure. *In vitro* studies of dispersed parathyroid cells in tissue culture have suggested that calcium-regulated PTH release is abnormal in parathyroid cells obtained from patients with chronic renal failure when compared to normal (19); thus, higher calcium levels may be required to achieve comparable reductions in PTH release in hyperplastic tissues (19). Several mechanisms could account for this upward shift in the set point for calcium-regulated PTH secretion in chronic renal failure. Calcitriol directly affects both the synthesis and release of PTH by the parathyroid cell, and reduced serum calcitriol levels may disrupt the normal inhibitory feedback regulation of PTH secretion *in vivo* (20). The observations by Slatopolsky et al. in a group of hemodialysis patients treated with intravenous doses of calcitriol are consistent with this concept (21); thus, calcitriol administration lowered serum PTH levels without an associated rise in serum ionized calcium early in the course of treatment in patients with moderate secondary hyperparathyroidism (Fig. 1).

A decrease in the number of receptors for vitamin D in the parathyroid cell may also contribute to alterations in calcium-mediated PTH secretion in chronic renal failure (22). Calcitriol is known to upregulate its own receptor in normal parathyroid tissue (23), but it is not known whether diminished vitamin D receptor expression in chronic renal failure is due to low circulating calcitriol levels, to the hyperplastic state of the parathyroid glands per se, or to differences in cell function that are a consequence of the uremic environment (24,25). Adenylate cyclase activity is abnormal in hyperplastic parathyroid tis-

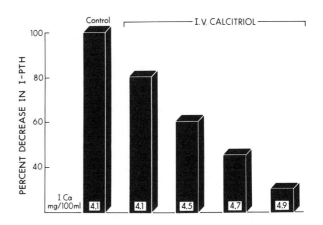

FIG. 1. The effect of intravenous calcitriol on serum ionized calcium and iPTH levels in 20 patients undergoing maintenance hemodialysis. Serum iPTH values decrease before changes in ionized calcium levels can be demonstrated. (Adapted from Slatopolsky, E., et al., *J Clin Invest* 74:21, 1984. Reproduced with permission.)

sues (26), and other disturbances in cell membrane function could also be involved.

Skeletal resistance to the calcemic action of PTH may also contribute to the development of hypocalcemia and secondary hyperparathyroidism in chronic renal failure. The calcemic response to infusions of parathyroid extract is subnormal in patients with moderate to advanced renal failure, and the correction of hypocalcemia is less rapid than in normal individuals (27). Disturbances in the metabolism of vitamin D appear to be largely responsible for these changes (28).

Low-Turnover Bone Disease (Osteomalacia and Adynamic Lesions of Bone)

In contrast to the high-turnover skeletal disorders of secondary hyperparathyroidism, osteomalacia and adynamic lesions account for most cases of low-turnover bone disease in patients with chronic renal failure. Bone formation and turnover are reduced in each, but osteomalacia is characterized by a further impairment in the mineralization of newly formed bone. Thus, unmineralized bone collagen, or osteoid, accumulates in osteomalacia, whereas the amount of osteoid is normal or reduced in the adynamic lesion.

In the past, aluminum toxicity was largely responsible for the development of these two disorders in patients with chronic renal failure, but the prevalence of aluminum-related bone disease has declined substantially in recent years. In contrast, the number of patients with adynamic lesions of bone without evidence of bone aluminum deposition has increased substantially (9,29,30). Recent observations suggest that 40–50% of those undergoing long-term dialysis have adynamic lesions of renal osteodystrophy, and the serum levels of PTH are either normal or only modestly elevated in most of these patients (30). Apart from other clinical disorders known to be associated with low-turnover skeletal lesions such as diabetes, corticosteroid therapy, and aluminum intoxication, the increased use of vitamin D sterols and oral calcium carbonate may be factors that contribute to parathyroid gland suppression and the development of adynamic bone in patients with chronic renal failure. The long-term consequences of this disorder in the absence of aluminum toxicity remain to be determined.

A number of factors can contribute to the development of osteomalacia in patients with advanced renal failure and in those treated with maintenance dialysis (3,8). Evidence of vitamin D deficiency, as judged by low serum levels of 25(OH)-vitamin D, was noted in some dialysis patients with osteomalacia in England (31), but this is an uncommon finding in the United States. It is likely that differences in sunlight exposure and in the amount of vitamin D in fortified foods and nutritional supplements accounts for this discrepancy. Long-term therapy with phenytoin and/or phenobarbital is associated with the development of osteomalacia in nonuremic patients, and a higher incidence of symptomatic bone disease has been observed in dialysis patients receiving these drugs (32). Nutritional deficiencies, particularly with respect to cal-

cium and phosphorus, can occasionally lead to osteomalacia in patients with chronic renal failure.

Before 1980, little was known about the biological consequences of aluminum accumulation in patients with renal failure. It is now apparent, however, that aluminum represented a major cause of osteomalacia and adynamic bone disease in patients undergoing regular dialysis during the past 10–12 yr (33). Early epidemiologic studies in Britain established an association between the occurrence of vitamin D resistant, fracturing osteomalacia and the neurologic syndrome, dialysis encephalopathy, or dialysis dementia (34). Contamination with aluminum of water that was used for the preparation of dialysis solutions was subsequently identified as the major source of aluminum loading in such patients, and the introduction of adequate water purification procedures markedly reduced the prevalence of this epidemic form of aluminum intoxication (35).

Nevertheless, dialysis encephalopathy and aluminum-related bone disease were also observed in adults and in children with chronic renal failure prior to the initiation of dialysis or in those treated with dialysis solutions that did not contain aluminum (36,37). In these patients, aluminum-containing phosphate-binding agents that were used for the control of hyperphosphatemia were the primary source of aluminum loading. Plasma aluminum levels, which reflect recent aluminum loading, were correlated with the amounts of aluminum ingested orally, and values decreased substantially following the withdrawal of aluminum-containing medications (38). These observations underscore the potential for aluminum absorption from the intestine when aluminum-containing compounds are given to patients with chronic renal failure.

Aluminum can influence the metabolism of bone in several ways. Deposits of aluminum are found within the mineralization front of bone in patients with aluminum-related renal osteomalacia or adynamic lesions (39). This site, which is located at the junction between surface osteoid seams and adjacent mineralized bone, is where the calcification of newly formed bone collagen is initiated. *In vivo* experiments indicate that aluminum can impede the mineralization process directly (40–42), at least in part by slowing the rate of formation and growth of hydroxyapatite crystals, the major structural component of mineralized bone (7,43). In addition to its effects on the calcification process, aluminum can adversely affect the osteoblast (6,44). Reductions in the number of osteoblasts are a characteristic finding in aluminum-related bone disease, and this change may be related to decreases in the rate of osteoblastic proliferation and/or in the differentiation of osteoblastic precursors into mature osteoblasts (6). Basal and hormone-stimulated osteoblastic functions have also been shown to be impaired by aluminum *in vitro* (45,46). Thus, collagen synthesis and mineralized bone formation are each markedly reduced by aluminum loading *in vivo*.

Whether patients with aluminum-related bone disease develop overt histologic osteomalacia or adynamic lesions is related to the severity of the respective impairments in collagen synthesis and skeletal mineralization. Although the rate of collagen synthesis is low in both lesions, the defect in skeletal mineralization is disproportionally more severe in patients with osteomalacia; thus, mineralization lags behind collagen synthesis, leading to osteoid accumulation and thickened osteoid seams. In contrast, the rates of mineralization and collagen synthesis are reduced to a similar degree in patients with adynamic lesions of bone; consequently, osteoid volume and osteoid seam thickness are normal or reduced in this form of aluminum-related bone disease.

Several clinical disorders increase the risk of aluminum-related bone disease in patients with chronic renal failure, including previous parathyroidectomy, a history of renal transplantation and graft failure, bilateral nephrectomy, and diabetes mellitus (47–49). In addition, citrate can form soluble complexes of aluminum in aqueous solutions; this compound markedly enhances intestinal aluminum absorption, and it can lead to aluminum intoxication when ingested together with aluminum-containing medications (50,51). In contrast, sustained elevations in serum PTH levels appear to partially offset the adverse effects of aluminum on bone; thus, aluminum-related bone disease may not be seen despite evidence of aluminum deposition in bone in some patients with persistent secondary hyperparathyroidism (42). This may account for the greater risk of aluminum-related bone disease in patients who have undergone parathyroidectomy or in those with diabetes since the serum levels of PTH are generally low in these two conditions. In this regard, marked increases in bone aluminum content and the development of overt aluminum-related osteomalacia have been noted after parathyroidectomy in patients undergoing regular dialysis (49,52).

HISTOLOGIC FEATURES OF RENAL OSTEODYSTROPHY

The use of bone biopsy has contributed greatly to our understanding of renal bone disease (8). Bone biopsies provide valuable information about various histologic features such as the amounts of mineralized and unmineralized tissue, the thickness of osteoid seams, the extent of resorption surfaces, the number of osteoblasts and osteoclasts, and the presence or absence of marrow fibrosis. Dynamic measurements of bone formation can also be obtained using the technique of double tetracycline labeling. These agents are deposited within bone at sites of active mineralization, and their presence can be demonstrated in thin sections of tissue by fluorescence microscopy. Where new bone is formed, double bands of tetracycline fluorescence can be seen, and the amount of bone formed during the labeling interval is circumscribed by the two labels. Consequently, the rate of bone formation can be determined (53). This information is often essential for the correct diagnostic interpretation of biopsy material from patients with renal osteodystrophy (53).

Procedures for achieving double tetracycline labeling of bone differ among laboratories, but the following approach is suitable for patients with chronic renal failure. Patients are given demeclocycline, 300 mg orally twice a day, for 2 or 3 days followed by a 10 to 20 day interval during which no tetracycline is given. A second course of oral tetracycline HCl, 500 mg twice a day, is then ad-

ministered for another 2 or 3 days. The bone biopsy should be obtained 3 to 7 days after completion of the second course of oral tetracycline (54). For pediatric patients, two-day courses of tetracycline are recommended for each label, and doses should not exceed 10 mg/kg/day (9).

In addition to histomorphometric assessments, histochemical staining procedures can be used to demonstrate deposits of aluminum and iron in bone, and the aluminum content of bone can be measured using atomic absorption spectroscopy in small samples obtained at the time of biopsy (39). Iliac crest bone biopsy can be done safely in the outpatient setting with minimal morbidity both in adults and in children (54).

High-Turnover Bone Disease

Osteitis fibrosa is the most common of the high-turnover lesions of renal osteodystrophy both in adults and in children (8,9). Overall, the disorder represents the response of bone to persistently high serum levels of parathyroid hormone. There is histologic evidence of active bone resorption with increases in the number and size of osteoclasts and an increase in the number of resorption bays, or Howship's lacunae, within cancellous bone. Fibrous tissue may be found immediately adjacent to bony trabeculae, or it may accumulate more extensively within the marrow space (Fig. 2); partial or complete fibrous replacement of individual bony trabeculae occurs in advanced cases.

Osteoblastic activity is also increased in patients with osteitis fibrosa (8,9), and the combined increase in osteoblastic and osteoclastic activity accounts for the high rate of bone remodeling and turnover in secondary hyperparathyroidism. Bone formation exceeds the normal range, and values often reach three to four times the upper limit of normal. The number of osteoblasts is substantially increased, and a greater proportion of the cancellous bone surface is covered with newly formed osteoid. Overall, the total amount of osteoid is moderately increased. Many osteoid seams exhibit a woven appearance similar to that of a woven straw basket; this finding is characteristic of skeletal disorders in which collagen synthesis and bone formation are markedly increased, and it is the result of changes in the arrangement of collagen fibrils within osteoid seams.

Patients who have more modest increases in osteoclastic activity and bone formation with little or no evidence of peritrabecular fibrosis are classified as having mild lesions of renal osteodystrophy. This disorder is a less severe manifestation of hyperparathyroid bone disease (8,9). Serum PTH levels are elevated, and other biochemical and roentgenographic manifestations of secondary hyperparathyroidism are also present. Because the histologic features are much less striking than those of overt osteitis fibrosa, tetracycline-based measurements of bone formation are useful for distinguishing this subgroup of patients from those with normal bone or adynamic lesions (8,9).

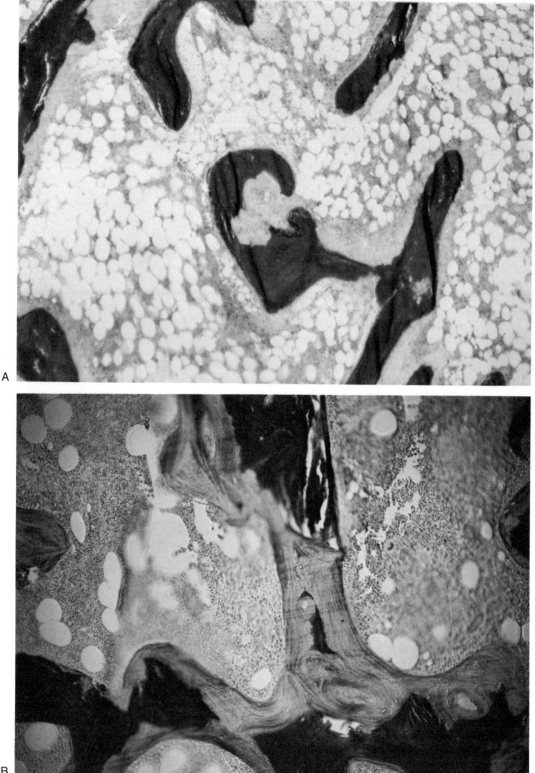

FIG. 2. A: Goldner-stained section of undecalcified bone from a hemodialysis patient with osteitis fibrosa; magnification 50×. Mineralized bone stains green (light), and osteoid appears red (dark). Fibrous tissue has accumulated within the marrow space immediately adjacent to bone, and the serrated margins along the bone surface represent sites of osteoclastic bone resorption. **B:** Goldner-stained section of undecalcified bone from a hemodialysis patient with osteomalacia; magnification 50×. Mineralized bone stains green (light), and osteoid appears red (dark). The total amount of osteoid is markedly increased; osteoid seams are wide, and they have a multilaminant appearance.

Low-Turnover Bone Disease

Osteomalacia is the most striking histologic manifestation of low-turnover bone disease. Excess osteoid, or unmineralized bone collagen, accumulates in bone due to a primary defect in mineralization (7). Osteoid seams are wide, and they often have a multilamellar appearance (Fig. 2); the extent of bone surfaces covered with osteoid is also increased. In contrast, osteoblastic activity is markedly reduced, and bone formation often cannot be measured because of the lack of tetracycline uptake into bone. In patients with aluminum-related osteomalacia, the bone aluminum content is elevated, and deposits of aluminum can be seen along trabecular bone surfaces using histochemical staining methods (8,9,33). The histologic severity of osteomalacia generally corresponds to the amount of surface-stainable aluminum in bone (55).

Bone biopsies from other patients with symptomatic bone disease exhibit normal or reduced amounts of osteoid, no tissue fibrosis, diminished numbers of osteoblasts and osteoclasts, and low or unmeasurable rates of bone formation (8,9,56). This disorder has been termed the adynamic, or aplastic, lesion of renal osteodystrophy, and aluminum deposition along bone surfaces is a common finding (56). *In vivo* experimental studies suggest that this disorder may be the forerunner of overt histologic osteomalacia when bone aluminum accumulation is the underlying cause (40,57); thus, bone aluminum levels are often not as high in this subgroup of patients compared to those with overt aluminum-related osteomalacia.

In recent years, a greater proportion of adult and pediatric dialysis patients with adynamic lesions of renal osteodystrophy have had no evidence of bone aluminum deposition, and the overall prevalence of this disorder in patients undergoing both hemodialysis and peritoneal dialysis appears to be increasing (9,58). It is now generally recognized that other factors, in addition to aluminum, can account for the development of adynamic lesions of bone in patients with chronic renal failure; these probably include the use of large doses of calcium-containing, phosphate-binding antacids and vitamin D sterols relatively early in the clinical course of secondary hyperparathyroidism in patients with chronic renal failure (30).

Occasionally patients demonstrate histologic evidence of both osteitis fibrosa and osteomalacia on bone biopsy. This pattern is termed the mixed lesion of renal osteodystrophy (59). Such patients usually have biochemical evidence of secondary hyperparathyroidism in conjunction with findings that are more characteristic of patients with impaired bone formation and mineralization. Persistent hypocalcemia is present in some patients, and this can contribute to defective skeletal mineralization (59). Mixed lesions of renal osteodystrophy may be seen in patients with osteitis fibrosa who are in the process of developing aluminum-related bone disease or in patients with aluminum-related osteomalacia who are undergoing treatment with deferoxamine (60). The mixed renal osteodystrophy can therefore represent a transitional state between the high-turnover lesions of secondary hyperparathyroidism and the low-turnover disorders of osteomalacia or adynamic bone (10).

CLINICAL MANIFESTATIONS

The signs and symptoms of renal osteodystrophy are rather nonspecific, and laboratory and roentgenographic abnormalities often do not correspond to the severity of the clinical manifestations (3). Common clinical features include bone pain, muscle weakness, skeletal deformities, and extraskeletal calcifications. In children, growth retardation is a particularly prominent feature.

Bone Pain

Bone pain is very common in patients with renal osteodystrophy; its onset is usually insidious, and symptoms progress gradually over many months. The pain is frequently diffuse and nonspecific, but it is often aggravated by weight bearing or by changes in posture. When localized, the lower back, hips, and legs are most often affected. The appendicular skeleton can also be involved, and pain in the heel or ankles may be a presenting complaint (3). Occasionally, the initial manifestation is that of an acute arthritis or periarthritis that is not relieved by massage or by application of local heat. Severe bone pain is more common in patients with aluminum-related bone disease than in those with osteitis fibrosa, and it is often a prominent clinical feature of this disorder (61). There is marked variation among patients, however, and some with advanced secondary hyperparathyroidism are severely incapacitated. The physical examination is generally unremarkable unless fractures or skeletal deformities are present.

Muscle Weakness

Proximal myopathy develops in some patients with advanced renal failure. Symptoms appear very slowly, and weakness and aching are the most common manifestations both in adults and in children (3). The physiologic basis of this disorder is not understood, and several factors may contribute. Favorable clinical responses have been noted after treatment with calcitriol or $25(OH)D_3$, following parathyroidectomy, after successful renal transplantation, and during the treatment of aluminum-related bone disease with deferoxamine (3). The role of abnormal vitamin D metabolism in the pathogenesis of uremic myopathy remains uncertain, but a careful evaluation must be done to exclude the presence of severe secondary hyperparathyroidism or aluminum toxicity. In patients with prominent symptoms of muscle pain and weakness, an empiric therapeutic trial of calcitriol or $25(OH)D_3$ is warranted.

Skeletal Deformities

Deformities of bone are a major manifestation of renal osteodystrophy, particularly in children with long-standing renal failure. The frequency of skeletal deformity in pediatric patients is probably related to the high rates of bone growth and skeletal modeling that characterize the immature skeleton. Bone deformities may affect either the axial or appendicular skeleton.

The pattern of bone deformity varies with age in children with chronic renal failure. In patients younger than 3 to 4 yr of age, the changes of secondary hyperparathyroidism most often resemble those of vitamin D deficiency rickets; characteristic features include rachitic rosary, Harrison grooves, and enlargement of the wrists and ankles due to a widening of the metaphysis beneath the growth plate in long bones. Craniotabes and frontal bossing of the skull occur in children who develop renal failure in the first 2 yr of life (62). The onset of overt renal failure before the age of 10 yr is often associated with deformities of the long bones; bowing is the most frequent change. Genu valgum is a common manifestation at any age, and ulnar deviation of hands, pes varus, "swelling" of the wrists, ankles, or medial ends of clavicles due to metaphyseal widening and pseudoclubbing are frequently observed. Despite regular treatment with vitamin D sterols, 20–25% of pediatric patients undergoing long-term dialysis may require corrective orthopedic procedures for skeletal deformities (63).

Slipped epiphyses are another common complication of renal bone disease in pediatric patients. The disorder usually occurs in association with severe secondary hyperparathyroidism (62), and the femoral epiphysis is most often affected. Dental abnormalities, including enamel defects and malformations of the teeth, are typical in children with congenital renal diseases due to disturbances in mineral metabolism that develop early in life (62).

In adults with aluminum-related bone disease, skeletal deformities are confined predominantly to the axial skeleton; changes include lumbar scoliosis, kyphosis, and distortion of the thoracic cage. Adult patients with severe osteitis fibrosa may develop rib deformities and pseudoclubbing.

Growth Retardation

Children with chronic renal failure almost invariably exhibit growth retardation; among the factors that contribute to this disturbance are chronic acidosis, malnutrition, renal bone disease, and abnormal somatomedin metabolism (64). Treatment with calcitriol has been shown to improve linear growth in some children (65), but similar responses have not been documented by other investigators. Consistent increases in growth rate have not been observed in the majority of children undergoing maintenance dialysis during treatment with vitamin D, 1α-hydroxyvitamin D, or calcitriol (66).

Extraskeletal Manifestations

Several types of soft tissue calcification can be detected by radiographic examination. Among the most frequent are tumoral or periarticular calcifications; these are occasionally associated with acute periarticular inflammation, and the clinical presentation may suggest an episode of acute arthritis. Soft tissue calcifications are common when serum phosphorus levels are greater than 8–9 mg/dl or when the calcium-phosphorus ion product exceeds 75. Soft tissue calcifications can regress substantially if sustained reductions in serum phosphorus levels can be achieved. Although extraskeletal calcifications are more common with advancing age, they can occur in children with end-stage renal disease.

The most frequent form of vascular calcification in patients with renal failure is localized to the medial layer of small and medium-sized arteries (Mockerberg's sclerosis); this type of calcification is diffuse and continuous along the vessel wall (Fig. 3). Involvement is most common in diabetic patients, and the roentgenographic appearance differs from the irregular pattern of calcified intimal plaques. Medial calcifications are usually asymptomatic, but palpation of the peripheral pulses and blood pressure measurements may be rendered difficult in affected limbs. Vascular calcifications are best detected by lateral views of the ankle or anterioposterior views of the hands or feet using magnification techniques with macroradioscopy (67). The importance of a high serum

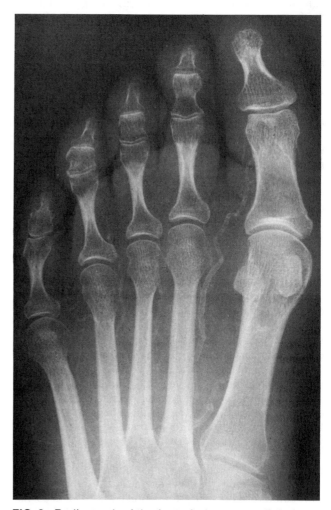

FIG. 3. Radiograph of the foot of a long-term dialysis patient demonstrating extensive medial calcification of the arteries.

calcium-phosphorus ion product in the development of vascular calcifications has been questioned, but a concerted effort should be made to avoid values above 65–70 (68).

In extreme cases, there may be ischemic necrosis of the skin, muscle and/or subcutaneous tissues; this syndrome is known as "calciphylaxis," but its pathogenesis is not understood. Most patients have evidence of advanced secondary hyperparathyroidism, and parathyroidectomy may result in significant clinical improvement. Calciphylaxis can be seen in patients with advanced renal failure, in those receiving regular dialysis, and in patients with functioning renal allografts (69).

Visceral calcifications are rather infrequent, and they may differ in chemical composition from vascular calcifications (70); the lungs, heart, kidneys, skeletal muscle, and stomach are mainly involved. Pulmonary calcifications can cause restrictive lung disease that may be severe and progressive, and the disorder often persists even after successful kidney transplantation or parathyroidectomy.

Amyloidosis in Patients with Chronic Renal Failure

Over the past several years clinicians have become increasingly aware of the association between bone cysts, pathologic fractures, scapulohumeral periarthritis, and the carpal tunnel syndrome in patients treated with long-term hemodialysis (71–75). These syndromes arise from the accumulation of a unique type of amyloid protein that is comprised of beta-2 microglobulin (B-2-M), a polypeptide with a molecular weight of 11,800 D that comprises the beta chain of the HLA Class I molecule (76,77). Although it is normally degraded by the kidney, B-2-M is retained in patients with renal failure, and serum levels are increased. Histologically, B-2-M amyloid fibrils exhibit features similar to those of amyloid AA, but they have a strong predilection to form deposits in tendons, periarticular structures, at the end of long bones and within intervertebral disks (77,78). Because the clinical syndromes associated with amyloid deposition commonly affect the musculoskeletal system, their manifestations may be confused with those of other forms of renal osteodystrophy.

The clinical manifestations of amyloid deposition almost never appear before 5 yr of dialysis therapy, but the disorder is more common in patients who begin regular dialysis after the age of 50 yr (2,79). Carpal tunnel syndrome is the most frequent clinical feature, but arthritic complaints and bone disease are not infrequent. Deposits of B-2-M are found in periarticular structures as well as in joints, bone, and tendon sheaths (Fig. 4). Far less commonly, the liver, spleen, rectal mucosa, or blood vessels are involved (2).

Skeletal manifestations include generalized arthritis, erosive arthritis, and joint effusions. Scapulohumeral involvement with shoulder pain is a common clinical presentation. Generalized arthritis can lead to pain and stiffness, decreased joint mobility, effusions, and even deformities. Erosive arthritis can involve the metacarpophalangeal joints, the interphalangeal joints, shoulders, wrists, and knees, and effusions may occur at these sites

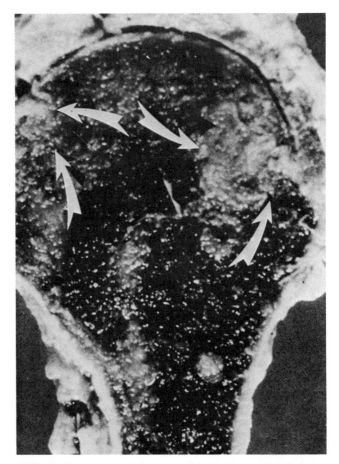

FIG. 4. Postmortem photograph showing extensive deposits of amyloid within the femoral head (*white arrows*); such areas often appear as cystic lesions on roentgenographs. (From van den Broucke, J.M., et al., *Kidney Int* 33:S-35, 1988. Reprinted with permission.)

(2). The cervical spine is commonly involved by destructive arthropathy (80).

Roentgenographically, bone cysts may be found in the hip, femoral neck, wrist, metacarpal, shoulder, knee, and acromioclavicular joint; the carpal bones, tibial plateau, symphysis pubis, and tarsal bones may also be affected. Cystic deposits of amyloid may resemble brown tumors, but their location and the presence of multiple rather than solitary cysts suggests that amyloid deposition is responsible. Cystic changes usually occur at the site of tendinous insertions, and pathologically these may represent "amyloidomas" that replace the bone. Fractures can develop in bones weakened by such cysts (71).

The fraction of patients afflicted with amyloidosis increases progressively with the duration of dialysis therapy; thus, 70–80% of patients treated with hemodialysis for 10 yr or more will have evidence of B-2-M accumulation in tissues (79). The distinction between this disorder and either severe secondary hyperparathyroidism or aluminum-related bone disease can be difficult, and thorough clinical, biochemical, and radiographic evaluations are required. B-2-M amyloidosis may coexist with either high-turnover or low-turnover lesions of renal osteodystrophy.

Overall, the management of amyloidosis in patients with chronic renal failure is unsatisfactory. The use of highly permeable dialysis membranes can lower serum B-2-M levels, but there is limited evidence that this has any effect on the progression of established disease. Nevertheless, patients treated from the onset of regular dialysis with polyacrilonitrile (PAN) dialysis membranes appear to have a lower incidence of the disease compared with those managed with conventional dialyzers (79). Renal transplantation provides the best prospect for symptomatic improvement, but bone cysts persist even after successful transplantation (77).

BIOCHEMICAL FEATURES OF RENAL OSTEODYSTROPHY

A progressive decline in glomerular filtration rate (GFR) is associated with marked changes in bone and mineral metabolism. When the GFR falls below 30% of normal, hyperphosphatemia is common, and phosphate-binding agents and dietary phosphorus restriction are often needed to correct and/or prevent this disorder (3). Although hemodialysis and continuous ambulatory peritoneal dialysis (CAPD) remove substantial amounts of phosphorus, additional efforts to control hyperphosphatemia are required in 80–90% of patients treated with dialysis.

Serum calcium levels are often subnormal in patients with advanced renal failure. With the initiation of hemodialysis, calcium levels usually increase, and they may return to normal. The magnitude of the rise in serum calcium values is partially related to the calcium concentration in dialysate. In patients treated with CAPD who are not receiving vitamin D supplements, serum calcium levels often remain at the lower limit of normal (81).

The development of hypercalcemia in patients undergoing regular dialysis warrants an immediate and thorough investigation. Conditions associated with hypercalcemia in this group of patients include marked hyperplasia of the parathyroid glands due to severe secondary hyperparathyroidism, aluminum-related bone disease, therapy with calcitriol or other vitamin D sterols, the administration of calcium carbonate or other calcium-containing compounds, immobilization, malignancy, and granulomatous disorders such as sarcoidosis or tuberculosis with extrarenal production of $1,25(OH)_2D_3$ (3).

In advanced renal failure, serum magnesium levels often increase due to reduced renal magnesium excretion, but they remain within the upper range of normal or become only slightly elevated when dialysate magnesium concentrations are maintained between 0.5–0.8 mEq/L (82). The use of magnesium-containing laxatives or antacids can abruptly raise serum magnesium levels in patients with renal failure (83); such agents should be avoided in patients with diminished renal function, and serum magnesium levels must be measured frequently and regularly if magnesium-containing medications are used.

Plasma alkaline phosphatase values are fair markers of the severity of secondary hyperparathyroidism in patients with renal failure. Osteoblasts normally express large amounts of the bone isoenzyme of alkaline phosphatase, and serum levels are usually elevated when osteoblastic activity and bone formation are increased. Elevated levels generally correspond to the degree of histologic change in patients with high-turnover lesions of renal osteodystrophy, and values frequently correlate with serum PTH levels (84). Measurements of serum alkaline phosphatase are also useful for monitoring the response of bone to treatment with vitamin D sterols in patients with osteitis fibrosa; values that decrease over weeks or months usually indicate histologic improvement. Serum alkaline phosphatase levels may also increase early in the course of treatment with the chelating agent deferoxamine in patients with aluminum-related bone disease.

Serum alkaline phosphatase levels are less useful for differentiating between patients with high-turnover and low-turnover lesions of bone. Although the serum levels of alkaline phosphatase are usually high in patients with secondary hyperparathyroidism, values can also be elevated in those with aluminum-related osteomalacia (85). Normal alkaline phosphatase levels are more common in patients with severe aluminum toxicity resulting from aluminum contamination of dialysis fluids. In pediatric patients undergoing peritoneal dialysis, plasma alkaline phosphatase levels have been a poor predictor of bone histology, and values can be elevated in patients with either osteitis fibrosa or osteomalacia (9).

Increases in isoenzymes of alkaline phosphatase that originate in nonskeletal tissues, particularly liver, can account for high plasma levels in patients with renal failure; consequently, confirmation of a skeletal source of alkaline phosphatase activity should be obtained. This can be achieved by measuring the heat labile fraction of the enzyme if valid and reliable techniques are available. In clinical practice, measurements of other liver enzymes that reflect biliary tract dysfunction, such as gamma glutamyltranspeptidase or 5′-nucleotidase, are of value in excluding hepatic disturbances as the cause of high serum alkaline phosphatase levels.

Serum osteocalcin levels, or bone Gla-protein, can also be used as an index of osteoblastic activity in patients with chronic renal failure (86). Absolute values are increased in patients with chronic renal failure, but measurements can be useful in separating patients with high-turnover lesions of secondary hyperparathyroidism from those with low-turnover lesions such as osteomalacia and adynamic bone (86,87).

Serum PTH levels are elevated in most patients with advanced renal failure (14,88,89), and values are often used to gauge the severity of secondary hyperparathyroidism and bone disease in patients with chronic renal failure or those receiving regular dialysis. In the past, most radioimmunoassays for parathyroid hormone utilized antisera directed against epitopes located in the carboxy-terminal or midportions of the PTH molecule. Results obtained using these methods were often difficult to interpret, however, in patients with chronic renal failure due to the retention in plasma of biologically inactive peptide fragments that cross-reacted with carboxy- and mid-region antisera (90). Because the sequence of the initial 34 amino acids of PTH determines its receptor-binding and hormonal actions, more recently developed assays for PTH have utilized measurements of the amino-terminal portion of the molecule or the intact hormone (91,92). Numerous assays for PTH are currently available commercially, but the relationship between the histologic findings in bone and the serum levels of immunoreactive PTH in patients with renal bone disease has been examined in relatively few of them; proper interpretation of PTH measurements must be made, therefore, with a knowledge about its value as an indicator of bone histology.

Using a mid-carboxy-terminal assay in patients with chronic renal failure, Hruska et al. found moderate correlations between serum immunoreactive PTH levels and several parameters of bone histology including osteoblastic osteoid surface, osteoclastic bone surface, osteoclast count, and trabecular bone surface adjacent to areas of marrow fibrosis (84). The same PTH assay was less useful, however, in evaluating pediatric patients undergoing CCPD, and it was of limited value in distinguishing among the various histologic subtypes of renal bone disease in pediatric patients (9).

Andress et al. measured serum PTH levels using both an amino-terminal and a carboxy-terminal antisera in adult patients treated with hemodialysis (93). Amino-terminal measurements provided good discrimination between patients with osteitis fibrosa and those with either osteomalacia or mild lesions of secondary hyperparathyroidism, and the degree of marrow fibrosis corresponded more closely with amino-terminal than with carboxy-terminal PTH values (93). Amino-terminal PTH values were also lower in patients with aluminum-related bone disease than in patients with other histologic subtypes of renal osteodystrophy, but values remained elevated in some patients with evidence of bone aluminum toxicity (93). Thus, although patients with aluminum-related bone disease generally have lower serum PTH levels than those with osteitis fibrosa (Fig. 5), bone aluminum deposition must be documented by bone biopsy, and a high serum PTH value does not exclude this diagnostic possibility.

The more widespread availability of immunoradiometric assays (IRMA) for intact parathyroid hormone may in the future make it possible to distinguish more reliably among patients with various histologic subtypes of renal osteodystrophy (94–96). Cohen-Solal et al. recently reported that measurements of intact PTH were superior for separating patients with secondary hyperparathyroidism from those with adynamic lesions of bone (94). Moreover, it is now apparent that many patients with advanced renal failure have normal or minimally elevated serum PTH levels in association with adynamic lesions of bone that are not due to bone aluminum deposition (30). Although the long-term consequences of this disturbance are unknown, such patients may have a state of relative hypoparathyroidism for their degree of renal failure. Currently available evidence indicates that serum values 1–2 times above the upper limit of normal using assays for intact PTH correspond to relatively normal histologic findings on bone biopsy in patients with chronic renal failure (94,95).

Plasma aluminum levels are often elevated in patients with chronic renal failure and in those treated with maintenance dialysis (35,37,97). It should be noted, however, that the reported normal range for plasma aluminum in man varies considerably among different laboratories, in part due to variations in methodology. The use of elec-

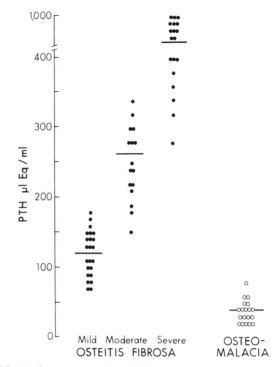

FIG. 5. Serum parathyroid hormone levels in adult dialyzed patients with mild, moderate, and severe osteitis fibrosa. Patients with osteomalacia have low values for iPTH.

trothermal atomic absorption spectrometry provides an accurate and reproducible method for measuring aluminum in tissues and plasma, and values from reliable reference laboratories in normal subjects are generally less than 10 µg/L. Levels of 20–40 µg/L are relatively common in patients undergoing regular dialysis (98,99), whereas values above 50 µg/L suggest some degree of aluminum loading. Aluminum levels in plasma probably reflect recent loads of aluminum entering the body either from contaminated dialysate or from aluminum-containing medications taken as phosphate-binding agents. Thus, plasma aluminum levels should be monitored at regular intervals in patients treated by maintenance dialysis and particularly in those with chronic renal failure who continue to ingest aluminum-containing medications (100).

Although plasma aluminum levels may correspond to the amount of aluminum ingested orally from phosphate-binding agents (Fig. 6), they frequently do not accurately reflect tissue stores of aluminum (101). Bone and liver represent major sites of aluminum deposition within the body (102), but the degree of aluminum retention in these tissues does not correspond with measurements in plasma. Deferoxamine is a metal-chelating agent that binds to aluminum, and infusions of deferoxamine can markedly increase plasma aluminum levels in patients with aluminum-related bone disease. This agent has been used to treat patients with aluminum intoxication, often with dramatic clinical results (103,104), and a diagnostic test has also been developed to assist in the noninvasive assessment of aluminum loading in patients with chronic renal failure (98).

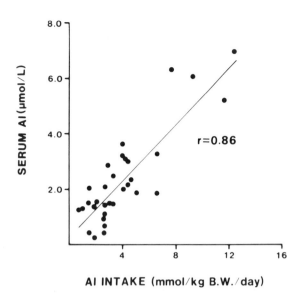

FIG. 6. Relationship between oral aluminum intake from aluminum hydroxide and serum aluminum levels in pediatric patients undergoing CAPD. (From Salusky, I.B., et al., *J Pediatrics* 105:717, 1984. Reprinted with permission.)

The deferoxamine infusion test is completed as follows: Patients are given a standardized intravenous dose of deferoxamine, 40 mg/kg in 100 ml of 5% dextrose solution, during the 2 hr immediately after a hemodialysis procedure; plasma aluminum levels are measured before and 24–48 hr after the infusion. An increase in plasma aluminum greater than 300 μg/L above baseline values is often a better predictor of high bone aluminum levels in individual cases than basal plasma aluminum values (98).

The deferoxamine infusion test has been evaluated as a diagnostic tool for aluminum-related bone disease in patients with renal osteodystrophy. Malluche et al. noted that the magnitude of the rise in plasma aluminum after deferoxamine was not specific in all cases (105). In addition, Hodsman et al. demonstrated that dialysis patients with secondary hyperparathyroidism may have substantial increases in plasma aluminum following infusions of deferoxamine despite little evidence of stainable aluminum in bone biopsy specimens (99). Thus, some patients with osteitis fibrosa have high tissue levels of aluminum and a positive deferoxamine infusion test without overt histologic evidence of bone aluminum toxicity. Such patients may be at increased risk, however, for the development of aluminum-related bone disease after parathyroidectomy or following prolonged treatment with maintenance dialysis.

ROENTGENOGRAPHIC FEATURES OF RENAL OSTEODYSTROPHY

Osteitis Fibrosa

The presence of subperiosteal erosions is one of the most consistent findings in patients with secondary hyper-

parathyroidism, and the extent of this change often corresponds to the serum levels of PTH and alkaline phosphatase (106). Patchy osteosclerosis is also common, and this accounts for the classic appearance of the "rugger jersey" spine on lateral views of the thoracic vertebrae and the "salt and pepper" appearance of the skull. Skeletal roentgenographs may be normal, however, in patients with mild to moderate osteitis fibrosa. In addition, subperiosteal erosions can be present in patients with established aluminum-related bone disease and osteomalacia (107); this finding emphasizes the need for independent biochemical or histologic confirmation of the diagnosis of secondary hyperparathyroidism.

Subperiosteal erosions can be detected at the surfaces of the digital phalanges (Fig. 7), at the distal ends of the clavicles, beneath the surfaces of the ischium and pubis, at the sacroiliac joints, and at the junction of the metaphysis and diaphysis of long bones. Meema and Schatz have utilized fine-grain films and a hand lens of 6–7× magnification to detect the presence of erosions on radiographs of the hands (108). In pediatric patients, metaphyseal changes—i.e., growth zone lesions—are common and have been described as ricketslike lesions. Mehls demonstrated that this radiographic finding of secondary hyperparathyroidism differs from that of true vitamin D deficiency (62). Both subperiosteal erosions of the digits and growth zone lesions are best demonstrated by examining x-ray films of the hands; the presence of growth zone changes is the best indicator of the severity of secondary hyperparathyroidism in children as judged by serum PTH and alkaline phosphatase levels (106).

Slipped epiphyses are among the most striking clinical and radiographic manifestations of renal osteodystrophy in children; this complication is a consequence of advanced osteitis fibrosa in uremic children (62). The age of the patient often determines the site affected. In preschool children, epiphyseal slippage occurs either in the upper or lower femoral region or in the distal tibial epiphysis, but not in the distal radius or distal ulna. In contrast, the upper femoral epiphysis and the distal epiphyses of the forearm are affected most often in older children. Severe epiphyseal slippage can lead to gross deformities of the skeleton with ulnar deviation of the hands and abnormalities in gait.

Osteomalacia

The roentgenographic features of osteomalacia are less specific than those of secondary hyperparathyroidism. Indeed, pseudofractures are the only pathognomonic finding in adult patients. These are straight, wide radiolucent bands in the cortex oriented perpendicular to the longitudinal axis of the bone. Fractures of the ribs and hips and compression fractures of the vertebral bodies are more common in dialyzed patients with osteomalacia than in those with osteitis fibrosa (61).

Ricketslike lesions have also been described in pediatric patients with aluminum-related bone disease and osteomalacia, and these changes may resolve after treatment with deferoxamine (109). Rachitic lesions in

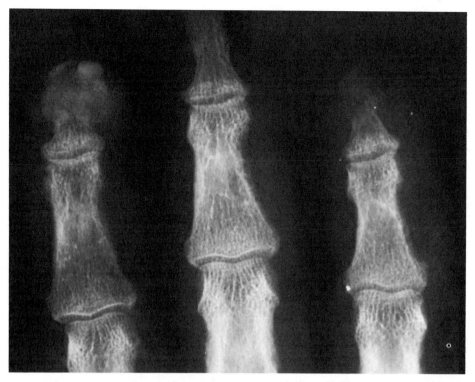

FIG. 7. Radiograph of the left hand showing abundant subperiosteal erosions of the phalanges in a patient with severe secondary hyperparathyroidism. The abnormalities are more pronounced on the radial surfaces.

pediatric patients are not pathognomonic of any particular histologic lesion, however, and bone biopsies are usually needed to determine the type of bone disease in pediatric patients with end-stage renal failure.

Amyloidosis

Cystic changes in bone, particularly if they are large, suggest the possibility of amyloidosis of bone. Cysts most commonly involve the metacarpals and regions immediately adjacent to large joints near the site of tendon insertions; the hip, wrist, proximal humerus, pubic ramus, and proximal tibia are most commonly affected, but the carpal and tarsal bones may also be involved (Fig. 8). X-rays may demonstrate fractures at the site of cyst formation (2). The finding of multiple bone cysts suggests the presence of amyloidosis, whereas brown tumors more often occur as isolated cysts, usually located in the ribs or jaw.

Bone Scan

The compounds used most frequently for skeletal scintigraphy are technetium-labeled bisphosphonates, mainly ^{99}Tc-methylene diphosphonate. Bone scans may be useful for evaluating the severity of skeletal disease in patients with advanced renal failure, and they can help in the assessment of responses to therapy. Bone scintigraphy may reveal pseudofractures or extraskeletal calcifications, and

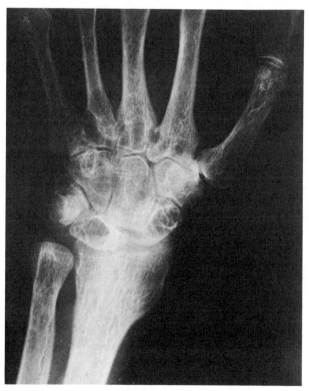

FIG. 8. Radiograph of the hand of a long-term hemodialysis patient showing cystic lesions due to B$_2$-microglobulin amyloidosis. (From Grateau, G., et al., *Am J Kidney Dis* 11:231, 1988. Reprinted with permission.)

local increases in the uptake of tracer can occur in areas of amyloid deposition. Patients with osteitis fibrosa often exhibit symmetrical increases in isotope activity in the skull, mandible, sternum, shoulders, vertebral bodies, and distal portions of the femur and tibia; these findings have been termed the "super scan." In contrast, the uptake of isotopic tracers into bone is less in patients with aluminum-related osteomalacia than in those with osteitis fibrosa (110). Despite these general trends, Hodson et al. noted that the findings on bone scan did not agree closely with those obtained by histologic assessment in patients with chronic renal failure (111); thus, it was impossible to predict the type of bone disease using this noninvasive radiographic technique. Although bone scans offer supportive information, they are currently not sufficient to be of diagnostic value in the assessment of renal bone disease.

TREATMENT OF RENAL OSTEODYSTROPHY

The successful management of patients with renal osteodystrophy must include interventions designed to correct or to counteract several major pathogenic factors. Important objectives of long-term clinical management include (A) the maintenance of normal serum calcium and phosphorus levels to prevent further hyperplasia of the parathyroid glands; (B) the prevention of extraskeletal calcifications; (C) the avoidance of exposure to toxic agents such as aluminum and excess iron; (D) the judicious use of vitamin D sterols; and (E) the appropriate administration of chelating agents such as deferoxamine to treat aluminum intoxication.

Dietary Adjustments

Adequate control of serum phosphorus levels is important for the prevention of soft tissue calcifications and for the management of secondary hyperparathyroidism in patients with advanced renal failure and in those receiving regular dialysis. Dietary phosphorus restriction may also reduce serum PTH levels in patients with moderate renal failure (14). The daily dietary intake of phosphorus ranges from 1.0–1.8 g in normal adults, but it must be lowered to 400–800 mg/day to prevent hyperphosphatemia in patients with chronic renal failure. Such diets are generally unpalatable, and long-term compliance is difficult to achieve (112). Consequently, the administration of phosphate-binding antacids is usually required to adequately control hyperphosphatemia when the glomerular filtration rate decreases to 25–30% of normal.

Phosphate-Binding Agents

Phosphate-binding antacids lower intestinal phosphate absorption by forming poorly soluble complexes of phosphorus within the intestinal lumen, thereby lowering phosphorus absorption. In the past, aluminum-containing, phosphate-binding gels were widely used to control

serum phosphorus levels in patients with advanced renal failure; this can result in aluminum loading and aluminum toxicity, however, due largely to reductions in the renal excretion of absorbed aluminum (101). Both the duration of treatment and the daily dose of aluminum ingested are important determinants of the degree of aluminum retention in tissues, but guidelines for the use of aluminum-containing medications in patients with renal failure have not been established (113–115). Generally, these compounds should be avoided to limit the potential for aluminum intoxication. If aluminum-containing agents are to be given, the duration of treatment should be limited, doses must be kept as low as possible, and the concurrent administration of citrate-containing compounds must be carefully avoided. Aluminum levels in plasma should also be monitored at regular intervals.

Calcium carbonate can reduce intestinal phosphorus absorption, but its use in dialysis patients was associated with multiple episodes of hypercalcemia, diarrhea, and metabolic alkalosis when originally evaluated (116). Subsequent studies both in adult and in pediatric patients have demonstrated that calcium carbonate can adequately control serum phosphorus levels in those undergoing maintenance dialysis (Fig. 9), although hypercalcemia remains a major side effect (117,118). The regular use of dialysate containing 2.5 mEq/L rather than 3.5 mEq/L of calcium can reduce the frequency of episodes of hypercalcemia in dialyzed patients ingesting calcium carbonate (119,120).

When used as a phosphate-binding agent, calcium carbonate should be ingested with meals to increase the efficiency of phosphate binding and to minimize intestinal calcium absorption. Doses in individual patients range from 4–14 g/day. Some patients require combined therapy with aluminum hydroxide and calcium carbonate to achieve adequate control of serum phosphorus levels. Indeed, Fournier et al. noted that only 50% of adult patients undergoing long-term dialysis attained adequate control of serum phosphorus levels when calcium carbonate was given as the sole phosphate-binding agent (121). The long-term side effects of calcium carbonate therapy are un-

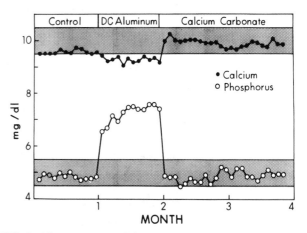

FIG. 9. Mean serum calcium and phosphorus levels in 20 adult dialyzed patients during the three phases of the 4-mo study. (From Slatopolsky, E., et al., *N Engl J Med* 315: 157, 1986. Reprinted with permission.)

known, but no increase in vascular calcifications was found in adult patients treated for as long as 3 yr (122).

Calcium acetate has recently been used as a phosphate-binding agent in patients with chronic renal failure (123,124). *In vitro* studies and short-term *in vivo* evaluations indicate that this compound is a more potent phosphate-binding agent than either calcium carbonate or aluminum hydroxide. Only limited data are yet available using calcium acetate in patients undergoing long-term dialysis; in one recent report, the frequency of hypercalcemic episodes did not differ in patients given calcium acetate compared with those receiving calcium carbonate (125).

Other phosphate-binding agents have been used in limited numbers of patients with chronic renal failure with variable results. Calcium citrate is a useful phosphate-binding agent, but the effect of citrate to enhance intestinal aluminum absorption is a major concern in patients who may be given other medications that contain aluminum (50,126). Generally, the use of calcium citrate should be avoided in patients with chronic renal failure. Magnesium oxide was reported to be ineffective or poorly tolerated in two studies (127), whereas magnesium carbonate was effective when utilized in conjunction with magnesium-free dialysate in patients undergoing regular hemodialysis (128).

Vitamin D Sterols

Despite dietary phosphate restriction, maintenance of an adequate dietary calcium intake, the use of appropriate levels of calcium in dialysate, and the regular use of phosphate-binding agents, a substantial proportion of patients receiving regular dialysis develop secondary hyperparathyroidism. Consequently, the administration of active vitamin D sterols such as 1,25 dihydroxyvitamin D_3, 1α-hydroxyvitamin D, dihydrotachysterol, or even large doses of vitamin D_3 or D_2 is required in many patients with advanced renal failure.

Calcifediol, or $25(OH)D_3$, can be effective for the control of secondary hyperparathyroidism both in adults and in children treated with maintenance dialysis (129,130). In a multicenter study of patients undergoing regular dialysis, musculoskeletal symptoms improved, serum alkaline phosphatase levels decreased, and the histologic severity of osteitis fibrosa diminished following treatment with calcifediol. Hypercalcemia may develop, however, when serum 25-hydroxyvitamin D_3 levels exceed the normal range.

Several clinical trials have documented the efficacy of calcitriol for the treatment of patients with symptomatic renal osteodystrophy (131,132). Bone pain often diminishes, muscle strength and gait-posture frequently improve, and the histologic features of osteitis fibrosa commonly undergo partial or complete resolution (133); when measured using reliable assays, serum PTH levels also decrease in patients who respond favorably to treatment. Increases in growth velocity have been reported in some uremic children (65). Findings similar to these have been reported in patients treated with oral 1α-hydroxyvitamin

D, which undergoes 25-hydroxylation in the liver to form calcitriol (134,135). Overall, calcitriol and 1α-hydroxyvitamin D appear to be similarly effective in the treatment of secondary hyperparathyroidism in patients with advanced renal failure.

Doses of oral calcitriol in most clinical trials have ranged from 0.25–1.5 µg/day; hypercalcemia is the most common side effect, but most patients tolerate daily doses of 0.25–0.50 µg without marked increases in serum calcium levels. The appearance of hypercalcemia during treatment with calcitriol may help to predict the underlying type of renal bone disease. When hypercalcemia occurs after many weeks or months of calcitriol therapy and previously elevated serum alkaline phosphatase levels have returned to normal, it is likely that the skeletal changes of osteitis fibrosa have substantially resolved. In contrast, the development of hypercalcemia within the first several weeks of treatment is commonly seen in patients with aluminum-related bone disease or in those with severe secondary hyperparathyroidism and marked parathyroid gland hyperplasia (133). If there is evidence of autonomous hyperparathyroidism, parathyroidectomy may be required. Ideally, the dose of oral calcitriol should be adjusted to maintain serum calcium levels between 10.5 mg/dl and 11.0 mg/dl, an approach that leads to effective PTH suppression in most patients undergoing regular dialysis (106). The shorter biological half-life of calcitriol compared with calcifediol facilitates the management of hypercalcemia if it develops, and serum calcium levels usually decrease within several days after withdrawal of treatment.

There has been considerable recent interest in the use of parenteral calcitriol for the management of secondary hyperparathyroidism in patients undergoing regular dialysis. Slatopolsky et al. demonstrated that the intravenous administration of calcitriol three times weekly markedly lowered serum PTH levels in adult hemodialysis patients (21). A portion of this response appears to be independent of changes in serum ionized calcium, findings that suggest that calcitriol may have direct *in vivo* effects to reduce PTH synthesis and/or release. Delmez et al. found that intraperitoneal calcitriol administration could also lower serum PTH levels in patients undergoing continuous ambulatory peritoneal dialysis (136).

Considerably higher serum calcitriol levels can be achieved after intravenous doses of the sterol, and a larger cumulative weekly dose can be administered when calcitriol is given two or three times per week rather than every day (137). These factors may increase the delivery of calcitriol to the parathyroid glands and enhance its suppressive effect on PTH secretion. Intermittent, or pulse, therapy with oral rather than intravenous calcitriol has also been used in patients with established secondary hyperparathyroidism (138,139). Indeed, Fukagawa et al. reported that the size of the parathyroid glands, measured by ultrasound, decreased in dialyzed patients during intermittent oral calcitriol therapy (138). Thus, the use of an intermittent, rather than a daily, schedule of calcitriol administration may improve its therapeutic efficacy in patients with established secondary hyperparathyroidism.

Parathyroidectomy

The development of certain clinical findings in patients with advanced secondary hyperparathyroidism indicates the need for parathyroid surgery. In all instances, aluminum-related bone disease must be excluded prior to parathyroidectomy, and the diagnosis of severe secondary hyperparathyroidism must be documented by biochemical, radiographic, and bone histologic criteria (3). Specific indications for parathyroidectomy include (A) persistent hypercalcemia with serum calcium levels above 11.5–12.0 mg/dl; (B) intractable pruritus that does not respond to intensive dialysis or to other medical treatments; (C) progressive extraskeletal calcifications and/or persistent hyperphosphatemia despite continued and appropriate use of dietary phosphorus restriction and phosphate-binding agents; (D) severe skeletal pain or skeletal fractures; and (E) the development of calciphylaxis (140). Other causes of hypercalcemia, such as sarcoidosis, malignancy, and excessive calcium or vitamin D intake, must also be considered and excluded. Because the risk of aluminum toxicity may increase following parathyroidectomy, aluminum hydroxide should be avoided after parathyroid surgery, and calcium carbonate should be used as the sole phosphate-binding agent.

Management of Aluminum Intoxication

After initial reports about the use of deferoxamine for the treatment of aluminum toxicity, others documented significant improvements in the clinical manifestations and histologic features of aluminum-related bone disease during deferoxamine therapy in patients undergoing regular dialysis (103,105). After intravenous doses of deferoxamine, aluminum removal during both hemodialysis and peritoneal dialysis is substantially greater than that achieved with dialysis alone (141,142). Subcutaneous deferoxamine administration also enhances aluminum removal during dialysis procedures.

After 4 to 10 mo of treatment with deferoxamine, clinical improvement has been observed in a large proportion of patients with severe bone disease (103,143). Analgesic use decreased, and patients who had been confined to bed or wheelchair were able to resume walking without assistance. Typical biochemical changes after deferoxamine treatment include reductions in serum calcium levels and increases in serum alkaline phosphatase levels, findings consistent with an improvement in the mineralization of bone. Modest increments in serum PTH levels occur in most patients, but it is not known whether this change is due to aluminum removal from the parathyroid glands or to decreases in serum calcium levels. Repeat bone biopsies generally show increases in bone formation and improved mineralization; indeed, some patients with low-turnover lesions of bone may develop osteitis fibrosa (103). The amount of surface-stainable aluminum in bone decreases in most patients who improve with treatment, but the response to deferoxamine may be less marked in patients who have undergone a previous parathyroidectomy (103). Thus, restoration of parathyroid function may

be important for skeletal recovery in patients with aluminum intoxication.

Unfortunately, serious and often lethal infections with Rhizopus and Yersinia species have been documented in a number of dialysis patients receiving deferoxamine (144–148). In one series, 6 of 131 patients given deferoxamine over a 3-yr period were affected (144). These observations raise serious questions about the appropriate use of deferoxamine for the treatment of aluminum intoxication in patients undergoing regular dialysis. Deferoxamine should be given only to patients with symptomatic aluminum intoxication, and evidence of tissue toxicity should be documented before therapy is begun. Doses of deferoxamine should not exceed 0.5–1.0 g/week, and plasma aluminum levels should be measured regularly. In asymptomatic patients with aluminum accumulation in bone, improvements in bone histology and bone formation have been demonstrated without the use of deferoxamine after the complete withdrawal of aluminum-containing medications and utilization of calcium carbonate as the sole phosphate-binding agent (149).

BONE AND MINERAL METABOLISM IN RENAL TRANSPLANT RECIPIENTS

Although the restoration of kidney function after successful renal transplantation corrects many of the disturbances that lead to renal osteodystrophy, disorders of bone and mineral metabolism remain a major clinical problem in renal transplant recipients. Indeed, as many as 80–90% of patients have histologic evidence of bone disease 5 yr after transplantation (150,151). In these patients, alterations in bone and mineral homeostasis can be a manifestation of preexisting renal osteodystrophy or the result of changes peculiar to the posttransplant setting.

Hypercalcemia is not uncommon after renal transplantation; its frequency corresponds to the duration of previous dialysis treatment and, probably, to the degree of parathyroid gland hyperplasia at the time of transplantation (152). Several other factors also contribute. The presence of a functioning renal allograft rapidly corrects the deficit in renal 1,25-dihydroxyvitamin D production that is characteristic of chronic renal failure, and calcitriol synthesis is further enhanced by the resolution of hyperphosphatemia. Since the reversal of parathyroid gland hyperplasia may take many months or years, most patients exhibit persistently high serum PTH levels in the immediate posttransplant period, and this change also promotes renal calcitriol production. Overall, these factors lead to increased intestinal calcium absorption, enhanced calcium mobilization from bone, and increased renal tubular calcium reabsorption, each of which can contribute to the development of hypercalcemia.

Hypercalcemia during the first several months after renal transplantation can be quite severs, and serum calcium levels may reach 15 mg/dl. Hypercalcemia can lead to allograft dysfunction, and peripheral ischemia may develop on rare occasion owing to extensive vascular calcification—i.e., calciphylaxis (69). Those with advanced secondary hyperparathyroidism prior to transplantation are at greatest risk. More often, the degree of hypercalcemia after renal transplantation is less severe. Serum calcium levels usually range from 10.5–12.0 mg/dl in such cases, and episodes of hypercalcemia are intermittent and of short duration; the disorder usually resolves within 12 mo (153). In 4–10% of patients, mild to moderate hypercalcemia can persist for more than 1 yr and as long as 5 yr. Serum calcium levels between 10.5 mg/dl and 12.0 mg/dl are usually well tolerated without adverse effects on renal allograft function (154), but elective parathyroidectomy should be considered when serum calcium levels persistently exceed 12.5 mg/dl more than 1 yr after renal transplantation (155).

Hypophosphatemia is common in the early postoperative period after renal transplantation. Persistent secondary hyperparathyroidism is the major contributor, leading to reduced renal tubular phosphate reabsorption and increased renal phosphate excretion. Primary defects in the tubular reabsorption of phosphorus occasionally occur, however, and some patients may excrete large amounts of phosphorus in the urine despite normal levels of PTH in serum (156–158). Pharmacologic doses of glucocorticoids also increase renal phosphorus excretion, and this may further aggravate renal phosphate wasting (159).

The clinical manifestations of hypophosphatemia are quite variable; some patients complain of malaise, fatigue, and proximal muscle weakness (160). Although hypophosphatemia can persist for many months, osteomalacia rarely develops (161). Symptomatic patients with serum phosphorus levels below 1.0 mg/dl should be given oral phosphorus supplements, and the serum phosphorus level should be monitored regularly. In those who require supplemental phosphorus, potassium rather than sodium salts should be used to avoid extracellular volume expansion, which increases renal phosphate excretion by lowering phosphate reabsorption in the proximal nephron (162).

Osteopenia is common following renal transplantation, and evidence of reduced bone mass is found in nearly all patients within 5 yr (150,151,163). Substantial decreases in bone mass have been documented within the first 6–18 mo after renal transplantation; these changes are associated with histologic evidence of diminished bone formation and turnover, findings consistent with the known effects of glucocorticoids on bone (164). The development of osteopenia is not confined, however, to renal transplant recipients, and reductions in bone mass have been demonstrated in patients undergoing cardiac and hepatic transplantation (165).

The use of large, immunosuppressive doses of corticosteroids is generally considered to be a major contributor to the development of osteopenia in transplant recipients. Glucocorticoids directly inhibit osteoblastic activity and collagen synthesis (166,167), and they impede the differentiation of progenitor cells into fully mature osteoblasts (168). Glucocorticoids also accelerate bone resorption by lowering intestinal calcium absorption, thereby inducing a mild state of secondary hyperparathyroidism (169).

The effects of cyclosporine on human bone have not been well characterized. Movsowitz et al. demonstrated increases in bone remodeling with reductions in cancellous bone volume, but there was no change in the serum levels of calcium, magnesium, $1,25(OH)_2D_3$, or PTH in rats given cyclosporine (170). Stewart and coworkers reported that cyclosporine inhibited in vitro bone resorption in a dose-dependent manner during incubations with PTH, $1,25(OH)_2D_3$, and interleukin-1 (171). Although preliminary data in humans suggest that cyclosporine may decrease the incidence of osteonecrosis in renal transplant recipients by lowering the dose of prednisone required for adequate immunosuppression (172), the effects of this immunosuppressive agent on bone and mineral metabolism require further investigation.

Measures that are effective for the prevention of bone loss in transplant recipients have yet to be identified, but few studies have been done. Newer synthetic derivatives of prednisolone, such as deflazacort, are effective immunosuppressive agents, and they appear to have fewer adverse effects on bone and mineral metabolism (173,174). Such agents may be of benefit for the management of transplant recipients in the future, but they await fuller clinical evaluation.

Osteonecrosis, or avascular necrosis, is by far the most debilitating skeletal complication associated with transplantation surgery. Approximately 15% of patients will develop osteonecrosis within 3 yr of renal transplantation (175,176). The occurrence of osteonecrosis in patients undergoing cardiac, hepatic, and bone marrow transplantation as well as in those with systemic lupus erythematosus given high doses of corticosteroids strongly suggests that glucocorticoids play a critical pathogenic role (177,178).

The mechanism by which corticosteroids contribute to the development of osteonecrosis has not been established. These agents may promote the accumulation of fat cells within the marrow space, thereby increasing intraosseous hydrostatic pressure and altering blood flow within bone (179). Alternatively, corticosteroids may interfere with the process of microfracture repair, leading to a loss of the structural integrity of bone.

Osteonecrosis usually begins in weight-bearing areas; the femoral head and femoral neck are the sites most commonly affected in adults, but the distal femur, proximal tibia, and humeral head can also be affected (180). Osteonecrosis can occur at several sites in an individual patient. Thus, Ibels et al. found two sites of involvement in 85% of renal transplant recipients, whereas three or more areas were affected in 27% of patients (181). Risk factors for osteonecrosis include the cumulative dose of corticosteroids, advanced age, and the duration of dialysis prior to transplantation.

ACKNOWLEDGMENTS

Support was provided in part by USPHS grants DK-35423 and RR00865.

REFERENCES

1. Goodman WG: Aluminum metabolism and the uremic patient. In: Simpson DJ (ed), *Nutrition and Bone Development*, Oxford University Press, New York, 269–294 1990
2. Kleinman KS, Coburn JW: Amyloid syndrome associated with hemodialysis. *Kidney Int* 35:567–575, 1989
3. Coburn JW, Slatopolsky E: Vitamin D, parathyroid hormone,

and renal osteodystrophy. In: Brenner B, Rector F (eds), *The Kidney.* WB Saunders, Philadelphia, 1657–1729 1986

4. Holick MF: Vitamin D and the kidney. *Kidney Int* 32:912–929, 1987

5. Morrissey J, Rothstein M, Mayor G: Suppression of parathyroid hormone secretion by aluminum. *Kidney Int* 23:699–704, 1983

6. Sedman AB, Alfrey AC, Miller NL, Goodman WG: Tissue and cellular basis for impaired bone formation in aluminum-related osteomalacia in the pig. *J Clin Invest* 79:86–92, 1987

7. Blumenthal NC, Posner AS: In vitro model of aluminum-induced osteomalacia: inhibition of hydroxyapatite formation and growth. *Calcif Tissue Int* 36:439–441, 1984

8. Sherrard DJ, Ott SM, Maloney NA, Andress DL, Coburn JW: Uremic osteodystrophy: classification, cause and treatment. In: Frame B, Potts J (eds), *Clinical Disorders of Bone and Mineral Metabolism.* Excerpta Medica, Amsterdam, 254–259 1984

9. Salusky IB, Coburn JW, Brill J, et al.: Bone disease in pediatric patients undergoing dialysis with CAPD or CCPD. *Kidney Int* 33:975–982, 1988

10. Goodman WG, Leite Duarte ME: Aluminum: effects on bone and role in the pathogenesis of renal osteodystrophy. *Miner Electrolyte Metab* 17:221–232, 1991

11. Delmez JA, Slatopolsky E: Hyperphosphatemia: its consequences and treatment in patients with chronic renal disease. *Am J Kidney Dis* 19:303–317, 1992

12. Slatopolsky E, Caglar S, Pennell JP, et al.: On the pathogenesis of hyperparathyroidism in chronic experimental renal insufficiency in the dog. *J Clin Invest* 50:492–499, 1971

13. Llach F, Massry SG: On the mechanism of secondary hyperparathyroidism in moderate renal insufficiency. *J Clin Endocrinol Metab* 61:601–606, 1985

14. Portale AA, Booth BE, Halloran BP, Morris RD Jr: Effect of dietary phosphorus on circulating concentrations of 1,25-dihydroxyvitamin D and immunoreactive parathyroid hormone in children with moderate renal insufficiency. *J Clin Invest* 73:1580–1589, 1984

15. Reiss E, Canterbury JM, Bercovitz MA, Kaplan EL: The role of phosphate in the secretion of parathyroid hormone in man. *J Clin Invest* 49:2146–2149, 1970

16. Kumar R: Metabolism of 1,25-dihydroxyvitamin D3. *Physiol Rev* 64:478–504, 1984

17. Lopez-Hilker S, Galceran T, Chan Y-L, Rapp N, Martin KJ, Slatopolsky E: Hypocalcemia may not be essential for the development of secondary hyperparathyroidism in chronic renal failure. *J Clin Invest* 78:1097–1102, 1986

18. Lopez-Hilker S, Rapp N, Martin K, et al.: On the mechanism of the prevention of secondary hyperparathyroidism by phosphate retention (abstract). *Kidney Int* 29:164, 1986

19. Brown EM, Wilson RE, Eastmen RC, Pallotta J, Marynick S: Abnormal regulation of parathyroid hormone release by calcium in secondary hyperparathyroidism due to chronic renal failure, *J Clin Endocrinol Metab* 54:172–179, 1982

20. Silver J, Naveh-Many T, Mayer H, Schmelzer HJ, Popovtzer MM: Regulation by vitamin D metabolites of parathyroid hormone gene transcription in vivo in the rat. *J Clin Invest* 78:1296–1301, 1986

21. Slatopolsky E, Weerts C, Thielan J, Horst RL, Harter H, Martin KJ: Marked suppression of secondary hyperparathyroidism by intravenous administration of 1,25-dihydroxycholecalciferol in uremic patients. *J Clin Invest* 74:2136–2143, 1984

22. Korkor AB: Reduced binding of 3H-1,25-dihydroxyvitamin D in the parathyroid glands of patients with renal failure. *N Engl J Med* 316:1573–1577, 1987

23. Strom M, Sandgren ME, Brown TA, DeLuca HF: 1,25-Dihydroxyvitamin D3 up-regulates the 1.25-dihydroxyvitamin D3 receptor *in vivo. Proc Natl Acad Sci USA* 86:9770–9773, 1989

24. Merke J, Hugell U, Zlotkoswki A, et al.: Diminished parathyroid 1,25(OH)2D3 receptors in experimental uremia. *Kidney Int* 32:350–353, 1987

25. Szabo A, Merke J, Beier E, et al.: 1,25(OH)2 vitamin D3 inhibits parathyroid cell proliferation in experimental uremia. *Kidney Int* 35:1049–1056, 1989

26. Bellorin-Font E, Martin KJ, Freitag JJ, et al.: Altered adenylate cyclase kinetics in hyperfunctioning human parathyroid glands. *J Clin Endocrinol Metab* 52:499–507, 1981

27. Massry SG, Coburn JW, Lee DBN, Jowsey J, Kleeman CR: Skeletal resistance to parathyroid hormone in renal failure. *Ann Intern Med* 78:357–364, 1973

28. Massry SG, Tuma S, Dua S, Goldstein DA: Reversal of skeletal resistance to parathyroid hormone in uremia by vitamin D metabolites. *J Lab Clin Med* 94:152–157, 1979

29. Julian B, Quarles D, Niemann K: Musculoskeletal complications after renal transplantation: pathogenesis and treatment. *Am J Kidney Dis* 19:99, 1992

30. Pei Y, Hercz G, Greenwood C,et al.: Non-invasive prediction of aluminum bone disease in hemo- and peritoneal dialysis patients. *Kidney Int* 41:1374–1382, 1992

31. Eastwood JB, Harris E, Stamp TCB, de Wardener HE: Vitamin D deficiency in the osteomalacia of chronic renal failure. *Lancet* 2:1209–1211, 1976

32. Pierides AM, Ellis HA, Ward M, et al.: Barbiturate and anticonvulsant treatment in relation to osteomalacia with haemodialysis and renal transplantation. *Br Med J* 1:190, 1976

33. Llach F, Felsenfeld AJ, Coleman MD, Pederson JA: Prevalence of various types of bone disease in dialysis patients. In: Robinson RR (ed), *Nephrology, Proceedings of the Ninth International Congress of Nephrology.* Springer-Verlag, New York, 2:1375–1382, 1984

34. Platts MM, Goods GC, Hislop JS: Composition of the domestic water supply and the incidence of fractures and encephalopathy in patients on home dialysis. *Br Med J* 2:657–660, 1977

35. Pierides AM, Edwards WG Jr, Cullu US Jr, McCall JT, Ellis HA: Hemodialysis encephalopathy with osteomalacic fractures and muscle weakness. *Kidney Int* 18:115–124, 1980

36. Andreoli SP, Bergstein JM, Sherrard DJ: Aluminum intoxication from aluminum-containing phosphate binders in children with azotemia not undergoing dialysis. *N Engl J Med* 310:1079–1084, 1984

37. Felsenfeld AJ, Gutman RA, Llach F, Harrelson JM: Osteomalacia in chronic renal failure: a syndrome previously reported only with maintenance dialysis. *Am J Nephrol* 2:147–154, 1982

38. Salusky IB, Coburn JW, Paunier L, Sherrard DJ, Fine RN: Role of aluminum hydroxide in raising serum aluminum levels in children undergoing continuous ambulatory peritoneal dialysis. *J Pediatr* 105:717–720, 1984

39. Maloney NA, Ott SM, Alfrey AC, Miller NL, Coburn JW, Sherrard DJ: Histological quantitation of aluminum in iliac bone from patients with renal failure. *J Lab Clin Med* 99:206–216, 1982

40. Goodman WG, Henry DA, Horst R, Nudelman RK, Alfrey AC, Coburn JW: Parenteral aluminum administration in the dog. II. Induction of osteomalacia and effect on vitamin D metabolism. *Kidney Int* 25:370–375, 1984

41. Robertson JA, Felsenfeld AJ, Haygood CC, Wilson P, Clarke C, Llach F: Animal model of aluminum-induced osteomalacia: role of chronic renal failure. *Kidney Int* 23:327–335, 1983

42. Ellis HA, McCarthy JH, Herrington J: Bone aluminum in haemodialysed patients and in rats injected with aluminum chloride: relationship to impaired bone mineralisation. *J Clin Pathol* 32:832–844, 1979

43. Meyer JL, Thomas WC Jr: Aluminum and aluminum complex. Effect of calcium phosphate precipitation. *Kidney Int* 29 (suppl 18):S20–S23, 1986

44. Goodman WG, Gilligan J, Horst R: Short-term aluminum administration in the rat: effects on bone formation and relationship to renal osteomalacia. *J Clin Invest* 73:171–181, 1984

45. Lieberherr M, Grosse B, Cournot-Witmer G, Hermann-Erlee MP, Balsan S: Aluminum action on mouse bone cell metabolism and response to PTH and 1,25(OH)2D3, *Kidney Int* 31:736–743, 1987

46. Kasai K, Hori MT, Goodman WG: Transferrin enhances the anti-proliferative actions of aluminum in osteoblast-like cells. *Am J Physiol* 260:E537–E543, 1991

47. Andress DL, Kopp JB, Maloney NA, Coburn JW, Sherrard DJ: Early deposition of aluminum in bone in diabetic patients on hemodialysis. *N Engl J Med* 316:292–296, 1987

48. Norris KC, Crooks PW, Nebeker HG, et al.: Clinical and laboratory features of aluminum-related bone disease: differences between sporadic and "epidemic" forms of the syndrome. *Am J Kidney Dis* 6:342–347, 1985

49. de Vernejoul MC, Marchais S, London G, Morieux C, Bielakoff J, Miravet L: Increased bone aluminum deposition after subtotal parathyroidectomy in dialyzed patients. *Kidney Int* 27:785–791, 1985

50. Molitoris BA, Froment DH, Mackenzie TA, Huffer WH, Alfrey AC: Citrate: a major factor in the toxicity of orally administered aluminum compounds. *Kidney Int* 36:949–953, 1989

51. Froment DPH, Molitoris BA, Buddington B, Miller A, Alfrey AC: Site and mechanism of enhanced gastrointestinal absorption of aluminum by citrate. *Kidney Int* 36:978–984, 1989

52. Felsenfeld AJ, Harrelson JM, Gutman RA, Wells SA, Drezner MK: Osteomalacia after parathyroidectomy in patients with uremia. *Ann Intern Med* 960:34–39, 1982

53. Parfitt AM: The physiologic and clinical significance of bone histomorphometric data. In: Recker RR (ed), *Bone Histomorphometry: Techniques and Interpretation*. CRC Press, Boca Raton, 143–223, 1983

54. Norris KC, Goodman WG, Howard N, Nugent ME, Coburn JW: The iliac crest bone biopsy for the diagnosis of aluminum toxicity and a guide to the use of deferoxamine. *Semin Nephrol* 6 (suppl 1):27–34, 1986

55. Hodsman AB, Sherrard DJ, Alfrey AC, et al.: Bone aluminum and histomorphometric features of renal osteodystrophy. *J Clin Endocrinol Metab* 54:539–546, 1982

56. Andress DL, Maloney NA, Endres DB, Sherrard DJ: Aluminum-associated bone disease in chronic renal failure: high prevalence in a long-term dialysis population. *J Bone Miner Res* 1:391–398, 1986

57. Goodman WG: Short-term aluminum administration in the rat: reductions in bone formation without osteomalacia. *J Lab Clin Med* 103:749–757, 1984

58. Parisien M, Charhon SA, Arlot M, et al.: Evidence for a toxic effect of aluminum on osteoblasts: a histomorphometric study in hemodialysis patients with aplastic bone disease. *J Bone Miner Res* 3:259–267, 1988

59. Sherrard DJ, Baylink DJ, Wergedal JE, Maloney NA: Quantitative histological studies on the pathogenesis of uremic bone disease. *J Clin Endocrinol Metab* 39:119–135, 1974

60. Sherrard DJ: Renal osteodystrophy. *Semin Nephrol* 6:56–67, 1986

61. Llach F, Felsenfeld AJ, Coleman MD, Keveney JJ Jr, Pederson JA, Medlock TR: The natural course of dialysis osteomalacia. *Kidney Int* 29:S74–S79, 1986

62. Mehls O: Renal osteodystrophy in children: etiology and clinical aspects. In: Fine RN, Gruskin AB (eds), *Endstage Renal Disease in Children*. WB Saunders, Philadelphia, 227–250, 1984

63. Salusky IB, Brill J, Oppenheim W, Goodman WG: Features of renal osteodystrophy in pediatric patients receiving regular peritoneal dialysis. *Semin Nephrol* 9:37–42, 1989

64. Stickler GB, Bergen BJ: A review: short stature in renal disease. *Pediatr Res* 7:978–982, 1973

65. Chesney RW, Moorthy AV, Eisman JA, Tax DK, Mazess RB, De Luca HF: Increased growth after long-term oral 1,25-vitamin D3 in childhood renal osteodystrophy. *N Engl J Med* 298:238–242, 1978

66. Chantler C, Donckerwolcke RA, Brunner FP, et al.: Combined report on regular dialysis and transplantation of children in Europe. *Proc EDTA* 16:74–104, 1979

67. Meema HE, Oreopoulos DG, Rapoport A: Serum magnesium and arterial calcification in end-stage renal disease. *Kidney Int* 32:388–394, 1987

68. Ibels LS, Alfrey AC, Huffer WE, Craswell PW, Anderson JT, Well R III: Arterial calcification and pathology in uremic patients undergoing dialysis. *Am J Med* 66:790–796, 1979

69. Gipstein RM, Coburn JW, Adams JA, et al.: Calciphylaxis in man: a syndrome of tissue necrosis and vascular calcification in 11 patients with chronic renal failure. *Arch Intern Med* 136:1273–1280, 1976

70. Alfrey AC, Solomons CC, Ciricillo J, Miller NL: Extraosseous calcification. Evidence for abnormal pyrophosphate metabolism in uremia. *J Clin Invest* 57:692–699, 1976

71. DiRaimondo CR, Casey TT, DiRaimondo CV, Stone WJ: Pathologic fractures associated with idiopathic amyloidosis of bone in chronic hemodialysis patients. *Nephron* 43:22–27, 1986

72. Fenves AZ, Emmett M, White MG, Greenway G, Michaels DB: Carpal tunnel syndrome with cystic bone lesions secondary to amyloidosis in chronic hemodialysis patients. *Am J Kidney Dis* 7:130–134, 1986

73. Bardin T, Kuntz D, Zingraff J, Voisin MC, Zelmer A, Lansaman J: Synovial amyloidosis in patients undergoing long-term hemodialysis. *Arthritis Rheum* 28:1052–1058, 1985

74. Munoz-Gomez J, Bergada-Barado E, Gomez-Perez R, et al.: Amyloid arthropathy in patients undergoing periodical haemodilaysis for chronic renal failure: a new complication. *Ann Rheum Dis* 44:729–733, 1985

75. Kachel HG, Altmeyer P, Baldamus CA, Koch KM: Deposition of an amyloid-like substance as a possible complication of regular dialysis treatment. *Contrib Nephrol* 36:127–132, 1983

76. Gorevic PD, Munoz PC, Casey TT, et al.: Polymerization of intact beta 2-microglobulin tissue causes amyloidosis in patients on chronic hemodialysis. *Proc Natl Acad Sci USA* 83:7908–7912, 1986

77. Zingraff J, Drueke T: Can the nephrologist prevent dialysis-related amyloidosis? *Am J Kidney Dis* 18:1–11, 1991

78. Koch KM: Dialysis-related amyloidosis. *Kidney Int* 41:1416–1429, 1992

79. van Ypersele de Strihou C, Jadoul M, Malghem J, Maldague B, Jamart J: The working party on dialysis amyloidosis: effect of dialysis membrane and patient's age on signs of dialysis-related amyloidosis. *Kidney Int* 39:1012–1019, 1991

80. Ohashi K, Hara M, Kawai R, et al.: Cervical discs are most susceptible to beta-2 microglobulin amyloid deposition in the vertebral column. *Kidney Int* 41:1646–1654, 1992

81. Buccianti G, Bianchi ML, Valenti G: Progress of renal osteodystrophy during continuous ambulatory peritoneal dialysis. *Clin Nephrol* 22:279–283, 1984

82. Stewart WK, Fleming LW: The effects of dialysate magnesium on plasma and erythocyte magnesium and postassium concentrations during maintenance haemodialysis. *Nephron* 10:221–231, 1973

83. Guillot AP, Hood VL, Runge CF, Gennari FJ: The use of magnesium-containing phosphate binders in patients with end-stage renal disease on maintenance hemodialysis. *Nephron* 30:114–117, 1982

84. Hruska KA, Teitelbaum SL, Kopelman R, et al.: The predictability of the histological features of uremic bone disease by non-invasive techniques. *Metab Bone Dis Rel Res* 1:39–44, 1978

85. Coburn JW, Norris KC: Diagnosis of aluminum-related bone disease and treatment of aluminum toxicity with deferoxamine. *Semin Nephrol* 6 (suppl 1): 12–21, 1986

86. Charhon SA, Delmas PD, Malaval L, et al.: Serum bone Gla-protein in renal osteodystrophy: comparison with bone histomorphometry. *J Clin Endocrinol Metab* 63:892–897, 1986

87. Epstein S, Traberg H, Raja R, et al.: Serum and dialysate osteocalcin levels in hemodialysis and peritoneal dialysis patients and after renal transplantation. *J Clin Endocrinol Metab* 60:1253–1256, 1985

88. Wilson L, Felsenfeld A, Drezner MK, Llach F: Altered divalent ion metabolism in early renal failure: role of 1,25(OH)2D. *Kidney Int* 27:565–573, 1985

89. Reichel H, Deibart B, Schmidt-Gayk H, Ritz E: Calcium metabolism in early chronic renal failure: implications for the pathogenesis of hyperparathyroidism. *Nephrol Dial Transplant* 6:162–169, 1991

90. Freitag J, Martin KJ, Hruska KA, et al.: Impaired parathyroid hormone metabolism in patients with chronic renal failure. *N Eng J Med* 298:29–32, 1978

91. Segre GV: Amino-terminal radioimmunoassays for parathyroid hormone. In: Frame B, Potts JT Jr (eds), *Clinical Disorders of Bone and Mineral Metabolism*. Excerpta Medica, Amsterdam, 14–17, 1983

92. Nussbaum SR, Zahradnik RJ, Lavigne JR, et al.: Highly sensitive two-site immunoradiometric assay of parathyrin, and its

clinical utility in evaluating patients with hypercalcemia. *Clin Chem* 33:1364, 1987

93. Andress DL, Endres DB, Ott SM, Sherrard DJ: Parathyroid hormone in aluminum bone disease: a comparison of parathyroid hormone assays. *Kidney Int* 29 (suppl 18):S87–S90, 1986

94. Cohen Solal ME, Sebert JL, Boudailliez B, et al.: Comparison of intact, midregion, and carboxy terminal assays for parathyroid hormone for the diagnosis of bone disease in hemodialyzed patients. *J Clin Endocrinol Metab* 73:516–524, 1991

95. Quarles LD, Lobaugh B, Murphy G: Intact parathyroid hormone overestimates the presence and severity of parathyroid-mediated osseous abnormalities in uremia. *J Clin Endocrinol Metab* 75:145–150, 1992

96. Mathias RS, Harmon WH, Emans J, Segre GV, Salusky IB, Goodman WG: Immuno-radiometric assay for PTH: correlation with bone histology in children undergoing hemodialysis (abstract). *J Am Soc Nephrol* 1:1572, 1990

97. Coburn JW, Nebeker HG, Hercz G, et al.: Role of aluminum accumulation in the pathogenesis of renal osteodystrophy. In: Robinson RR (ed): *Nephrology, Vol. II*. Springer-Verlag, New York, 2:1380–1395, 1984

98. Milliner DS, Nebeker HG, Ott SM, et al.: Use of the deferoxamine infusion test in the diagnosis of aluminum-related osteodystrophy. *Ann Intern Med* 101:775–779, 1984

99. Hodsman AB, Hood SA, Brown P, Cordy PE: Do serum aluminum levels reflect underlying skeletal aluminum accumulation and bone histology before or after chelation by deferoxamine? *J Lab Clin Med* 106:674–681, 1985

100. Winney RJ, Cowie JF, Robson JS: What is the value of plasma/serum aluminum in patients with chronic renal failure? *Clin Nephrol* 24 (suppl 1):S2–S8, 1985

101. Alfrey AC: Aluminum metabolism. *Kidney Int* 29 (suppl 18):S8–S11, 1986

102. Alfrey AC, Hegg A, Craswell P: Metabolism and toxicity of aluminum in renal failure. *Am J Clin Nutr* 33:1509–1516, 1980

103. Ott SM, Andress DL, Nebeker HG, et al.: Changes in bone histology after treatment with desferrioxamine. *Kidney Int* 29 (suppl 18):S108–S113, 1986

104. Ackrill P, Ralston AJ, Day JP, Hodge KC: Successful removal of aluminum from a patient with dialysis encephalopathy. *Lancet* 2:692–693, 1980

105. Malluche HH, Smith AJ, Abreo K, Faugere MC: The use of deferoxamine in the management of aluminum accumulation in bone in patients with renal failure. *N Engl J Med* 311:140–144, 1984

106. Salusky IB, Fine RN, Kangarloo H, et al.: "High-dose" calcitriol for control of renal osteodystrophy in children on CAPD. *Kidney Int* 32:89–95, 1987

107. Shimada H, Nakamura M, Marumo F: Influence of aluminum on the effect of 1-alpha-(OH)D3 on renal osteodystrophy. *Nephron* 35:163–170, 1983

108. Meema HE, Schatz DL: Simple radiologic demonstration of cortical bone loss in thyrotoxicosis. *Radiology* 97:9–15, 1970

109. Andreoli SP, Smith JA, Bergstein JM: Aluminum bone disease in children: radiographic features from diagnosis to resolution. *Radiology* 156:663–667, 1985

110. Karsenty G, Vigneron N, Jorgetti V, et al.: Value of the 99-mTc-methylene diphosphonate bone scan in renal osteodystrophy. *Kidney Int* 29:1058–1065, 1986

111. Hodson EM, Howman-Gilles RB, Evans RB, et al.: The diagnosis of renal osteodystrophy: a comparison of technitium99 pyrophosphate bone scintigraphy with other techniques. *Clin Nephrol* 16:24–28, 1981

112. Barsotti G, Guiducci A, Ceardella G, Giovannetti S: Effects on renal function of a low-nitrogen diet supplemented with essential amino acids and ketoanalogues and of hemodialysis and free protein supply in patients with chronic renal failure. *Nephron* 27:113–117, 1981

113. Sedman AB, Miller NL, Warady BA, Lum GM, Alfrey AC: Aluminum loading in children with chronic renal failure. *Kidney Int* 26:201–201, 1984

114. Winney RJ, Cowie JF, Robson JS: The role of plasma aluminum in the detection and prevention of aluminum toxicity. *Kidney Int* 29 (suppl 18)S91–S95, 1986

115. Salusky IB, Foley J, Nelson P, Goodman WG: Aluminum accumulation during treatment with aluminum hydroxide and dialysis in children and young adults with chronic renal disease. *N Engl J Med* 324:527–531, 1991

116. Meyrier A, Marsac J, Richet G: The influence of a high calcium carbonate intake on bone disease in patients undergoing hemodialysis. *Kidney Int* 4:146–153, 1973

117. Salusky IB, Coburn JW, Foley J, Nelson P, Fine RN: Effects of oral calcium carbonate on control of serum phosphorus and changes in plasma aluminum levels after discontinuation of aluminum-containing gels in children receiving dialysis. *J Pediatr* 108:767–770, 1986

118. Slatopolsky E, Weerts C, Lopez-Hilker S, et al.: Calcium carbonate is an effective phosphate binder in patients with chronic renal failure undergoing dialysis. *N Engl J Med* 315:157–161, 1986

119. Mactier RA, Van Stone J, Cox A, Van Stone M, Twardowski Z: Calcium carbonate is an effective phosphate binder when dialysate calcium concentration is adjusted to control hypercalcemia *Clin Nephrol* 28:222–226, 1987

120. Slatopolsky E, Weerts C, Norwood K, et al.: Long-term effects of calcium carbonate and 2.5 mEq/liter calcium dialysate on mineral metabolism. *Kidney Int* 36:897–903, 1989

121. Fournier A, Moriniere PH, Sebert JL, et al.: Calcium carbonate, an aluminum-free agent for control of hyperphosphatemia, hypocalcemia and hyperparathyroidism in uremia. *Kidney Int* 29:S115–S119, 1986

122. Renaud H, Atik A, Herve M, et al.: Evaluation of vascular calcinosis risk factors in patients on chronic hemodialysis: lack of influence of calcium carbonate. *Nephron* 48:28–32, 1988

123. Schiller LR, Santa Ana CA, Sheikh MS, Emmett M, Fordtran JS, Effect of the time of administration of calcium acetate on phosphorus binding. *N Engl J Med* 320:1110–1113, 1989

124. Mai ML, Emmett M, Sheikh MS, Santa Ana CA, Schiller L, Fordtran JS: Calcium acetate, an effective phosphorus binder in patients with renal failure. *Kidney Int* 36:690–695, 1989

125. Schaefer K, Scheer J, Asmus G, Umlauf E, Hagemann J, von Herrath D: The treatment uraemic hyperphosphataemia with calcium acetate and calcium carbonate: a comparative study. *Nephrol Dial Transplant* 6:171–175, 1991

126. Bakir AA, Hryhorczuk DO, Berman E, Dunea G: Acute fatal hyperaluminemic encephalopathy in undialyzed and recently dialyzed uremic patients. *Trans Am Soc Artif Intern Organs* 32:171–176, 1986

127. Oe PL, Lips P, van der Muelen J et al.: Long-term use of magnesium hydroxide as a phosphate binder in patients on hemodialysis. *Clin Nephrol* 28:180–185, 1987

128. O'Donovan R, Baldwin D, Hammer M, et al.: Substitution of aluminum salts by magnesium salts in control of dialysis hyperphosphatemia. *Lancet* 1:880–882, 1986

129. Witmer G, Margolis A, Fontaine O, et al.: Effects of 25-hydroxycholecalciferol on bone lesions of children with terminal renal failure. *Kidney Int* 10:395–408, 1976

130. Recker R, Schoenfeld P, Letteri J, Slatopolsky E, Goldsmith R, Brickman AS: The efficacy of calcifediol in renal osteodystrophy. *Arch Intern Med* 138:857, 1978

131. Baker LR, Muir JW, Sharman VL, et al.: Controlled trial of calcitriol in hemodialysis patients. *Clin Nephrol* 26:185–191, 1986

132. Berl T, Berns AS, Huffer WE, et al.: 1,25-dihydroxycholecalciferol effects in chronic dialysis. A double-blind controlled study. *Ann Intern Med* 88:774–780, 1978

133. Ott SM, Maloney NA, Coburn JW, Alfrey AC, Sherrard DJ: The prevalence of bone aluminum deposition in renal osteodystrophy and its relation to the response to calcitriol therapy. *N Engl J Med* 307:709–713, 1982

134. Pierides AM, Simpson W, Ward MK, Ellis HA, Dewar JH, Kerr DNS: Variable response to long-term 1α-hydroxycholecalciferol in hemodialysis osteodystrophy. *Lancet* 1:1092–1095, 1976

135. Kanis JA, Henderson RG, Heynen G, et al.: Renal osteodystrophy in nondialysed adolescents: long term-treatment with 1α-hydroxycholecalciferol. *Arch Dis Child* 52:573–481, 1977

136. Delmez JA, Dougan CS, Gearing BK, et al.: The effects of

intraperitoneal calcitriol on calcium and parathyroid hormone. *Kidney Int* 31:795–799, 1987

137. Salusky IB, Goodman WG, Horst R, et al.: Pharmakokinetics of calcitriol in CAPD/CCPD patients. *Am J Kidney Dis* 16:126–132, 1990

138. Fukagawa M, Kitaoka M, Kaname S, et al.: Suppression of parathyroid gland hyperplasia by 1,25(OH)$_2$D$_3$ pulse therapy. *N Engl J Med* 315:421–422, 1990

139. Martin KJ, Bullal HS, Domoto DT, Blalock S, Weindel M: Pulse oral calcitriol for the treatment of hyperparathyroidism in patients on continuous ambulatory peritoneal dialysis: preliminary observations. *Am J Kidney Dis* 19:540–545, 1992

140. Llach F: Parathyroidectomy in chronic renal failure: indications, surgical approach, and the use of calcitriol. *Kidney Int* 38 (suppl 29):S29, 1990

141. Hercz G, Salusky IB, Norris KC, Fine RN, Coburn JW: Aluminum removal by peritoneal dialysis: intravenous vs. intraperitoneal deferioxamine. *Kidney Int* 30:944–948, 1986

142. Milliner DS, Hercz G, Miller JH, Shinaberger JH, Nissenson AR, Coburn JW: Clearance of aluminum by hemodialysis: effect of deferoxamine. *Kidney Int* 29(suppl 18):S100–S103, 1986

143. Coburn JW, Norris NC, Nebeker HG: Osteomalacia and bone disease arising from aluminum. *Semin Nephrol* 6:68–89, 1986

144. Windus DW, Stokes TJ, Julian BA, Fenves AZ: Fatal rhizopus infections in hemodialysis patients receiving deferoxamine. *Ann Intern Med* 107:678–680, 1987

145. Boelaert JR, Valcke YL, Vanderbroucke DH: Yersinia enterocolitica bacteraemia in hemodialysis. *Proc EDTA* 22:283, 1985

146. Gallant T, Freedman MH, Vellend H, Francombe WH: Yersinia sepsis in patients with iron overload treated with deferoxamine. *N Engl J Med* 314:1643, 1986

147. Hoen B, Renoult E, Jonon B, Kessler M: Septicemia due to Yersinia enterocolitica in a long-term hemodialysis patient after a single desferrioxamine administration. *Nephron* 50:378–379, 1988

148. Segal R, Zoller KA, Sherrard DJ, Coburn JW: Mucormycosis: a life-threatening complication of deferoxamine therapy in long-term dialysis patients (abstract). *Kidney Int* 33:238, 1988

149. Hercz G, Andress DL, Nebeker HG, Shinaberger JH, Sherrard DJ, Coburn JW: Reversal of aluminum-related bone disease after substituting calcium carbonate for aluminum hydroxide. *Am J Kidney Dis* 11:70–75, 1988

150. Kober M, Schneider H, Reinold HM, et al.: Development of renal osteodystrophy after kidney transplantation. *Kidney Int* 28:378, 1985

151. Bonomini V, Felelli C, DiFelice A, Buscaroli A: Bone remodeling after renal transplantation. *Adv Exp Med Biol* 178:207–216, 1984

152. Conceicao SC, Wilkinson R, Feest TJ, et al.: Hypercalcemia following renal transplantation: causes and consequences. *Clin Nephrol* 16:235–244, 1981

153. Diethelm AG, Edwards RP, Whelchel JD: The natural history and surgical treatment of hypercalcemia before and after renal transplantation. *Surg Gynecol Obstet* 154:481–490, 1982

154. Deierhoi MH, Diethelm AG: Management of hyperparathyroidism following renal transplantation. *Transplant Management* 2:3–10, 1991

155. D'Alessandro AM, Melzer JS, Pirsch JD, et al.: Tertiary hyperparathyroidism after renal transplantation: operative indications. *Surgery* 106:1049–1056, 1989

156. Parfitt AM: Are bone problems of dialysis patients always solved by renal transplantation? In: Zackson DA (ed), *CPC Series: Cases in Metabolic Bone Disease*. Education in Practice, New York, 1–12, 1986

157. Rosenbaum RW, Hruska KA, Korkor A, et al.: Decreased phosphate reabsorption after renal transplantation: evidence for a mechanism independent of calcium and parathyroid hormone. *Kidney Int* 19:568–578, 1981

158. Parfitt AM, Kleerekoper M, Cruz C: Reduced phosphate reabsorption unrelated to parathyroid hormone after renal transplantation: implications for the pathogenesis of hyperparathyroidism in chronic renal failure. *Miner Electrolyte Metab* 12:356, 1986

159. Ingbar S, Kon E, Burnett C, et al.: The effects of cortisone on the renal tubular transport of uric acid, phosphorus, and electrolytes in patients with normal renal and adrenal function. *J Lab Clin Med* 38:533–541, 1951

160. Goodman M, Solomons CC, Miller PD: Distinction between the common symptoms of the phosphate-depletion syndrome and glucocorticoid-induced disease. *Am J Med* 65:868–872, 1978

161. Felsenfeld AJ, Gutman RA, Drezner M, Llach F: Hypophosphatemia in long-term renal transplant recipients: effects on bone histology and 1,25-dihydroxycholecalciferol. *Miner Electrolyte Metab* 12:333–341, 1987

162. Lentz RD, Brown DM, Kjellstrand CM: Treatment of severe hypophosphatemia. *Ann Intern Med* 89:941–944, 1978

163. Nielsen HE, Melsen F, Christensen MS: Aseptic necrosis of bone following renal transplantation. *Acta Med Scand* 202:27, 1977

164. Julian BA, Laskow DA, Dubovsky J, Dubovsky EV, Curtis JJ, Quarles LD: Rapid loss of vertebral mineral density after renal transplantation. *N Engl J Med* 325:544–550, 1991

165. McDonald JA, Dunstan CR, Dilworth P, et al.: Bone loss after liver transplantation. *Hepatology* 14:613–619, 1991

166. Lukert BP, Raisz LG: Glucocorticoid-induced osteoporosis: pathogenesis and management. *Ann Intern Med* 112:352–364, 1990

167. Pocock NA, Eisman JA, Dunstan CR, et al.: Recovery from steroid-induced osteoporosis. *Ann Intern Med* 107:319–323, 1987

168. Peck WA, Brandt J, Miller I: Hydrocortisone-induced inhibition of protein synthesis and uridine incorporation in isolated bone cells in vitro. *Proc Natl Acad Sci USA* 57:1599–1606, 1967

169. Avioli LV: Effects of chronic corticosteroid therapy on mineral metabolism and calcium absorption. *Adv Exp Med Biol* 171:81–89, 1984

170. Movsowitz C, Epstein S, Fallon M, Ismail F, Thomas S: Cyclosporin A in vivo produces severe osteopenia in the rat: effect of dose and duration of administration. *Endocrinology* 123:2571–2577, 1988

171. Stewart PJ, Green OC, Stern PH: Cyclosporin A inhibits calcemic hormone-induced bone resorption in vitro. *J Bone Miner Res* 1:285–291, 1986

172. Landmenn J, Renner N, Gacher A, et al.: Cyclosporin A and osteonecrosis of the femoral head. *J Bone Joint Surg* 69A:1226–1228, 1987

173. Gray RES, Doherty SM, Galloway J, et al.: A double-blind study of deflazacort and prednisone in patients with chronic inflammatory disorders. *Arthritis Rheum* 34:287–295, 1991

174. Montecucco C, Baldi F, Fortina A, et al.: Serum osteocalcin (bone Gla-protein) following corticosteroid therapy in postmenopausal women with rheumatoid arthritis. Comparison of the effect of prednisone and deflazacort. *Clin Rheumatol* 7:366–371, 1988

175. Slatopolsky E, Martin K: Glucocorticoids and renal transplant osteonecrosis. *Adv Exp Med Biol* 171:353–359, 1984

176. Parfrey PS, Farge D, Parfrey NA, et al.: The decreased incidence of aseptic necrosis in renal transplant recipients: a case control study. *Transplantation* 41:182–187, 1986

177. Isono SS, Woolson ST, Schurman DJ: Total joint arthroplasty for steroid-induced osteonecrosis in cardiac patients. *Clin Orthop* 217:201–208, 1987

178. Enright H, Haake R, Weisorf D: Avascular necrosis of bone: a common serious complication of allogeneic bone marrow transplantation. *Am J Med* 89:733–738, 1990

179. Ficat RP: Idiopathic bone necrosis of the femoral head. Early diagnosis and treatment. *J Bone Joint Surg* 67B:3–9, 1985

180. Van Damme-Lombaerts R, Pirson Y, Squifflet JB, et al.: The avascular necrosis of bone after renal transplantation in children. *Tranplant Proc* 17:184–186, 1985

181. Ibels LS, Alfrey AC, Huffer WE, et al.: Aseptic necrosis of bone following renal transplantation: experience in 194 transplant recipients and review of the literature. *Medicine* (Baltimore) 57:25–45, 1978

SECTION VI

Genetic, Developmental, and Dysplastic Skeletal Disorders

Introduction

Physicians are confronted with a great diversity of rare genetic, developmental, and dysplastic skeletal disorders (1). Some are simply radiologic curiosities; others are challenging clinical problems. Some cause focal bony abnormalities; others result in generalized disturbances of bone growth or modeling or osteosclerosis or osteopenia. A few are associated with overt derangements in mineral homeostasis. Several are important because they offer clues concerning normal mechanisms of skeletal remodeling and mineral metabolism. Cumulatively, the number of affected subjects is substantial.

This section provides a concise overview of a number of the more common or more revealing of these entities, beginning with a description of some of the conditions that are traditionally grouped together as sclerosing bone dysplasias (2). A discussion of several additional important heritable or sporadic developmental and dysplastic skeletal disorders follows (1).

REFERENCES

1. Wynne-Davies R, Hall CM, Apley AG: Atlas of Skeletal Dysplasias. Churchill Livingstone, Edinburgh, 1985
2. Frame B, Honasoge M, Kottamasu SR: Osteosclerosis, Hyperostosis, and Related Disorders, Elsevier, New York, 1987

75. Sclerosing Bone Dysplasias

Michael P. Whyte, M.D.

*Metabolic Research Unit, Shriners Hospital for Crippled Children, and
Division of Bone and Mineral Diseases, The Jewish Hospital of St. Louis,
Washington University School of Medicine; St. Louis, Missouri*

In addition to a variety of dietary, metabolic, endocrine, hematologic, infectious, and neoplastic disorders, many rare (primarily hereditary) dysplastic conditions can cause focal or generalized osteosclerosis (Table 1). The following sections discuss the principal entities among the "sclerosing bone dysplasias."

OSTEOPETROSIS

Osteopetrosis (marble bone disease) was first described in 1904 by Albers-Schönberg (1); more than 300 cases have been reported. Two major clinical forms are well delineated—the autosomal dominant or "benign" type that is associated with few or no symptoms (2) and the autosomal recessive or "malignant" type that, if untreated, is typically fatal during infancy or early childhood (3). A rarer autosomal recessive "intermediate" form presents during childhood with some of the signs and symptoms of malignant osteopetrosis, but its impact on life expentancy is not well characterized (4). A fourth clinical type, the autosomal recessive syndrome of osteopetrosis with renal tubular acidosis and cerebral calcification is an inborn error of metabolism, carbonic anhydrase II deficiency (see the following section). Neuronal storage disease with malignant osteopetrosis has been reported in several subjects and seems to reflect a fifth clinical form (5). There also appear to be especially rare "lethal," "transient infantile," and "postinfectious" osteopetroses (6).

Although the diversity of clinical/hereditary types makes it apparent that several different genetic defects and mechanisms cause osteopetrosis in humans, the pathogenesis of all true forms is expressed through defective osteoclast function that impairs skeletal resorption. As a result, primary spongiosa (calcified cartilage deposited during endochondral bone formation) can persist during adult life and cause characteristic histological changes (see the following) (7). For some conditions, the term osteopetrosis has been incorrectly used "generically" to refer to a skeleton that appears diffusely sclerotic on radiographic study, yet where these histologic features are absent. Accordingly, it is important to recognize that some therapeutic approaches for true forms of osteopetrosis for which the pathogenesis is partly elucidated may be completely inappropriate for these generally less well understood disorders.

Clinical Presentation

Malignant osteopetrosis presents during infancy (3). An increased incidence of parental consanguinity and occurrence within sibships indicate that this form is transmitted as an autosomal recessive trait. Nasal "stuffiness" that results from malformation of mastoid and paranasal sinuses is often an early symptom. Cranial foramina do not widen fully and this defect can gradually causes palsies of the optic, oculomotor, and facial nerves. There is failure to thrive. Eruption of the dentition is delayed. Bones may appear to be dense on radiologic study, but are actually fragile and may fracture. Some subjects develop hydrocephalus; sleep apnea can occur. Retinal degeneration is another cause of blindness. Recurrent infection with spontaneous bruising and bleeding are common problems and appear to reflect myelophthisis from dense bone, many osteoclasts, and abundant fibrous tissue that crowd bone marrow spaces. Hypersplenism and hemolysis can also worsen the associated anemia. Physical examination shows short stature, frontal bossing, a large head, "adenoid appearance," nystagmus, hepatosplenomegaly, and *genu valgum*. Untreated children usually die during the first decade of life from hemorrhage, pneumonia, severe anemia, or sepsis (3).

Intermediate osteopetrosis causes short stature. Some affected individuals develop cranial nerve deficits, macrocephaly, ankylosed teeth that predispose to osteomyelitis of the jaw, mild or occasionally moderately severe anemia, and recurrent fracture (4).

Benign (autosomal dominant) osteopetrosis can be a developmental condition in which radiologic abnormalities become apparent during childhood. In some kindreds, "skip generations" occur such that carriers show no radiologic abnormalities. Although most affected subjects are asymptomatic (2), the long bones are brittle and fractures may occur. Facial palsy, deafness, osteomyelitis of the mandible, compromised vision or hearing, psychomotor delay, carpal-tunnel syndrome, and osteoarthritis are additional clinical problems. Studies from Denmark suggest that there are at least two types of benign osteopetrosis (8). They are distinguishable by their radiologic appearance and have somewhat different clinical expression and biochemical findings.

Neuronal storage disease with osteopetrosis has the additional features of epilepsy and neurodegenerative disease (5). Lethal osteopetrosis results in stillbirth (6). Transient infantile osteopetrosis resolves during the first few years of life (6).

Radiologic Features

Generalized osteosclerosis is the principal radiologic finding in the osteopetroses (9). In the severe forms, abnormal skeletal growth, modeling, and remodeling are as-

327

TABLE 1. *Disorders that cause osteosclerosis*

1. Dysplasias
   A. Craniodiaphyseal dysplasia
   B. Craniometaphyseal dysplasia
   C. Dysosteosclerosis
   D. Endosteal hyperostosis
      van Buchem disease
      sclerosteosis
   E. Frontometaphyseal dysplasia
   F. Infantile cortical hyperostosis (Caffey disease)
   G. Melorheostosis
   H. Metaphyseal dysplasia (Pyle disease)
   I. Mixed sclerosing bone dystrophy
   J. Oculodento-osseus dysplasia
   K. Osteodysplasia of Melnick and Needles
   L. Osteoectasia with hyperphosphatasia (hyperostosis corticalis)
   M. Osteopathia striata
   N. Osteopetrosis
   O. Osteopoikilosis
   P. Progressive diaphyseal dysplasia (Engelmann disease)
   Q. Pycnodysostosis
2. Metabolic
   A. Carbonic anhydrase II deficiency
   B. Fluorosis
   C. Heavy metal poisoning
   D. Hypervitaminosis A,D
   E. Hyper-, hypo-, and pseudohypoparathyroidism
   F. Hypophosphatemic osteomalacia
   G. Milk-alkali syndrome
   H. Renal osteodystrophy
3. Other
   A. Axial osteomalacia
   B. Fibrogenesis imperfecta osseum
   C. Ionizing radiation
   D. Lymphomas
   E. Mastocytosis
   F. Multiple myeloma
   G. Myelofibrosis
   H. Osteomyelitis
   I. Osteonecrosis
   J. Paget's disease
   K. Sarcoidosis
   L. Skeletal metastases
   M. Tuberous sclerosis

Reproduced with permission from Whyte MP and Murphy WA: Osteopetrosis and Other Sclerosing Bone Disorders. In: Avioli LV, Krane SM (eds), *Metabolic Bone Disease*, 2nd edition, WB Saunders, Philadelphia, 1990.

sociated with a symmetrical increase in bone mass. The skeleton may be uniformly dense, but alternating dense and lucent bands are commonly noted in the pelvis and near the ends of the long bones whose diaphyses and metaphyses are typically broadened and may have an "Ehrlenmeyer flask" deformity (Fig. 1). The distal phalanges rarely are eroded (a finding more characteristic of pycnodysostosis). Pathologic fracture of the long bones is not uncommon. Rachitic changes may occur (10). In the axial skeleton, the cranium is usually thickened and dense, especially at the base, and the paranasal and mastoid sinuses are underpneumatized (Fig. 2). Vertebrae may show, on

lateral view, a "bone-in-bone" (endobone) configuration caused by areas of apparent radiolucency.

The two heritable types of benign osteopetrosis manifest progressive osteosclerosis from childhood with either (A) marked sclerosis and thickening of the cranial vault and diffusely increased density of the spine without endobone formation (Type I), or (B) selective thickening of the base of the skull together with typical vertebral endplate sclerosis that causes an endobone or a "rugger-jersey" appearance of the spine (Type II) (8). In both types, skeletal modeling defects are absent.

In the various forms of osteopetrosis, skeletal scintigraphy will show fractures, osteomyelitis, and so on (11). Magnetic resonance imaging may help to monitor patients with severe disease who undergo bone marrow transplantation, since successful engraftment will enlarge marrow spaces (12) (see the following sections). The cranial CT and MRI findings of infants and children have been characterized (13).

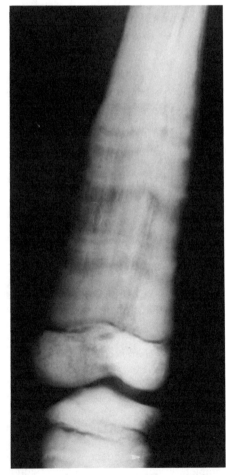

FIG. 1. *Osteopetrosis.* Anteroposterior radiograph of the distal femur of a 10-year-old boy shows a widened metadiaphyseal region with characteristic alternating dense and lucent bands. (Reproduced with permission from Whyte MP, Murphy WA: Osteopetrosis and other sclerosing bone disorders. In: Avioli LV, Krane SM (eds), *Metabolic Bone Disease, 2nd ed.* WB Saunders, Philadelphia, 1990.)

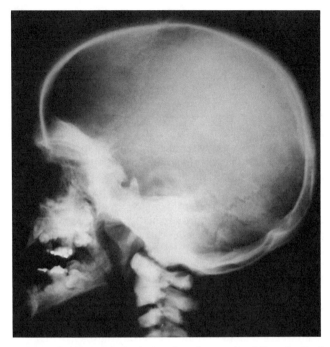

FIG. 2. *Osteopetrosis.* Lateral radiograph of the skull of a 13-year-old boy shows osteosclerosis, especially apparent at the base. (Reproduced with permission from Whyte MP, Murphy WA: Osteopetrosis and other sclerosing bone disorders. In: Avioli LV, Krane SM (eds), *Metabolic Bone Disease, 2nd ed.* WB Saunders, Philadelphia, 1990.)

Laboratory Findings

In malignant osteopetrosis, serum calcium levels generally reflect the dietary intake (14). Hypocalcemia can occur and may be severe enough to cause rickets. Secondary hyperparathyroidism with increased serum levels of calcitriol is commonly present (15). Acid phosphatase and creatine kinase activity in serum, which apparently originate from osteoclasts, are typically increased.

In the benign form, standard biochemical indices of mineral homeostasis have usually been described as unremarkable. However, recent studies indicate that serum immunoreactive PTH levels and acid phosphatase activity are often increased in subjects with type II disease (8).

Histopathologic Findings

The radiologic features of the osteopetroses can be considered diagnostic in most cases (9). However, the pathogenetic failure of osteoclasts to resorb skeletal tissue also provides a histologic finding that is pathognomonic (16); i.e., remnants of mineralized primary spongiosa that persist as "islands" of calcified cartilage within mature bone (Fig. 3). Recent studies of benign osteopetrosis indicate, however, that these structures may not always be found in adults on iliac crest biopsy (8).

In osteopetrosis, osteoclasts may be present in increased, normal, or decreased numbers. In the malignant form, these multinucleated cells are usually abundant and are found at bone surfaces, but their nuclei are especially numerous, and characteristic "ruffled borders" or "clear zones" are absent (17). Fibrous tissue often crowds the marrow spaces (17). Benign osteopetrosis may show increased amounts of osteoid, and osteoclasts can be few and lack ruffled borders or can be especially numerous and large (18). Woven osseous tissue in areas of trabecular and cortical bone seems to be a common histologic finding (8,16).

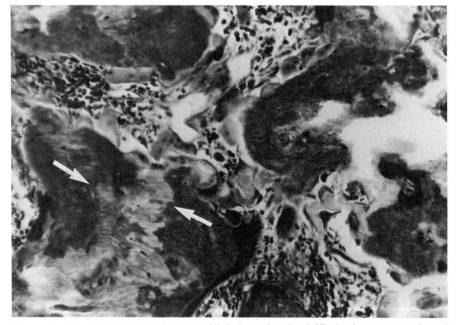

FIG. 3. *Osteopetrosis.* A characteristic area of lightly-stained calcified primary spongiosa (*arrows*) is found within darkly-stained mineralized bone (magnification × 150).

Etiology and Pathogenesis

Although most forms of human osteopetrosis appear to be heritable as autosomal traits, the molecular defects or gene loci are unknown, except for carbonic anhydrase II deficiency (see later section) (6). Diminished osteoclast-mediated bone resorption is characteristic of all clinical types (6). Abnormalities in its microenvironment or in the osteoclast stem cell itself, in the mature osteoclast, or in the bone tissue could be at fault (6,7). Leukocyte function studies in the malignant form have revealed abnormalities in circulating monocytes and granulocytes (19,20). In the few cases of osteopetrosis with neuronal storage disease (characterized by accumulation of ceroid lipofuscin), a primary lysosomal defect may be present (5). Viral-like inclusions have been found in some of the osteoclasts of a few sporadic cases of benign osteopetrosis, but their significance is uncertain (21). Synthesis of an abnormal parathyroid hormone (22), or defective production of interleukin-2 (23) or superoxide (compounds necessary for bone resorption), may also be pathogenetic defects (20). Ultimately these factors impair bone resorption, and skeletal fragility may be attributed to the presence of a paucity of collagen fibrils that normally connect osteons, as well as to defective remodeling of woven bone to compact bone (7).

Treatment

Since the etiology, pathogenesis, prognosis, and even pattern of inheritance for the various forms of osteopetrosis differ, a correct diagnosis of the particular subtype is especially important before therapy is attempted. Intermediate osteopetrosis is relatively benign. Infants or young children with carbonic anhydrase II deficiency (see later section) may have radiologic features consistent with malignant osteopetrosis, yet serial studies can show spontaneous gradual resolution of their osteosclerosis. Distinction among the various forms may require investigation of the family and careful evaluation of the patient's disease progression.

Marrow Transplantation

Bone marrow transplantation has remarkably improved a few cases of malignant osteopetrosis (24). Transplanted osteoclasts, but not osteoblasts, were shown to be of donor origin in one affected infant (25)—an observation that supported the hypothesis that osteopetrosis is caused by defective osteoclast-mediated bone resorption, and that the progenitor cell for the osteoclast is normally derived from the marrow (25). Patients with severely crowded marrow spaces appear less likely to benefit from this procedure. Accordingly, histomorphometric studies of bone may help to prognosticate the outcome of marrow transplantation. Use of marrow from HLA-*non*identical donors warrants continued study (26). It is understandable that marrow transplantation may not benefit all patients (6), since it seems that a variety of defects (not all of which are intrinsic to osteoclasts) may cause osteopetrosis.

Hormonal/Dietary Treatment

Some success in the treatment of osteopetrosis was reported with a calcium-deficient diet alone. However, supplementation of dietary calcium may be necessary for symptomatic hypocalcemia and rickets in some severely affected infants or children.

Massive oral doses of calcitriol together with limited dietary calcium intake to prevent hypercalciuria/hypercalcemia occasionally improves malignant osteopetrosis as dramatically as does successful marrow transplantation (27). Calcitriol appears to be helpful by stimulating dormant osteoclast activity. Long-term infusion of parathormone was helpful for one infant (22) perhaps by stimulating calcitriol synthesis. Recently, the observation that leukocytes from severely affected cases have diminished production of superoxide has led to short-term success using recombinant human interferon treatment (20).

High-dose glucocorticoid therapy stabilizes patients with pancytopenia and hepatomegaly from malignant osteopetrosis. Prednisone and a low-calcium/high-phosphate diet may be an alternative treatment to marrow transplantation for this form of the disorder (28).

Other

Hyperbaric oxygenation can be an important adjunctive treatment for osteomyelitis of the jaw. Surgical decompression of the optic and facial nerves may benefit some patients.

Early prenatal diagnosis of osteopetrosis by ultrasound has been unsuccessful. A conventional radiographic study failed to diagnose malignant osteopetrosis at 20 weeks gestation.

REFERENCES

1. Albers-Schönberg H: Rontgenbilder einer seltenen, Knochenerkrankung. *Meunch Med Wochenschr* 51:365, 1904
2. Johnston CC Jr, Lavy N, Lord T, et al.: Osteopetrosis: a clinical, genetic metabolic, and morphologic study of the dominantly inherited, benign form. *Medicine* 47:149–167, 1968
3. Loria-Cortes R, Quesada-Calvo E, Cordero-Chaverri E: Osteopetrosis in children: a report of 26 cases. *J Pediat* 91:43–47, 1977
4. Kahler SG, Burns JA, Aylsworth AS: A mild autosomal recessive form of osteopetrosis. *Am J Med Genet* 17:451–464, 1984
5. Jagadha V, Halliday WC, Becker LE, Hinton D: The association of infantile osteopetrosis and neuronal storage disease in two brothers. *Acta Neuropathol* 75:233–240, 1988
6. Whyte MP: Recent advances in osteopetrosis. In: Cohn DV, Gennari C, Tashian AH (eds) *Calcium Regulating Hormones and Bone Metabolism* Elsevier, Amsterdam, pp. 420–430, 1992
7. Marks SC Jr: Osteopetrosis—multiple pathways for the interception of osteoclast function. *Appl Pathol* 5:172–183, 1987
8. Bollerslev J: Autosomal dominant osteopetrosis: bone metabolism and epidemiological, clinical and hormonal aspects. *Endocr Rev* 10:45–67, 1989

9. Resnick D, Niwayama G: *Diagnosis of Bone and Joint Disorders 2nd ed.* WB Saunders, Philadelphia, 1988
10. Oliveira G, Boechat MI, Amaral SM, et al.: Osteopetrosis and rickets: an intriguing association. *Am J Dis Child* 140:377–378, 1986
11. Park H-M, Lambertus J: Skeletal and reticuloendothelial imaging in osteopetrosis: case report. *J Nucl Med* 18:1091–1095, 1977
12. Rao VM, Dalinka MK, Mitchell DG, et al.: Osteopetrosis: MR characteristics at 1.5T'. *Radiology* 161:217–220, 1986
13. Elster AD, Theros EG, Key LL, Chen MYM: Cranial imaging in autosomal recessive osteopetrosis (parts I & II). *Radiol* 183:129–144, 1992
14. Key LL, Carnes D, Holtrop M, et al.: Treatment of congenital osteopetrosis with high dose calcitriol. *N Engl J Med* 310:409–415, 1984
15. Cournot G, Trubert-Thil CL, Petrovic M, Boyle A, Cormier C, Girault D, Fischer A, Garabedian M: Mineral metabolism in infants with malignant osteopetrosis: heterogeneity in plasma 1,25-dihydroxyvitamin D levels and bone histology. *J Bone Min Res* 7:1–10, 1992
16. Revell PA: *Pathology of Bone.* Springer-Verlag, Berlin, 1986
17. Helfrich MH, Aronson DC, Everts V, Mieremet RHP, Gerritsen EJA, Eckhardt PG, Groot CG, Scherft JP: Morphologic features of bone in human osteopetrosis. *Bone* 12:411–419, 1991
18. Bollerslev J, Steiniche T, Melsen F, Mosekilde L: Structural and histomorphometric studies of iliac crest trabecular and cortical bone in autosomal dominant osteopetrosis: a study of two radiological types. *Bone* 10:19–24, 1989
19. Beard CJ, Key L, Newburger PE, et al.: Neutrophil defect associated with malignant infantile osteopetrosis. *J Lab Clin Med* 108:498–505, 1986
20. Key LL Jr, Ries WL, Rodriguiz RN, Hatcher HC: Recombinant human interferon gamma therapy for osteopetrosis. *J Peds* 121:119–124, 1992
21. Mills BG, Yabe H, Singer FR: Osteoclasts in human osteopetrosis contain viral-nucleocapsid-like nuclear inclusions. *J Bone Min Res* 3:101–106, 1988
22. Glorieux FH, Pettifor JM, Marie PJ, et al.: Induction of bone resorption by parathyroid hormone in congenital malignant osteopetrosis. *Metab Bone Dis Rel Res* 3:143–150, 1981
23. Key LL, Ries WL, Schiff R: Osteopetrosis associated with interleukin-2 deficiency. *J Bone Min Res* 2(Suppl II):85, 1987
24. Kaplan FS, August CS, Fallon MD, et al.: Successful treatment of infantile malignant osteopetrosis by bone-marrow transplantation: a case report. *J Bone Joint Surg* (Am) 70:617–623, 1988
25. Coccia PF, Krivit W, Cervenka J, et al.: Successful bone-marrow transplantation for infantile malignant osteopetrosis. *N Engl J Med* 302:701–708, 1980
26. Orchard PJ, Dickerman JD, Mathews CHE, et al.: Haploidentical bone marrow transplantation for osteopetrosis. *Am J Ped Hematol* Oncol 9:335–340, 1987
27. Key LL Jr: Osteopetrosis: a genetic window into osteoclast function. In: *Cases in Metabolic Bone Disease,* 2(3), Triclinica Communications, New York, pp. 1–12, 1987
28. Dorantes LM, Mejia AM, Dorantes S: Juvenile osteopetrosis: effects of blood and bone of prednisone and low calcium, high phosphate diet. *Arch Dis Child* 61:666–670, 1986

CARBONIC ANHYDRASE II DEFICIENCY

In 1983, the autosomal recessive syndrome of osteopetrosis with renal tubular acidosis (RTA) and cerebral calcification was discovered to be a new inborn error of metabolism caused by deficiency of the carbonic anhydrase II (CA II) isoenzyme (1).

Clinical Presentation

Descriptions of more than 25 patients with CA II deficiency demonstrate that there is considerable clinical variability among affected families (2,3). The perinatal history is typically unremarkable, but then in infancy or early childhood affected subjects may fracture or show failure to thrive, developmental delay, or short stature. Mental subnormality is common but not invariable. Compression of the optic nerves and dental malocclusion are additional complications. RTA may explain the hypotonia, apathy, and muscle weakness that troubles some affected individuals. Periodic hypokalemic paralysis has been described. Although fracture is unusual, recurrent breaks in long bones may cause significant morbidity (1). Life expectancy does not appear to be shortened, but to date the oldest subjects reported have been young adults (2,3).

Radiologic Features

CA II deficiency resembles other forms of osteopetrosis on radiologic study, except that cerebral calcification develops during childhood and the defects in skeletal modeling and the osteosclerosis may diminish spontaneously (rather than increase) over years (4). Radiologic abnormalities of the skeleton have been present at diagnosis in all cases, though one subject had only subtle findings at birth. Computed tomography reveals that the cerebral calcification is developmental and appears between 2–5 years of age, increases during childhood, affects gray matter of the cortex and basal ganglia, and is similar if not identical to that of idiopathic hypoparathyroidism or pseudohypoparathyroidism.

Laboratory Findings

Bone marrow examination is unremarkable. If anemia is present, it is generally mild and likely to be of nutritional origin. Metabolic acidosis occurs as early as the neonatal period. Both proximal and distal RTA have been described (5); however, occurrence of distal (Type I) RTA seems to be better documented. Additional studies are required to clarify the pathogenesis of the abnormality in acid/base homeostasis (5). Aminoaciduria and glycosuria are absent (2).

Autopsy studies have not been reported (3). Histopathologic examination of bone from four individuals who represented two affected families revealed characteristic areas of unresorbed calcified primary spongiosa (4).

Etiology and Pathogenesis

The CA isoenzymes accelerate the first step in the reaction $CO_2 + H_2O \rightarrow H_2CO_3 \rightarrow H^+ + HCO_3^-$. Accordingly, they function importantly in acid/base regulation. CA II is widely distributed; e.g., in brain, kidney, erythrocytes, cartilage, lung, and gastric mucosa (6). The other CA isoenzymes have a more limited tissue distribution.

All of 21 patients from 12 unrelated kindreds of diverse ethnic and geographic origin were shown to have selective deficiency of CA II in erythrocytes (2). Autosomal recessive inheritance for CA II deficiency is supported by the observation that red cell CA II levels are approximately half-normal in parents of affected subjects (2,3).

Although deficiency of CA II remains to be shown in tissues other than erythrocytes, the presence of osteopetrosis, RTA, and cerebral calcification in subjects with this disorder suggests that there is a global deficiency of CA II and that this isoenzyme has an important function in bone, kidney, and perhaps brain (2,3). Defects in the CA II gene, which is localized on the short arm of chromosome 8 in humans (6), have recently been identified in several patients (7).

Treatment

RTA in CA II deficiency has been treated by bicarbonate supplementation, but the long-term impact of this therapy is unknown. Transfusion of CA II-replete erythrocytes to one affected individual did not correct her systemic acidosis (8).

REFERENCES

1. Sly WS, Hewett-Emmett D, Whyte MP, et al.: Carbonic anhydrase II deficiency identified as the primary defect in the autosomal recessive syndrome of osteopetrosis with renal tubular acidosis and cerebral calcification. *Proc Natl Acad Sci USA* 80: 2752–2756, 1983
2. Sly WS, Whyte MP, Sundaram V, et al.: Carbonic anhydrase II deficiency in 12 families with the autosomal recessive syndrome of osteopetrosis with renal tubular acidosis and cerebral calcification. *N Engl J Med* 313:139–145, 1985
3. Sly WS: Carbonic anhydrase II deficiency syndrome: osteopetrosis with renal tubular acidosis and cerebral calcification. In: Scriver CR, Beaudet AL, Sly WS, Valle D (eds), *The Metabolic Basis of Inherited Disease, 6th ed.* McGraw-Hill Inc., New York, 2857–2868, 1989
4. Whyte MP, Murphy WA, Fallon MD, et al.: Osteopetrosis, renal tubular acidosis and basal ganglia calcification in three sisters. *Am J Med* 69:64–74, 1980
5. Sly WS, Whyte MP, Krupin T, et al.: Positive renal response to acetazolamide in carbonic anhydrase II–deficient patients. *Pediatr Res* 19:1033–1036, 1985
6. Dodgson SJ, Tashian RE, Gros G, Carter ND: The Carbonic Anhydrases, Plenum Press, New York, 1991
7. Roth DE, Venta PJ, Tashian RE, Sly WS: Molecular basis of human carbonic anhydrase II deficiency. *Proc Natl Acad Sci USA* 89:1804–1808, 1992
8. Whyte MP, Hamm LL III, Sly WS: Transfusion of carbonic anhydrase-replete erythrocytes fails to correct the acidification defect in the syndrome of osteopetrosis, renal tubular acidosis, and cerebral calcification (carbonic anhydrase II deficiency). *J Bone Miner Res* 3:385–388, 1988

PYCNODYSOSTOSIS

Pycnodysostosis is the skeletal dysplasia that is believed to have affected the French impressionist painter Henri de Toulouse-Lautrec (1864–1901) (1). More than 100 cases from 50 kindreds have been described since the condition was delineated in 1962 (2). It is transmitted as an autosomal recessive trait; parental consanguinity has been reported for about 30% of cases. Most descriptions have come from Europe or the United States, but the disorder has been found in Israel, Indonesia, Asian Indians, and Africans; pycnodysostosis appears to be especially common in Japanese (3).

Clinical Presentation

Pycnodysostosis is generally diagnosed during infancy or early childhood because of disproportionate short stature and dysmorphic features that include fronto-occipital prominence, relatively large cranium, obtuse mandibular angle, small facies and chin, high-arched palate, dental malocclusion with retained deciduous teeth, proptosis, bluish sclerae, and a beaked and pointed nose (4). The anterior fontanel and other cranial sutures are usually open. Fingers are short and clubbed from acro-osteolysis or aplasia of terminal phalanges, the fingernails are hypoplastic, and the hands are small and square. The thorax is narrow and there may be *pectus excavatum*, kyphoscoliosis, and increased lumbar lordosis. Recurrent fractures usually involve the lower limbs and cause *genu valgum* deformity. Patients are, however, usually able to walk independently. Atypical subjects with visceral manifestations and with rickets have been described. Mental retardation affects about 10% of cases (4). Adult height ranges from 4′3″ to 4′11″. Recurrent respiratory infections and right heart failure from chronic upper airway obstruction due to micrognathia occur in some affected individuals.

Radiologic Features

Pycnodysostosis shares many radiologic features with osteopetrosis; e.g., both disorders cause generalized osteosclerosis and are associated with recurrent fractures. The osteosclerosis is developmental, is uniform, first becomes apparent in childhood, and increases with age. However, the marked modeling defects of the severe forms of osteopetrosis do not occur in pycnodysostosis, although long bones have thick cortices and narrow medullary canals. Additional findings that help to differentiate pycnodysostosis from osteopetrosis include delayed closure of cranial sutures and fontanels (prominently the anterior) (Fig. 4), obtuse mandibular angle, wormian bones, gracile clavicles that are hypoplastic at their lateral segments, hypoplasia or aplasia of the distal phalanges and ribs, and partial absence of the hyoid bone (5). Endobones and radiodense striations are also absent (6). The calvarium and base of the skull are sclerotic, and the orbital ridges are radiodense. Hypoplasia of facial bones, sinuses, and terminal phalanges are characteristic. Vertebrae are sclerotic, yet their transverse processes are uninvolved; anterior and posterior concavities occur. Lumbosacral spondylolithesis is not uncommon, and lack of segmentation of the atlas and axis may be present. Madelung deformity can affect the forearms.

Laboratory Findings

Serum calcium and inorganic phosphate levels and alkaline phosphatase activity are usually unremarkable. Ane-

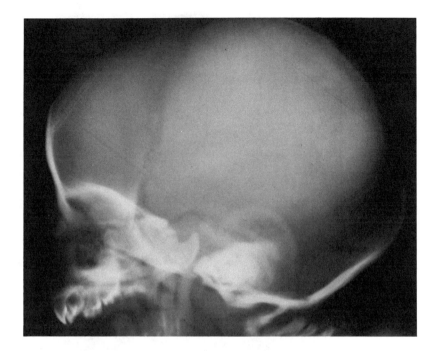

FIG. 4. *Pycnodysostosis.* Lateral radiograph of the skull of an infant shows that the cranial sutures are markedly widened. The base is sclerotic. (Reproduced with permission from Whyte MP, Murphy WA: Osteopetrosis and other sclerosing bone disorders. In: Avioli LV, Krane SM (eds). *Metabolic Bone Disease, 2nd ed.* WB Saunders, Philadelphia, 1990.)

mia is not a problem. Histopathologic study of bone shows cortical bone structure that appears to be normal despite the appearance of decreased osteoclastic and osteoblastic activity (7). Skeletal turnover may be decreased. Electron microscopy of bone from two affected subjects suggested that degradation of collagen could be defective, perhaps from an abnormality in the bone matrix or in the osteoclast itself (8). In chondrocytes, abnormal inclusions have been described.

Etiology and Pathogenesis

The genetic basis for pycnodysostosis is unknown. Absorption of dietary calcium has been noted to be markedly increased. Both the rate of bone accretion and the size of the exchangeable calcium pool may be reduced (9). Accordingly, diminished rates of bone resorption may explain the osteosclerosis. Virus-like inclusions were found in the osteoclasts of two affected brothers (10).

Treatment

There is no effective medical therapy for pycnodysostosis. Fractures of the long bones are typically transverse. They usually heal at a satisfactory rate, although delayed union and massive callus formation have been reported. Internal fixation of long bones is formidable because of their hardness. Extraction of teeth is similarly difficult; fracture of the jaw has occurred in several instances (4). Osteomyelitis of the mandible may require treatment by a combined antibiotic and surgical approach.

REFERENCES

1. Maroteaux P, Lamy M: The malady of Toulouse-Lautrec. *JAMA* 191:715–717, 1965

2. Maroteaux P, Lamy M: La pycnodysostose. *Presse Med* 70:999, 1962
3. Sugiura Y, Yamada Y, Koh J: Pycnodysostosis in Japan: report of six cases and a review of Japanese literature. *Birth Defects Orig Art Ser X* (12):78–98, 1974
4. Elmore SM: Pycnodysostosis: a review. *J Bone Joint Surg* 49A: 153–162, 1967
5. Wolpowitz A, Matisson A: A comparative study of pycnodysostosis, cleidocranial dysostosis, osteopetrosis and acro-osteolysis. *S Afr Med J* 48:1011, 1974
6. Resnick D, Niwayama G: *Diagnosis of Bone and Joint Disorders, 2nd ed.* WB Saunders, Philadelphia, 1988
7. Soto TJ, Mautalen CA, Hojman D, et al.: Pycnodysostosis, metabolic and histologic studies. In: *Birth Defects: Original Article Series.* V(4):109–115, 1969
8. Everts V, Aronson DC, Beertsen W: Phagocytosis of bone collagen by osteoclasts in two cases of pycnodysostosis. *Calcif Tissue Int* 37:25–31, 1985
9. Cabrejas ML, Fromm GA, Roca JF: Pycnodysostosis: some aspects concerning kinetics of calcium metabolism and bone pathology. *Am J Med Sci* 271(2):215, 1976
10. Beneton MNC, Harris S, Kanis JA: Paramyxovirus-like inclusions in two cases of pycnodysostosis. *Bone* 8:211–217, 1987

PROGRESSIVE DIAPHYSEAL DYSPLASIA (CAMURATI-ENGELMANN DISEASE)

Progressive diaphyseal dysplasia was characterized by Cockayne in 1920 (1). Camurati reported that the condition was heritable. Engelmann described the severe typical form in 1929 (2). This is a developmental disorder that is transmitted as an autosomal dominant trait. Descriptions of more than 100 cases show that the clinical and radiologic penetrance is quite variable (3). The characteristic feature is new bone formation that occurs gradually on both the periosteal and endosteal surfaces of the long bones. All races appear to be affected. In severe cases, osteosclerosis is widespread and the skull and axial skeleton are also involved. Some carriers have no radiologic abnormalities.

Clinical Presentation

Progressive diaphyseal dysplasia typically presents during childhood with limping or a broad-based and waddling gait, leg pain, muscle wasting, and decreased subcutaneous fat in the extremities. The condition may be mistaken for a form of muscular dystrophy (4). Severely affected subjects have a characteristic body habitus that includes an enlarged head with prominent forehead, proptosis, and thin limbs with thickened bones but with little muscle mass. Cranial nerve palsies may develop when the skull is affected. Puberty is sometimes delayed. Raised intracranial pressure can occur. Physical findings include palpable bony enlargement and skeletal tenderness. Some patients have hepatosplenomegaly, Raynaud's phenomenon, and other findings suggestive of vasculitis (5). Although radiologic studies typically show progressive disease, the clinical course is variable, and remission of symptoms seems to occur in some subjects during adulthood (6).

Radiologic Features

The principal radiologic feature of progressive diaphyseal dysplasia is cortical hyperostosis of major long bone diaphyses that is due to proliferation of new bone on both the periosteal and endosteal surfaces (7). The sclerosis is fairly symmetrical and gradually spreads to involve metaphyses as well—epiphyses are spared (Fig. 5). The tibiae and femora are the bones that are most commonly involved; less frequently, the radii, ulnae, humeri, and occasionally the short tubular bones are affected. The scapulae, clavicles, and pelvis may also become involved. Typically, the shafts of long bones gradually widen and develop irregular surfaces. The age of onset, rate of progression, and degree of osteosclerosis are very variable. With relatively mild disease, especially in adolescents or young adults, radiographic and scintigraphic abnormalities may be confined to the long bones of the lower limbs. Maturation of the new bone increases the osteosclerosis. In severely affected children, some areas of the skeleton can appear osteopenic.

Bone scanning generally reveals focally increased radionuclide accumulation in affected areas (8). Clinical, radiologic, and scintigraphic findings are generally concordant. In some affected subjects, however, bone scans can be unremarkable despite considerable radiologic abnormality. This association seems to reflect advanced but "quiescent" disease (8). Markedly increased radioisotope accumulation with minimal radiologic findings can reflect early and active skeletal disease (8). MR and CT findings for cranial involvement have recently been described (9).

Laboratory Findings

Routine biochemical parameters of bone and mineral metabolism are typically normal, although serum alkaline phosphatase activity, urinary hydroxyproline levels, and

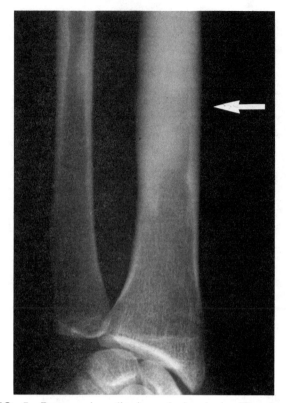

FIG. 5. *Progressive diaphyseal dysplasia (Engelmann disease).* The distal radius of this 20-year-old woman has a characteristic area of patchy thickening (*arrow*) of the periosteal and endosteal surface of the diaphysis.

the erythrocyte sedimentation rate are elevated in some individuals. Modest hypocalcemia and significant hypocalciuria occur in some affected subjects who have severe disease and appear to reflect their positive calcium balance (6). Mild anemia and leukopenia may also be present (5).

New bone formation is the characteristic feature of progressive diaphyseal dysplasia. Peripheral to the original bony cortex, disorganized newly formed woven bone undergoes centripetal maturation and then incorporation into the cortex (3). Electron microscopy of muscle has shown myopathic changes and vascular abnormalities (4).

Recently, aberrant differentiation of monocytes/macrophages to fibroblasts, and hence to osteoblasts, has been explored as a fundamental pathogenetic feature (10).

Etiology and Pathogenesis

Progressive diaphyseal dysplasia is caused by an autosomal gene defect that remains to be mapped and characterized. Some especially mild cases were reported to be an autosomal recessive condition; i.e., "Ribbing's disease" (11). However, sporadic cases do occur, and mild clinical forms can be transmitted as an autosomal dominant trait with variable penetrance.

The clinical and laboratory features of the disease when severe, together with its responsiveness to glucocorticoid treatment, have led some to suggest that progressive diaphyseal dysplasia is a systemic condition (i.e., an inflammatory connective tissue disease) (5).

Treatment

Progressive diaphyseal dysplasia is a chronic and somewhat unpredictable disorder (12). Symptoms may remit during adolescence or adulthood. Since its initial use in 1967 for this disorder, glucocorticoid therapy (typically prednisone given in small doses on an alternate day schedule) has become a well-documented effective treatment that can not only relieve bone pain but also normalize histologic abnormalities in affected bone (13). Complete relief of localized pain has followed surgical removal of the affected area of diaphysis by a "cortical window" (14).

REFERENCES

1. Cockayne EA: A case for diagnosis. *Proc R Soc Med* 13: 132–136, 1920
2. Engelmann G: Ein fall von osteopathia hyperostotica (sclerotisans) multiplex infantilis. *Fortschr Geb Roentgen* 39:1101–1106, 1929
3. Hundley JD, Wilson FC: Progressive diaphyseal dysplasia: review of the literature and report of seven cases in one family. *J Bone Joint Surg* 55(A):461–474, 1973
4. Naveh Y, Ludatshcer R, Alon U, et al.: Muscle involvement in progressive diaphyseal dysplasia. *Pediatrics* 76:944–949, 1985
5. Crisp AJ, Brenton DP: Engelmann's disease of bone—a systemic disorder? *Ann Rheum Dis* 41:183–188, 1982
6. Smith R, Walton RJ, Corner BD, et al.: Clinical and biochemical studies in Engelmann's disease (progressive diaphyseal dysplasia). *Q J Med* 46:273–294, 1977
7. Resnick D, Niwayama G: *Diagnosis of Bone and Joint Disorders 2nd ed.* WB Saunders, Philadelphia, 1988
8. Kumar B, Murphy WA, Whyte MP: Progressive diaphyseal dysplasia (Engelmann's disease): scintigraphic-radiologic-clinical correlations. *Radiology* 140:87–92, 1981
9. Applegate LJ, Applegate GR, Kemp SS: MR of multiple cranial neuropathies in a patient with Camurati-Engelmann disease: case report. *Am Soc Neuroradiol* 12:557–559, 1991
10. Labat ML, Bringuier AF, Séébold C, Moricard Y, Meyer-Mula C, Laporte P, Talmage RV, Grubb SA, Simmons DJ, Milhaud G: Monocytic origin of fibroblasts: spontaneous transformation of blood monocytes into neo-fibroblastic structures in osteomyelosclerosis and Engelmann's disease. *Biomed Pharmacother* 45:289–299, 1991
11. Shier CK, Krasicky GA, Ellis BI, Kottamasu SR: Ribbing's disease: radiographic-scintigraphic correlation and comparative analysis with Engelmann's disease. *J Nucl Med* 28:244–248, 1987
12. Kaftori JK, Kleinhaus U, Neveh Y: Progressive diaphyseal dysplasia (Camurati-Engelmann): radiographic follow-up and CT findings. *Radiology* 164:777–782, 1987
13. Naveh Y, Alon U, Kaftori JK, et al.: Progressive diaphyseal dysplasia: evaluation of corticosteroid therapy. *Pediatrics* 75: 321–323, 1985
14. Fallon MD, Whyte MP, Murphy WA: Progressive diaphyseal dysplasia (Engelmann's disease): report of a sporadic case of the mild form. *J Bone Joint Surg* 62(A):465–472, 1980

ENDOSTEAL HYPEROSTOSIS

In 1955, van Buchem and colleagues first described the entity *hyperostosis corticalis generalisata* (1). This report subsequently led to characterization of the disorders that are considered endosteal hyperostoses.

van Buchem Disease

This is an autosomal recessive, clinically severe condition (1) that is differentiated from an autosomal dominant, more mild, benign form of endosteal hyperostosis (Worth type) (1,2). Nevertheless, van Buchem disease is considerably less common than the cumulative number of reports in the literature might suggest (3).

Clinical Presentation

Van Buchem disease has been described in children and adults; sex distribution seems to be equal. Progressive asymmetrical enlargement of the jaw occurs during puberty. The mandibles of affected adults are markedly thickened with wide angles, but there is no prognathism, and dental malocclusion is uncommon. Affected subjects may be symptom-free; however, recurrent facial nerve palsy, deafness, and optic atrophy from narrowing of cranial foramina are common and can begin as early as infancy. Long bones may become painful with applied pressure, but they are not fragile, and joint range of motion is generally normal. Sclerosteosis had, until recently (4), been differentiated from van Buchem disease because affected subjects are excessively tall and have syndactyly (see later sections).

Radiologic Features

Endosteal cortical thickening that produces a dense and homogeneous diaphyseal cortex and narrows the medullary canal is the major radiologic feature of van Buchem disease. The hyperostosis is selectively endosteal; long bones are properly modeled. Generalized osteosclerosis also includes the base of the skull, facial bones, vertebrae, pelvis, and ribs. The mandible becomes enlarged (Fig. 6). Cranial CT findings have been reported (5).

Laboratory Findings

Alkaline phosphatase activity in serum is primarily of skeletal origin and may be increased; calcium and inorganic phosphate levels are unremarkable.

Van Buchem and colleagues suggested that the excessive bone was of essentially normal quality.

Etiology and Pathogenesis

Recently, evidence has been summarized that indicates that van Buchem disease and sclerosteosis reflect the same genetic defect so that their clinical/radiologic differences are explained by the epistatic effects of modifying genes (4).

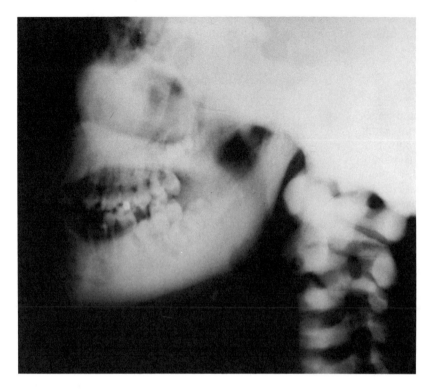

FIG. 6. *Endosteal hyperostosis.* Lateral radiograph of the mandible and facial bones of a 9-year-old boy with van Buchem disease shows dense sclerosis of all osseous structures. (Reproduced with permission from Whyte MP, Murphy WA: Osteopetrosis and other sclerosing bone disorders. In: Avioli LV, Krane SM (eds), *Metabolic Bone Disease, 2nd ed.* WB Saunders, Philadelphia, 1990.)

Treatment

There is no specific medical therapy. Surgical decompression of narrowed foramina may help to alleviate cranial nerve palsies (6). Surgery has also been used to recontour the mandible (7).

Sclerosteosis

Sclerosteosis (cortical hyperostosis with syndactyly), like van Buchem disease (see the preceding section), is an autosomal recessive form of endosteal hyperostosis. It occurs primarily in the Afrikaners of South Africa. Affected subjects who live elsewhere are also often of Dutch ancestry (4). Initially, sclerosteosis was distinguished from van Buchem disease by some radiographic differences and presence of syndactyly, but more recent studies suggest that both disorders are caused by the same primary gene defect (4).

Clinical Presentation

At birth, only syndactyly may be noted (8). During early childhood, there is overgrowth and attendant sclerosis of the skeleton that involves especially the skull and causes facial disfigurement. Affected subjects are tall and heavy beginning in childhood. Understandably, "gigantism" has been used to refer to their appearance. Deafness and facial palsy due to nerve entrapment are also presenting problems. The mandible has a rather square configuration.

Raised intracranial pressure and headache may be sequellae of a small cranial cavity. The brain stem can become compressed. Syndactyly from either cutaneous or bony fusion of the middle and index fingers is typical, but of variable severity. The fingernails are dysplastic. Patients are not prone to fracture and their intelligence is normal. Life expectancy may be shortened (9).

Radiologic Features

Except when syndactyly is present, the skeleton of sclerosteosis is normal in early childhood. The principal radiologic feature is progressive bony thickening that causes widening of the skull and prognathism (10). In the long bones, modeling defects occur and the cortices are thickened. Syndactyly, most often involving the index and long fingers, is common. The vertebral pedicles, ribs, pelvis, and tubular bones may also become somewhat dense. Computed tomography has shown fusion of the ossicles and narrowing of the internal auditory canals and cochlear aqueducts that can explain the associated deafness (5).

Histopathologic Findings

In an American kindred with sclerosteosis, histomorphometric analysis of the calvarium of an affected subject following *in vivo* tetracycline labeling showed dense thickened trabeculae and osteoidosis where the rate of bone formation was increased; osteoclastic bone resorption appeared to be quiescent (10).

Etiology and Pathogenesis

Enhanced osteoblast activity with failure of osteoclasts to compensate for the increased bone formation appears to explain the osteosclerosis of sclerosteosis (11). No abnormality of calcium homeostasis or of pituitary gland function has been documented (12). The pathogenesis of the neurological defects has been described in detail (11). A recent comparison of sclerosteosis and van Buchem disease suggests that both disorders are caused by abnormalities in the same gene and that the phenotypic variation results from epistatic effects of modifying genes (4).

Treatment

There is no specific medical treatment for sclerosteosis. Surgical correction of syndactyly is especially difficult if there is bony fusion; correction of syndactyly is especially difficult if there is bony fusion; correction of prognathism is complicated by dense mandibular bone. Management of associated neurological dysfunction has been reviewed (11).

REFERENCES

1. van Buchem FSP, Prick JJG, Jaspar HHJ: *Hyperostosis Corticalis Generalisata Familiaris* (Van Buchem's Disease). Excerpta, Amsterdam, 1976
2. Perez-Vicente Jr, Rodriguez de Castro E, Lafuente J, et al.: Autosomal dominant endosteal hyperostosis. Report of a Spanish family with neurological involvement. *Clin Genet* 31: 161–169, 1987
3. Eastman JR, Bixler D: Generalized cortical hyperostosis (van Buchem disease): nosologic considerations. *Radiology* 125: 297–304, 1977
4. Beighton P, Barnard A, Hamersma H, et al.: The syndromic status of sclerosteosis and van Buchem disease. *Clin Genet* 25: 175–181, 1984
5. Hill SC, Stein SA, Dwyer A, Altman J, Dorwart R, Doppman J: Cranial CT findings in sclerosteosis. *Am J Neuroradiol* 7: 505–511, 1986
6. Ruckert EW, Caudill RJ, McCready PJ: Surgical treatment of van Buchem disease. *J Oral Maxillofac Surg* 43:801–805, 1985
7. Schendel SA: van Buchem disease: surgical treatment of the mandible. *Ann Plast Surg* 20:462–467, 1988
8. Beighton P, Durr L, Hamersma H: The clinical features of sclerosteosis: a review of the manifestations in twenty-five affected individuals. *Ann Intern Med* 84:393–397, 1976
9. Barnard AH, Hamersma H, Kretzmar JH, et al.: Sclerosteosis in old age. *S Afr Med J* 58:401–403, 1980
10. Beighton P, Cremin BJ, Hamersma H: The radiology of sclerosteosis. *Br J Radiol* 49:934–939, 1976
11. Stein SA, Witkop C, Hill S, et al.: Sclerosteosis, neurogenetic and pathophysiologic analysis of an American kinship. *Neurology* 33:267–277, 1983
12. Epstein S, Hamersma H, Beighton P: Endocrine function in sclerosteosis. *S Afr Med J* 55:1105–1110, 1979

OSTEOPOIKILOSIS

Osteopoikilosis literally translated means "spotted bones." This condition is a radiologic curiosity that is transmitted as an autosomal dominant trait with a high degree of penetrance (1). Affected subjects in some kindreds may also have a form of connective tissue nevus called *dermatofibrosis lenticularis disseminata;* the disorder is then called the Buschke-Ollendorff syndrome (2). Although the bony lesions of osteopoikilosis are asymptomatic, incorrectly diagnosed patients may be subjected to rigorous and expensive studies for other important disorders including metastatic disease to the skeleton (3).

Clinical Presentation

Osteopoikilosis is typically an incidental discovery that follows a radiologic study. Musculoskeletal pain is described in many cases but is probably coincidental. The nevi usually involve the lower trunk or extremities and present before puberty; occasionally they are congenital. This dermatosis characteristically appears as small asymptomatic papules; however, they are sometimes yellow or white disks or plaques, deep nodules, or streaks (2).

Radiologic Features

The characteristic radiologic finding is numerous small foci of bony sclerosis in cancellous bone that are of variable shape (usually round or oval) (4). Commonly affected areas are the ends of the short tubular bones, the metaepiphyseal regions of the long bones, and the tarsal, carpal, and pelvic bones (Fig. 7). The foci are unchanged in shape and size for decades, but may mimic metastatic lesions. Radionuclide accumulation is not increased on bone scintigraphy (3).

Histopathologic Studies

Dermatofibrosis lenticularis disseminata is characterized by excessive amounts of unusually broad, markedly branched, interlacing elastin fibers in the dermis; the epidermis is normal (3).

The foci of osteosclerosis are thickened trabeculae that merge with surrounding normal bone, or islands of cortical bone that include Haversian systems. Mature lesions seem to be remodeling slowly (5).

Treatment

Osteopoikilosis does not require treatment. Nevertheless, family members at risk should be screened with a radiograph of the hand/wrist and knee after childhood and educated concerning the disorder.

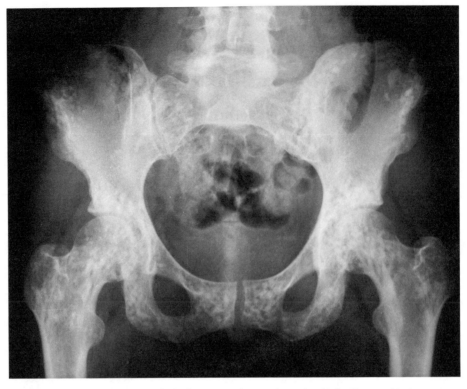

FIG. 7. *Osteopoikilosis.* Characteristic features shown here include the spotted appearance of the pelvis and metaepiphyseal regions of the femora. (Reproduced with permission from Whyte MP: Rare disorders of skeletal formation and homeostasis. In: Becker KN (ed), *Principles and Practice of Endocrinology and Metabolism,* JB Lippincott, Philadelphia, 1990.)

REFERENCES

1. Berlin R, Hedensio B, Lilja B, et al.: Osteopoikilosis—a clinical and genetic study. *Acta Med Scand* 18:305–314, 1967
2. Uitto J, Starcher BC, Santa-Cruz DJ, et al.: Biochemical and ultrastructural demonstration of elastin accumulation in the skin of the Buschke-Ollendorff syndrome. *J Invest Derm* 76:284–287, 1981
3. Whyte MP, Murphy WA, Seigel BA: 99m Tc-pyrophosphate bone imaging in osteopoikilosis, osteopathia striata, and melorheostosis. *Radiology* 127:439–443, 1978
4. Resnick D, Niwayama G: *Diagnosis of Bone and Joint Disorders, 2nd ed.* WB Saunders, Philadelphia, 1988
5. Lagier R, Mbakop A, Bigler A: Osteopoikilosis: a radiological and pathological study. *Skeletal Radiol* 11:161–168, 1984

OSTEOPATHIA STRIATA

Osteopathia striata is characterized by linear striations at the ends of long bones and in the ileum (1). Like osteopoikilosis, it is a radiographic curiosity when the skeletal findings occur alone. However, osteopathia striata is also a feature of a variety of clinically important syndromes including osteopathia striata with cranial sclerosis (2) and osteopathia striata with focal dermal hypoplasia (3).

Clinical Presentation

When osteopathia striata occurs alone, it is benign. This form can be transmitted as an autosomal dominant trait.

The musculoskeletal symptoms that may have led to the radiologic studies are probably unrelated. When there is cranial sclerosis, however, cranial nerve palsies are common (2). This clinical type is also inherited as an autosomal dominant trait.

Osteopathia striata with focal dermal hypoplasia (Goltz's syndrome) is a serious X-linked recessive condition in which affected boys have widespread linear areas of dermal hypoplasia through which adipose tissue can herniate. They also have a variety of additional bony defects in the limbs (3).

Radiologic Features

Gracile linear striations in the cancellous regions of the skeleton, particularly in the metaepiphyseal portions of the long bones and in the periphery of the iliac bones, is the characteristic radiologic finding (Fig. 8) (1). The carpal, tarsal, and tubular bones of the hands and feet are less commonly and more subtly affected. The striations will remain unchanged in appearance for years. Radionuclide accumulation is not increased during bone scintigraphy (4).

Histopathologic Findings

Histopathologic studies have not been described.

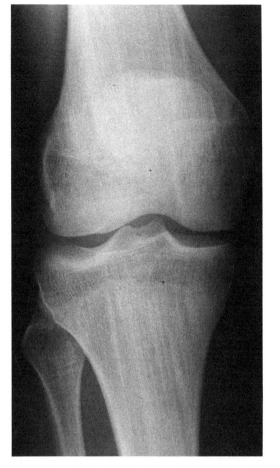

FIG. 8. *Osteopathia striata.* Characteristic longitudinal striations are present in the femur and tibia of this 17-year-old girl.

Treatment

Medical treatment for the osteopathia striata per se is not necessary. Although the characteristic skeletal findings are unlikely to be misdiagnosed, radiologic screening of individuals at risk would seem prudent after childhood.

In one family with osteopathia striata and cranial sclerosis, the diagnosis was reportedly made prenatally by ultrasound examination (5).

REFERENCES

1. Resnick D, Niwayama G: *Diagnosis of Bone and Joint Disorders 2nd ed.* WB Saunders, Philadelphia, 1988
2. Rabinow M, Unger F: Syndrome of osteopathia striata, macrocephaly, and cranial sclerosis. *Am J Dis Child* 138:821–823, 1984
3. Happle R, Lenz W: Striation of bones in focal dermal hypoplasia: manifestation of functional mosaicism? *Brit J Dermatol* 96:133–138, 1977
4. Whyte MP, Murphy WA, Seigel BA: 99m Tc-pyrophosphate bone imaging in osteopoikilosis, osteopathia striata, and melorheostosis. *Radiology* 127:439–443, 1978
5. Kornreich L, Grunebaum M, Ziv N, Shuper A, Mimouni M: Osteopathia striata, cranial sclerosis with cleft palate and facial nerve palsy. *Eur J Pediatr* 147:101–103, 1988

MELORHEOSTOSIS

Melorheostosis, from the Greek, refers to flowing hyperostosis of the limbs. The radiologic findings in the skeleton have been likened to the appearance of melted wax that has dripped down the side of a candle. Since its initial description in 1922 (1), about 200 cases have been reported (2,3). No Mendelian basis has been found; the disorder occurs sporadically.

Clinical Presentation

Melorheostosis typically manifests during childhood. Usually there is monomelic involvement; bilateral disease, when it occurs, is generally asymmetric. Cutaneous changes that overlie affected skeletal regions are not uncommon. Of 131 patients reported in one investigation, 17% had linear scleroderma-like areas and hypertrichosis. Fibromas, fibrolipomas, capillary hemangiomas, lymphangiectasis, and arterial aneurysms also occur (4,5). Soft tissue abnormalities are often noted before the hyperostosis is discovered. Pain and stiffness are the major symptoms. Affected joints may become contracted and deformed. In affected children, leg length inequality occurs from soft tissue contractures and premature fusion of epiphyses. The skeletal changes appear to progress most rapidly during childhood. During the adult years, melorheostosis may gradually extend or not progress (6). Nevertheless, pain is a more frequent symptom in adults because of subperiosteal new bone formation.

Radiologic Features

Irregular, dense, eccentric hyperostosis that affects both the cortex and the adjacent medullary canal of a single bone, or several adjacent bones, is the characteristic radiologic finding in melorheostosis (Fig. 9) (3,7). Any anatomic region or bone may be affected, but the lower extremities are most commonly involved. Bone tissue may also develop in soft tissues that are adjacent to involved skeletal areas, particularly near joints. Melorheostotic bone has increased blood flow and avidly accumulates radionuclide during bone scintigraphy (8).

Laboratory Findings

Routine laboratory studies—e.g., serum calcium and inorganic phosphate levels and alkaline phosphatase activity—are normal in melorheostosis.

Histologic Findings

The skeletal lesion in melorheostosis is characterized by endosteal thickening during infancy and childhood and then periosteal new bone formation during adulthood (3). Bony lesions are sclerotic with thickened irregular lamellae that may occlude Haversian systems. Marrow fibrosis

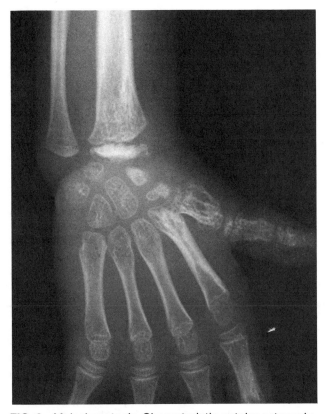

FIG. 9. *Melorheostosis.* Characteristic patchy osteosclerosis is most apparent in the radius and second metacarpal of this 8-year-old girl.

may also be present (3). Unlike in true scleroderma, the collagen of the sclerodermatous skin lesions of melorheostosis is normal appearing. Thus, this dermatosis has been called "linear melorheostotic scleroderma" (4,9).

Etiology and Pathogenesis

The distribution of melorheostosis and its associated soft tissue lesions in sclerotomes, myotomes, and dermatomes suggests that a segmentary embryogenetic defect explains this sporadic condition (4,9). The linear scleroderma may reflect the primary abnormality that extends deep into the skeleton to cause the hyperostosis.

Treatment

Surgical correction of contractures has been difficult; recurrent deformity is common. Recently, distraction techniques have given promising results (10).

REFERENCES

1. Léri A, Joanny J: Une affection non decrite des os. Hyperostose "en coulée" sur toute la longueur d'un membre ou "melorheostose." *Bul Mem Soc Hop Paris* 46:1141–1145, 1922

2. Murray RO, McCredie J: Melorheostosis and sclerotomes: a radiological correlation. *Skeletal Radiol* 4:57–71, 1979
3. Campbell CJ, Papademetriou T, Bonfiglio M: Melorheostosis: a report of the clinical, roentgenographic, and pathological findings in fourteen cases. *J Bone Joint Surg.* 50(A):1281–1304, 1968
4. Miyachi Y, Horio T, Yamada A, et al.: Linear melorheostotic scleroderma with hypertrichosis. *Arch Dermatol* 115:1233–1234, 1979
5. Applebaum RE, Caniano DA, Sun C-C, et al.: Synchronous left subclavian and axillary artery aneurysms associated with melorheostosis. *Surgery* 99:249–253, 1986
6. Colavita N, Nicolais S, Orazi C, Falappa PG: Melorheostosis: presentation of a case followed up for 24 years. *Arch Orthop Trauma Surg.* 106:123–125, 1987
7. Resnick D, Niwayama G: *Diagnosis of Bone and Joint Disorders, 2nd ed.* WB Saunders, Philadelphia, 1988
8. Davis DC, Syklawer R, Cole RL: Melorheostosis on three-phase bone scintigraphy: case report. *Clin Nuc Med* 17:561–564, 1992
9. Wagers LT, Young AW Jr, Ryan SF: Linear melorheostotic scleroderma. *Br J Dermatol* 86:297–301, 1972
10. Atar D, Lehman WB, Grant AD, Strongwater AM: The Ilizarov apparatus for treatment of melorheostosis: case report and review of the literature. *Clin Orthop* 281:163–167, 1992

MIXED SCLEROSING BONE DYSTROPHY

Mixed sclerosing bone dystrophy is a rare skeletal dysplasia in which radiologic features of osteopoikilosis, osteopathia striata, melorheostosis, cranial sclerosis, and additional skeletal defects occur together in various combinations in one individual (1).

Clinical Presentation

Patients may experience the symptoms and complications that are typically associated with the individual patterns of osteosclerosis; e.g., cranial sclerosis with skull enlargement may result in cranial nerve palsy, and melorheostosis can cause bone pain, etc. (1).

Radiologic Features

Two or more patterns of osteosclerosis—i.e., osteopoikilosis, osteopathia striata, melorheostosis, cranial sclerosis, generalized cortical hyperostosis, focal osteosclerosis, or progressive diaphyseal dysplasia—occur in one individual. Just a portion of the skeleton may be affected. Bone scanning shows increased radionuclide uptake in the areas where osteosclerosis is greatest (1,2).

Histopathologic Findings

Although the term "osteopetrosis" has been used to describe the generalized osteosclerosis in some subjects, histopathologic study has failed to show remnants of calcified primary spongiosa (see the Osteopetrosis section) (1,2).

Etiology and Pathogenesis

Delineation of mixed sclerosing bone dystrophy suggests a common pathogenesis for the individual component osteosclerotic patterns. However, osteopoikilosis and most forms of osteopathia striata are clearly heritable, whereas mixed sclerosing bone dystrophy in its most florid presentation, like melorheostosis, appears to be a sporadic disorder (1,2).

Treatment

There is no specific medical treatment. Contractures or neurovascular compression by osteosclerotic lesions may require surgical intervention.

REFERENCES

1. Whyte MP, Murphy WA, Fallon MD, et al.: Mixed-sclerosing-bone-dystrophy: report of a case and review of the literature. *Skeletal Radiol* 6:95–102, 1981
2. Pacifici R, Murphy WA, Teitelbaum SL, Whyte MP: Mixed-sclerosing-bone-dystrophy: 42-year follow-up of a case reported as osteopetrosis. *Calcif Tissue Int* 38:175–185, 1986

AXIAL OSTEOMALACIA

Axial osteomalacia is characterized radiologically by coarsening of the trabecular pattern of the axial but not appendicular skeleton (1). Fewer than 20 patients have been described. Most affected subjects appear to have been sporadic cases, but dominant transmission has been reported (2); thus, additional family studies are necessary.

Clinical Presentation

Most subjects with axial osteomalacia have been middle-aged or elderly men; a few middle-aged women have been described. Radiologic manifestations, however, are likely to be detectable much earlier (2). The majority of cases have presented with dull, vague, and chronic axial skeletal pain (often in the cervical region) that prompts radiologic study. Family histories are usually negative for skeletal disease.

Radiologic Features

Abnormalities are limited essentially to the spine and pelvis, where trabeculae are coarsened and form a pattern like in other types of osteomalacia (3). However, Looser's zones (a radiologic hallmark of osteomalacia) have not been reported. The cervical spine and ribs seem most severely affected; the lumbar spine is abnormal to a lesser degree. Two affected subjects had features of ankylosing spondylitis (4). Radiologic survey of the appendicular skeleton is unremarkable.

Laboratory Studies

In four patients, serum inorganic phosphate levels tended to be low (4). In others osteomalacia occurred despite normal serum levels of calcium, inorganic phosphate, 25OHD, and 1,25(OH)$_2$D. Serum alkaline phosphatase activity (bone isoenzyme) may be increased.

Histopathologic Findings

Iliac crest specimens have distinct corticomedullary junctions, but the cortices can be especially wide and porous. Trabeculae are of variable thickness; total bone volume may be increased. Collagen has a normal lamellar pattern on polarized-light microscopy. There is increased width and extent of osteoid seams on trabecular bone surfaces and in cortical spaces. Tetracycline labeling confirms the defective skeletal mineralization and results in fluorescent "labels" that are single, irregular, and wide (2). Osteoblasts are flat and inactive-appearing "lining" cells with reduced Golgi zones, and rough endoplasmic reticulum and increased amounts of cytoplasmic glycogen, but they do stain intensely for alkaline phosphatase activity. Changes of secondary hyperparathyroidism are absent (2).

Etiology and Pathogenesis

Axial osteomalacia has been postulated to result from an osteoblast defect (5). Electron microscopic studies of iliac crest bone from one affected subject (2) revealed osteoblasts that had an inactive appearance but were able to form matrix vesicles within abundant osteoid.

Treatment

Effective medical therapy has not been reported. The natural history for axial osteomalacia, however, seems relatively benign. Methyltestosterone and stilbestrol has been tested unsuccessfully (5). Vitamin D$_2$ (as much as 20,000 units/day for three years) was similarly without beneficial effect (5). Slight improvement in skeletal histology, but not in symptoms, was reported for calcium and vitamin D$_2$ therapy in a study of four cases (4). Long-term follow-up of one patient showed that symptoms and radiologic findings did not change (5).

REFERENCES

1. Frame B, Frost HM, Ormond RS, et al.: Atypical axial osteomalacia involving the axial skeleton. *Ann Int Med* 55:632–639, 1961
2. Whyte MP, Fallon MD, Murphy WA, et al.: Axial osteomalacia: clinical, laboratory and genetic investigation of an affected mother and son. *Am J Med* 71:1041–1049, 1981
3. Christman D, Wenger JJ, Dosch JC, et al.: L'osteomalacie axiale: analyse compare avec la fibrogenese imparfaite. *J Radiol* 62: 37–41, 1981
4. Nelson AM, Riggs BL, Jowsey JO: Atypical axial osteomalacia:

report of four cases with two having features of ankylosing spondylitis. *Arthritis Rheum* 21:715–722, 1978

5. Condon JR, Nassim JR: Axial osteomalacia. *Postgrad Med* 47: 817–820, 1971

FIBROGENESIS IMPERFECTA OSSIUM

Fibrogenesis imperfecta ossium was first described in 1950 (1). Fewer than 10 cases have been reported (2,3). Although radiologic studies suggest that there is generalized osteopenia, the coarse and dense appearance of trabecular bone explains why it is included among the osteosclerotic disorders. The clinical, biochemical, radiologic, and histopathologic features of fibrogenesis imperfecta ossium and axial osteomalacia have been carefully contrasted (1).

Clinical Presentation

Fibrogenesis imperfecta ossium typically presents during middle-age or later. Both sexes are affected. Gradual onset of intractable skeletal pain that rapidly progresses is the characteristic symptom that precedes a debilitating course with progressive immobility. Spontaneous fractures are also a prominent clinical feature. Patients generally become bedridden. Physical examination typically shows marked bony tenderness.

Radiologic Features

Radiologic changes are noted throughout the skeleton, except in the skull. Initially, there may be only osteopenia and a slightly abnormal appearance of trabecular bone (3). Subsequently, the changes become more consistent with osteomalacia; i.e., further alterations of the trabecular bone pattern, heterogeneous bone density, and thinning of cortical bone. The corticomedullary junctions become indistinct as cortices are replaced by an abnormal pattern of trabecular bone. Areas of the skeleton may have a mixed lytic and sclerotic appearance (1–3). The generalized osteopenia causes the remaining trabeculae to appear coarse and dense in a "fish-net" pattern. Pseudofractures may develop. Deformities secondary to fractures can be present, although bony contours are typically normal. Some patients have a "rugger-jersey" spine that should not be confused with a similar radiographic finding in osteopetrosis or in renal osteodystrophy. The shafts of long bones may show periosteal reaction. In fibrogenesis imperfecta ossium and axial osteomalacia, the distribution of the radiographic abnormalities (generalized versus axial) helps to distinguish the two conditions. However, the histopathologic features are also clearly different (1).

Laboratory Findings

Serum calcium and inorganic phosphate levels are normal, but alkaline phosphatase activity is increased. Acute agranulocytosis and macroglobulinemia have been reported. Hydroxyproline levels in urine may be normal or increased (3). Typically, there is no aminoaciduria or other evidence of renal tubular dysfunction.

Histopathologic Findings

The bony lesion is a form of osteomalacia, although the amount of affected bone varies considerably from area to area (3). Aberrant collagen is found in regions with abnormal mineralization patterns but is unremarkable in other tissues. Cortical bone in the shaft of the femora and tibiae may demonstrate the least abnormality. Osteoid seams are thick. Osteoblasts and osteoclasts can be abundant. Polarized-light microscopy shows that the abnormal bone collagen fibrils lack birefringence. Electron microscopy reveals that the collagen fibrils are thin and randomly organized in a "tangled pattern." In some regions, peculiar circular matrix structures of 300–500 nm diameter have been noted (3). Unless bone specimens are viewed with polarized-light or electron microscopy, fibrogenesis imperfecta ossium can be mistaken for osteoporosis or other forms of osteomalacia (3).

Etiology and Pathogenesis

The etiology is unknown. Genetic factors have not been implicated, since this condition has been reported only sporadically. It seems to be an acquired disorder of collagen synthesis in lamellar bone. Subperiosteal bone formation and collagen synthesis in nonosseous tissues appears to be normal.

Treatment

There is no specific medical therapy. Temporary clinical improvement may occur (3). Treatment with vitamin D_2 (or an active metabolite) together with calcium supplementation has been tried without significant benefit. Indeed, ectopic calcification occurred with high-dose vitamin D_2 therapy in one affected subject. Synthetic salmon calcitonin, sodium fluoride, and $24,25(OH)_2D$ have also been tested, but without apparent benefit (3). Treatment with melphalan and prednisolone appeared to benefit one patient (4).

REFERENCES

1. Christman D, Wenger JJ, Dosch JC, et al.: L'osteomalacie axiale analyse compare avec la fibrogenese imparfaite. *J Radiol* 62: 37–41, 1981
2. Swan CHJ, Shah K, Brewer DB, et al.: Fibrogenesis imperfecta ossium. *Q J Med* 45:233–253, 1976
3. Lang R, Vignery AM, Jenson PS: Fibrogenesis imperfecta ossium with early onset: observations after 20 years of illness. *Bone* 7: 237–246, 1986
4. Ralphs JR, Stamp TCB, Dopping-Hepenstal PJC, Ali SY: Ultrastructural features of the osteoid of patients with fibrogenesis imperfecta ossium. *Bone* 10:243–249, 1989

PACHYDERMOPERIOSTOSIS

Pachydermoperiostosis (hypertrophic osteoarthropathy: primary or idiopathic) causes clubbing of the digits, hyperhydrosis and thickening of the skin of especially the face and forehead, and periosteal new bone formation that occurs prominently in the distal limbs. Autosomal dominant inheritance with variable expression is established (1), but autosomal recessive transmission also seems to occur (2).

Clinical Presentation

Men appear to be more severely affected than women, and blacks more commonly than whites. The age at presentation is variable, but symptoms typically first manifest during adolescence (1,2). All three principal features (pachydermia, *cutis verticis gyrata,* periostitis) are present in some affected individuals; others have just one or two of these findings. Clinical expression develops during the course of a decade, but the disorder then becomes quiescent (3). Progressive gradual enlargement of the hands and feet can result in a "pawlike" appearance. Some patients are described as acromegalic. Arthralgias of the ankles, knees, wrists, and elbows are common. Occasionally, the small joints are also painful. Acroosteolysis has also been reported. Symptoms of pseudogout can occur. Chondrocalcinosis, with calcium pyrophosphate crystals in synovial fluid, has been found in one affected subject. Stiffness and limited mobility of both the appendicular and the axial skeleton can develop. Compression of cranial or spinal nerves has been described. Cutaneous changes include coarsening, thickening, furrowing, pitting, and oiliness of especially the scalp and face. Fatigue is not uncommon. Myelophthisic anemia with extramedullary hematopoiesis may occur. Life expectancy is normal (3).

Radiologic Features

Severe periostitis that thickens and scleroses the distal portions of the tubular bones—typically the tibia, fibula, radius, and ulna—is the principal radiologic abnormality (Fig. 10). The metacarpals, tarsal/metatarsals, clavicles, pelvis, base of the skull, and phalanges may also be affected. Clubbing is obvious, and acroosteolysis can occur. The spine is rarely involved. Ankylosis of joints, especially in the hands and in the feet, may occur in older affected individuals (4).

The principal consideration in the differential diagnosis for pachydermoperiostosis is secondary hypertrophic osteoarthropathy (pulmonary or otherwise). The radiologic features of this condition are, however, somewhat different. In secondary hypertrophic osteoarthropathy, the periosteal reaction typically has a smooth, undulating appearance (5). In pachydermoperiostosis, periosteal proliferation is more exuberant, has an irregular appearance, and often involves epiphyses. Bone scanning in either

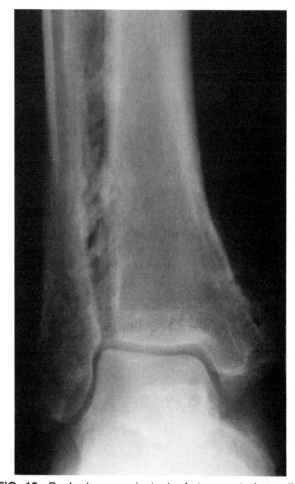

FIG. 10. *Pachydermoperiostosis.* Anteroposterior radiograph of the ankle shows ragged periosteal reaction along the interosseous membrane between the tibia and fibula (note also the proliferative bone formation along the medial malleolus). (Reproduced with permission from Whyte MP: Rare disorders of skeletal formation and homeostasis. In: Becker KN (ed), *Principles and Practice of Endocrinology and Metabolism,* JB Lippincott, Philadelphia, 1990.)

condition reveals symmetrical, diffuse, regular uptake along the cortical margins of long bones, especially in the legs. This feature results in a "double stripe" sign.

Laboratory Findings

Synovial fluid examination typically does not reveal evidence of inflammation.

Periosteal new bone formation roughens the surface of cortical bone (6). This newly formed osseous tissue undergoes cancellous compaction and can accordingly be difficult to distinguish from the original cortex (6). However, there may be osteopenia of trabecular bone from quiescent formation (4). Mild cellular hyperplasia and thickening of subsynovial blood vessels is found near synovial membranes (7). Electron microscopy demonstrates layered basement membranes.

Etiology and Pathogenesis

No gene defects have been identified. A controversial hypothesis suggests that some unknown circulating factor acts on the vasculature initially to cause hypermia and thereby alters soft tissues, but later blood flow is reduced (2).

Treatment

There is no established medical treatment. Painful synovial effusions may respond to nonsteroidal antiinflammatory drugs (8). Colchicine was reported to be an effective medication for arthralgias, clubbing, folliculitis, and pachyderma in one affected subject (9). Contractures or neurovascular compression by osteosclerotic lesions may require surgical intervention.

REFERENCES

1. Rimoin DL: Pachydermoperiostosis (idiopathic clubbing and periostosis). Genetic and physiologic considerations. *N Engl J Med* 272:923–931, 1965
2. Matucci-Cerinic M, Lott T, Jajic IVO, Pignone A, Bussani C, Cagnoni M: The clinical spectrum of pachydermoperiostosis (primary hypertrophic osteoarthropathy). *Medicine* 79:208–214, 1991
3. Herman MA, Massaro D, Katz S: Pachydermoperiostosis—clinical spectrum. *Arch Intern Med* 116:919–923, 1965
4. Resnick D, Niwayama G: *Diagnosis of Bone and Joint Disorders, 2nd ed.* WB Saunders, Philadellphia, 1988
5. Ali A, Tetalman M, Fordham EW: Distribution of hypertrophic pulmonary osteoarthropathy. *Am J Roentgenol* 134:771–780, 1980
6. Vogl A, Goldfischer S: Pachydermoperiostosis: primary or idiopathic hypertrophic osteoarthropathy. *Am J Med* 33:166–187, 1962
7. Lauter SA, Vasey FB, Hüttner I, et al.: Pachydermoperiostosis: studies on the synovium. *J Rheumatol* 5:85–95, 1978
8. Cooper RG, Freemont AJ, Riley M, Holt PJL, Anderson DC, Jayson MIV: Bone abnormalities and severe arthritis in pachydermoperiostosis. *Ann Rheum Dis* 51:416–419, 1992
9. Matucci-Cerinic M, Fattorini L, Gerini G, Lombardi A, Pignone A, Petrini N, Lotti T: Cochicine treatment in a case of pachydermoperiostosis with acroosteolysis. *Rheumatol Int* 8:185–188, 1988

OTHER SCLEROSING BONE DYSPLASIAS

Table 1 lists the relatively large number of conditions that cause focal or generalized increases in skeletal mass (1). Of note, sarcoidosis characteristically causes cysts within coarsely reticulated bone; occasionally, however, sclerotic areas are found in the axial skeleton or in long tubular bones. These skeletal changes may occur well after the pulmonary disease is arrested. Although multiple myeloma typically presents with generalized osteopenia or with discrete osteolytic lesions, widespread osteosclerosis can occur. Lymphoma, myelosclerosis, and mastocytosis are additional hematologic causes of increased bone mass. Metastatic carcinoma, primarily prostatic, commonly causes osteosclerosis. Diffuse osteosclerosis is also a relatively frequent radiologic finding in secondary hyperparathyroidism (as with renal disease), but it can occur in primary hyperparathyroidism as well. Intoxication with vitamin A or vitamin D, heavy metal poisoning, milk-alkali syndrome, ionizing radiation, osteomyelitis, and osteonecrosis are additional etiologies for increased bone mass (1).

REFERENCE

1. Frame B, Honasoge M, Kottamasu SR: *Osteosclerosis, Hyperostosis, and Related Disorders.* Elsevier, New York, 1987

76. Fibrous Dysplasia

Michael P. Whyte, M.D.

Metabolic Research Unit, Shriners Hospital for Crippled Children, and Division of Bone and Mineral Diseases, The Jewish Hospital of St. Louis, Washington University School of Medicine; St. Louis, Missouri

Fibrous dysplasia is a sporadic developmental condition that is characterized by a unifocal or multifocal expanding fibrous lesion of bone-forming mesenchyme. The disorder affects either sex and often results in fracture and/or deformity.

McCune-Albright syndrome refers to subjects with fibrous dysplasia (generally polyostotic) and café-au-lait spots who also have hyperfunction of one or more endocrine glands. Recently, somatic mosaicism for "activating" mutations in the Gsα subunit of the receptor/adenylate cyclase-coupling G protein was discovered to cause this form of fibrous dysplasia (see the following).

Clinical Presentation

Mono-ostotic fibrous dysplasia characteristically develops during the second or third decade of life; polyostotic disease typically manifests before 10 yr of age (1). Mono-ostotic fibrous dysplasia is more common than the polyostotic variety. Typically, an expansile bony lesion causes fracture or deformity and may occasionally entrap nerves. The skull and long bones are affected most often. Sarcomatous degeneration of involved skeletal sites occurs with somewhat increased frequency (incidence <1%), especially when the facial bones or femora are involved (2). Pregnancy may "reactivate" previously quiescent lesions (3).

In the McCune-Albright syndrome, café-au-lait spots are characteristic hyperpigmented macules with a rough border (Fig. 1), as opposed to a smooth border in neurofibromatosis (i.e., "Coast-of-Maine" versus "Coast-of-California," respectively). Typically, the endocrinopathy is pseudoprecocious puberty in girls. Less commonly, thyrotoxicosis, Cushing's syndrome, acromegaly, hyperprolactinemia, hyperparathyroidism, or pseudoprecocious puberty in boys can occur (4). In rare individuals who have very widespread bony lesions, renal phosphate wasting causes hypophosphatemic bone disease and, therefore, resembles "oncogenic" forms of rickets or osteomalacia (5).

Radiologic Features

The femora, tibiae, ribs, and facial bones are involved most frequently, but any skeletal site can be affected (6). Small bones show radiographic features in about 50% of individuals who have polyostotic disease. In the long bones, the lesions may be found either in the metaphysis or in the diaphysis. They are typically well defined and are characterized by thin cortices and a "ground glass" appearance (Fig. 2). Occasionally, they are lobulated with trabeculated areas of radiolucency.

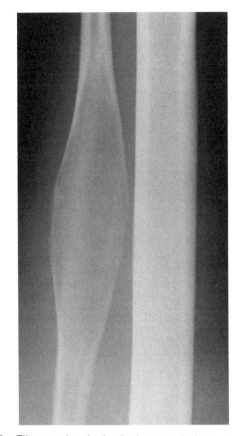

FIG. 2. *Fibrous dysplasia.* A characteristic expansile lesion with ground glass appearance has caused thinning of the cortex in the mid-diaphyseal region of the right fibula of this young man.

Laboratory Findings

Although serum alkaline phosphatase activity may be elevated, calcium and inorganic phosphate levels are typically normal.

Both mono-ostotic and polyostotic lesions have a similar histological appearance. They are anatomically well defined but are not encapsulated. Characteristically, spindle-shaped fibroblasts occur in a "swirled" formation within marrow spaces. Haphazardly arranged trabeculae are composed of woven bone. Cartilaginous tissue is found within lesions more often when there is polyostotic involvement. Cystic regions, which are lined by multinucleated giant cells, may also be present. These findings resemble the histopathologic changes found in hyperparathyroidism (osteitis fibrosa cystica), but an important distinction is that osteoblasts are absent in fibrous dysplasia rather than plentiful as in hyperparathyroid bone disease.

Etiology and Pathogenesis

Whether fibrous dysplasia is caused by the same "activating" mutation in the Gsα subunit discovered in 1991 in the McCune-Albright syndrome (7) should soon be known. The skeletal lesion appears to result from the for-

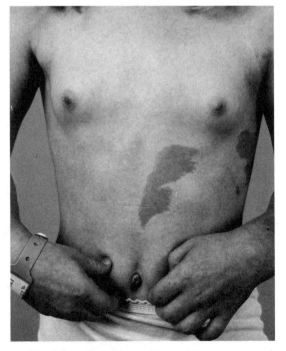

FIG. 1. *McCune-Albright syndrome.* Characteristic café-au-lait spots (rough border) are present on the left abdomen and chest of this $3^{10}/_{12}$ year old girl who also has obvious precocious breast development.

mation of imperfect bone because mesenchymal cells do not fully differentiate to osteoblasts. Endocrine hyperfunction in the McCune-Albright syndrome has been ascribed to end-organ hyperactivity (4,8). Recent studies of growth hormone and prolactin hypersecretion in this syndrome suggest that some affected subjects have abnormal hypothalamic regulation and/or an embryological abnormality in pituitary cell differentiation and function (8).

Treatment

There is no specific medical treatment for the skeletal disease of fibrous dysplasia; spontaneous healing of the bone lesions does not occur. In most subjects with mild disease, the radiologic appearance of bone defects does not change. In more severe cases, individual lesions may progress, and new ones can appear. Fractures generally mend well. Nevertheless, stress or fissure fractures may be difficult to detect and treat. When the skull is involved, neurological assessment and careful follow-up is necessary since nerve compression may require surgical intervention. In the McCune-Albright syndrome, the aromatase inhibitor testolactone appears to control the precocious puberty of affected girls (9). Calcitriol and inorganic phosphate supplementation has not been thoroughly evaluated for the rare occurrence of hypophosphatemic bone disease.

REFERENCES

1. Harris WH, Dudley HR Jr, Barry RJ: The natural history of fibrous dysplasia: an orthopedic, pathological and roentgenographic study. *J Bone Joint Surg* 44(A):207–233, 1962
2. Johnson CB, Gilbert EF, Gottlieb LI: Malignant transformation of polyostotic fibrous dysplasia. *South Med J* 72:353–356, 1979
3. Kaplan FS, Fallon MD, Boden SD, Schmidt R, Senior M, Haddad JG: Estrogen receptors in bone in a patient with polyostotic fibrous dysplasia (McCune-Albright Syndrome). *N Engl J Med* 319:241–245, 1988
4. Harris RI; Polyostotic fibrous dysplasia with acromegaly. *Am J Med* 78:538–542, 1985
5. Lever EG, Pettingale KW: Albright's syndrome associated with a soft-tissue myxoma and hypophosphatemic osteomalacia. Report of a case and review of the literature. *J Bone Joint Surg* 65(B):621–626, 1983
6. Resnick D, Niwayama G: *Diagnosis of Bone land Joint Disorders, 2nd ed.* WB Saunders, Philadelphia, 1988
7. Weinstein LS, Shenker A, Gejman PV, Merino MJ, Friedman E, Spiegel AM: Activating mutations of the stimulatory G protein in the McCune-Albright syndrome. *New Engl J Med* 325:1688–1695, 1991
8. Cuttler L, Jackson JA, Saeed uz-Zafar M, Levitsky LL, Mellinger RC, Frohman LA: Hypersecretion of growth hormone and prolactin in McCune-Albright Syndrome. *J Clin Endocrinol Metab* 68:1148–1154, 1989
9. Feuillan PP, Foster CM, Pescovitz OH, Hench KD, Shawker T, Dwyer A, Malley JD, Barnes K, Loriaux DL, Cutler GB Jr: Treatment of precocious puberty in the McCune-Albright syndrome with the aromatose inhibitor testolactone. *N Engl J Med* 315:1115–1119, 1986

77. Osteogenesis Imperfecta

Michael P. Whyte, M.D.

Metabolic Research Unit, Shriners Hospital for Crippled Children, and Division of Bone and Mineral Diseases, The Jewish Hospital of St. Louis, Washington University School of Medicine; St. Louis, Missouri

Osteogenesis imperfecta ("brittle bone disease") is a heritable disorder of connective tissue in which the pathogenesis of nearly all clinical types (Table 1) appears to involve an abnormality in the synthesis or structure of type I collagen (1,2). Type I collagen is the most abundant protein in bone matrix but is also found in ligaments, skin, sclerae, teeth, and elsewhere (1). The cardinal clinical feature of osteogenesis imperfecta is osteopenia that is associated with recurrent fracture and skeletal deformity (3). However, many affected subjects also have dental disease caused by defects in the formation of dentin (dentinogenesis imperfecta), as well as abnormalities of other tissues that contain type I collagen. The severity of clinical expression is extremely variable, however, and ranges from stillbirth to lifelong absence of symptoms (1,3). The classification system devised by Sillence according to clinical/hereditary types has been useful in providing a framework for prognostication and a foundation for further biochemical/molecular studies (4). However, this nosology proved to have significant limitations, and recent molecular findings provide important new interpretations for the modes of inheritance. The clinical heterogeneity of osteogenesis imperfecta is now being better understood by identification of a great variety of molecular defects within the genes that encode the two protein components (the pro-α_1 and pro-α_2 chains) of the type I collagen heterotrimer (1,2). These genetic studies have altered our understanding of the transmission patterns for especially the severe clinical forms (1,5).

Clinical Presentation

The severity of clinical expression of osteogenesis imperfecta (Table 1) is extremely variable (1,3). This diversity can be manifested even among affected individuals in a single family or kindred. The cardinal feature is generalized osteopenia that predisposes to recurrent fracture of long bones and vertebrae, often with subsequent deformity. Generalized osteopenia during childhood may be

TABLE 1. *Clinical heterogeneity and biochemical defects in osteogenesis imperfecta[a]*

OI type	Clinical features	Inheritance[b]	Biochemical defects
I	Normal stature, little or no deformity, blue scleras, hearing loss in about 50% of individuals; dentinogenesis imperfecta is rare and may distinguish a subset.	AD	Decreased production of type I procollagen Substitution for residue other than glycine in triple helix of $\alpha 1(I)$
II	Lethal in the perinatal period, minimal calvarial mineralization, beaded ribs, compressed femurs, marked long bone deformity, platyspondyly.	AD (new mutation)	Rearrangements in the COL1A1 and COL1A2 genes Substitutions for glycyl residues in the triple-helical domain of the $\alpha 1(I)$ $\alpha 2(I)$ chain
		AR (rare)	Small deletion in $\alpha 2(I)$ on the background of a null allele
III	Progressively deforming bones, usually with moderate deformity at birth. Scleras variable in hue, often lighten with age. Dentinogenesis imperfecta common, hearing loss common. Stature very short.	AR	Frameshift mutation that prevents incorporation of pro$\alpha 2(I)$ into molecules (Noncollagenous defects)
		AD	Point mutations in the $\alpha 1(I)$ or $\alpha 2(I)$ chain
IV	Normal scleras, mild to moderate bone deformity and variable short stature, dentinogenesis imperfecta is common, and hearing loss occurs in some.	AD	Point mutations in the $\alpha 2(I)$ chain Rarely, point mutations in the $\alpha 1(I)$ chain Small deletions in the $\alpha 2(I)$ chain

[a] Reproduced with permission from Byers PH: Disorders of collagen biosynthesis and structure. In: Scriver CR, Beaudet AL, Sly WS, Valle D (eds), *The Metabolic Basis of Inherited Disease,* 6th edition, McGraw Hill, New York, 2805–2842, 1989.

[b] AD, autosomal dominant; AR, autosomal recessive.

due to idiopathic juvenile osteoporosis, Cushing's disease, and a variety of other conditions. The differential diagnosis of multiple fractures in infants and children includes child abuse and congenital indifference to pain. However, because of the underlying biochemical defect that affects type I collagen biosynthesis, subjects with osteogenesis imperfecta can usually be distinguished readily by clinical features. They may manifest ligamentous laxity with joint hypermobility, excessive diaphoresis, easy bruisability, dentinogenesis imperfecta that causes fragile and discolored teeth, and hearing loss that occurs in about 50% of affected individuals younger than age 30 yr and in nearly all patients who are older (6). Deafness is typically from conductive or mixed pathogenesis but less commonly results from sensorineural disease (6). Often the sclerae have a blue or grey tint (Fig. 1). Other signs and symptoms that reflect relatively severe disease include a high-pitched voice, short stature, scoliosis, herniae, a head that appears to be disproportionately large compared to body size, and a triangular-shaped face. Thoracic deformity results in predisposition to pulmonary infection that can be life-threatening in severe cases. Mitral valve clicks are not uncommon, but cardiac disease is unusual. Subjects with even the most deforming skeletal disease are generally of normal intelligence.

Clinical Types

The classification scheme for osteogenesis imperfecta devised by Sillence was based upon the clinical phenotype

and apparent mode of inheritance (4). This nosology remains useful but has been greatly clarified by revelations concerning the heterogeneous biochemical/molecular lesions and modes of transmission, especially for the more severe types (Table 1).

Type I patients typically have bluish coloration of the sclerae that is especially prominent during childhood, relatively mild osteopenia with recurrent fracture (deformity is uncommon or mild), and deafness that first manifests during early adulthood (30% incidence). They are typically of normal height. Elderly women with this mild form of osteogenesis imperfecta can be mistaken as having postmenopausal or "involutional" osteoporosis if they present with fracture during late adult life since radiologic findings are unlikely to distinguish the two disorders. Undecalcified specimens of bone, however, may reveal increased numbers of cortical osteocytes compared to specimens obtained from patients with osteoporosis (7,8). This form of osteogenesis imperfecta has been subdivided into type I-A and type I-B depending upon the absence or (more rarely) the presence, respectively, of dentinogenesis imperfecta. Type I osteogenesis imperfecta is transmitted as an autosomal dominant disorder. However, approximately one-third of cases are new mutations.

Type II disease is often fatal within the first few days or weeks of life from respiratory complications. Affected newborns are often premature and small for gestational age and have short bowed limbs, numerous fractures, markedly soft skulls, and a small thoracic cavity.

Type III disease is characterized by progressive skeletal deformity from recurrent fracture (4). These patients often have dental manifestations and short stature.

Type IV disease is transmitted as an autosomal dominant trait and, until recently, was considered rare. However, it may frequently account for instances of multigeneration disease (1). The sclerae are of normal color, but skeletal deformity, dental disease, and hearing loss can occur.

Radiologic Features

Characteristic findings are found in severely affected subjects (9). The cardinal features are modeling defects of long bones and deformity from fractures due to generalized osteopenia. The modeling defect involves defective periosteal bone formation that retards circumferential growth of bone and produces characteristic thin cortices. Multiple and recurrent fractures deform vertebrae as well as long bones (Fig. 2). In some severely affected infants, there is severe micromelia in which the major long bones appear short but "thick" in their external diameter from recurrent fracture and marked bowing deformity. Wormian bones (Fig. 3) of significant number and size in the skull are a common but not pathognomonic feature of osteogenesis imperfecta (10). Platybasia and excessive pneumatization of the frontal and mastoid sinuses are commonly found in severely affected subjects (10). The pelvis can have a triradiate-shaped appearance. Radiologic abnormalities may evolve markedly during growth—a feature that helps to define especially the progressively deforming type III disease. "Popcorn calcifications" are unusual developmental defects in the epiphyses and metaphyses of major long bones (predominantly in the ankles and knees) that occur most often in type III patients (11). This feature is believed to result from traumatic fragmentation and then disordered maturation of growth plate cartilage that may severely limit long bone growth and thereby contribute importantly to short stature. Popcorn calcifications develop during childhood but "resolve" after puberty when the growth plates fuse as their cartilage is fully mineralized. When fractures occur in osteogenesis imperfecta they are often transverse but heal at normal rates. Occasionally, there is exuberant callus formation that has been mistaken for skeletal malignancy. Platybasia may progress to basilar impression. Osteoarthritis is also a common problem for ambulatory adults with skeletal deformity.

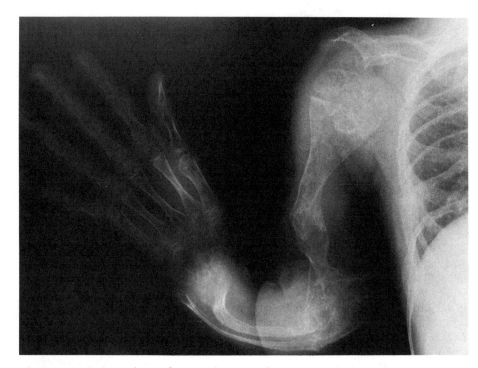

FIG. 1. *Osteogenesis imperfecta.* Severe changes of osteogenesis imperfecta are noted in the upper extremity of this 14-year-old boy, including marked osteopenia with characteristic thinning of bony cortices, evidence of old fractures, gracile ribs, and limb deformities. (Reproduced with permission from Whyte MP: Hereditary disorders of bone and mineral metabolism. In: Monolagas SC, Olefsky JM (eds), *Metabolic Bone and Mineral Disorders,* Churchill Livingston, New York, 1988.)

Etiology and Pathogenesis

Table 1 summarizes the types of biochemical/molecular defects that have been identified in the various clinical types of osteogenesis imperfecta (1). They include abnormalities that lead to low levels of type I collagen synthesis as well as numerous mutations affecting either, and rarely both, the pro-α 1 and pro-α 2 chains for type I collagen. Nearly all affected families have "private" mutations (14). The interested reader is referred elsewhere for detailed discussion (14).

Treatment

Although there has been considerable progress in the elucidation of the biochemical and molecular (genetic) defects that cause osteogenesis imperfecta, there is no established medical therapy. Treatment remains supportive and may require expert orthopedic, rehabilitative, and dental intervention to care for recurrent fractures, limb deformities, kyphoscoliosis, dental sequellae, etc. The management of osteogenesis imperfecta has been reviewed (15). Use of some bisphosphonate compounds seems promising for increasing bone mass but requires much further study (16). Support groups (e.g., Osteogenesis Imperfecta Foundation, Inc.) are important sources of information and comfort for patients and their families.

Genetic counseling should be made available and should be periodically updated when appropriate, since progress in this area is now quite rapid. Recent studies have shown that although some rare cases of type II osteogenesis imperfecta may represent homozygosity for an autosomal recessive trait or reflect germline mosaicism, most cases result from new dominant mutations (1). Thus, the overall recurrence risk is now estimated to be 5%–10% for this type of osteogenesis imperfecta (1). Prenatal diagnosis of severe disease by a variety of techniques, particularly ultrasound examination at 14–18 weeks gestation, has been quite successful (1).

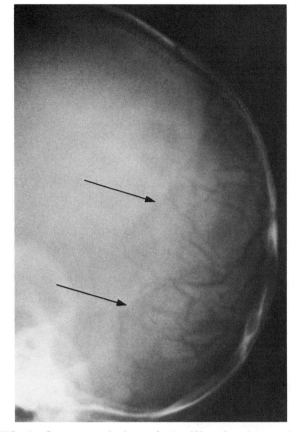

FIG. 2. *Osteogenesis imperfecta.* Wormian bones (*arrows*), although not pathognomonic of this disorder, may be found in the lambdoidal sutures of the posterior occiput. (Reproduced with permission from Whyte MP: Rare disorders of skeletal formation and homeostasis. In: Becker KN (ed), *Principles and Practice of Endocrinology and Metabolism,* JB Lippincott, Philadelphia, 1990.)

Laboratory Findings

Routine biochemical studies are typically unremarkable; elevations in serum alkaline phosphatase activity and urinary levels of hydroxyproline occur in some individuals. Recently, hypercalciuria has been found to be relatively common in children with osteogenesis imperfecta—especially those who are severely affected (12).

Specimens of bone often have findings that reflect the abnormal skeletal matrix, especially in severely affected individuals. Polarized-light microscopy may reveal an abundance of disorganized ("woven") bone and abnormally thin collagen bundles in lamellar bone. Numerous osteocytes are found in the cortical bone of some individuals. This finding appears to reflect a decreased rate of bone production by individual osteoblasts, yet many of these cells are active at one time. Subsequently, the overall rate of skeletal turnover can be rapid, as shown by *in vivo* tetracycline labeling (13).

REFERENCES

1. Byers PH: Disorders of collagen biosynthesis and structure. In: Scriver CR, Beaudet AL, Sly WS, Valle D, (eds), *The Metabolic Basis of Inherited Disease, 6th ed.* McGraw-Hill, New York, 2805–2842, 1989
2. Hollister DW: Molecular basis of osteogenesis imperfecta. Curr Probl Dermatol 17:76–94, 1987
3. Albright JA, Millar EA: Osteogenesis Imperfecta (Symposium).

Clinical Orthopaedics. JB Lippincott Company, Philadelphia, 159:1–156, 1981

4. Sillence D: Osteogenesis imperfecta: an expanding panorama of variants. *Clin Orthop* 159:11–25, 1981
5. Byers PH, Tsipouras P, Bonadio JF, Starman BJ, Schwartz RC: Perinatal lethal osteogenesis imperfecta (OI Type II): a biochemically heterogeneous disorder usually due to new mutations in the genes for type I collagen. *Am J Hum Genet* 42:237–248, 1988
6. Pedersen U: Hearing loss in patients with osteogenesis imperfecta. *Scand Audiol* 13:67–74, 1984
7. Revell PA: *Pathology of Bone.* Springer-Verlag, Berlin, 1986
8. Falvo KA, Bullough PG: Osteogenesis imperfecta: a histometric analysis. *J Bone Joint Surg* (Am) 55:275–286, 1973
9. Resnick D, Niwayama G: *Diagnosis of Bone and Joint Disorders, 2nd ed.* WB Saunders, Philadelphia, 1988
10. Cremin B, Goodman H, Prax M, Spranger J, Beighton P: Wormian bones in osteogenesis imperfecta and other disorders. *Skeletal Radiol* 8:35–38, 1982
11. Goldman AB, Davidson D, Pavlor H, Bullough PG: "Popcorn" calcifications: a prognostic sign in osteogenesis imperfecta. *Radiology* 136:351–358, 1980
12. Chines A, Petersen DJ, Schranck FW, Whyte MP: Hypercalciuria in children severely affected with osteogenesis imperfecta. *J Pediatr* 119:51–57, 1991
13. Baron R, Gertner JM, Lang R, Vighery A: Increased bone turnover with decreased bone formation by osteoblasts in children with osteogenesis imperfecta tarda. *Pediatr Res* 17:204–207, 1983
14. Byers PH, Wallis GA, Willing MC: Osteogenesis imperfecta: translation of mutation to phenotype. *J Med Genet* 28:433–442, 1991
15. Marini JC: Osteogenesis imperfecta: comprehensive management. *Adv Pediatr* 35:391–426, 1988
16. Devogelaer JP, Malghem J, Maldague B, Nagant de Deuxchaisnes C: Radiological manifestations of bisphosphonate treatment with ADP in a child suffering from osteogenesis imperfecta. *Skeletal Radiol* 16:360–363, 1987

78. Chondrodystrophies and Mucopolysaccharidoses

Michael P. Whyte, M.D.

Metabolic Research Unit, Shriners Hospital for Crippled Children, and Division of Bone and Mineral Diseases, The Jewish Hospital of St. Louis, Washington University School of Medicine; St. Louis, Missouri

Beginning in the 1960s, vigorous attempts to classify the skeletal dysplasias led to recognition of more than 80 distinct entities (1). Understandably, the nomenclature for these disorders has been unsatisfactory since the biochemical and molecular basis is poorly understood for nearly all forms. Accordingly, the most commonly used method for differentiating skeletal dysplasias is based on the parts of the skeleton that appear to be most involved after radiologic study (1).

The osteochondrodysplasias constitute one group of conditions among the skeletal dysplasias and are characterized by abnormal growth or development of cartilage and/or bone. The reader is referred to reference 1 for a brief description and review of the nomenclature for these conditions. In turn, osteochondrodysplasias are subdivided further into several groups of disorders, some of which are characterized by defects of growth of tubular bones and/or the spine. These conditions are frequently referred to as chondrodysplasias. The region of the long bones that is most affected (epiphysis, metaphysis, or diaphysis) constitutes the basis for subclassification; e.g., epiphyseal, metaphyseal, or diaphyseal dysplasia (2,3). When the vertebrae are also deformed, they are further subdivided (e.g., spondyloepiphyseal, dysplasia, etc.) (Fig. 1).

For the purposes of this primer, it should be noted that in those chondrodysplasias that have primarily metaphyseal defects (metaphyseal dysplasia and spondylometaphyseal dysplasia), the radiologic appearance of the growth plates may be confused with metabolic bone disease (i.e., rickets) (Fig. 2). However, serum biochemistries are not abnormal, the skeleton is otherwise generally well mineralized, and the configuration of the metaphyseal defects can often be correctly identified by an experienced radiologist. When abnormalities of the spine are present (Fig. 3), the correct diagnosis should be especially apparent.

The mucopolysaccharidoses constitute a group of inborn errors of metabolism that result from diminished activity of the lysosomal enzymes that degrade glycosaminoglycans (acid mucopolysaccharides). Accumulation of these complex carbohydrates in marrow spaces results in skeletal dysplasia that is sometimes referred to generically as "dysostosis multiplex." However, the degree of severity and precise bony manifestations vary according to the specific inborn error of metabolism (1–4). Reference 4

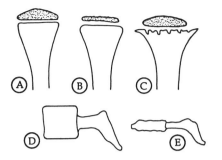

Involvement	Disease Category
A+D	Normal
B+D	Epiphyseal dysplasia
C+D	Metaphyseal dysplasia
B+E	Spondyloepiphyseal dysplasia
C+E	Spondylometaphyseal dysplasia
B+C+E	Spondyloepimetaphyseal dysplasia

FIG. 1. *Chondrodysplasias.* Classification based on radiologic involvement of long bones and vertebrae (1). Reproduced with permission from Churchill Livingstone, Edinburgh.

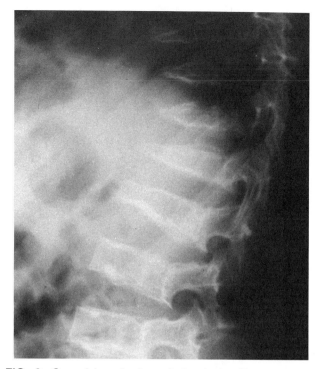

FIG. 3. *Spondylometaphyseal dysplasia.* Characteristic dysplastic changes in the vertebrae are present in this radiograph of the spine taken of the patient shown in Fig. 2 at 11 years of age and distinguish spondylometaphyseal from metaphyseal dysplasia.

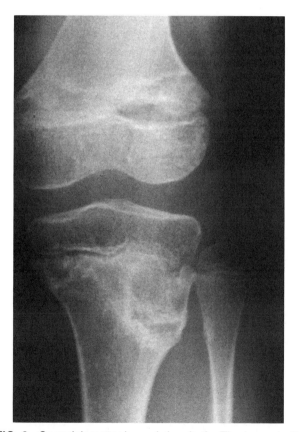

FIG. 2. *Spondylometaphyseal dysplasia.* The irregularity of the metaphyses in the knees of this 8%₁₂-year-old girl are sometimes mistaken for rachitic disease.

provides a recent and detailed description of this group of conditions.

Dysostosis multiplex is characterized by the following general radiographic features that help to distinguish the mucopolysaccharidoses from other disorders that affect the skeleton: osteoporosis with coarsened trabeculae, macrocephaly, dyscephaly, a *J*-shaped sella turcica, oar-shaped ribs, widened clavicles, oval-shaped or hooked-shaped vertebral bodies, dysplasia of the capital femoral epiphyses, coxa valga, epiphyseal and metaphyseal dysplasia, proximal tapering of the 2nd and 5th metacarpals, and dysplasia of long tubular bones (2,3).

REFERENCES

1. Rimoin DL, Lachman RS: The chondrodysplasias. In: Emery AEH, Rimoin DL (eds), *Principles and Practice of Medical Genetics,* Churchill Livingstone, London, 1983
2. Wynne-Davies R, Hall CM, Apley AG: *Atlas of Skeletal Dysplasias,* Churchill Livingstone, Edinburgh, 1985
3. Resnick D, Niwayama G: *Diagnosis of Bone and Joint Disorders, 2nd ed.* WB Saunders, Philadelphia, 1988
4. Neufeld EF, Muenzer J: The mucopolysaccharidoses. In: Scriver CR, Beaudet AL, Sly WS, Valle D (eds), *The Metabolic Basis of Inherited Disease, 6th ed.* McGraw-Hill, New York, 1565–1588, 1989

Acquired Disorders of Cartilage and Bone

Introduction

Physicians who specialize in the care of patients with metabolic bone diseases encounter a considerable number and variety of acquired disorders of cartilage and bone. Among these conditions are skeletal neoplasms, problems that result from disruption of the vascular supply to the skeleton, and diseases that are characterized by infiltration of the marrow spaces. Furthermore, in certain "metabolic" bone diseases and some skeletal dysplasias there is predisposition to neoplastic transformation (e.g., Paget's disease, fibrous dysplasia), metabolic disturbances can cause skeletal ischemia (e.g., Cushing's syndrome, storage diseases), and infiltrative marrow disorders may be associated with aberrant mineral homeostasis (e.g., sarcoidosis). This section provides an overview of some of the principal acquired disorders of cartilage and bone.

79. Skeletal Neoplasms

Michael P. Whyte, M.D.

Metabolic Research Unit, Shriners Hospital for Crippled Children, and
Division of Bone and Mineral Diseases, The Jewish Hospital of St. Louis,
Washington University School of Medicine; St. Louis, Missouri

GENERAL CONSIDERATIONS

Among the acquired disorders of cartilage and bone are a variety of neoplasms. Some are malignant and cause considerable morbidity and may metastasize and cause death; others are benign and can even heal spontaneously. Rarely, some behave as though "transitional" with both benign and malignant characteristics. Diagnosis and treatment of bone tumors is a complex discipline. Only a brief overview is provided here. The reader may also refer to several recent reviews of this subject (1–5).

The histopathological classification of skeletal tumors is based upon the cell or tissue type from which they appear to have originated (Table 1). The source of the neoplasm is usually revealed by the kind of tissue that the tumor cells make; e.g., osteoid, cartilage, etc. However, in some instances (e.g., giant cell tumor of bone) the origin is unknown (1–5).

The classification of bone tumors also depends importantly on their "biologic behavior" (see below). Even within the major distinctions (i.e., benign vs malignant) there are neoplasms with different degrees of aggressivity. Biologic behavior reflects the capacity of the tumor to exceed its natural barriers. Such barriers may include a tumor capsule which is a shell of fibrous tissue or bone around the neoplasm, its "reactive zone" composed in part of either fibrous tissue or bone that forms between the capsule and normal tissue, and any adjacent articular cartilage, cortical bone, or periosteum (1–6).

Skeletal neoplasms will be properly managed only if there is a thorough understanding of their clinical presentation and natural history, as well as use of current staging procedures that often require histopathologic examination (6). Proper choice of therapy may include medical and/or surgical approaches (1–8). Optimum patient management requires multidisciplinary expertise. Better radiologic imaging studies, histopathologic methods, surgical techniques, and chemotherapeutic regimens have all led to improved survival and function of patients with skeletal sarcomas. Chemotherapy can often improve the treatment of early metastatic deposits (4,9–11). Consequently, aggressive limb-salvaging procedures are now possible and are associated with survival rates that were previously achieved only by radical amputation (1,4,7,10,12,14).

Benign Bone Tumors

Benign skeletal tumors, with only rare exception, do not metastasize. Nevertheless, as a group, their biological behavior can still be rather variable and may range from completely inactive to quite aggressive. Fortunately, this behavior can often be predicted by examining the clinical and radiologic features of the individual neoplasm (15,16); sometimes histopathologic inspection is essential as well (2,4,6). Each tumor can be classified generally as "inactive," "active," or "aggressive" (3).

Inactive benign bone tumors are also sometimes called "latent" or "static." They are encapsulated by mature fibrous tissue or by cortical bone-like material and do not expand or deform surrounding skeletal tissue. Each will have only a minimal (if any) reactive zone, and their histopathologic appearance is that of a benign neoplasm; i.e., a low cell-to-matrix ratio, a well-differentiated matrix, and no cellular hyperchromasia, anaplasia, or pleomorphism. Inactive benign tumors are usually asymptomatic (1–4).

Active benign bone tumors can deform or destroy adjacent cortical bone or joint cartilage as they grow, but they do not metastasize. They are encapsulated within fibrous tissue, though a thin reactive zone can develop. These lesions generally cause mild symptoms but may lead to pathological fracture (1–4).

Aggressive benign bone tumors are not uncommon in children. They demonstrate invasive properties like those of low-grade malignancies. Their reactive zone forms a capsule or pseudocapsule that prevents the tumor itself from extending directly into normal tissue, but the neoplasm can resorb and destroy adjacent bone and spread to nearby skeletal compartments. Despite their aggressive behavior, the cytologic features are benign—including a well-differentiated matrix. These tumors cause symptoms and can result in pathological fracture (1–4).

Malignant Bone Tumors

Malignant bone tumors can metastasize. Nevertheless, as a group, their biologic behavior also varies considerably (1–3). Some grow slowly with a low probability of spreading, such that there may be a long interval between the discovery of the primary neoplasm and the development and recognition of metastases. Others are biologically very aggressive and not only cause rapid and extensive local tissue destruction, but also have a high incidence of metastases so that primary and metastatic lesions are frequently recognized together. The biologic behavior of malignant skeletal tumors can usually be predicted by their clinical, radiologic (15,16), and histopathologic features (2). Indeed, assessment of the histopathologic type and "grade" is the best predictor of biologic activity and of paramount importance for successful treatment and accurate prognostication (see below) (1–5).

Low-grade sarcomas invade local tissues but grow

355

TABLE 1. *Common skeletal neoplasms (1-5)*

Tissue origin	Benign	Malignant
Osseous		Classic osteosarcoma Parosteal osteosarcoma Periosteal osteosarcoma
Cartilaginous	Enchondroma Exostosis	Primary chondrosarcoma Secondary chondrosarcoma
Fibrous	Nonossifying fibroma	Fibrosarcoma Malignant fibrous histiocytoma
Reticuloendothelial		Ewing's sarcoma Multiple myeloma
Unknown	Giant cell tumor in bone	

slowly and have a low risk of metastasizing. They are usually asymptomatic and manifest as gradually growing masses. Nevertheless, the histopathologic features of malignancy are present, such as anaplasia, pleomorphism, and hyperchromasia together with a few mitotic cells. The tumor capsule can be disrupted in many areas, and there may be an extensive reactive zone that forms a pseudocapsule and contains satellite tumor nodules that slowly erode the various natural barriers. Over time and after repeatedly unsuccessful surgical excision with tumor recurrence, there is a risk of transformation to a high-grade sarcoma (1–5).

High-grade sarcomas readily extend beyond their reactive zone. They seem to have minimal pseudoencapsulation. Their margins are poorly demarcated. Metastases may appear in seemingly uninvolved areas of the same bone and often in the medullary canal. Extension to nearby tissues destroys cortical bone, joint capsules, articular cartilage, etc. These tumors show all of the histopathologic features that typify malignancy and produce a poorly differentiated (immature) matrix (1–5).

Diagnosis of Bone Tumors

A thorough history and complete physical examination is the foundation for successful diagnosis and management of skeletal neoplasms. The patient's age, presence or absence of predisposing conditions (e.g., Paget's disease), and anatomic site of the lesion will provide important clues to the precise diagnosis (see the following).

Radiologic studies should be chosen both to establish the tumor type and to provide staging information that will be critical for choosing treatment and for understanding the patient's prognosis (1–5,17). The tumor "stage" reflects the neoplasm's location and extent as well as biologic activity or "grade" and is based in part on the presence or absence of metastases (6). Radiographs establish the tumor location, often suggest the underlying histopathologic type (15,16), help to evaluate its extent, and guide the selection of additional staging studies. Clinical

and radiologic examination is completed prior to biopsy or other surgical procedures (6).

Bone scintigraphy will help to determine if multiple areas of neoplasm are present and if the extent of skeletal involvement exceeds that indicated by conventional radiographs. This procedure can also suggest the tumor's biologic activity (15,16,18). Avidity for radionuclide uptake generally reflects biologic activity.

Computed tomography is very useful for precisely defining the anatomic extent of the primary, lesion, detecting destruction of spongy or cortical bone, assessing compartmental changes, and locating neurovascular structures that may be impinged upon by tumor or are located near planned surgery (19). This technique also supplements conventional radiography for detecting pulmonary metastases.

Magnetic resonance imaging is especially helpful for defining tumor soft tissue extension and for showing any disruption of the marrow spaces (18–21).

Angiography can help plan limb-salvage procedures, since this study may show involvement of major neurovascular bundles (3,4).

Arthrography will help to demonstrate joint involvement and thus be useful for determining whether a cartilagenous tumor is of intraarticular or extraarticular origin (3,4).

Biopsy and histopathologic study are essential for successful staging and treatment of many skeletal neoplasms (1–6). Open incisional biopsy is typically the technique of choice if a malignant lesion is suspected since it secures sufficient tissue for study (3). However, this technique carries a greater risk of tumor contamination of uninvolved tissues (e.g., by dissecting hematoma) than closed biopsy and could therefore compromise a limb-salvage procedure because of added risk of local recurrence. Accordingly, careful attention must be paid to where the incision for biopsy is made and the surgical technique (1–6). Accessible benign tumors may be removed by incisional biopsy as they are intracapsular, or with *en bloc* marginal incision (1,4,7).

INDIVIDUAL TYPES OF SKELETAL NEOPLASIA

Benign and Transitional Bone Tumors

Benign skeletal neoplasms occasionally originate from marrow elements, but most often they are derived from cartilage or bone itself. Typically, they develop before skeletal maturation is complete or during the early adult years and are most prevalent in areas of rapid bone growth and cellular metabolism; i.e., the epiphyses and metaphyses of the major long bones (1–4,22). In some individuals or families with particular heritable disorders, benign skeletal tumors (e.g., enchondromas and exostoses) are multiple and have a significantly increased risk of malignant transformation. Most benign skeletal tumors, however, are solitary lesions and are associated with a good prognosis (1–4,22). Principal types are discussed as follows:

Nonossifying fibroma is the most common bone tumor (23). This lesion is often called a "fibrous cortical defect." Each is the outcome of a focal developmental abnormality in periosteal bone formation that results in an area of failure of ossification. Nonossifying fibromas most commonly occur in the metaphyses of the distal femur or distal tibia and are located eccentrically in or near the bony cortex (15,16). They are somewhat more common in boys than in girls, develop during childhood or adolescence, and are active lesions that enlarge throughout childhood yet typically do not cause symptoms. However, when more than 50% of the diameter of a long bone is involved, pathologic fracture can occur (23). Radiologic study may show a well-demarcated radiolucent zone with apparent trabecularization that results in a multilocular or even septated appearance (Fig. 1). Some cortical bone erosion may be present. The radiologic pattern can be considered diagnostic, and further staging is typically unnecessary (15,16). At puberty with skeletal maturation, nonossifying fibromas become inactive or latent and ultimately ossify. Surgical intervention is usually unnecessary unless pathologic fracture is a significant risk. Intracapsular curettage is effective, but bone grafting or other stabilizing techniques for fracture prevention or treatment may be required (1–4,23).

Enchondroma is a benign and typically asymptomatic tumor of cartilage that results from focal disruption in otherwise orderly endochrondral bone formation. It can be considered a dysplasia of the central growth plate (24). Enchondromas appear to arise in the metaphysis but may eventually become incorporated into the diaphysis. Solitary lesions are noted typically in adolescence or during early adulthood. They most commonly involve small tubular bones of the hands or feet or the proximal humerus, but they can occur in any bone. Several distinct disorders are characterized by multiple enchondromas (enchondromatosis, Ollier's disease, and Maffucci's syndrome). Single lesions rarely become chondrosarcomas, but when multiple the incidence of malignant degeneration is considerably increased (1–4,22,24).

Radiographs show a medullary radiolucent lesion with a well-defined but only slightly thickened bony margin

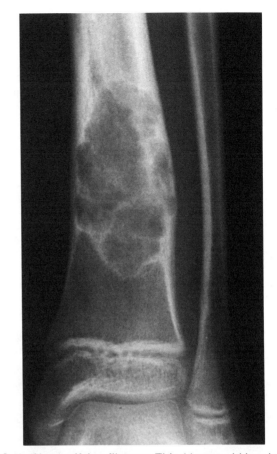

FIG. 1. *Nonossifying fibroma.* This 11-year-old boy has a typical benign-appearing lesion of his distal left tibia. It is an ovoid, radiolucent fibrous tumor located at the metadiaphyseal junction that is slightly expansile and has a multiloculated appearance with regions of cortical scalloping and thinning.

(Fig. 2) (15,16). This lesion may enlarge slowly during its active phase in adolescence, but when it becomes latent during the adult years it calcifies to produce a diffusely punctate or stippled appearance (Fig. 3). In time, enchondromas become surrounded by dense reactive osseous tissue. Skeletal scintigraphy typically reflects the tumor's biological activity and shows increased radioisotope uptake in the reactive zone (greatly increased uptake suggests malignant transformation). Accordingly, it is prudent to secure for young adults with multiple enchondromas a baseline bone scan and radiographs. Biopsy is often not necessary since the lesion's identity is revealed by conventional radiography (15,16). Histopathologic examination may be required, however, to distinguish benign from low-grade malignant enchondromas. Here the patient's age is an especially important consideration (24).

Solitary asymptomatic enchondromas are generally benign and require no treatment, although periodic follow-up is indicated. If they become symptomatic and begin to enlarge, careful surveillance is necessary (24). Imaging techniques may be helpful to search for evidence of malignancy (18). Surgical treatment would then be indicated.

Fewer than 1% of asymptomatic solitary tumors undergo malignant transformation. However, with enchondromatosis the risk of malignant degeneration has been estimated to be 10% (24).

Osteocartilaginous exostosis (osteochondroma) is a common developmental dysplasia of cartilage within the peripheral region of a growth plate (22,24). It can arise in any bone that derives from cartilage but usually involves long bone. Typically either end of a femur, proximal humerus or tibia, pelvis, or scapula is affected. Exostoses present as hard painful masses that are fixed to bone. They enlarge during childhood but become latent in adulthood. These lesions can irritate overlying soft tissues and may form a fluid-filled bursa. Generally they are solitary, but multiple hereditary exostoses is a well-characterized entity that can cause significant angular deformity of the lower limbs, clubbing of the radius, and short stature. A painful and enlarging exostosis in an adult, especially in the pelvis or shoulder girdle, should suggest malignant transformation to a chondrosarcoma (22,24).

Radiologic study may show either a flat, sessile, or pe-

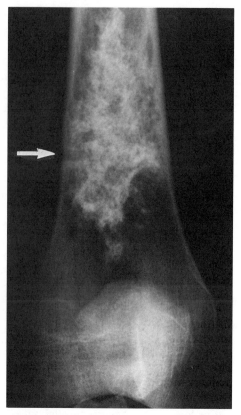

FIG. 3. *Enchondroma.* This 43-year-old woman has an extensively calcified lesion of the metadiaphyseal region of her distal femur. The calcification is amorphous and dense with little radiolucent component (the arrow indicates a biopsy needle track). This lesion is differentiated from bone infarction, which should have a dense, linearly marginated periphery.

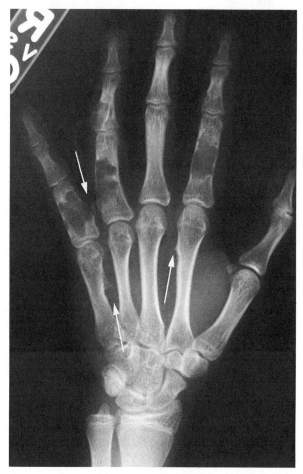

FIG. 2. *Enchondromatosis.* This 13-year-old girl has multiple lucent benign-appearing lesions of the phalanges. Each has produced expansion of the bone as well as cortical scalloping and thinning. Several periosteum-based chondromas are present that show reactive bone formation at their margins (*arrows*).

dunculated metaphyseal bony lesion of variable density that is typically well defined and covered by a radiolucent cartilaginous cap (Fig. 4). A characteristic feature of an exostosis is continuity of the tumor bone with metaphyseal bone (15,16). The diagnosis is rarely difficult. Following malignant transformation, there may be a soft tissue mass on computed tomography or magnetic resonance imaging, and skeletal scintigraphy will demonstrate a sudden increase in, or great amount of, tracer uptake.

The cartilagenous cap of an exostosis appears histopathologically like a poorly organized growth plate. The trabeculae are not remodeled and thus contain cartilage cores (primary spongiosum) like in the various forms of osteopetrosis (see Section VI).

Excisional treatment of an active exostosis should include the cartilagenous cap and overlying perichondrium to minimize the risk of recurrence (1,3,4,24). There is about a 5% recurrence rate following marginal excision of a solitary lesion. Malignant degeneration occurs in fewer than 1% of solitary lesions, but the risk is almost 10% for multiple hereditary exostoses (24).

Giant cell tumor of bone (osteoclastoma) is a common benign bone neoplasm. The cellular origin, however, is unknown (1–4). Men are more frequently affected than women; typically at 20–40 years of age. These tumors cause chronic and deep pain that mimics an arthropathy. Pathologic fracture or effusion into the knee is not an infrequent first clinical sign. The epiphysis of a distal femur or proximal tibia is frequently affected. However, the distal radius, proximal humerus, distal tibia, and sacrum are also commonly involved. Often, giant cell tumors enlarge to occupy most of the epiphysis and portions of the adjacent metaphysis, and they can penetrate into subchondral bone and may even invade articular cartilage. In contrast to other benign skeletal neoplasms, they occasionally metastasize. Accordingly, giant cell tumors of bone are sometimes referred to as "transitional" neoplasms (3).

Radiologic studies show a relatively large lucent abnormality that is surrounded by an obvious reactive zone (15,16). The cortex can appear eroded from the endosteal surface (Fig. 5). A trabecular bone pattern may fill in the tumor cavity. Skeletal scintigraphy may demonstrate decreased tracer uptake at the center of the lesion ("doughnut sign"). Histopathologic examination shows numerous, scattered, multinucleated giant cells in a proliferative stroma; mitoses are occasionally present (2).

Curettage with bone grafting or use of cement is the treatment of less advanced lesions. Recurrent or advanced tumors are removed with *en bloc* wide excision and reconstructive surgery (1–4,7).

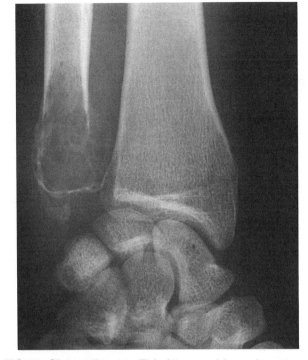

FIG. 5. *Giant cell tumor.* This 25-year-old man has an expansile, destructive, lucent lesion of the distal ulna. The lesion extends to the end of the bone.

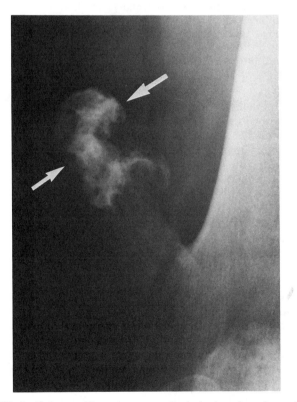

FIG. 4. *Osteocartilagenous exostosis (osteochondroma).* This 51-year-old woman has a typical pedunculated exostosis of her distal femur. The cortex and trabecular components of the exostosis are continuous with the host bone. Note how the exostosis slants away from the knee joint. The osteocartilagenous cap (*arrows*) is densely mineralized.

Malignant Bone Tumors

The most common cancer of the skeleton, myeloma, is a tumor of bone marrow origin. Nevertheless, a considerable variety of malignant neoplasms commonly arise from bone, cartilage, fibrous tissue, histiocytes, and perhaps endothelial tissue in the skeleton (1–4,23,24). Malignant bone tumors typically cause skeletal pain that is especially prominent at night. Accordingly, this symptom, particularly in adolescents or young adults, is reason for evaluation. The treatment of malignant lesions is complex and is primarily based on the tumor grade and staging (3–6).Only general comments are provided in this subsection; principal types among these neoplasms are discussed as follow:

Multiple myeloma typically develops during middle age and affects multiple skeletal sites. Constitutional symptoms can include bone pain, fever, malaise, fatigue, and weight loss. There is often anemia, thrombocytopenia, and renal failure (25). Hypercalcemia due to the elaboration of osteoclast-activating factors (Chapter 41) occurs at some time in the disease course of about 20–40% of patients (26). The diagnosis is made by conventional examination of the bone marrow for plasmacytosis and demonstration of paraproteinemia by serum and urine immunoelectrophoresis (25).

Radiologic findings may include classic discrete osteolytic lesions, but generalized osteopenia actually is a more common presentation. Bone scintigraphy findings can be unexpected because of little tracer uptake in foci of osteolysis (15,16).

Myeloma is radiation sensitive and treatable by chemotherapy. Reossification of tumor sites can occur within several months of therapy. Prevention of pathologic fractures may require surgical stabilization (25).

Osteosarcoma (osteogenic sarcoma) is the most common primary malignancy of the skeleton (1–4,27–31). There are about 1,100–1,500 new cases in the United States yearly. Typically, this bone cancer develops before age 30 and affects men somewhat more frequently than women. Although most are the "classic" variety, there are variants of osteosarcoma that include parosteal, periosteal, and telangiectatic types (see the following) that have somewhat different presentations and prognoses (27–31).

Classic osteosarcoma characteristically arises in the metaphysis of a long bone where there is the most rapid growth velocity. It primarily affects teenagers. In about 50% of cases, these tumors develop near the knee in the distal femur or proximal tibia. Other commonly involved sites are the humerus, proximal femur, and pelvis, but they can occur *de novo* anywhere in the skeleton. They also occur from malignant transformation of Paget's disease (Section VIII) (27–31).

Typically, an osteosarcoma presents as a tender bony mass. Its pain is severe and unremitting. Pathologic fracture can occur. Osteosarcomas are aggressive neoplasms that readily penetrate metaphyseal cortical bone, and the majority have already infiltrated surrounding soft tissue at diagnosis. At presentation, about 50% of affected adolescents show penetration of their growth plates with epiphyseal involvement, about 20% have metastases elsewhere in the affected bone, and in approximately 10% tumor has spread to lymph nodes or lung (27–31).

Radiologic study shows a destructive lesion that is comprised of amorphous osseous tissue with poorly defined margins (15,16,32). Some tumors are predominately osteoblastic and radiologically dense; others are predominately osteolytic and radiolucent. Some have a mixed pattern (15,16). Cortical bone destruction is often apparent (Fig. 6). A characteristic "sunburst" pattern results from spicules of amorphous neoplastic bone that form perpendicular to the affected bone's long axis. This is in distinct contrast to the parallel or "onion skin" appearance of reactive periosteal new bone. Codman's triangle results from periosteal reaction and elevation that demarcates a triangular area of cortical bone (see Fig. 8 for illustration). Bone scintigraphy shows intense uptake of tracer and may disclose more widespread disease than is indicated by conventional radiographs. Computed tomography, magnetic resonance imaging, and angiography are helpful as discussed previously. Microscopic examination typically shows a very malignant stroma that produces an amorphous and immature osteoid in a trabecular pattern (1–4).

Use of chemotherapy preoperatively (4,9–11,27,28) has significantly improved the prognosis for this malignancy and has enabled many osteosarcomas to be managed by limb-salvage procedures instead of radical amputation (7,12,14).

Parosteal osteosarcomas are juxtacortical (i.e., they develop between the bony cortex and soft tissue as a surface neoplasm). Adolescents and young adults are most commonly affected by these slowly growing, low-grade

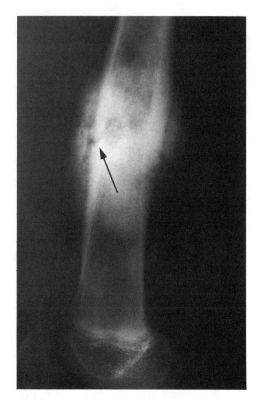

FIG. 6. *Central (medullary) osteosarcoma.* This 12-year-old boy has a sclerotic diaphyseal lesion that arose in the medullary cavity. It has penetrated the cortex and produced a densely mineralized mass surrounding the femur. Portions of the cortex appear to have been destroyed (*arrow*), whereas other regions are thickened.

tumors that typically occur as a fixed and painless mass posteriorly on the distal femur or medially on the proximal humerus. They are less aggressive than classic osteosarcomas and can be separated for a considerable length of time from the parent bone by a narrow radiolucent region of soft tissue. Eventually, they may extend into underlying bone and degenerate into a high-grade osteosarcoma (1–4,27).

Radiologic study typically reveals a densely ossified, broad-based, fusiform mass that seems to encircle the metaphyseal region of a long bone (Fig. 7) (15,16). Reactive tissue initially separates the neoplasm from the underlying bone that is destroyed once the normal cortex is penetrated and the medullary canal becomes involved. Parosteal osteosarcomas have mature trabeculae with cement lines similar to those seen in Paget's disease; however, a low-grade malignant stroma is present. This tumor is often misdiagnosed as benign. Limb-salvage with wide marginal excision is the usual treatment for less advanced disease. The prognosis is good. Chemotherapy is typically not used unless there has been dedifferentiation (1–4,27).

Periosteal osteosarcoma often presents as a painless growing mass that extends from the surface of a bone into soft tissue (1–4,27). This is an uncommon variant of classic osteosarcoma that principally affects young adults. On radiologic study, it is poorly mineralized and found primarily on a bone surface in an area of cortical

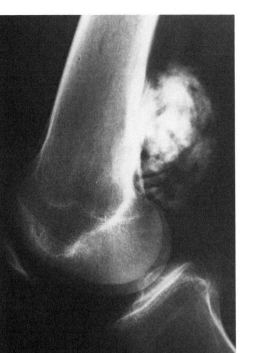

FIG. 7. *Parosteal osteosarcoma.* This 30-year-old woman has a very densely mineralized mass arising from the periosteal surface of the distal femoral metaphysis posteriorly. This tumor has lobular calcification and is attached to the femur by a broad pedicle.

erosion. The craterlike region has irregular margins and is associated with periosteal reaction (15,16). Penetration by this neoplasm through cortical bone into the medullary canal is more rapid than for parosteal osteosarcoma. When this occurs the frequency of pulmonary metastasis is greater—a feature that contributes to its poorer prognosis. Bone scintigraphy shows seemingly avid tracer uptake for this radiolucent tumor. Computed tomography reveals a mass that fills a shallow cortical bone defect and contains minimal calcification. Malignant mesenchymal stroma with neoplastic osteoid occurs in and around areas of mature cartilage (2,3).

Periosteal osteosarcoma is often treated by excision with a wide margin (3,4,7,11,14,27). Adjuvant chemotherapy is used when the tumor has regions of high-grade malignancy (1–4,9,11).

Chondrosarcoma occurs most often between 40–60 years of age when it is a primary tumor (1–5,24,33). In about 25% of affected subjects, malignant transformation has occurred in a preexisting enchondroma or osteocartilaginous exostosis. This neoplasm usually involves the pelvis, proximal femur, or shoulder girdle. There is a persistent dull ache that may mimic arthritis as the initial symptom. Variants of the classic form include a high-grade dedifferentiated tumor, an intermediate-grade clear cell type, and a low-grade juxtacortical tumor. The particular designation depends on the histopathologic pattern and anatomic location (1–3,24,33).

Radiographs show a subtle radiolucent lesion that contains hazy or speckled calcification in a diffuse "salt and pepper" or "popcorn" pattern (15,16). Primary chondrosarcomas can develop either within the medullary canal or on the surface of a bone where they can cause cortical bone destruction and a mass. On histopathologic examination of chondrosarcomas, it can be difficult to demonstrate that high-grade tumors are cartilaginous in origin or that low-grade tumors are actually malignant (2,24,33).

Treatment depends on the tumor stage. Limb amputation may be necessary for higher grade tumors. Adjuvant chemotherapy or radiation therapy has been disappointing (1–4,24).

Ewing sarcoma is a very malignant neoplasm that arises from nonmesenchymal cells in the bone marrow (2,3,34). Recently, this type of cancer was found to harbor a t(11;12) (q24;q12)translocation (35,36). It typically presents in children aged 10–15 years and is more common in boys than in girls (37,38). Initial manifestations are an enlarging and tender soft tissue swelling together with weight loss, malaise, fever, and lethargy. The erythrocyte sedimentation rate may be elevated, and there can be leukocytosis and anemia. The diaphysis of the femur is most commonly involved, but an ilium, tibia, fibula, or rib is often affected. When the tumor occurs in the pelvis it is usually found late and therefore has an especially poor prognosis (34).

Radiologic study typically reveals a diaphyseal lesion of patchy density that destroys cortical bone and frequently causes an "onion skin" appearance of reactive periosteum (Fig. 8) (15,16). Bone scintigraphy may show intense tracer uptake that extends considerably beyond the radiographic abnormality.

Preliminary chemotherapy may be followed by wide excision or radiation therapy depending on, among other factors, the anatomic site. Newer therapeutic approaches have reduced the incidence of pulmonary metastases and markedly improved survival (1–4,34,37,38).

Malignant fibrous histiocytoma occurs more frequently in soft tissues than in the skeleton and is less common than benign fibrous tumors (1–5,23). It affects adults and often originates in Paget's disease or at the site of a bone infarct. Typically, this is an aggressive sarcoma that readily spreads in the lymphatics. Bone is infiltrated early on, and pathologic fracture is a common presenting symptom.

Radiologic study reveals a poorly defined radiolucent lesion that causes cortical bone erosion (15,16). The histopathologic pattern is variable from area to area; extremely large and bizarre histiocytic cells are found in some sections, and undifferentiated cells that resemble histiocytic lymphoma are noted in others. Areas that contain fibrous tissue may suggest that the tumor is a fibrosarcoma. Special stains and electron microscopy may be required to establish the correct diagnosis (2,3,23). Staging studies direct the therapy, which may require radical resection or amputation and perhaps chemotherapy (3,4). The prognosis is guarded (23).

Fibrosarcoma is a painful neoplasm that typically arises in a major long bone of an adolescent or young adult (1–4,23). Radiologic study reveals a poorly defined and destructive lucent lesion in a metaphysis (15,16). Low-

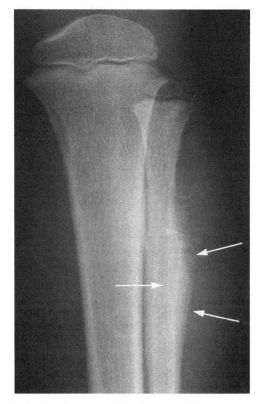

FIG. 8. *Ewing sarcoma.* This 5-year-old boy has a subtle permeative lesion of the proximal diaphysis of his fibula. The tumor is characterized by layered (onion-skin) periosteal reaction forming a Codman's triangle (*arrows*) and by "sunburst" new bone formation more proximally that is oriented perpendicularly to the long axis of the fibula. A large soft tissue mass is associated with the skeletal abnormalities.

grade and high-grade fibrosarcomas have similar radiologic and histopathologic appearances. Accordingly, electron microscopy may be necessary to reveal the collagenous composition of the matrix of a high-grade tumor (2,3,23). Therapy depends upon the staging results (6,23).

Metastatic bone tumors are considerably more common than primary skeletal malignancies (about 25 to 1) (1–5). Prostate, breast, thyroid, lung, and kidney are the sources of tumors that commonly metastasize to bone. There is a predelection for deposition of malignant cells within blood-forming marrow spaces in the spine, ribs, skull, pelvis, and metaphyses of long bones (particularly the femur and humerus). In children, metastases to the skeleton usually reflect a neuroblastoma, leukemia, or Ewing sarcoma. In teenagers or young adults, lymphomas are the predominant source. After age 30, an adenocarcinoma is the likely primary. Osteoblastic metastases are most commonly carcinoma of the prostate or breast. Osteolytic metastases may come from the lung, thyroid gland, kidney, or gastrointestinal tract (15,16). In a significant number of subjects, a primary neoplasm is not evident and, therefore, staging studies with biopsy are performed to exclude a primary skeletal sarcoma (1–5).

REFERENCES

1. Mirra JM, Picci P, Gold RH: *Bone Tumors: Clinical, Radiologic, and Pathologic Correlations.* Lea & Febiger, Philadelphia, 1989
2. Unni KK: *Bone Tumors.* Churchill Livingstone, New York, 1988
3. Enneking WF, Conrad EU III: *Common Bone Tumors. Clinical Symposia,* Pharmaceuticals Division, Ciba-Geigy Corp, Summit, NJ, 41:1–32, 1989
4. Lewis MM (Ed): *Musculoskeletal Oncology: A Multidisciplinary Approach.* WB Saunders, Philadelphia, 1992
5. Moser RP Jr (Ed): *Cartilaginous Tumors of the Skeleton.* Hanley and Belfus, Philadelphia, 1990
6. Heare TC, Enneking WF, Heare MM: Staging techniques and biopsy of bone tumors. *Orthop Clin North Am* 20:273–285, 1989
7. Lewis MM: *Bone Tumor Surgery: Limb Sparing Techniques.* Lippincott, Philadelphia. Gower Medical Publishers, New York, 1988
8. Mankin HJ, Springfield DS, Gebhardt MC, Tomford WW: Current status of allografting for bone tumors. *Orthopedics* 15: 1147–1154, 1992
9. Jaffe N: Chemotherapy for malignant bone tumors. *Orthop Clin North Am* 20:487–503, 1989
10. Sweetnam R: Malignant bone tumor management: 30 years of achievement. *Clin Orthop Rel Res* 247:67–73, 1989
11. Eilber FR, Rosen G: Adjuvant chemotherapy for osteosarcoma. *Semin Oncol* 16:312–323, 1989
12. Langlais F, Tomeno B (eds): *Limb Salvage: Major Reconstruction in Oncologic and Nontumoral Conditions.* Springer-Verlag, Berlin, 1991
13. Springfield DS, Schmidt R, Graham-Pole J, Marcus RB Jr, Spanier S, Enneking WF: Surgical treatment of osteosarcoma. *J Bone Joint Surg* 70A:1124–1130, 1988
14. Simon MA: Limb salvage for osteosarcoma. *J Bone Joint Surg* 70A:307–310, 1988
15. Edeiken J, Dalinka M, Karasick D: *Edeiken's Roentgen Diagnosis of Diseases of Bone, 4th ed.* Williams and Wilkins, Baltimore, 1990
16. Resnick D, Niwayama G: *Diagnosis of Bone and Joint Disorders, 2nd ed.* WB Saunders, Philadelphia, 1988
17. Moser RP Jr, Madewell JE: An approach to primary bone tumors. *Radiol Clin North Am* 25:1049–1093, 1987
18. Murphy WA Jr: Imaging bone tumors in the 1990s. *Cancer* (Feb 15 suppl) 67:1169–1176, 1991
19. Sundaram M, McGuire MH: Computed tomography or magnetic resonance for evaluating the solitary tumor or tumor-like lesion of bone? *Skeleton Radiol* 17:393–401, 1988
20. Redmond OM, Stack JP, Dervan PA, Hurson BJ, Carney DN, Ennis JT: Osteosarcoma: use of MR imaging and MR spectroscopy in clinical decision making. *Radiology* 172:811–815, 1989
21. DeSchepper AMA, Degryse HRM: *Magnetic Resonance Imaging of Bone and Soft Tissue Tumors and Their Mimics: A Clinical Atlas.* Kluwer Academic Publishers, Boston, 1989
22. Schubiner JM, Simon MA: Primary bone tumors in children. *Orthop Clin North Am* 18:577–595, 1987
23. Marks KE, Bauer TW: Fibrous tumors of bone. *Orthop Clin North Am* 20:377–393, 1989
24. Greenspan A: Tumors of cartilage origin. *Orthop Clin North Am* 20:347–366, 1989
25. Osserman EF, Merlini G, Butler VP Jr: Multiple myeloma and related plasma cell dyscrasias. *JAMA* 258:2930–2937, 1987
26. Mundy GR: Calcium Homeostasis: *Hypercalcemia and Hypocalcemia.* Martin Dunitz, London, 1989
27. Meyers PA: Malignant bone tumors in children: osteosarcoma. *Hematol Oncol Clin North Am* 1:655–665, 1987
28. Taylor WF, Ivins JC, Unni KK, Beabout JW, Golenzer HJ, Black LE: Prognostic variables in osteosarcoma: multi-institutional study. *J Natl Cancer Inst* 81:21–30, 1989
29. Dahlin D, Coventry MB: Osteogenic sarcoma: a study of six hundred cases. *J Bone Joint Surg* 49A:101–110, 1967
30. Klein MJ, Kenan S, Lewis M: Osteosarcoma: clinical and pathological considerations. *Orthop Clin North Am* 20:327–345, 1989
31. Eckardt JJ (ed): Newest knowledge of osteosarcoma (symposium). *Clin Orthop Rel Res* 270, 1991

32. Edeiken-Monroe B, Edeiken J, Jacobson HG: *Osteosarcoma.* *Semin Roentgenol* 24:153–173, 1989
33. Welkerling H, Dreyer T, Delling G: Morphological typing of chondrosarcoma: a study of 92 cases. *Virchows Arch A Pathol Anat Histopathol* 418:419–425, 1991
34. Meyers PA: Malignant bone tumors in children: Ewing's sarcoma. *Hematol Oncol Clin North Am* 1:667–673, 1987
35. Womer RB: The cellular biology of bone tumors. *Clin Orthop Rel Res* 262:12–21, 1991
36. Selleri L, Hermanson GG, Eubanks JH, Lewis KA, Evans GA: Molecular localization of the t (11;22) (q24;q12) translocation of Ewing sarcoma by chromosomal in situ suppression hybridization. *Proc Natl Acad Sci USA* 88:887–891, 1991
37. Horowitz ME, Tsokos MG, DeLaney TF: Ewing's Sarcoma. CA *Cancer J Clin* 42:300–320, 1992
38. O'Connor MI, Pritchard DJ: Ewing's sarcoma. *Clin Orthop Rel Res* 262:78–87, 1991

80. Ischemic Bone Disease

Michael P. Whyte, M.D.

Metabolic Research Unit, Shriners Hospital for Crippled Children and
Division of Bone and Mineral Diseases, The Jewish Hospital of St. Louis,
Washington University School of Medicine; St. Louis, Missouri

Regional interruption of blood flow to the skeleton causes an important group of acquired disorders of cartilage and bone (1–3). Ischemia, if sufficiently severe and prolonged, will kill osteoblasts and chrondrocytes. Clinical problems may subsequently arise because reparative resorption of necrotic areas of bone and cartilage compromises skeletal strength and predisposes to fracture (4). A change in bone density is the principal radiologic finding (2,3). Characteristic radiologic signs of osteonecrosis also include crescent subchondral radiolucencies, patchy areas of sclerosis and lucency, bony collapse, diaphyseal periostitis, and preservation of joint space despite an affected epiphyseal region. These changes may take several months to appear.

There are a number of conditions that cause ischemic bone disease (Table 1) and a great variety of clinical presentations based primarily on the affected anatomic region. Legg-Calvé-Perthes Disease is discussed in some detail here since it represents an archetype form of ischemic bone disease. A few additional important clinical presentations are reviewed subsequently.

LEGG-CALVÉ-PERTHES DISEASE

Legg-Calvé-Perthes Disease (LCPD) is a complex and controversial pediatric disorder of the hip that can be defined as idiopathic ischemic necrosis (osteonecrosis) of the capital femoral epiphysis in children (5–7). It is a common problem that affects boys more frequently than girls (4:1 to 5:1). Typically, it presents between 2–12 years of age; the mean age at diagnosis is 7 years. When it first manifests later in life, the term "adolescent ischemic necrosis" is used to indicate the same poorer prognosis that occurs in affected adults (see the following). Usually one hip is involved but bilateral disease troubles about 20% of patients. Increased familial incidence varies from 1–20% (5–7).

Although the precise etiology of LCPD is unknown, the pathogenesis seems to be fairly well understood. Interruption of blood flow to the capital femoral epiphysis appears to be the fundamental skeletal insult. Ischemia may occur at this site in children from raised intracapsular pressure due to congenital or developmental abnormalities, episodes of synovitis, venous thrombosis, or perhaps increased blood viscosity (5–7). Consequently, most if not all of the capital femoral epiphysis is rendered ischemic. As a result marrow cells, osteoblasts, and osteocytes may die. Endochondral ossification ceases temporarily because blood flow to chondrocytes in the growth plate is impaired. Articular cartilage, however, initially remains intact because it depends instead on the synovial fluid for nourishment. Revascularization then follows and proceeds from the periphery to the center of the capital femoral epiphysis. New bone is deposited on the surface of dead subchondral cortical or central trabecular bone. Subsequently, the critical process of removal of necrotic bone begins, during which time the rate of bone resorption exceeds the rate of reparative new bone formation. As a result, the subchondral bone becomes weak. If there is no resulting fracture, the child may remain asymptomatic, and there is eventual healing. However, if fracture does occur the first symptoms manifest. Furthermore, trabecular bone collapse can also cause a second episode of ischemia (5–7). Longitudinal growth of the proximal femur can be stunted since the disrupted blood flow disturbs the physis and metaphysis. Premature closure of the growth plate may occur. As reossification of the capital femoral epiphysis takes place, the femoral head will remodel and remold its shape according to mechanical forces acting on it (2,3,5–7).

Children with LCPD typically limp, complain of pain in a knee or anterior thigh, and demonstrate limited mobility of the hip, especially with abduction or internal rotation. The Trendelenburg sign may be positive. If unsuccessfully treated, adduction and flexion contractures of the hip can develop, and thigh muscles can atrophy.

Laboratory investigation may show a slightly elevated erythrocyte sedimentation rate. Radiologic examination, which should include anteroposterior and "frog" lateral views for diagnosis and follow-up, often reveals a bone age that is 1–3 yr delayed (2,3). Sequential studies typi-

TABLE 1. *Causes of ischemic necrosis of cartilage and bone (2, 3)*

Endocrine/metabolic
 Glucocorticoid therapy
 Cushing's disease
 Alcoholism
 Gout
 Osteomalacia
Storage diseases (e.g., Gaucher's disease)
Hemoglobinopathies (e.g., Sickle cell disease)
Trauma (e.g., dislocation, fracture)
Dysbaric conditions
Collagen vascular disorders
Irradiation
Pancreatitis
Renal transplantation
Idiopathic, familial

cally demonstrate cessation of growth of the capital femoral epiphysis, resorption of necrotic bone, subchondral fracture, reossification, and finally healing (Fig. 1). Magnetic resonance imaging (MRI) is a helpful technique. Since signal intensity patterns change with circulatory compromise, MRI shows changes not only in bone but also in soft tissues and can assess containment of the femoral head (8).

The short-term prognosis for LCPD depends on the severity of femoral head deformity at completion of the healing phase. The long-term outcome is conditioned by how much secondary degenerative osteoarthritis develops. In general, the more extensive the involvement of the capital femoral epiphysis, the worse the prognosis. Girls appear to fare more poorly than boys, since they tend to have greater involvement of the capital femoral epiphysis and mature earlier. Earlier sexual maturation means less time for proper femoral head modeling before closure of the growth plates. Onset at 2–6 years of age is associated with the least femoral head deformity; onset after 10 years of age has a poor outcome (5–9).

Treatment for LCPD is directed principally by the orthopedic surgeon. Prevention of femoral head deformity is a primary goal. Significant deformity, not mild, predisposes to osteoarthritis. This complication seems to be greatest in those children in whom there is "loss of containment" of the femoral head by the acetabulum. Hip subluxation or loss of motion from muscle spasm and contractures disproportionately increases mechanical stresses on some regions of the femoral head. Prevention of subluxation of the femoral head with elimination of irritability and restoration and maintenance of range of motion of the hip are major therapeutic goals (5–7). Recent studies indicate that bedrest does not substantially decrease compressive forces that may actually stimulate the healing and modeling process if properly distributed (6). The goal is to increase the coverage of the femoral head by the acetabulum, thus allowing it to act as a mold during reparative reossification. Appropriate manage-

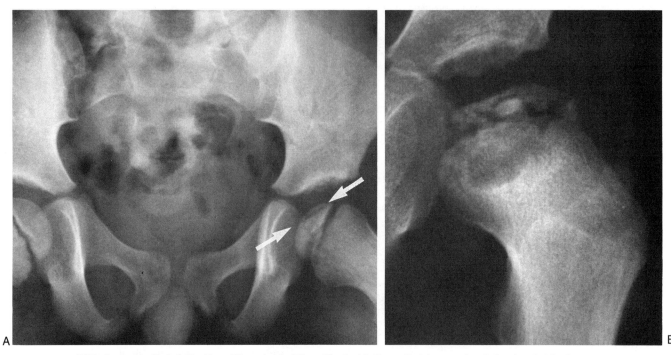

FIG. 1. *Legg-Calvé-Perthes Disease.* **A:** The affected left capital femoral epiphysis of this 4-year-old boy is denser and smaller than the contralateral normal side and shows a radiolucent area that forms the "crescent sign" (*arrows*) indicative of subchondral bone collapse. **B:** Seven months later, there is flattening of the capital femoral epiphysis with widening and irregularity of the femoral neck.

ment may be observation alone, intermittent treatment of symptoms with periodic bedrest, stretching exercises to maintain hip range of motion, and early or late surgical prevention or correction of deformity (10,11). Casts, orthoses, or a "stirrup" crutch may achieve containment. Operative approaches may include osteotomy. Late surgical procedures for deformities include muscle release and abduction casting, osteotomy, and partial excision of the femoral head (5–7,10,11). Periodic radiographic follow-up is essential; arthrography, bone scintigraphy, and especially MRI may be useful (6,8).

The long-term results of these treatments remain controversial. Whether containment is useful and which method of achieving containment is best are clinical questions that are being actively studied (5–7,10,11).

OTHER CLINICAL PRESENTATIONS

Numerous other clinical presentations for ischemic bone disease occur in children and adults (Table 2) (1–3). The specific condition depends on the patient's age, anatomic site, and size of the area of bone where there is interruption of blood flow. LCPD is an excellent illustration that the microvascular anatomy of the skeleton predisposes especially subchondral regions of bone to infarction. Several mechanisms for vascular insuffi-

TABLE 2. *Common sites of osteochondrosis and ischemic necrosis of bone*[a]

Adult skeleton
  Osteochondritis dissecans (König)
  Osteochondrosis of lunate (Kienböck)
  Fractured head of femur (Axhausen, Phemister)
  Proximal fragment of fractured carpal scaphoid
  Fractured head of humerus
  Fractured talus
  Osteonecrosis of the knee (spontaneous or idiopathic ischemic necrosis)
  Idiopathic ischemic necrosis of the femoral head
Developing skeleton
  Osteochondrosis of femoral head (Calvé-Legg-Perthes)
  Slipped femoral epiphysis
  Vertebral epiphysitis affecting secondary ossification centers (Scheuermann)
  Vertebral osteochondrosis of primary ossification centers (Calvé)
  Osteochondrosis of tibial tuberosity (Osgood-Schlatter)
  Osteochondrosis of tarsal scaphoid (Köhler)
  Osteochondrosis of medial tibial condyle (Blount)
  Osteochondrosis of primary ossification center of patella (Köhler) and of secondary ossification center (Sinding Larsen)
  Osteochondrosis of os calcis (Sever)
  Osteochondrosis of head of second metatarsal (Freiberg) and of other metatarsals and metacarpals
  Osteochondrosis of the humeral capitellum (Panner)

[a] Reproduced with permission from Edeiken J, Dalinka M, Karasic D (eds): *Edeiken's Roentgen Diagnosis of Diseases of Bone*, 4th ed. Williams & Wilkins, Baltimore, 937, 1990.

ciency—traumatic rupture, obstruction, or external pressure—may lead to ischemic bone disease. A variety of conditions can cause this group of disorders (Table 1). Arteries, veins, or sinusoids may be directly affected, or there may be extrasinusoidal occlusion. The resulting ischemic bone disease has been referred to as "avascular," "aseptic," "ischemic," or "idiopathic" necrosis (1–3). Symptoms result primarily from skeletal disintegration.

The pathogenesis of disrupted blood flow in ischemic bone disease is incompletely understood (1–3). For many types of nontraumatic ischemic necrosis, the predisposed sites of the skeleton seem to recapitulate the conversion of red marrow to fatty marrow with aging (2). This process occurs from distal to proximal in the appendicular skeleton. As the transition occurs, there is a decrease in marrow blood flow. Accordingly, disorders that increase the size and/or number of fat cells within critical areas of marrow space (e.g., alcoholism, Cushing's syndrome) may ultimately compress sinusoids and infarct bone. However, fat embolization, hemorrhage, and/or abnormalities in the quality of susceptible bone tissue may also be pathogenetic factors in some types of traumatic or nontraumatic ischemic bone disease (2).

The radiologic manifestations of all forms of ischemic necrosis depend on the variable amounts of skeletal revascularization, reossification, and resorption of infarcted bone that may occur (2,3). Revascularization occurs within 6–8 wk of the ischemic event and may cause trabecular bone resorption (radiolucent bands near necrotic areas). New bone formation then occurs on dead bone surfaces. Over months or years, dead bone may, or may not, be slowly resorbed. Osteosclerosis will occur if new bone encases dead bone and/or if there is bony collapse. Histopathologic study is consistent with the pathogenesis that is suggested radiographically. It demonstrates that these various processes are focal and may occur simultaneously (Fig. 2) (4).

Following infarction, affected bone does not change density for at least 10 days (2). MRI is currently the most sensitive way to detect ischemic necrosis of the skeleton and therefore is particularly useful early on, although occasionally false negatives do occur (8,12,13). Bone scintigraphy with ^{99m}technetium diphosphonate, although not specific, can also detect osteonecrosis before x-ray changes are apparent (14,15). Prior to the process of revascularization, the infarcted area will show decreased radioisotope uptake. Later, increased tracer accumulation will occur. Computed tomography is especially helpful for detecting ischemic necrosis of the proximal femur, since the bony anatomy normally has an "asterisk" shape at the center of the femoral head that is distorted by new bone formation (16).

The various clinical presentations of ischemic bone disease (Table 2) may also be divided into two major anatomic categories: diaphysometaphyseal and epiphysometaphyseal (2).

Diaphysometaphyseal ischemia can be caused by dysbaric disorders, hemoglobinopathies, collagen vascular diseases, thromboembolic conditions, gout, storage disorders (e.g., Gaucher disease), acute or chronic pancreatitis, pheochromocytoma, and other conditions.

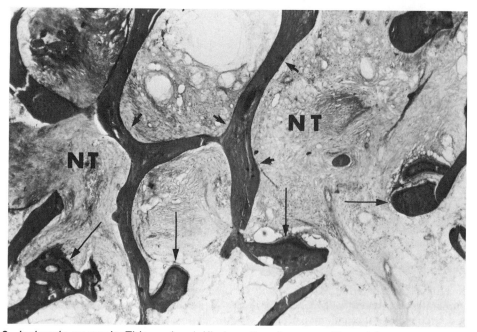

FIG. 2. *Ischemic necrosis.* This undecalcified section from an affected femoral head shows a typical area of dead bone (*arrows*) with a smooth acelluar surface. A band of necrotic tissue (NT) is visible. Reparative bone formation is occurring in adjacent areas where darkly stained, newly synthesized osteoid is covered by osteoblasts (*arrowheads*) [Goldner stain, ×160].

Typically, this category refers to large bones (especially the distal femur or proximal tibia) where radiologic studies show changes that extend into the metaphysis. Such lesions are often symmetrical; however, the size of involved areas can vary considerably. Small bones may be affected; e.g., in the hands and feet of infants with sickle cell anemia. New bone deposition delineates infarcted bone especially well on radiographic study.

Epiphysometaphyseal infarcts can result from trauma, storage problems, dysbaric conditions, Cushing's syndrome, gout, sickle cell disease, and other disorders. When the lesions are small, they are typically found in children or young adults and occur without a history of injury, though occult trauma may actually be important in their pathogenesis. Thrombosis, disease of arterial walls, or abnormalities within adjacent bone such as those occurring in Gaucher's disease or histiocytosis-X (see Chapter 81) may cause this category of ischemic bone disease. The term "osteochondrosis" refers to atraumatic ischemic necrosis that typically affects a growth or ossification center of a growing child (2). Osteochondritis dissecans describes a small epiphysometaphyseal infarct that can cause fracture immediately adjacent to a joint space. The lesion appears as a small button of osseous tissue of increased density that is separated from normal bone by a radiolucent band. This fragment can become loose and enter the joint, but it may also heal. Larger infarcts are often also idiopathic, occur frequently in adults, and typically involve the hip and the femoral condyles. Large fragments of ischemic bone can collapse, thus flattening joint surfaces and destroying articular cartilage. Ultimately, this will lead to osteoarthritis (Fig. 3). Very extensive epiphysometaphyseal infarction results from trauma or sys-

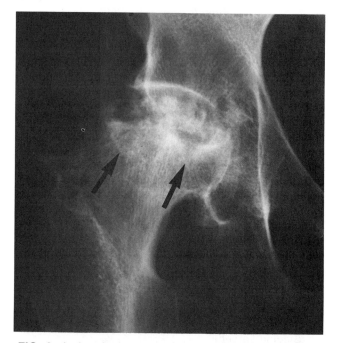

FIG. 3. *Ischemic (avascular) necrosis.* This 50-year-old man has advanced avascular necrosis of the femoral head. Note that much of the femoral head has been resorbed, with resultant collapse of the articular surface. The necrotic area is fragmented. A sclerotic zone of reparative tissue (*arrows*) indicates the interface between viable and necrotic tissues. The acetabular cartilage is focally thin. This finding indicates that he is developing secondary osteoarthritis.

temic disease and frequently involves the femoral head. LCPD is an example (2).

Eponyms for discrete types of osteochondrosis or ischemic necrosis of the skeleton are numerous (e.g., Blount's disease, Scheuermann disease) and are widely used. However, nosology according to the involved anatomic site offers an understandable system of classification. Table 2 matches the eponym with the affected skeletal region and helps to illustrate that the subject's age is an important factor for determining which skeletal sites are predisposed (2).

Treatment of ischemic bone disease will vary according to the site, size, and patient's age. This care is traditionally provided by the orthopedic surgeon and may include conservative or surgical approaches (1,17).

REFERENCES

1. Eicat P, Arlet J, Hungerford DS: *Ischemia and Necroses of Bone.* Williams and Wilkins, Baltimore, 1980
2. Edeiken J, Dalinka M, Karasick D: *Edeiken's Roentgen Diagnosis of Diseases of Bone, 4th ed.* Williams and Wilkins, Baltimore, 1990
3. Resnick D, Niwayama G: *Diagnosis of Bone and Joint Disorders, 2nd ed.* WB Saunders, Philadelphia, 1988
4. Revell PA: *Pathology of Bone.* Springer-Verlag, Berlin, 1986
5. Katz JE: *Legg-Calvé-Perthes Disease.* Praeger, New York, 1984
6. Thompson GH, Salter RB: Legg-Calvé-Perthes disease: current concepts and controversies. *Orthop Clin North Am* 18:617–635, 1987
7. Wenger DR, Ward WT, Herring JA: Current concepts review: Legg-Calvé-Perthes disease. *J Bone Joint Surg* 73A:778–788, 1991
8. Rush BH, Bramson RT, Ogden JA: Legg-Calvé-Perthes disease: detection of cartilaginous and synovial changes with MR imaging. *Radiology* 167:473–476, 1988
9. Mukherjee A, Fabry G: Evaluation of the prognostic indices in Legg-Calvé-Perthes disease: statistical analysis of 116 hips. *J Pediatr Orthop* 10:153–158, 1990
10. Kruse RW, Guille JT, Bowen JR: Shelf arthroplasty in patients who have Legg-Calvé-Perthes disease. *J Bone Joint Surg* 73A: 1338–1347, 1991
11. Paterson DC, Leitch JM, Foster BK: Results of innominate osteotomy in the treatment of Legg-Calvé-Perthes disease. *Clin Orthop Rel Res* 266:96–103, 1991
12. Mitchell MD, Kundel HL, Steinberg ME, Kressel HY, Alavi A, Axel L: Avascular necrosis of the hip: comparison of MR, CT, and scintigraphy. *Am J Roentgenol* 147:67–71, 1986
13. Mitchell DG, Rao VM, Dalinka MK, et al.: Femoral head avascular necrosis: correlation of MR imaging, and clinical findings. *Radiology* 162:709–715, 1987
14. Bonnarens F, Hernandez A, D'Ambrosia RD: Bone scintigraphic changes in osteonecrosis of the femoral head. *Orthop Clin North Am* 16:697–703, 1985
15. Spencer JD, Maisey M: A prospective scintigraphic study of avascular necrosis of bone in renal transplant patients. *Clin Orthop Rel Res* 194:125–135, 1985
16. Dihlmann W: CT analysis of the upper end of the femur: the asterisk sign and ischemic bone necrosis of the femoral head. *Skeletal Radiol* 8:251–258, 1982
17. Crenshaw AH: *Campbell's Operative Orthopaedics, 7th ed.* CV Mosby, St. Louis, 1987

81. Infiltrative Disorders of Bone

Michael P. Whyte, M.D.

Metabolic Research Unit, Shriners Hospital for Crippled Children and Division of Bone and Mineral Diseases, The Jewish Hospital of St. Louis, Washington University School of Medicine; St. Louis, Missouri

An important and interesting variety of skeletal conditions is associated with infiltration or proliferation of abnormal cell types within the marrow spaces. Reviewed briefly here are two major entities: systemic mastocytosis and histiocytosis-X.

SYSTEMIC MASTOCYTOSIS

Systemic mastocytosis is characterized by increased numbers of mast cells in the viscera: principally the liver, spleen, gastrointestinal tract, and lymph nodes. The skin may show numerous hyperpigmented macules that reflect dermal mast cell accumulation—a manifestation called urticaria pigmentosa (Fig. 1). The bone marrow is typically involved, which appears to lead to the skeletal changes. The etiology is unknown (1,2). Recent observations concerning mast cell disease in subjects who have undergone bone marrow transplantation (for other disorders) are of interest (4,5).

Symptoms of systemic mastocytosis are largely attributable to release of mediator substances from mast cells and include generalized pruritis, urticaria, flushing, episodic hypotension, diarrhea, weight loss, peptic ulcer, and syncope. With cutaneous involvement, there will be urtication on stroking of the skin (Darier's sign) because of histamine release. Skeletal symptoms occur relatively infrequently in this condition but typically include bone pain or tenderness from deformity due to fracture (1,2,5–8).

Radiologic abnormalities of the skeleton are common and are found in approximately 70% of affected individuals. They have been thoroughly characterized (9,10). Radiographs typically show diffuse, poorly demarcated, sclerotic, and lucent areas that involve predominantly the axial skeleton (Fig. 2). However, circumscribed lesions can occur especially in the skull and in the extremities. These focal lesions can be mistaken for metastatic disease. Lytic lesions are often small and have a surrounding rim of osteosclerosis from new bone formation. Progression may be observed as focal involvement becomes generalized. Radiologic abnormalities in the skeleton can

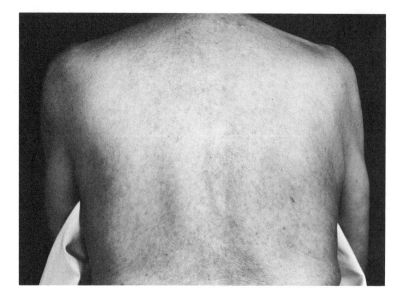

FIG. 1. *Systemic mastocytosis.* Numerous characteristic hyperpigmented macules (urticaria pigmentosa) are present on the back of this 61-year-old woman.

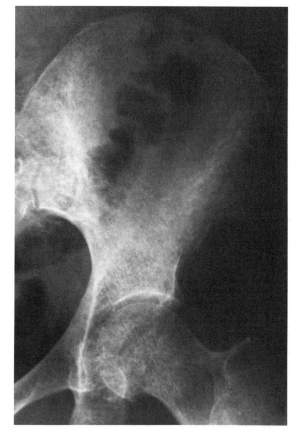

FIG. 2. *Systemic mastocytosis.* This 81-year-old woman has characteristic diffuse punctuate radiolucencies of her pelvis and hip that indicate a permeative process in the bone marrow.

occur without more generalized disease (9,10). Focal bony changes may also be absent even though there is extensive accumulation of mast cells in the skeleton. Recently, it has been emphasized that generalized osteopenia (without focal bony abnormalities) may be a common presentation (5,6,8). Bone scintigraphy is an effective way to detect affected skeletal areas (11).

The histopathologic correlates of systemic mastocytosis in bone have been well documented (5,12). Indeed, examination of nondecalcified sections of bone, can be a particularly effective way to establish the diagnosis. Iliac crest biopsy may be superior to bone marrow aspiration or biopsy for diagnosis (5,12). Undecalcified sections of iliac crest show multiple nodules of 150–450 micron diameter that resemble granulomas. Within the granulomas are characteristic oval or spindle-shaped cells, eosinophils, lymphocytes, and plasma cells. The spindle-shaped cells resemble histiocytes or fibroblasts, but contain granules that stain metachromatically and are a type of mast cell (Fig. 3) (5,12). In addition, the marrow also contains increased numbers of these mast cells individually or in smaller aggregates (5,12).

The treatment of systemic mastocytosis is discussed elsewhere (1,2,13–16).

HISTIOCYTOSIS-X

Histiocytosis-X is the term first used in 1953 to unify what had been considered to be the three distinct entities of Letterer-Siwe disease. Hand-Schüller-Christian disease, and eosinophilic granuloma (17–19). The presence of the Langerhans cell was recognized as a consistent and pathognomonic feature that appeared to link these three syndromes. This disorder seems to result from some poorly understood dysfunction of the immune system. However, histiocytosis-X is an extremely heterogeneous condition. The tripartite distinction continues to be used because of the generally different clinical courses and prognoses for each of the three subtypes (17–19).

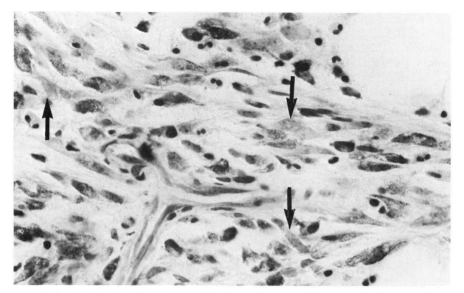

FIG. 3. *Mast cell granuloma.* A nondecalcified specimen of iliac crest shows a characteristic mast cell granuloma that contains (*arrows*) numerous spindle-shaped mast cells (toluidine blue stain, ×220).

About 1,200 cases of histiocytosis-X are diagnosed yearly in the United States. Sex incidence is equal. Northern Europeans are affected more commonly than hispanics, and the condition is rare in blacks. Many tissues and organs can be diseased, including brain, lung, oropharynx, gastrointestinal tract, skin, and bone marrow. Diabetes insipidus is common in affected children and adults. Prognosis is age related. The signs and symptoms of the three principal clinical forms are described briefly here. Infants and the elderly have poor outcomes.

Letterer-Siwe disease presents between several weeks and 2 years of age with hepatosplenomegaly, lymphadenopathy, anemia, a tendency to hemorrhage, fever, failure to grow, and skeletal lesions. It may end fatally after just several weeks (17–19).

Hand-Schüller-Christian disease is a chronic disorder that begins in early childhood, although symptoms may not manifest until the third decade of life (17–19). The classic triad is exophthalmos, diabetes insipidus, and bony lesions; however, they occur together in only 10% of cases. The most common skeletal manifestation is osteolytic lesions in the skull with overlying soft tissue nodules (Fig. 4) (20). Proptosis is associated with destruction of orbital bones. There may by spontaneous remissions and exacerbations. Soft tissue nodules may remit without treatment.

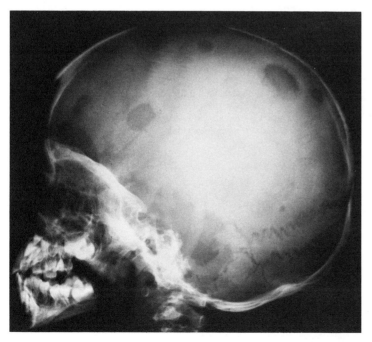

FIG. 4. *Hand-Schüller-Christian Disease.* This 2⁴/₁₂-year-old boy has multiple, well-defined, beveled-edge, lucent lesions of the skull. Note the extensive destruction of the paranasal sinuses and at the base of the skull.

Eosinophilic granuloma occurs most frequently in children between 3–10 years of age, and is rare past the age of 15 years (17–19). A solitary and painful lesion in a flat bone is the most common finding (20). There may be a soft tissue mass. The calvarium is usually affected, although any bone may show involvement. The prognosis is excellent with the monostotic lesions responding well to X-ray therapy or healing spontaneously.

The radiologic findings in the skeleton are similar in the three disorders (9,10,20). Single bony lesions are most common. Nevertheless, multiple affected areas can occur and show progressive enlargement. Individual lesions are well defined, punched-out-appearing, osteolytic, and destructive with scalloped edges. They vary from a few milimeters to several centimeters in diameter. Fewer than half of these radiolucencies show marginal reactive osteosclerosis. Membranous bone as well as long bones can be affected. In the long bones, lesions occur in the medullary canal where there is erosion of the endosteal cortex (commonly in the metaphyseal or epiphyseal regions). Periosteal reaction is frequent and causes a solid layer of new bone formation. In the skull, bone tables can be eroded. Destruction of orbital bones may or may not be associated with exophthalmos. Vertebra plana (i.e., flattened vertebrae) can result from spinal involvement in young children. Radionuclide accumulation is poor during bone scanning (9,10). Biochemical parameters of mineral homeostasis are usually normal.

Histiocytosis-X tends to be benign and self-limiting when there is no systemic disease (9–12,21). Treatment modalities for severe disease include chemotherapy, radiation therapy, and immunotherapy (19). Methylprednisolone injected into lesions is an effective treatment (22). Central nervous system involvement is often treated by radiation therapy. Recently, allogeneic bone marrow transplantation was reported to have been successful in a severe case with poor prognosis (23).

REFERENCES

1. Travis WD, Li CY, Bergstrahl EJ, Yam LI, Swee RG: Systemic mast cell disease: analysis of 58 cases and literature review. *Medicine* 67:345–368, 1988
2. Friedman BS, Metcalfe DD: Mastocytosis. *Prog Clin Biol Res* 297:163–173, 1989
3. Ronnov-Jessen D, Nielsen PL, Horn T: Persistence of systemic mastocytosis after allogeneic bone marrow transplantation in spite of complete remission of the associated myelodysplastic syndrome. *Bone Marrow Transplant* 8:413–415, 1991
4. Van Hoof A, Criel A, Louwagie A, Vanvuchelen J: Cutaneous mastocytosis after autologous bone marrow transplantation. *Bone Marrow Transplant* 8:151–153, 1991
5. Fallon MD, Whyte MP, Teitelbaum SL: Systemic mastocytosis associated with generalized osteopenia: histopathological characterization of the skeletal lesion using undecalcified bone from two patients. *Hum Pathol* 12:813–820, 1981
6. Harvey JA, Anderson HC, Borek D, Morris D, Lukert BP: Osteoporosis associated with mastocytosis confined to bone: report of two cases. *Bone* 10:237–241, 1989
7. Cook JV, Chandy J: Systemic mastocytosis affecting the skeletal system. *J Bone Joint Surg* 71B:536, 1989
8. Lidor C, Frisch B, Gazit D, Gepstein R, Hallel T, Mekori YA: Osteoporosis as the sole presentation of bone marrow mastocytosis. *J Bone Miner Res* 5:871–876, 1990
9. Edeiken J, Dalinka M, Karasick D: *Edeiken's Roentgen Diagnosis of Diseases of Bone, 4th ed.* Williams and Wilkins, Baltimore, 1990
10. Resnick D, Niwayama G: *Diagnosis of Bone and Joint Disorders, 2nd ed.* WB Saunders, Philadelphia, 1988
11. Arrington ER, Eisenberg B, Hartshorne MF, Vela S, Dorin RI: Nuclear medicine imaging of systemic mastocytosis. *J Nucl Med* 30:2046–2048, 1989
12. De Gennes C, Kuntz D, De Vernejoul MC: Bone mastocytosis: a report of nine cases with a bone histomorphometric study. *Clin Orthop Rel Res* 279:281–291, 1992
13. Gasior-Chrzan B, Falk ES: Systemic mastocytosis treated with histamine H_1 and H_2 receptor antagonists. *Dermatology* 184: 149–152, 1992
14. Metcalfe DD: The treatment of mastocytosis: an overview. *J Invest Derm* 96:55S–59S, 1991
15. Póvoa P, Ducla-Soares J, Fernandes A, Palma-Carlos AG: A case of systemic mastocytosis; therapeutic efficacy of ketotifen. *J Intern Med* 229:475–477, 1991
16. Kluin-Nelemans HC, Jansen JH, Breukelman H, Wolthers BG, Kluin PM, Kroon HM, Willemze R: Response to interferon alfa-2b in a patient with systemic mastocytosis. *N Engl J Med* 326: 619–623, 1992
17. Osband ME, Pochedley C: Histiocytosis X. *Hematol Oncol Clin North Am* 1:1–165, 1987
18. Raney RB Jr, D'Angio GJ: Langerhans' cell histiocytes (histiocytosis X): experience at the Children's Hosptial of Philadelphia, 1970–1984. *Med Pediatr Oncol* 17:20–28, 1989
19. Osband ME: Histiocytosis X: Langerhans' cell histiocytosis. *Hematol Oncol Clin North Am* 1:737–751, 1987
20. Bollini G, Jouve JL, Gentet JC, Jacquemier M, Bouyala JM: Bone lesions in histiocytosis X. *J Pediatr Orthop* 11:469–477, 1991
21. Alexander JE, Seibert JJ, Berry DH, Glasier CM, Williamson SL, Murphy J: Prognostic factors for healing of bone lesions in histiocytosis X. *Pediatr Radiol* 18:326–332, 1988
22. Greenberger JS, Crocker AC, Vawter G, Jaffe N, Cassady JR: Results of treatment of 127 patients with systemic histiocytosis (Letterer-Siwe syndrome, Schüller-Christian syndrome and multifocal eosinophilic granuloma). *Medicine* 60:311–388, 1981
23. Ringdén O, Aohström L, Lönnqvist B, Boaryd I, Svedmyr E, Gahrton G: Allogeneic bone marrow transplantation in a patient with chemotherapy-resistant progressive histiocytosis X. *N Engl J Med* 316:733–735, 1987

82. Sarcoidosis

Michael P. Whyte, M.D.

*Metabolic Research Unit, Shriners Hospital for Crippled Children and
Division of Bone and Mineral Diseases, The Jewish Hospital of St. Louis,
Washington University School of Medicine; St. Louis, Missouri*

This systemic disease of unknown etiology affects the skeleton in about 5–25% of cases (1–3). When bone is involved, 80–90% of patients have pulmonary, mediastinal, or supraclavicular nodal pathology; only rarely are there no skin lesions. Blacks have skeletal involvement more frequently than whites.

Radiologic evaluation of the skeleton shows that the small bones of the hands and feet are affected most frequently, especially the middle and distal phalanges (2–4). However, skeletal involvement may be assessed best by bone scintigraphy (5). Characteristically there is a reticular trabecular pattern in the phalanges. This finding reflects perivascular disease that in the Haversian canals thins bony cortices but also destroys fine trabeculae. Occasionally, cystlike lesions of various size are also present (Fig. 1). In advanced disease, the phalanges may be almost completely destroyed and have pathologic fractures. The cystlike lesions may heal with filling in by fibrous tissue. Periosteal proliferation and new bone formation are infrequent. Isolated vertebral involvement, characterized by areas of destruction with a sclerotic margin, occurs most often in the lower thoracolumbar spine. Diffuse sclerosis of single or multiple vertebrae can also occur. Scattered osteosclerotic changes may also be noted in the skull, long bones, ribs, and pelvis (2–4).

Mild to severe hypercalcemia appears transiently in about 10–20% of patients (6,7). Hypercalciuria is even more common, and together with hypercalcemia may cause nephrocalcinosis or nephrolithiasis. Tuberculosis, silicosis, and berylliosis are among additional granulomatous diseases that are associated with hypercalcemia (see Chapter 37).

The abnormal calcium homeostasis that occurs in sarcoidosis appears to result from increased plasma concentrations of $1,25(OH)_2D(6–9)$. Elevated plasma $1,25(OH)_2D$ levels increase dietary absorption of calcium and perhaps enhance bone resorption (10). Excessive $1,25(OH)_2D$ synthesis occurs in diseased lymph nodes (8) and pulmonary alveolar macrophages (9). Understandably, patients are sensitive to vitamin D. This complication responds to treatment with glucocorticoids and chloroquine (11).

The diagnosis and treatment of sarcoidosis is discussed elsewhere (Chapter 34) (1,9,12).

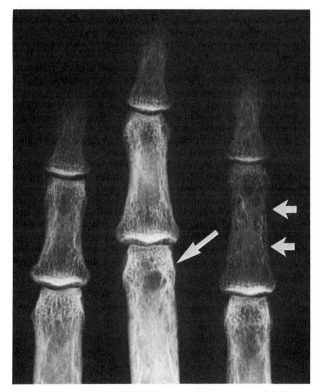

FIG. 1. *Sarcoidosis.* This 57-year-old woman, with known sarcoidosis affecting several organs including skeletal involvement, has a rounded lucency of the head of the proximal phalanx of the long finger (*long arrow*) and a lacy permeative destruction of the middle phalanx of her ring finger (*short arrows*).

REFERENCES

1. Lieberman J: *Sarcoidosis.* Grune and Stratton, Orlando, 1985
2. Edeiken J, Dalinka M, Karasick D: *Edeiken's Roentgen Diagnosis of Diseases of Bone, 4th ed.* Williams and Wilkins, Baltimore, 1990
3. Resnick D, Niwayama G: *Diagnosis of Bone and Joint Disorders, 2nd ed.* WB Saunders, Philadelphia, 1988
4. Abdelwahab IF, Norman A: Osteosclerotic sarcoidosis. *Am J Roentgenol* 150:161–162, 1988
5. Rohatgi PK: Radioisotope imaging in osseous sarcoidosis. *Am J Roentgenol* 134:189–191, 1980
6. Stern PH, De Olazabal J, Bell NH: Evidence for abnormal regulation of circulating $1\alpha,25$-dihydroxyvitamin D in patients with sarcoidosis and normal calcium metabolism. *J Clin Invest* 66:852–855, 1980
7. Singer FR, Adams JS: Abnormal calcium homeostasis in sarcoidosis. *N Engl J Med* 315:755–757, 1986
8. Mason RS, Frankel T, Chan Y-L, Lissner D, Posen S: Vitamin D conversion by sarcoid lymph node homogenate. *Ann Intern Med* 100:59–61, 1984
9. Adams JS: Vitamin D metabolite-mediated hypercalcemia. *Endocrinol Metab Clin North Am* 18:765–778, 1989
10. Meyrier A, Valeyre D, Bouillon R, Paillard F, Battesti J-P, Georges R: Resorptive versus absorptive hypercalciuria in sarcoidosis: correlations with 25-hydroxyvitamin D_3 and 1,25-dihydroxyvitamin D_3 and parameters of disease activity. *Q J Med* 54:269–281, 1985
11. Adams JS, Diz MM, Sharma OP: Effective reduction in the serum 1,25-dihydroxyvitamin D and calcium concentration in sarcoidosis-associated hypercalcemia with short-course chloroquine therapy. *Ann Intern Med* 111:437–438, 1989
12. Bia MJ, Insogna K: Treatment of sarcoidosis-associated hypercalcemia with ketoconazole. *Am J Kidney Dis* 18:702–705, 1991

SECTION VIII

Paget's Disease

83. Paget's Disease of Bone

Ethel S. Siris, M.D.

Department of Medicine, College of Physicians and Surgeons, Columbia University, New York, New York

Paget's disease of bone is a localized disorder of bone remodeling. The process is initiated by increases in osteoclast-mediated bone resorption, with subsequent compensatory increases in new bone formation, resulting in a disorganized mosaic of woven and lamellar bone at affected skeletal sites. This structural change produces bone that is expanded in size, less compact, more vascular, and more susceptible to deformity or fracture than normal bone. Clinical signs and symptoms will vary from one patient to the next depending on the number and location of affected skeletal sites as well as the rapidity of the abnormal bone turnover. It is believed that most patients are asymptomatic, but a substantial minority may experience a variety of symptoms, including bone pain, secondary arthritic problems, bone deformity, excessive warmth over bone from hypervascularity, and a variety of neurological complications due in most instances to compression of neural tissues adjacent to pagetic bone.

ETIOLOGY

The etiology of Paget's disease remains unknown. However, existing data from several different areas of investigation have provided some useful working hypotheses. First, Paget's disease appears to have a significant genetic component. Fifteen to 30% of patients with Paget's disease from several clinical series have positive family histories of the disorder. Genetic analyses of multiple affected kindreds support an autosomal dominant pattern of inheritance. There are data indicating that Paget's disease may be linked to HLA, and Singer has reported an increased frequency of HLA-DQW 1 antigen in pagetic subjects with either positive or negative family histories of the disease. Familial aggregation studies suggest that the risk of a first-degree relative of a pagetic subject developing the condition is 7 times greater than is the risk for someone who does not have an affected relative. Moreover, the risk increases if the first-degree relative has more severe disease and an early age at diagnosis. The data suggest that the predicted cumulative incidence to age 90 is about 2% in people without affected first-degree relatives and over 9% in people with one or more affected first-degree relatives.

Ethnic and geographic clustering of Paget's disease has also been described, with the intriguing observation that the disorder is quite common in some parts of the world but relatively rare in others. Clinical observations indicate that the disease is most common in Europe, North America, Australia, and New Zealand. Studies surveying radiologists have computed prevalence rates in hospitalized patients over age 55 in several European cities and have found the highest percentages in England (4.6%) and

France (2.4%), with other Western European countries reporting slightly lower prevalences (0.7–1.7% in Ireland, 1.3% in Spain and West Germany, 0.5% in Italy and Greece). There is a remarkable focus of Paget's disease in Lancashire, England, where 6.3–8.3% of people over age 55 in several Lancashire towns had x-rays revealing Paget's disease.

Prevalence rates appear to decrease when moving north to south in Europe, except for the finding that Norway and Sweden have a particularly low rate (0.3%). Few data are available from Eastern Europe, but Russian colleagues indicate that Paget's disease is not uncommon in that country. The disorder is seen in Australia and in New Zealand at rates of 3–4%. Paget's disease is distinctly rare in Asia, particularly in China, India, and Malaysia, although occasional cases of Indians living in the United States have been documented. Similar radiographic studies have described 0.01–0.02% prevalences in several areas of sub-Saharan Africa. Dolev has described the characteristics of 278 cases in Israel, of which all patients were Jewish and none Arabs. Mautalen has recently noted a relatively high frequency of Paget's disease in Argentina, restricted to an area surrounding Buenos Aires and predominantly occurring in patients descended form European immigrants.

It is estimated—based on very little data—that up to 3% of people over the age of 55 living in the United States have Paget's disease, making it second only to osteoporosis in terms of numbers of people with the disorder. It is believed that most Americans with Paget's disease are caucasian, of Anglo-Saxon or European descent. The disorder is described in African Americans, and most clinical series from hospitals in major American cities report having black patients.

In addition to the geographic, ethnic, and genetic data, data support a viral etiology for Paget's disease. It has been proposed that the changes in bone remodeling occur as a result of a viral infection of osteoclasts in pagetic bone. Inclusions that resemble viral nucleocapsids have been described in the nuclei and cytoplasm of osteoclasts at pagetic sites, but not in nonpagetic osteoclasts from the same patients or from normal subjects. The viruslike particles resemble members of the paramyxovirus family, but debate has continued for over a decade as to whether the putative virus is respiratory syncytial, measles, canine distemper, some mutation of one or more of these, or some other paramyxovirus. It has been shown that this family of viruses promotes the fusion of infected cells and the formation of multinucleated giant cells. Recent studies have suggested that interleukin-6 may play a role in regulating the behavior of the osteoclast line in Paget's disease. A current "unifying" hypothesis suggests that the large, functionally hyperactive osteoclasts in pagetic bone are a product of a virus-mediated increase in cell fusion between osteoclasts and osteoclast progenitor cells that migrate to pagetic sites. Despite the lack of definitive proof of a viral etiology, many investigators believe that a common viral infection, perhaps early in life, in a gentically susceptible host predisposes to an osteoclast lesion that is manifested in adulthood (typically in the fifth or sixth decade) as the abnormality that produces Paget's disease.

PATHOLOGY

Histopathologic Findings in Paget's Disease

The initiating lesion in Paget's disease is an increase in bone resorption. This occurs in association with an abnormality in the osteoclasts found at affected sites, as previously described. Pagetic osteoclasts are more numerous than normal and contain substantially more nuclei than do normal osteoclasts, with up to 100 nuclei per cell noted by some investigators.

In response to the increase in bone resorption, numerous osteoblasts are recruited to pagetic sites where active and rapid new bone formation occurs. Although some ultrastructural variation in morphology of these osteoblasts is occasionally seen, no inclusion bodies are found, and it is believed by many investigators that the osteoblasts are inherently normal.

In the earliest phases of Paget's disease, increased osteoclastic bone resorption dominates, a picture appreciated radiographically by an advancing lytic wedge or "blade of grass" lesion in a long bone or by osteoporosis circumscripta as seen in the skull. At the level of the bone biopsy, the structurally abnormal osteoclasts are abundant. Following this is a combination of increased resorption and relatively tightly coupled new bone formation, produced by the large numbers of osteoblasts present at these sites. During this phase and presumably due to the accelerated nature of the process, the new bone that is made is abnormal. Newly deposited collagen fibers are laid down in a haphazard rather than linear fashion, creating more primitive woven bone. The woven bone pattern is not specific for Paget's disease, but it reflects a high rate of bone turnover. The end product is the so-called mosaic pattern of woven bone plus irregular sections of lamellar bone linked in a disorganized way by numerous cement lines representing the extent of previous areas of bone resorption. The bone marrow becomes infiltrated by excessive fibrous connective tissue and by an increased number of blood vessels, explaining the hypervascular state of the bone.

Bone matrix at pagetic sites is usually normally mineralized, and tetracycline labeling shows increased calcification rates. It is not unusual, however, to find areas of pagetic biopsies in which widened osteoid seams are apparent, perhaps reflecting inadequate calcium-phosphorus products in localized areas where rapid bone turnover heightens mineral demands.

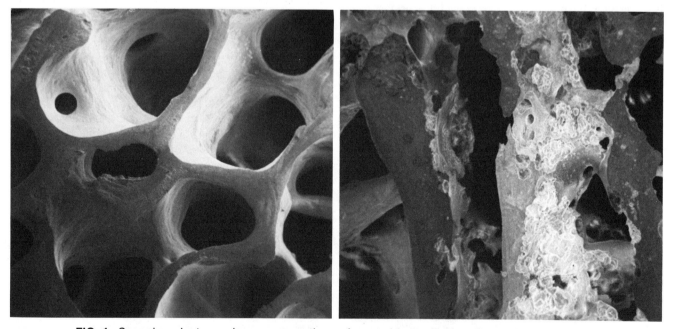

FIG. 1. Scanning electron microscope sections of normal bone (*left*) and pagetic bone (*right*). Both samples were taken from the iliac crest. The normal bone shows the plates and marrow spaces to be well preserved, whereas the pagetic bone has totally lost this architectural appearance. Extensive pitting of the pagetic bone is apparent, due to dramatically increased osteoclastic bone resorption. (Photographs courtesy of Dr. David Dempster; reproduced, with permission, from Siris ES, Canfield RE: Paget's disease of bone. In: Becker KL (ed), *Principles and Practice of Endocrinology and Metabolism,* JB Lippincott, Philadelphia, 1990.)

In time, the hypercellularity at a locus of affected bone may diminish, leaving the end product of a sclerotic, pagetic mosaic without evidence of active bone turnover. This is so-called "burned-out" Paget's disease. Typically, all phases of the pagetic process can be seen at the same time at different sites in a particular subject.

Scanning electron microscopy affords an excellent view of the chaotic architectural changes that occur in pagetic bone and provides the visual imagery that makes the loss of structural integrity comprehensible. Figure 1 compares the appearance of normal and pagetic bone utilizing this technique. Similarly, a view of the mosaic bone pattern of Paget's disease contrasted with an apparent early restoration toward normal following treatment can be seen in Fig. 2.

Biochemical Parameters of Paget's Disease

Increases in the urinary excretion of total hydroxyproline reflect the primary lesion in Paget's disease, the increase in bone resorption. Increases in osteoblastic activity are associated with elevated levels of serum alkaline phosphatase. In untreated patients, the values of these two markers rise in proportion to each other, offering a reflection of the preserved coupling between resorption and formation. From the clinical perspective, the degree of elevation of these indices offers an approximation of the extent or severity of the abnormal bone turnover, with higher levels reflecting a more active, ongoing localized metabolic process. Interestingly, the patients with the highest levels of alkaline phosphatase elevation (e.g., 10 times the upper limit of normal or greater) typically have involvement of the skull as at least one site of the disorder.

Active monostotic disease (other than skull) may have lower biochemical values than polyostotic disease. Lower values (e.g., less than 3 times the upper limit of normal) may reflect a lesser extent of involvement (i.e., fewer sites on bone scans or radiographs) or a burned-out form of Paget's disease, especially in a very elderly person known to have had extensive polyostotic disease in the past. However, minimal elevations in a patient with highly localized disease (e.g., the proximal tibia) may be associated with symptoms and clear progression of disease at the affected site over time.

In addition to offering some estimate of the degree of abnormal bone turnover, the hydroxyproline and alkaline phosphatase measurements are useful in observing the disorder over time and especially for monitoring the effects of treatment. Currently approved therapies generally reduce these parameters by about 50% in up to two-thirds of patients, and these measurements provide the physician with an indication of the efficacy of a particular regimen. As newer treatments become available (see the following sections), urinary markers such as hydroxyproline or pyridinium cross-links may serve as rapid predictors of eventual pharmacologic response, as dramatic decreases in bone resorption may quickly occur with some of the potent new bisphosphonates. The serum alkaline phosphatase may decrease into the normal range after a period of several weeks to 2–3 mo or more as an indication of true "remission" with some of these agents.

Several investigators have examined the usefulness of serum osteocalcin measurements in Paget's disease. This test appears to be substantially less sensitive than serum alkaline phosphatase in this disorder and has not yet shown utility in the monitoring of these patients. As improved assays of serum bone-specific alkaline phospha-

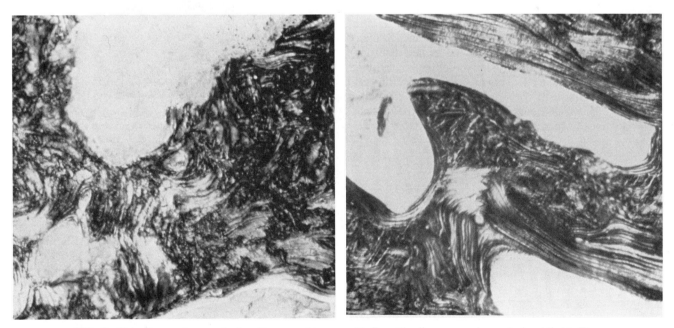

FIG. 2. This figure demonstrates iliac crest bone with Paget's disease under polarized light. The view at the left shows typical woven bone; the one on the right is a section from the same area 6 mo after treatment with EHDP, showing a more lamellar pattern after treatment. (Courtesy of Dr. Pierre Meunier.)

tase emerge, such measurements may prove to have considerable value in this condition.

Serum calcium levels are typically normal in Paget's disease. Clinical experience indicates that the serum calcium may occasionally become elevated in two types of situations. First, if a patient with active, usually extensive Paget's disease is immobilized, the loss of the weight-bearing stimulus to new bone formation may transiently uncouple resorption and accretion, so that increasing hypercalciuria and hypercalcemia may occur. Alternatively, when a raised serum calcium is discovered in an otherwise healthy, ambulatory patient with Paget's disease, coexistent primary hyperparathyroidism may be the cause. Inasmuch as increased levels of parathyroid hormone (PTH) can drive the intrinsic pagetic remodeling abnormality to even higher levels of activity, correction of primary hyperparathyrodism in such cases is indicated. It is currently believed that the coexistence of these two common disorders is a clinical coincidence.

Several investigators have commented on the 15–20% prevalence of secondary hyperparathyroidism (associated with normal levels of serum calcium) in Paget's disease, typically seen in patients with very high levels of serum alkaline phosphatase. The increase in PTH is believed to reflect the need to increase calcium availability to bone during phases of very active pagetic bone formation, particularly in subjects in whom dietary intake of calcium is inadequate. Secondary hyperparathyroidism and transient decreases in serum calcium may be found in some patients being treated with potent new bisphosphonates, reflecting an effective and rapid suppression of bone resorption in the setting of ongoing new bone formation. As restoration of coupling occurs with time, PTH levels fall. In these cases of secondarily increased PTH, it is desirable to be certain that the patient's intake of calcium is at least 1 g/day.

Elevations in serum uric acid and serum citrate have been described in Paget's disease and are of unclear clinical significance. Gout has been noted in this disorder, but it is uncertain whether it is more common in pagetic patients than in nonpagetic subjects. Hypercalciuria may occur in some patients with Paget's disease, presumably due to the increased bone resorption, and kidney stones are occasionally found as a consequence of this abnormality.

CLINICAL FEATURES

Paget's disease affects both men and women, with most series describing a slight male predominance. It is rarely observed to occur below the age of 25, is thought to develop after the age of 40 in most instances, and is most commonly diagnosed in people in their 50s. In a survey of over 800 selected patients, 600 of whom had symptoms, the average age at diagnosis was 58. It seems likely that many patients have the disorder for a period of time before any diagnosis is made, especially since it is often an incidental finding.

It is important to emphasize the localized nature of Paget's disease. It may be monostotic, affecting only a single

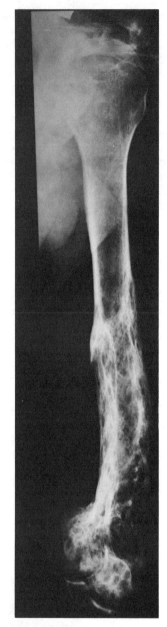

FIG. 3. X-ray of a humerus showing typical pagetic change in the distal half, with cortical thickening, expansion, and mixed areas of lucency and sclerosis, contrasted with normal bone in the proximal half.

bone or portion of a bone (see Fig. 3), or may be polyostotic, involving two or more bones. Sites of disease are often asymmetrical. A patient might have a pagetic right femur with a normal left, involvement of only half the pelvis, or involvement of several noncontiguous vertebral bodies. Clinical observation suggests that in most instances, sites affected with Paget's disease when the diagnosis is made are the only ones that will show pagetic change over time. Although progression of disease within a given bone may occur, the sudden appearance of new sites of involvement years after the initial diagnosis is uncommon. This information can be very reassuring for patients who often worry about extension of the disorder to new areas of the skeleton as they age.

The most common sites of involvement include the pelvis, femur, spine, skull, and tibia. The bones of the upper extremity, as well as the clavicles, scapulae, ribs, and facial bones, are less commonly involved, and the hands and feet are only rarely affected. It is generally believed that most patients with Paget's disease are asymptomatic and that the disorder is most often diagnosed when an elevated serum alkaline phosphatase is noted on routine screening or when a radiograph taken for an unrelated problem reveals typical skeletal changes. The development of symptoms or complications of Paget's disease is influenced by the particular areas of involvement, the interrelationships between affected bone and adjacent structures, and the extent of metabolic activity.

Signs and Symptoms

Bone pain from a site of pagetic involvement, experienced either at rest or with motion, is probably the most common symptom. The direct cause of the pain may be difficult to characterize and requires careful evaluation. Pagetic bone has an increased vascularity, leading to a warmth of the bone that some patients perceive as an unpleasant sensation. Small transverse lucencies along the expanded cortices of involved weight-bearing bones or advancing, lytic, blade of grass lesions may occasionally cause pain. It is postulated that microfractures frequently occur in pagetic bone and can cause discomfort for a period of days to weeks.

A bowing deformity of the femur or tibia, as shown in Fig. 4, can lead to pain for several possible reasons. A bowed limb is typically shortened, resulting in specific gait abnormalities that can lead to abnormal mechanical stresses. Clinically severe secondary arthritis can occur at joints adjacent to pagetic bone, (e.g., the hip, knee, or ankle). The secondary gait problems may also lead to arthritic changes on the contralateral nonpagetic side, particularly at the hip.

Back pain in pagetic patients is another difficult symptom to assess. Nonspecific aches and pains may emanate from enlarged pagetic vertebrae in some instances; vertebral compression fractures may also be seen. In the lumbar area spinal stenosis with neural impingement may arise, producing radicular pain and possibly motor impairment. Degenerative changes in the spine may accompany pagetic changes, and it is useful for the clinician to determine which symptoms arise as a consequence of the pagetic process and which result from degenerative disease of nonpagetic vertebrae. Kyphosis may occur, or there may be a forward tilt of the upper back, particularly when compression fractures or spinal stenosis are present. Treatment options will differ, depending on the basis of the symptoms. When Paget's disease affects the thoracic spine, there may rarely be syndromes of direct spinal cord compression with motor and sensory changes. Several cases of apparent direct cord compression with loss of neural function have now been documented to have resulted from a vascular steal syndrome, whereby hyper-

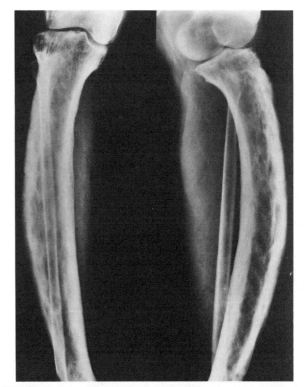

FIG. 4. Bowing deformity of the tibia on anteroposterior (L) and lateral views. The deformity leads to poor alignment at the knee and ankle and to a shortened limb.

vascular pagetic bone "steals" blood from the neural tissue.

Paget's disease of the skull, demonstrated radiographically in Fig. 5, may be asymptomatic, but common complaints in up to one-third of patients with skull involve-

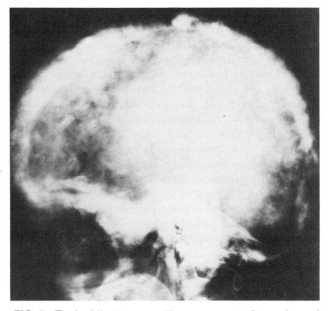

FIG. 5. Typical "cotton-wool" appearance of an enlarged pagetic skull with marked osteoblastic change. The patient had an increase in head size and deafness.

ment may include an increase in head size with or without frontal bossing or deformity, or headache, sometimes described as a bandlike tightening around the head. Hearing loss may occur due to isolated or combined conductive or neurosensory abnormalities. Other cranial nerve palsies (II, VI, VII, etc.) are described less often. With extensive skull involvement, a softening of the base of the skull may produce platybasia, or flattening, with the development of basilar invagination, so that the odontoid process begins to extend upward as the skull sinks downward upon it. This feature can be appreciated by various radiographic measures including skull x-rays and CT or MRI scans. Although many patients with severe skull changes may have radiographic evidence of basilar invagination, a relatively small number develop the very serious complications of direct brain stem compression or an obstructive hydrocephalus and increased intracranial pressure due to blockage of CSF flow. Pagetic involvement of the facial bones may cause facial deformity, dental problems, and, rarely, narrowing of the airway. Mechanical changes of these types may lead to a nasal intonation when the patient is speaking.

Fracture through pagetic bone is an occasional and serious complication. These fractures may be either traumatic or pathologic, particularly involving long bones with active areas of advancing lytic disease; the most common involve the femoral shaft or subtrochanteric area. The increased vascularity of actively remodeling pagetic bone (i.e., with a moderately increased serum alkaline phosphatase) may lead to substantial blood loss in the presence of fractures due to trauma. Fractures may also occur in the presence of areas of malignant degeneration, a rare complication of Paget's disease. Far more common are the small fissure fractures along the convex surfaces of bowed lower extremities, which may be asymptomatic, stable, and persistent for years, but sometimes a more extensive transverse lucent area extends medially from the cortex and may lead to a clinical fracture with time. As described in following sections, there are data indicating that blade of grass lytic areas as well as these larger transverse fractures may respond to treatment with calcitonin and heal. These types of lesions warrant radiographic follow-up over time. Conversely, the smaller fissure fractures typically do not change with treatment and, in the absence of new pain, rarely require extensive radiographic monitoring. In most cases, fracture through pagetic bone heals normally, although some groups have reported as high as a 10% rate of nonunion.

Neoplastic degeneration of pagetic bone is a relatively rare event, occurring with an incidence of less than 1%. This abnormality has a grave prognosis, typically manifesting itself as new pain at a pagetic site. The Mayo Clinic series reported that the most common site of sarcomatous change is the pelvis, with the femur and humerus next in frequency. Typically, these lesions are osteolytic. The majority of the tumors are classified as osteogenic sarcomas, although both fibrosarcomas and chondrosarcomas are also seen. Current treatment regimens emphasize maximal resection of tumor mass and chemotherapy (or sometimes radiotherapy), but death from massive local extension of disease or from pulmonary metastases occurs in the majority of cases in 1–3 yr.

Benign giant cell tumors may also occur in bone affected by Paget's disease. These lesions may present as localized masses at the affected site. Radiographic evaluation may disclose lytic changes. Biopsy reveals clusters of large osteoclasts, which some authors believe represent reparative granulomas. These tumors may show a remarkable sensitivity to glucocorticoids, so in many instances the mass will disappear following prednisone or dexamethasone.

Diagnosis

When Paget's disease is suspected, the diagnostic evaluation should include a careful medical history and physical examination. Gout, pseudogout, and arthritis are all possible complications of Paget's disease. Rarely, patients with underlying intrinsic heart disease may develop congestive heart failure in the presence of severe Paget's disease. There are also reports suggesting that patients may have an increased incidence of calcific aortic disease. Angioid streaks are seen on funduscopic examination of the eye in some patients with polyostotic Paget's disease. The possibility of a positive family history and a symptom history should be ascertained. The physical exam should also note the presence or absence of warmth, tenderness, or bone deformity in the skull, spine, pelvis, and extremities as well as evidence of loss of range of motion at major joints or leg length discrepancy.

Laboratory tests include measurement of serum alkaline phosphatase and 24-hr urinary hydroxyproline, as described earlier. Many investigators prefer to express the urinary hydroxyproline as a ratio to creatinine (mg/g) in order to have a more accurate and precise value. Radiographic studies (bone scans and conventional radiographs) complete the initial evaluation. Bone biopsy is not usually indicated, as the characteristic radiographic and laboratory findings are diagnostic in most instances.

Bone scans are the most sensitive means of identifying pagetic sites and are most useful for this purpose. Scans are nonspecific, however, and can also be positive in nonpagetic areas that have degenerative changes or, more ominously, may reflect metastatic disease. Plain radiographs of bones noted to be positive on the bone scan provide the most specific information, since the changes noted on the radiograph are usually characteristic to the point of being pathognomonic. Examples of these are shown in Figs. 3, 4, and 5. Enlargement or expansion of bone, cortical thickening, coarsening of trabecular markings, and typical lytic and sclerotic changes may be found. Radiographs also provide data on the status of the joints adjacent to involved sites, identify fissure fractures, indicate the degree to which lytic or sclerotic lesions predominate, and demonstrate the presence or absence of deformity or fracture.

Repeat scans or radiographs are usually unnecessary in observing patients over time, unless new symptoms develop or current symptoms become significantly worse. The possibility of an impending fracture or, rarely, of sarcomatous change should be borne in mind in these situations.

The characteristic radiographic and clinical features of Paget's disease usually eliminate problems with differential diagnosis. However, an older patient may occasionally present with severe bone pain, elevations of the serum alkaline phosphatase and urinary hydroxyproline, a positive bone scan, and less than characteristic radiographic areas of lytic or blastic change. Here the question of metastatic disease to bone or some other form of metabolic bone disease (e.g., osteomalacia with secondary hyperparathyroidism) must be considered. Old radiographs and laboratory tests are very helpful in this setting, as normal studies a year earlier would make a diagnosis of Paget's disease less likely. A similar dilemma occurs when someone with known and established Paget's disease develops multiple painful new sites; here, too, the likelihood of metastatic disease must be carefully considered, and bone biopsy for a tissue diagnosis may be indicated.

TREATMENT

Antipagetic Therapy

Specific antipagetic therapy consists of those agents capable of suppressing the activity of pagetic osteoclasts. Currently approved agents available by prescription in the Untied States include salmon and human calcitonin, both parenterally administered, and the orally administered bisphosphonate (or diphosphonate) etidronate disodium. Plicamycin (previously called mithramycin), although not specifically approved for use in Paget's disease by the Food and Drug Administration (it is FDA approved for the management of hypercalcemia) is available for use in Paget's disease and has value in certain situations. Other bisphosphonates, including pamidronate (aminohydroxypropylidene bisphosphonate) and clodronate (dichloromethylene bisphosphonate) have been successfully used in Europe for the past 15 yr for the management of Paget's disease. Pamidronate has recently been approved for use in the US in an intravenous formulation for cancer hypercalcemia and is being used by some clinicians for the management of Paget's disease. Third-generation bisphosphonates such as alendronate, risedronate, and tiludronate are currently in clinical trials in the United States. These newer bisphosphonates, as well as others such as aminohexane bisphosphonate and di-methyl APD that are being used in other parts of the world, are extremely potent inhibitors of bone resorption and are agents of great promise. Regimens for their use will presumably be developed over the next several years. Gallium nitrate is also being studied for efficacy in Paget's disease, and preliminary studies suggest that its use can lower pagetic indices in many patients. Other symptomatic treatment for Paget's disease, including analgesics, antiinflammatory drugs, and selected orthopedic and neurosurgical interventions, also have roles in management.

Indications for treatment and choices of therapeutic agents continue to be issues of debate among clinicians who treat Paget's disease. The potential benefits of antipagetic agents as a group should be understood as a preface to discussion of the advantages and disadvantages of each specific antipagetic medication currently available in the United States. (Hopefully this will allow the reader to appreciate the arguments regarding agents of choice). Two logical indications for treatment of Paget's disease would be to relieve symptoms and to prevent future complications. It has been clearly demonstrated that suppression of the pagetic process by any of the available classes of agents can effectively ameliorate certain symptoms in the majority of patients. Symptoms such as bone aches or pain (probably the most common complaints of Paget's disease), excessive warmth over bone, headache due to skull involvement, low back pain secondary to pagetic vertebral changes, and some syndromes of neural compression (e.g., radiculopathy and some examples of slowly progressive brain stem or spinal cord compression) are the most likely to be relieved. Pain due to a secondary arthritis from pagetic bone involving the spine, hip, knee, ankle, or shoulder may or may not respond to antipagetic treatment. Filling in of osteolytic blade of grass lesions in weight-bearing bones has been reported in some treated cases. Conversely, a bowed extremity or other bone deformity will not change after treatment, and deafness is unlikely to improve, although limited studies suggest progression of hearing loss may be slowed.

In the absence of potentially responsive symptoms, the indications for treatment are less clear. It has not been proved that a reduction in substantially elevated pagetic indices will prevent future complications. However, Meunier and others have demonstrated a restoration toward a more normal, lamellar pattern of bone in biopsy specimens after suppression of pagetic activity. It is also known that active, untreated disease may continue to undergo a persistent degree of abnormal bone turnover for many years. Thus, in the view of many investigators, the presence of moderately active asymptomatic disease (i.e., a serum alkaline phosphatase 3 to 4 times the upper limit of normal or more) at sites where the potential for later problems or complications exists (weight-bearing bones, areas near major joints, vertebral bodies, extensively involved skull) is an indication for treatment. Patients with monostotic disease of a tibia or femur with a minimal elevation of alkaline phosphatase are also treatment candidates, as progression of disease in such bones is likely over time. The need for treatment is particularly valid in patients who are young, for whom many years of coexistence with the disorder are likely. Although controlled studies are not available to prove efficaciousness, the use of antipagetic therapy prior to elective surgery on pagetic bone is recommended. The goal here is to reduce the hypervascularity associated with moderately active disease (e.g., a threefold or more elevation in serum alkaline phosphatase) to reduce the amount of blood loss at operation.

Calcitonin

The polypeptide hormones, salmon and human calcitonin, are each available therapeutically as synthetic formulations for parenteral administration. At present, the only forms commercially available in the United States must be injected subcutaneously or intramuscularly. Calcitonin preparations administered as a nasal spray are currently undergoing clinical trials and should become available soon.

Salmon calcitonin is available as Calcimar (Rhone-Poulenc-Rorer) or Miacalcin (Sandoz) in a 400 u vial (2 cc). The usual starting dose is 100 u (0.5 cc), generally self-injected subcutaneously, initially on a daily basis. Symptomatic benefit may be apparent in a few weeks, and the biochemical benefit is usually seen after 3–6 mo of treatment. After this period, many clinicians reduce the dose to 50–100 u every other day or three times weekly. Often maintenance with 50 u three times weekly after the first few months of therapy is quite satisfactory. Patients with moderate to severe disease may require indefinite treatment to maintain a 50% reduction in the biochemical indices and symptomatic relief, but milder or monostotic disease may allow discontinuation of treatment for prolonged periods of time.

Escape from the efficacy of salmon calcitonin may sometimes occur after a variable period of benefit. In some cases this may be due to a postulated downregulation of receptors, but in other instances it may be a consequence of the development of neutralizing antibodies to the salmon polypeptide. For this reason, human calcitonin, an agent somewhat less potent on a mass basis, was eventually developed and made available. The human calcitonin preparation, Cibacalcin (Ciba-Geigy), is provided in a prefilled syringe containing 0.5 mg, a dose probably equivalent to 150 to 200 u of Calcimar or Miacalcin.

Each of these agents has fairly similar effectiveness, although for individual patients one or the other may be preferred. Each may cause a slight decrease in serum calcium after the injection, usually of no clinical significance, during the early months of treatment. More troublesome in a small minority of patients is the development of nausea or queasiness, with or without flushing of the skin of the face and ears. These annoying side effects may last from a few minutes to several hours after each injection, though many patients can avoid them by experimenting with taking the agent at bedtime, with food, without food, etc. Some clinicians find that full doses of Cibacalcin are more likely to cause side effects, a problem significantly reduced by decreasing the daily dose. Although these side effects are unpleasant, they do not appear to be serious or harmful, and most patients develop tolerance to them. Despite the requirement for parenteral administration, many patients who are able to experience benefit from these agents gladly tolerate the need for injection.

Etidronate

The disodium salt of ethane-1,hydroxy-1,1-diphosphonic acid, or EHDP, generically referred to as etidronate disodium, is a pyrophosphate analog that may be given orally. It is commercially available as Didronel (Procter and Gamble) in a 200 or 400 mg tablet. Although only a small percentage of the administered dose is absorbed,

5 mg/kg/day will provide a 50% lowering of biochemical indices and a reduction in symptoms in perhaps two-thirds of patients, much as is observed with the calcitonins, and over similar time frames.

The dose of etidronate is limited by the fact that this agent, like other bisphosphonates, inhibits not only bone resorption but also new bone formation when high doses are administered for prolonged periods of time. For this reason, the recommended regimen for the agent is 5 mg/kg/day (i.e., 200 to 400 mg in most patients) for a 6-mo period, followed by at least 6 mo of no treatment. Over several years of repeated 6 mo on, 6 or more mo off cycles, long-term benefit with maintenance of lower levels of pagetic biochemical activity is possible in a majority of patients. A failure to adhere to a cyclic regimen can induce bone pain and, occasionally, fracture due to focal osteomalacia secondary to excessive etidronate effect. However, careful cyclic management is extremely well tolerated by the great majority of patients. Occasionally, mild transient diarrhea may occur with etidronate, but this does not usually require more than a day or two of withholding the agent, after which it may be taken again. Rarely, patients have some aches and pains, which are usually mild and transient as well. More severe new pain in patients taking etidronate warrants stopping the drug and evaluating the patient before continuing therapy to be certain that lytic disease or impending fracture—particularly in a weight-bearing extremity—has not been exacerbated.

The newer bisphosphonates such as pamidronate and those still under clinical investigation offer great promise for several reasons. First, they appear to be more potent and may permit normalization of pagetic indices rather than only partial suppression. Second, the effects may be longer lasting, so a limited course of treatment may provide many months of suppression. Third, all of the newer bisphosphonates have a much more favorable ratio of inhibition of resorption to inhibition of new bone formation, so the threat of focal osteomalacia should be markedly reduced if not eliminated.

Pamidronate

At the time of this writing, an optimal regimen for pamidronate remains controversial, and the literature is replete with numerous approaches. In my own experience, a small number of patients with relatively mild disease may experience a substantial reduction of alkaline phosphatase to normal or near normal with a single 60 mg infusion given over 3–4 h in 500 cc of 5% dextrose in water. Patients with more moderate to severe disease may require multiple infusions of 30–60 mg infused as described and given on a once weekly or biweekly basis. Total doses of 240–480 mg may be required in some cases, given over a number of weeks. Suppression of urinary markers can often be noted at once, but the serum alkaline phosphatase may take up to 3 mo to reach its nadir. Giving 3 to 4 doses and then reassessing at 3 mo with the possibility of more treatment is a reasonable approach until more is learned about the use of the agent. A successful course of therapy may result in up to 1 yr of continued disease suppression. Side effects may include a low-grade fever the day after the first dose, flulike symptoms in the first 24 h after an infusion (decreasing in likelihood with repeated dosing), and the possibility of mild and transient hypocalcemia, hypophosphatemia, and lymphopenia. Venous irritation may arise, especially if insufficient volume of fluid is used.

Plicamycin

Previously called mithramycin, this agent is a potent and somewhat toxic treatment of Paget's disease that is generally reserved by most investigators for severely affected or refractory patients or for individuals with syndromes of neural compression where rapid therapy is desirable. It is anticipated that pamidronate will replace plicamycin in most cases. At doses of 15–25 µg/kg per 6–8 h infusion, this agent can quickly lower pagetic indices over a few days. Regimens consisting of an infusion every second to third day for up to 5 to 10 infusions have been successfully utilized to reverse spinal cord compression. Even when full resolution of a serious neurological problem is not achieved, pretreatment with plicamycin (often together with dexamethasone) substantially reduces the hypervascularity associated with active pagetic bone turnover. If surgical decompression is then undertaken, there may be much less bleeding.

Plicamycin typically causes nausea and vomiting during the course of treatment, and elevations of hepatocellular enzymes and sometimes of blood urea nitrogen (BUN) are seen as toxic side effects. At the doses used in Paget's disease, marrow toxicity, particularly directed against platelets, is uncommon, but platelet counts should be monitored. Plicamycin also typically induces hypocalcemia after each infusion, with restoration toward normal in 24–36 h. Patients with very high levels of bone turnover may experience a rapid, marked suppression of bone resorption with the agent, but an inhibition of the compensatory new bone formation lags behind. Thus, calcium and phosphorus release from bone is stopped, but continued utilization of these ions by pagetic bone may precipitate 1–2 mg/dl decreases in total serum calcium and mild decreases in serum phosphorus. Calcium supplements and adequate vitamin D intake both during and for a few days after the treatment period can ameliorate this effect.

Selection of the Agent of Choice

In most instances etidronate is an appropriate first choice among the FDA-approved agents, primarily because it is an oral agent and is less expensive than either of the calcitonins. It also allows greater patient tolerance because it rarely causes annoying side effects. With the calcitonins, 10–20% of patients may have some nausea. However, when a patient has extensive lytic disease in a weight-bearing bone, a calcitonin is the drug of choice and is probably also the preferred drug when used prior to elective surgery on pagetic bone, as previously described.

If either etidronate or a calcitonin is initially chosen and is unsatisfactory, it may be discontinued and the other tried. Similarly, if after many years of treatment one agent fails to be effective any longer, one of the others should be initiated. A severely affected patient may have the best result by taking both etidronate and a calcitonin, each given according to the regimen described when it is used alone. Finally, after a course of plicamycin it is advisable to use etidronate, a calcitonin, or both as maintenance therapy. As previously noted, the optimal regimen for pamidronate is still evolving in the United States. The lack of an effective and safe oral formulation of the agent may limit its utility for many patients. Oral preparations of risedronate and alendronate may solve this problem in the future.

Other Therapies

Analgesics and nonsteroidal antiinflammatory agents (NSAIDs) may be tried empirically with or without antipagetic therapy to relieve pain. Pagetic arthritis (i.e., osteoarthritis caused by deformed pagetic bone at a joint space) may cause periods of pain often helped by the NSAIDs.

Surgery on pagetic bone may be necessary in the setting of established or impending fracture. Elective joint replacement, although more complex with Paget's disease than with osteoarthritis, is often very successful in relieving refractory pain. Rarely, osteotomy is performed to alter bowing deformity. Neurosurgical intervention is sometimes required in cases of spinal cord compression, spinal stenosis, or basilar invagination with neural compromise. Although medical management may be beneficial and adequate in some instances, all cases of serious neurologic compromise require immediate neurologic and neurosurgical consultation to allow the appropriate plan of management to be developed. As improved therapies emerge, long-term suppression of pagetic activity may have a preventive role in Paget's disease and may obviate the need for surgical management in many cases.

SELECTED REFERENCES

1. Paget J: On a form of chronic inflammation of bones. *Med Chir Trans* 60:37–63, 1877
2. Nagant de Deuxchaisnes CN, Krane S: Paget's disease of bone: clinical and metabolic observations. *Medicine* 43:233–266, 1964
3. Barry HC: *Paget's Disease of Bone.* Livingston, Edinburgh, 1969
4. Ryan WG, Schwartz TB, Perlia CP: Effects of mithramycin on Paget's disease of bone. *Ann Intern Med* 70:549–557, 1969
5. Smith R, Russell RGG, Bishop M: Diphosphonates and Paget's disease of bone. *Lancet* 1:945–957, 1971
6. Woodhouse NJY, Bordier Ph, Fisher M, Joplin G, Reiner M, Kalu D, Foster J, Macintyre I: Human calcitonin in the treatment of Paget's bone disease. *Lancet* 1:1139–1143, 1971
7. Altman RD, Johnston CC, Khairi MRA, Wellman H, Serafini AN, Sankey RR: Influence of disodium etidronate on clinical and laboratory manifestations of Paget's disease of bone (osteitis deformans). *N Engl J Med* 289:1379–1384, 1973
8. DeRose J, Singer F, Avramides A, Flores A, Dziadiw R, Baker R, Wallach S: Response of Paget's disease to porcine and salmon calcitonins. Effects of long term treatment. *Am J Med* 47:9–15, 1974

9. Canfield R, Rosner W, Skinner J, McWhorter J, Resnick L, Feldman F, Kammerman S, Ryan K, Kunigonis M, Bohne W: Diphosphonate therapy of Paget's disease of bone. *J Clin Endocrinol Metab* 44:96–106, 1977

10. Singer FR: *Paget's Disease of Bone.* New York, London, Plenum, 1977

11. Frijlink WB, TeVelde J, Bijvoet OLM, Heynen G: Treatment of Paget's disease of bone with (3-amino-1-hydroxypropylidene)-1,1-bisphosphonate (APD). *Lancet* 1:799–803, 1979

12. Siris ES, Canfield RE, Jacobs TP: Paget's disease of bone. *Bull NY Acad Med* 56:285–304, 1980

13. Altman RD, Singer F (eds): Proceedings of the Kroc Foundation Symposium of Paget's disease of bone. *Arthritis Rheum* 23:1073–1234, 1980

14. Meunier P, Coindre J, Edouard CM, Arlot ME: Bone histomorphometry in Paget's disease. *Arthritis Rheum* 23:1095–1103, 1980

15. Altman RD, Collins B: Musculoskeletal manifestations of Paget's disease of bone. *Arthritis Rheum* 23:1121–1127, 1980

16. Wick MR, Siegal GP, Unni KK, McLeod RA, Greditzer HB: Sarcomas of bone complicating osteitis deformans (Paget's disease.) *Am J Surg Pathol* 5:47–59, 1981

17. Siris ES, Canfield RE, Jacobs TP, Stoddart KE, Spector PJ: Clinical and biochemical effects of EHDP in Paget's disease of bone: patterns of response to initial treatment and to long-term therapy. *Metab Bone Dis Rel Res* 4,5:301–308, 1981

18. Hosking DJ: Calcitonin and diphosphonate in the treatment of Paget's disease of bone. *Metab Bone Dis Rel Res* 4,5:317–326, 1981

19. Delmas PD, Chapuy MC, Vignon E, Chantron S, Briancon D, Alexandre C, Edouard C, Meunier PJ: Long term effects of dichloromethylene diphosphonate in Paget's disease of bone. *J Clin Endocrinol Metab* 54:837–844, 1982

20. Johnston CC, Altman RD, Canfield RE, Finerman GAM, Taubee JD, Ebert ML: Review of fracture experience during treatment of Paget's disease of bone with etidronate disodium (EHDP). *Clin Orthop* 172:186–194, 1983

21. Barker DJ: The epidemiology of Paget's disease of bone. *Br Med Bull* 40:396–400, 1984

22. Altman R: Long term follow-up of therapy with intermittent etidronate disodium in Paget's disease of bone. *Am J Med* 79:583–590, 1985

23. El-Sammaa M, Linthicum FH, House HP, House JW: Calcitonin as treatment for hearing loss in Paget's disease. *Am J Otol* 7:241–243, 1986

24. Mills BG, Singer FR: Critical evalaution of viral antigen data in Paget's disease of bone. *Clin Orthop* 217:16–25, 1987

25. Harinck HIJ, Papapoulos SE, Blanksma HJ, Moolenaar BAI, Vermey P, Bijvoet OLM: Paget's disease of bone: early and late responses to three different modes of treatment with aminohydroxypropylidene bisphosphonate (APD). *Br Med J* 295:1301–1305, 1987

26. Delmas PD, Chapuy MC, Edouard DS, Meunier PJ: Beneficial effects of aminohexane diphosphonate in patients with Paget's disease of bone resistant to sodium etidronate. *Am J Med* 83:276–282, 1987

27. Thiebaud D, Jaeger P, Gobelet C, et al.: A single infusion of the bisphosphonate AHPrBP (APD) as treatment of Paget's disease of bone. *Am J Med* 85:207–212, 1988

28. Reginster JY, Jeugmans-Huynen AM, Albert A, Denis D, Deroisy R, Lecart MP, Fontaine MA, Collette J, Franchimont P: Biological and clinical assessment of a new bisphosphonate, (chloro-4 phenyl) thiomethylene bisphosphonate, in the treatment of Paget's disease of bone. *Bone* 9:349–354, 1988

29. Papapoulos SE, Hoekman K, Lowik CWGM, Vermeij P, Bijvoet OLM: Application of an in vitro model and a clinical protocol in the assessment of the potency of a new bisphosphonate. *J Bone Miner Res* 4:775–781, 1989

30. *Paget's Disease: An Annotated Bibliography.* National Arthritis and Musculoskeletal and Skin Diseases Information Clearing House. Bethesda, Maryland, 1990

31. O'Doherty DP, Bickerstaff DR, McCloskey EV, Hamdy NAT, Beneton MNC, Harris S, Mian M, Kanis JA: Treatment of Paget's disease of bone with aminohydroxybutylidene bisphosphonate. *J Bone Miner Res* 5:480–491, 1990

32. Siris ES, Ottman R, Flaster E, Kelsey JL: Familial aggregation of Paget's disease of bone. *J Bone Miner Res* 6:495–500, 1991

33. Singer FR, Wallach S (eds): *Paget's Disease of Bone: Clinical Assessment, Present and Future Therapy.* New York and Amsterdam, Elsevier, 1991

34. Kanis J: *Pathophysiology and Treatment of Paget's Disease of Bone.* Carolina Academic Press, Durham, 1991

35. Roodman GD, Kurihara N, Ohsaki Y, Kukita T, Hosking D, Demulder A, Singer FS: Interleukin-6: a potential autocrine/paracrine factor in Paget's disease of bone. *J Clin Invest* 89:46–52, 1992

Extraskeletal (Ectopic) Calcification and Ossification

Introduction

A significant number and variety of disorders cause extraskeletal deposition of calcium and phosphate (Table 1). In some, mineral is precipitated as amorphous calcium phosphate or as hydroxyapatite crystals; in others, bone tissue is formed. The pathogenesis of the ectopic mineralization in these conditions is generally ascribed to one of three mechanisms (Table 1). First, a supranormal "calcium-phosphate solubility product" in extracellular fluid can cause "metastatic" calcification. Alternatively, mineral may be deposited as "dystrophic" calcification into metabolically impaired or dead tissue despite normal serum levels of calcium and phosphate. Third, true bone formation occurs ectopically in a few disorders in which the pathogenesis is poorly understood.

Discussed briefly in this section are these three mechanisms for extracellular calcification or ossification; a description of three principal disorders follows that illustrates each pathogenesis.

MECHANISMS FOR EXTRACELLULAR CALCIFICATION AND OSSIFICATION

Calcium and inorganic phosphate are normally present in serum or extracellular fluid at concentrations that form a "metastable" solution; i.e., their levels are too low for spontaneous precipitation but sufficiently great to cause hydroxyapatite $[Ca_{10}(PO_4)_6(OH)_2]$ formation once crystal nucleation has begun (1). Normally, the presence of a variety of inhibitors of mineralization such as inorganic pyrophosphate helps to prevent ectopic calcification from occurring inappropriately in healthy tissues (2). The pathogenesis of metastatic and dystrophic calcification is partially understood at the cell level. The process typically involves mineral accumulation within matrix vesicles and sometimes within mitochondria (2). The pathogenesis of ectopic ossification is largely an enigma (see the following).

Metastatic calcification is a risk of significant hypercalcemia or hyperphosphatemia (especially both) of any etiology (Table 1). In fact, therapy with phosphate supplements during mild hypercalcemia, or treatment with vitamin D or calcium during mild hyperphosphatemia, may trigger this problem (3).

Direct precipitation of mineral occurs when the calcium-phosphate solubility product in extracellular fluid is exceeded. A value of 75 for this parameter (mg/dl $\times$ mg/dl) is commonly taken as the level which, if surpassed, is associated with mineral precipitation. However, the critical value at which renal calcification might occur is not precisely defined and may vary with age (3). In adults, some consider 70 to be the maximal safe value for the kidney. It is possible that children can tolerate a somewhat higher level, since they normally have higher serum phosphate levels compared to adults, but this is not well established (3). Mineral deposition can occur ectopically from hyperphosphatemia despite concomittant hypocalcemia.

TABLE 1. *Disorders associated with extraskeletal calcification or ossification*

A. Metastatic calcification
   I. Hypercalcemia
      a. Milk-alkali syndrome
      b. Hypervitaminosis D
      c. Sarcoidosis
      d. Hyperparathyroidism
      e. Renal failure
   II. Hyperphosphatemia
      a. Tumoral calcinosis
      b. Hypoparathyroidism
      c. Pseudohypoparathyroidism
      d. Cell lysis following chemotherapy for leukemia
      e. Renal failure
B. Dystrophic calcification
   I. Calcinosis (universalis or circumscripta)
      a. Childhood dermatomyositis
      b. Scleroderma
      c. Systemic lupus erythematosis
   II. Posttraumatic
C. Ectopic ossification
   I. Myositis ossificans (posttraumatic)
      a. Burns
      b. Surgery
      c. Neurologic injury
   II. Fibrodysplasia (myositis) ossificans progressiva

The mineral that is deposited in metastatic calcification may be amorphous calcium phosphate initially, but hydroxyapatite is formed soon after (2). The pattern of deposition varies somewhat between hypercalcemia and hyperphosphatemia but occurs irrespective of the specific underlying condition or mechanism for the disturbed mineral homeostasis. There is a predilection for precipitation into certain tissues.

Hypercalcemia is typically associated with mineral deposits in the kidneys, lungs, and fundus of the stomach. In these "acid-secreting" organs or tissues, a local alkaline milieu may account for the calcium deposition. In addition, the media of large arteries, elastic tissue of the endocardium (especially the left atrium), conjunctiva, and periarticular soft tissues are often affected. However, the predisposition for these sites is not well understood. In the kidney, hypercalciuria may cause calcium phosphate casts to form within the tubule lumen or calculi to develop in the calyces or pelvis. Furthermore, calcium phosphate may precipitate in peritubular tissues. In the lung, calcification affects the alveolar walls and the pulmonary venous system. Well-established causes of metastatic calcification mediated by hypercalcemia include the milk-alkali syndrome, hypervitaminosis D, sarcoidosis, and hyperparathyroidism (Table 1).

Hyperphosphatemia of sufficient severity to cause metastatic calcification occurs with idiopathic hypoparathyroidism or pseudohypoparathyroidism and with the massive cell lysis (release of cellular phosphate) that can follow chemotherapy for leukemia (Table 1). Renal insufficiency is commonly associated with metastatic calcification, in which the mechanism may involve hyperphosphatemia, hypercalcemia, or both. Of interest, but unexplained, is the fact that ectopic calcification is more common in pseudohypoparathyroidism (type I) than in idiopathic hypoparathyroidism despite comparable elevations in serum phosphate levels. Furthermore, the location of ectopic calcification in pseudohypoparathyroidism and hypoparathyroidism (e.g., cerebral basal ganglion) is different from that which occurs from hypercalcemia. With hyperphosphatemia, calcification of periarticular subcutaneous tissues is characteristic and may be related to tissue trauma from the movement of joints (see the following).

Dystrophic calcification occurs despite a normal serum calcium-phosphate solubility product. Injured tissue of any kind is predisposed to this type of extraskeletal calcification. Apparently, such tissue can release material that has nucleating properties. One example of this phenomenon is the caseous lesion of tuberculosis. What local factor predisposes to the precipitation of calcium salts is unknown. Indeed, several mechanisms seem likely. It is clear that mineral precipitation into injured tissue is even more striking and more severe when either the calcium or phosphate level in extracellular fluid is increased. The deposited mineral, as for metastatic calcification, may be either amorphorus calcium phosphate or crystalline hydroxyapatite.

The term "calcinosis" refers to an important type of dystrophic calcification that commonly occurs in or under the skin in connective tissue disorders—particularly in dermatomyositis (discussed in this section), scleroderma, and systemic lupus erythematosis. Other etiologies for calcinosis include metastases and trauma that produces necrotic tissue. As the symptoms of the acute connective tissue disease and the inflammatory process in the subcutaneous tissues subside, painful masses of calcium phosphate appear under the skin. Calcinosis may involve a relatively localized area with small deposits in the skin and subcutaneous tissues, especially over the extensor aspects of the joints and the fingertips (calcinosis circumscripta); or it may be widespread and not only in the skin and subcutaneous tissues, but deeper in periarticular regions and areas of trauma as well (calcinosis universalis). The lesions of calcinosis are small or medium-sized hard nodules that can cause muscle atrophy and contractures.

Ectopic bone formation is associated with two principal etiologies. It occurs with the fasciitis that follows neurologic injury, surgery, a burn, or trauma when it is called myositis ossificans. It also occurs as a principal feature of a separate, heritable entity—fibrodysplasia (myositis) ossificans *progressiva*—where the pathogenesis is especially unclear and controversial (see Chapter 86). Some consider the primary reason for the ectopic bone formation in this latter condition to be a muscle abnormality (myositis ossificans progressiva), whereas others favor a connective tissue defect (fibrodysplasia ossificans progressiva). In all of the preceding conditions, "true" bone tissue is formed. The bone is lamellar, actively remodeled by osteoblasts and osteoclasts, has Haversian systems, and sometimes contains marrow. Apparently, the injured or diseased tissue contains the necessary precursor cells and inductive signals to form bone.

Described in the following chapters are the major features of three conditions—tumoral calcinosis, dermatomyositis, and fibrodysplasia ossificans progressiva—that are principal examples of each type of ectopic mineralization.

REFERENCES

1. Fawthrop FW, Russell RGG: Ectopic calcification and ossification. In: Nordin BEC, Need AG, Morris HA (eds) *Metabolic Bone and Stone Disease, 3rd Edition*. Churchill Livingstone, Edinburgh, pp. 325–338, 1993
2. Anderson HC: Calcific diseases: a concept. *Arch Pathol Lab Med* 107:341–348, 1983
3. Harrison HE, Harrison HC: *Disorders of Calcium and Phosphate Metabolism in Childhood and Adolescence*. WB Saunders, Philadelphia, 291–304, 1979

84. Tumoral Calcinosis

Michael P. Whyte, M.D.

Metabolic Research Unit, Shriners Hospital for Crippled Children and
Division of Bone and Mineral Diseases, The Jewish Hospital of St. Louis,
Washington University School of Medicine; St. Louis, Missouri

Tumoral calcinosis, first described in 1899, is a heritable disorder that is characterized clinically by periarticular metastatic calcification (1). More than 2,000 cases have been described. Mineral deposition develops as soft tissue masses around the major joints. Vascular and visceral calcification does not occur. Typically, the shoulders and hips are affected, although additional joints may be involved (2). Hyperphosphatemia is a fundamental pathogenetic factor for many cases of this entity (3,4), but it is important to note that periarticular metastatic calcification also occurs in disorders in which hypercalcemia predominates (e.g., milk-alkali syndrome, sarcoidosis, and vitamin D intoxication).

Clinical Presentation

Most affected subjects in North America have been black. About one-third of reported cases are familial. Autosomal recessive inheritance is usually described, although autosomal dominant transmission has also been reported (1,2). There is no sex predominance. The condition may present in childhood, but characteristic masses have been noted first in infancy or in old age. This is a lifelong disorder. Hyperphosphatemic subjects more commonly are black, have a positive family history for tumoral calcinosis, manifest the disease before age 20 years, and have multiple lesions (4).

The soft tissue tumors of ectopic calcification are usually painless and grow at variable rates. After 1 or 2 yr, they may be the size of an orange or grapefruit; deposits may be 1 kg or more. Often each is hard, lobulated, and firmly attached to deep fascia. Occasionally, the masses infiltrate into muscles and tendons (4). Since the deposits are extracapsular, joint range of motion is not impaired unless the tumors are particularly large. However, compression of adjacent neural structures may occur. The lesions can also ulcerate the skin to form a sinus tract that drains a chalky fluid; this may lead to secondary infection. Other potential problems in tumoral calcinosis include anemia, low-grade fever, regional lymphadenopathy, and splenomegaly. Some affected subjects have features that resemble pseudoxanthoma elasticum; i.e., skin and vascular calcifications and angioid streaks in the retina. A dental abnormality, consisting of short bulbous roots and calcific deposits that often obliterate pulp chambers, is characteristic (2,5).

Radiologic Examination

The tumors typically appear as large aggregations of irregular, densely calcified lobules that are confined to soft tissues (Fig. 1). The presence of radiolucent fibrous septae accounts for the lobular appearance. Occasionally, fluid layers may be seen in the lobules. The joints per se are unaffected. Bone texture and density are also unremarkable. Periarticular masses that are radiologically indistinguishable from those of tumoral calcinosis also occur in chronic renal failure when mineral homeostasis is poorly controlled.

Recently, a "diaphysitis" has been recognized in some cases of tumoral calcinosis that may be confused with osteomyelitis or neoplasm (6); the new bone formation occurs along the medullary canal of the diaphysis, perhaps from calcific myelitis. When only calcific myelitis is present, computerized tomography and magnetic resonance imaging are excellent tools for diagnosis (6). Bone scanning, however, is the best method to detect and localize the masses.

Laboratory Findings

Serum calcium levels and alkaline phosphatase activity are usually normal. Hyperphosphatemia and increased serum calcitriol levels are present in some patients (4,7). The TmP/GFR may be supranormal, but renal function is otherwise unremarkable. Affected subjects are in positive calcium/phosphate balance. Renal studies reflect both the calcium and the phosphate retention, and some affected individuals are frankly hypocalciuric. The chalky fluid found in lesions is predominantly hydroxyapatite (8,9).

Histopathology

The masses that characterize tumoral calcinosis are essentially foreign body granuloma reactions that consist of multilocular, cystic structures. The cysts have tough connective tissue capsules and their fibrous walls contain numerous foreign body giant cells. They are filled with calcareous material in a viscous milky fluid. Occasionally, spicules of spongy bone and cartilage are found as well.

Etiology and Pathogenesis

The genetic basis for tumoral calcinosis is unknown (1). The precise pathogenesis is poorly understood, but it may lie within the renal tubule cell. Increased renal reclamation of filtered phosphate appears to be a fundamental pathogenetic factor. In hyperphosphatemic patients, enhanced renal tubular reabsorption of phosphate occurs independently of suppressed serum iPTH levels (4,7).

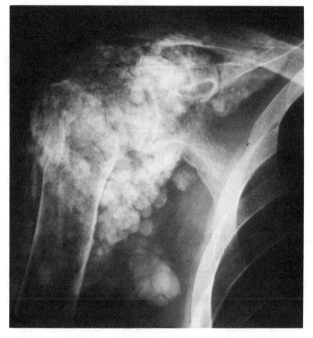

FIG. 1. *Tumoral calcinosis.* Typical lobular periarticular calcifications are present in the region of the right shoulder of this middle-aged man.

Furthermore, vitamin D bioactivation is deranged with defective regulation of the renal 25-hydroxyvitamin D, 1α-hydroxylase so that increased amounts of calcitriol are synthesized. In turn, there is enhanced absorption of dietary calcium and suppression of serum iPTH levels (4,7).

Since masses similar to those of tumoral calcinosis occur in disorders such as sarcoidosis, hypervitaminosis D, or milk-alkali syndrome, the ectopic mineralization of tumoral calcinosis is a nonspecific finding. The masses may begin as calcific bursitis but then extend into adjacent fascial planes as they grow. Tissue damage with fat necrosis can be a predisposing pathogenetic abnormality (9).

The major clinical complications of tumoral calcinosis are related to the metastatic calcifications that occur around joints and in skin, marrow, teeth, and blood vessels.

Treatment

Surgical removal of subcutaneous calcified masses may be helpful if they cause discomfort, interfere with function, or are cosmetically unacceptable. When surgical excision of a tumor is complete, apparently it will rarely reoccur.

Radiation therapy and cortisone treatment have not been effective. Use of phosphate-binding antacids together with dietary phosphate and calcium deprivation has been helpful (3,10,11). Although it might appear that if large apatite crystals were already in place, phosphate-binding antacid therapy alone might not be very effective, dissolution of calcific tumors after aluminum hydroxide therapy has been reported (3,10,11). Furthermore, use of such compounds to decrease extracellular fluid phosphate levels could help to prevent reformation of mineral deposits (3). Preliminary studies indicate that calcitonin therapy may also be efficacious, since this hormone helps to minimize the hyperphosphatemia by enhancing renal clearance of phosphate (12).

REFERENCES

1. McKusick VA: *Mendelian Inheritance in Man: Catalogs of Autosomal Dominant, Autosomal Recessive, and X-Linked Phenotypes, 10th ed.* The Johns Hopkins University Press, Baltimore, 1992
2. Lyles KW, Burkes EJ, Ellis GJ, et al.: Genetic transmission of tumoral calcinosis: autosomal dominant with variable clinical expressivity. *J Clin Endocrinol Metab* 60:1093–1096, 1985
3. Mozaffarian G, Lafferty FW, Pearson OH: Treatment of tumoral calcinosis with phosphorus deprivation. *Ann Intern Med* 77:741–745, 1972
4. Prince MJ, Schaefer PC, Goldsmith RS, Chausmer AB: Hyperphosphatemic tumoral calcinosis: association with elevation of serum 1,25-dihydroxy-cholecalciferol concentrations. *Ann Intern Med* 96:586–591, 1982
5. Burkes EJ Jr, Lyles KW, Dolan EA, Giammara B, Hanker J: Dental lesions in tumoral calcinosis. *J Oral Pathol Med* 20:222–227, 1991
6. Martinez S, Vogler JB, Harrelson JM, Lyles KW: Imaging of tumoral calcinosis: new observations. *Radiology* 174:215–222, 1990
7. Lyles KW, Halsey DL, Friedman NE, Lobaugh B: Correlations of serum concentrations of 1,25-dihydroxyvitamin D, phosphorus, and parathyroid hormone in tumoral calcinosis. *J Clin Endocrinol Metab* 67:88–92, 1988
8. Boskey AL, Vigorita VJ, Sencer O, Stuchin SA, Lane JM: Chemical, microscopic and ultrastructural characterization of mineral deposits in tumoral calcinosis. *Clin Orthop Rel Res* 178:258–270, 1983
9. Kindbolm L-G, Gunterberg B: Tumoral calcinosis: an ultrastructural analysis and consideration of pathogenesis. *APMIS* 96:368–376, 1988
10. Davies M, Clements MR, Mawer EB, Freemont AJ: Tumoral calcinosis: clinical and metabolic response to phosphorus deprivation. *Q J Med* 242:493–503, 1987
11. Gregosiewicz A, Warda E: Tumoral calcinosis: successful medical treatment. *J Bone Joint Surg* 71A:1244, 1989
12. Salvi A, Cerudelli B, Cimino A, Zuccato F, Giustina G: Phosphaturic action of calcitonin in pseudotumoral calcinosis (letter). *Horm Metabol Res* 15:260, 1983

85. Dermatomyositis

Michael P. Whyte, M.D.

Metabolic Research Unit, Shriners Hospital for Crippled Children and
Division of Bone and Mineral Diseases, The Jewish Hospital of St. Louis,
Washington University School of Medicine; St. Louis, Missouri

Dermatomyositis is a multisystem connective tissue disorder, due to small vessel vasculitis, that is characterized by nonsuppurative inflammation of especially skin and striated muscle (1,2).

Clinical Presentation

Females are affected more often than males. Two peak ages of disease incidence occur: childhood (5–15 yr) and adulthood (50–60 yr). When dermatomyositis presents before age 16 yr, it is designated as the "juvenile," or "childhood," form (1,2). The association of dermatomyositis with malignancy that is well documented for the adult form has not been found for the childhood disease.

In childhood dermatomyositis, the patient's sex or the age of onset of symptoms of myositis does not appear to influence the severity of calcinosis. Calcification typically occurs subsequent to the acute phase, and is generally noted 1–3 yr after the disease onset. New deposits of mineral develop for 1–3 yr. Although the dystrophic calcification then typically remains stable, some regression may occur, and spontaneous resolution of calcinosis has been reported (1,2).

In calcinosis universalis the mineral deposition takes place throughout the subcutaneous tissues, but primarily in periarticular regions or in areas that are subject to trauma (Fig. 1A). In calcinosis circumscripta the deposits are more localized and typically occur around joints. The ectopic calcification can cause pain, ulcerate the skin, limit mobility, and predispose to abscess formation.

Laboratory Findings

Hypercalcemia with hypercalciuria and hyperphosphaturia can occur. Elevated levels of gamma-carboxyglutamic acid have been found in the urine of children with dermatomyositis—especially if there is calcinosis (3).

Radiologic Findings

In childhood dermatomyositis, four types of dystrophic calcification occur (4):

1. Superficial masses (small circumscribed nodules or plaques) within the skin
2. Deep discrete subcutaneous nodular masses (Fig. 1B) near joints that can impair movement (calcinosis circumscripta)
3. Deep linear sheetlike deposits within intramuscular fascial planes (calcinosis universalis)
4. Lacy reticular subcutaneous deposits that encase the torso to form a generalized "exoskeleton"

Children with severe disease that is refractory to medical therapy seem to be especially prone to developing exoskeleton-like calcifications. The exoskeleton is in turn associated with severe calcinosis and poor physical function.

Etiology and Pathogenesis

Childhood dermatomyositis appears to be a form of complement-mediated microangiopathy (5). The precise cause of the dystrophic calcification, however, is unknown. Immune deficiencies may predispose the patient to this complication (6). Calcinosis seems to occur in the majority of long-term survivors and may reflect a scarring process. This hypothesis is supported by the observation that mineral deposition seems to occur primarily in the muscles that were most severely affected during the acute phase of the disease. Electron microscopy shows that the calcification consists of hydroxyapatite crystals.

A variety of mechanisms have been considered for the dystrophic calcification, including release of alkaline phosphatase or discharge of free fatty acids from diseased muscle that, in turn, directly precipitate calcium or first bind acid mucopolysaccharides. Increased urinary levels of gamma-carboxylated peptides suggest that calcium-binding proteins may be responsible for the mineral deposition.

Treatment

High-dose prednisone therapy soon after the onset of symptoms seems to be important for minimizing the risk of calcinosis and for ensuring good functional recovery (1,7). If the response is only incomplete, consideration is given to additional immunosuppressive agents. Accumulating evidence indicates that phosphate-binding antacid therapy may reverse the mineral deposition (8). In a small clinical trial, warfarin sodium treatment to decrease gamma-carboxylation was not associated with changes in calcium or phosphorus excretion or in a reduction of calcinosis (9). The calcium deposits can be removed surgically.

Prognosis

The clinical course of dermatomyositis in children is variable. Some have long-term relapsing or persistent dis-

391

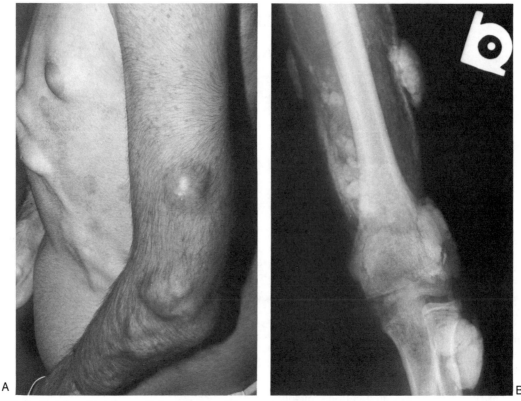

FIG. 1. *Calcinosis universalis in childhood dermatomyosis.* **A:** Characteristic subcutaneous nodules are apparent in the left arm and anterior chest wall of this 15-year-old boy. **B:** The nodules in this boy's arm are comprised of dense lobular calcifications. In addition, the muscles of the upper arm are encased in a characteristic calcified sheath.

ease, whereas others recover. When recovery is incomplete, there may be severe residual weakness, joint contractures, and calcinosis. The calcinosis may be the principal cause of long-term disability.

REFERENCES

1. Olson JC: Juvenile dermatomyositis. *Dermatologica* 11:57–64, 1992
2. Pachman LM, Maryjowski MC: Juvenile dermatomyositis and polymyositis. *Clin Rheum Dis* 10:95–115, 1984
3. Lian JB, Pachman LM, Gundberg CM, Partridge REH, Maryjowski MC: Gamma-carboxyglutamate excretion and calcinosis in juvenile dermatomyositis. *Arthritis Rheum* 25:1094–1100, 1982
4. Blane CE, White SJ, Braunstein EM, Bowyer SL, Sullivan DB: Patterns of calcification in childhood dermatomyositis. *Am J Roentgenol* 142:397–400, 1984
5. Kissel JT, Mendell JR, Rammohan KW: Microvascular deposition of complement membrane attack complex in dermatomyositis. *N Engl J Med* 314:329–334, 1986
6. Moore EC, Cohen F, Douglas SD, Gutta V: Staphylococcal infections in childhood dermatomyositis—association with the development of calcinosis, raised IgE concentrations and granulocyte chemotactic defect. *Ann Rheum Dis* 51(3):378–383, 1992
7. Bowyer SL, Blane CE, Sullivan DB, Cassidy JT: Childhood dermatomyositis: factors predicting functional outcome and development of dystrophic calcification. *J Pediatr* 103:882–888, 1983
8. Wang W-J, Lo W-L, Wong CK: Calcinosis cutis—juvenile dermatomyositis: remarkable response to aluminum hydroxide therapy (letter). *Arch Dermatol* 124:1721–1722, 1988
9. Moore SE, Jump AA, Smiley JD: Effect of warfarin sodium therapy on excretion of 4-carboxy-L-glutamic acid in scleroderma, dermatomyositis, and myositis ossificans progressiva. *Arthritis Rheum* 29:344–351, 1986

86. Fibrodysplasia (Myositis) Ossificans Progressiva

Michael P. Whyte, M.D.

*Metabolic Research Unit, Shriners Hospital for Crippled Children and
Division of Bone and Mineral Diseases, The Jewish Hospital of St. Louis,
Washington University School of Medicine; St. Louis, Missouri*

Fibrodysplasia ossificans progressiva (myositis ossificans progressiva) is a rare disorder that is characterized by two principal features: first, a variety of congenital skeletal abnormalities of the hands and feet; second, recurrent painful episodes of soft tissue swelling that lead to heterotopic mineralization (1,2). The ectopic calcification is not amorphous calcium phosphate or hydroxyapatite; instead, true bone is formed.

This condition is different from trauma-induced myositis ossificans. Posttraumatic myositis ossificans is characterized by a localized area of true bone formation in the connective tissue of muscle that has been severely traumatized, especially by a crush injury. It presents as a tumorlike mass of heterotopic bone and cartilage in soft tissue (typically muscle, but also in tendon, ligaments, joint capsules, and fascia). It may also occur, however, about the knees, thighs, and hips in paraplegics several months after spinal cord injury. Early on the mass may be painful and warm and of doughy consistency. About 4–6 wk after the injury, calcification is apparent on routine radiographs. Later, the bony mass will attach to soft tissue or bone. It is sometimes mistaken for an osteosarcoma on biopsy. Conversely, true malignancy may rarely occur within these masses. The ectopic calcification that follows hip replacement and that occurs in the hematomas formed by hemophiliacs is also true bone.

Fibrodysplasia ossificans progressiva is a distinct condition. It was first described in 1962; more than 600 cases have been reported (1,2). Although Caucasian subjects have been described most commonly, the disorder has been reported in all ethnic groups. The majority of cases appear to develop sporadically; however, autosomal dominant transmission with variable expressivity is established (3).

Clinical Presentation

The diagnosis of fibrodysplasia ossificans progressiva can be strongly suspected at birth, before swellings begin, if typical congenital skeletal anomalies are investigated (1,2). The most characteristic of these is shortened big toes, often with *hallux valgus* deformity (Fig. 1). However, the thumbs may also be strikingly short. Synostosis and hypoplasia of the phalanges are typical. Nevertheless, the anomalies are not pathognomonic for this disorder, and the diagnosis is made when swellings and radiologic evidence of ectopic bone formation are noted.

The severity of this disorder differs considerably from patient to patient (1,2). Typically, however, episodes of

soft tissue swelling begin during the first decade of life (4–6). Occasionally, they present as late as early adulthood, yet there are also reports in which involvement occurred *in utero*. Painful, tender, and rubbery soft tissue induration, which sometimes appears to be precipitated by minor trauma, develops during the course of several days. Typically, it occurs in paraspinal muscles of the back or in the limb girdles and may last for several weeks. Aponeuroses, fascia, tendons, ligaments, and connective tissue of voluntary muscles may be affected by the ectopic bone formation. Not all indurated masses will ossify. Usually, however, there is calcification within the swellings that gradually develops into true heterotopic bone. The episodes of induration recur at unpredictable frequency. Some affected subjects will seem to enter periods of disease quiescence.

Complications of the recurrent swellings include torticollis when there is (as often occurs) involvement of a sternocleidomastoid muscle. Fever may occur during periods of induration and can mistakenly suggest an infectious process. Gradually, the bony masses immobilize joints and cause muscle contractures and deformity, particularly in the neck and shoulders. Ossifications around the hips may prevent ambulation. Involvement of the muscles of mastication can severely limit movement of the jaw and ultimately impair nutrition. Ankylosis of the spine and rib cage further limit mobility. The incidence of scoliosis is increased. The thorax often becomes deformed (Figs. 1 and 2) and thereby causes restrictive lung disease and predisposes the patient to pneumonia. Although secondary amenorrhea is not uncommon, successful reproduction has been reported. Deafness beginning in adolescence or early adult life and alopecia also occur with increased frequency.

Radiologic Features

Skeletal anomalies together with soft tissue ossification comprise the characteristic radiologic features of fibrodysplasia ossificans progressiva (7). Among the principal anomalies are disturbances of formation of the great toe, although many other deformities occur in the extremities. The long bones may also be abnormally shaped, and exostoses occur frequently. A remarkable feature of this condition is developmental fusion of cervical vertebrae that may be confused with Still's disease.

The progressive heterotopic ossification of fibrodysplasia ossificans progressiva involves fascia, tendons, aponeuroses, and other tissues. Bony masses may appear

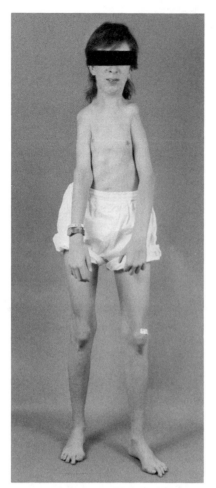

FIG. 1. *Fibrodysplasia (myositis) ossificans progressiva.* Severe underdevelopment of the chest has occurred from ectopic bone formation in the thorax of this 16-year-old boy. Note also the feet with characteristic hallux valgus deformity.

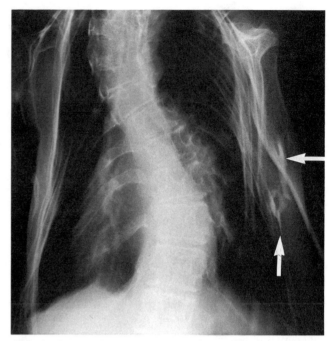

FIG. 2. The thorax of the boy shown in Fig. 1 is markedly narrowed by the ectopic bone within the chest wall (*arrows*) at 15 years of age. Scoliosis is also present and contributed to his restrictive lung disease that soon after proved lethal.

to penetrate deeply into muscle and replace the fascial structure. The neck and shoulders tend to be involved early in the course of the disease; the lower extremities may become affected relatively late. Paraspinal muscles, as noted, are especially prone to ossification. The bones are well mineralized; however, during episodes of severe inflammatory swelling, portions of the skeleton may become osteopenic. Immobilization may also lead to osteoporosis.

Computerized tomography to look for soft tissue calcification appears to be the best radiologic technique to detect an early lesion (8). Increased uptake of radiolabeled diphosphonate will also occur during skeletal scintigraphy before ossification can be demonstrated by conventional radiographs (9). MR of early lesions has also been described (10).

Laboratory Findings

Routine biochemical studies of mineral metabolism are usually normal in fibrodysplasia ossificans progressiva,

although alkaline phosphatase activity in serum may be increased, especially in the active phase (1,2). Recently, serum procollagen-III-peptide levels were found to be elevated in one patient (11).

Histopathology

The palpable soft tissue masses in fibrodysplasia ossificans progressiva are initially comprised of one or more edematous skeletal muscles. Ligaments, tendons, and joint capsules may also be affected. Edema of fascial planes is, in particular, actually one of the earliest histopathologic abnormalities. Subsequently, multifocal interconnecting nodules of fibroblasts are formed. Later, osteoid, bone, or sometimes cartilage develops in the center of a matrix of fibrous connective tissue (6). Endochondral ossification appears to be the mechanism of the new bone formation (12). The osseous lesions then have the appearance of mature bone with Haversian systems. They are macroscopically dense, flat, and irregular, lie within the connective tissue of facial planes, and partly or completely surround a muscle. Cancellous bone that contains hematopoietic tissue will eventually appear. Muscle fibers may secondarily degenerate and atrophy. Of interest is the fact that smooth muscle is not susceptible to the ectopic ossification.

Etiology and Pathogenesis

The autosomal gene defect that causes fibrodysplasia ossificans progressiva has not been mapped within the human genome. Most cases appear to be sporadic. Paternal age seems to contribute importantly to the occurrence of new mutations (13).

The pathogenesis of this disorder is poorly understood. In fact, there is still debate as to whether it primarily affects connective tissue and secondarily muscle or whether the fundamental abnormality is in muscle itself. The term "fibrodysplasia ossificans progressiva" is used by those who believe that connective tissue is primarily involved; "myositis ossificans progressiva" is favored by those who suspect a basic muscle disorder. In support of a connective tissue abnormality, computerized tomography has demonstrated that the first swellings occur within the facial planes of muscle. Subsequently, multiple areas of new bone formation occur adjacent to and encompass individual muscles (8). However, those who favor a primary abnormality in muscle emphasize that electromyographic and histologic abnormalities in muscle occur prior to connective tissue proliferation (14). Similarities between fibrodysplasia ossificans progressiva and the decapentaplegia mutation of *Drosophila* provide clues concerning a potential etiology (12).

Treatment

There is no established medical treatment for fibrodysplasia ossificans progressiva (1,2). The rarity of the disorder, its variable severity, and the fluctuating clinical course pose significant difficulties for evaluating potential therapies. Adrenocorticotrophic hormone, corticosteroids, binders of dietary calcium, and intravenous infusion of EDTA have seemed ineffective. In follow-up of reports that disodium etidronate may be helpful in the prevention of ectopic bone formation after hip replacement surgery, oral administration of this bisphosphonate was tested for fibrodysplasia ossificans progressiva. Unfortunately, it was associated with a variable and inconclusive therapeutic response. Use of warfarin to inhibit gamma-carboxylation of osteocalcin also does not appear to be helpful (15). Accordingly, medical intervention is currently supportive.

Physical therapy to maintain joint mobility appears to be beneficial. Surgical release of joint contractures is generally unsuccessful and presents the risk of new, trauma-induced swellings. Fracture of ectopic bone to mobilize a joint is usually of only temporary benefit. In some cases in which nutrition is becoming impaired, surgical release of an ankylosed jaw has improved mandibular range of motion. Because mobility of the jaw may become limited, dental work should be completed relatively early in life. If surgical intervention is contemplated at any site, computerized tomography can help to identify soft tissue abnormalities and/or ossifications that are not apparent by conventional radiography. Removal of lesions is often followed by their recurrence. In the exceptional case, it is possible that a brief course of high-dose disodium etidronate therapy immediately before and after critical surgery might help to minimize ossification of swellings (16). Intramuscular injections should be avoided. Guidelines for general anesthesia have been reported (17). Measures against recurrent pulmonary infections are important and might include antipneumococcal and antiinfluenza vaccines.

Prognosis

Despite widespread ectopic ossification, some subjects live into the fifth decade. Most, however, die earlier in life from pulmonary complications secondary to restricted ventilation due to chest wall involvement (5).

REFERENCES

1. Connor JM: Fibrodysplasia ossificans progressiva. In: Royce PM, Steinmann B (eds), *Connective Tissue and Its Heritable Disorders.* Wiley-Lyss, New York, 603–611, 1993
2. Beighton P: Fibrodysplasia ossificans progressiva. In: Beighton P (ed), *Heritable Disorders of Connective Tissue.* Mosby, St. Louis, 501–518, 1993
3. McKusick VA: *Mendelian Inheritance in Man: Catalogs of Autosomal Dominant, Autosomal Recessive, and X-Linked Phenotypes, 10th ed.* The Johns Hopkins University Press, Baltimore, 1992
4. Rogers JG, Geho WB: Fibrodysplasia ossificans progressiva: a survey of forty-two cases. *J Bone Joint Surg* 61A:909–914, 1979
5. Connor JM, Evans DAP: Fibrodysplasia ossificans progressiva: the clinical features and natural history of 34 patients. *J Bone Joint Surg* 64B:76–83, 1982
6. Sumiyoshi K, Tsuneyoshi M, Enjoji M: Myositis ossificans: a clinicopathologic study of 21 cases. *Acta Pathol Jpn* 35:1109–1122, 1985
7. Cremin B, Connor JM, Beighton P: The radiological spectrum of fibrodysplasia ossificans progressiva. *Clin Radiol* 33:499–508, 1982
8. Reinig JW, Hill SC, Fang M, et al.: Fibrodysplasia ossificans progressiva: CT appearance. *Radiology* 159:153–157, 1986
9. Fang MA, Reinig JW, Hill SC, et al.: Technitium-99m MDP demonstration of heterotopic ossification in fibrodysplasia ossificans progressiva. *Clin Nucl Med* 11:8–9, 1986
10. Caron KH, DiPetro MA, Aisen AM, Heidelberger KP, Phillips WA, Martel W: MR imaging of early fibrodysplasia ossificans progressiva. *J Comput Assist Tomogr* 14:318–321, 1990
11. Kullich W, Klein G: Elevated procollagen-III-peptide in myositis ossificans progressiva. *Clin Rheumatol* 8:542–543, 1989
12. Kaplan F, Tabas JA, Zasloff MA: Fibrodysplasia ossificans progressiva: a clue from the fly? *Calcif Tissue Int* 47:117–125, 1990
13. Rogers JG, Chase GA: Paternal age effect in fibrodysplasia ossificans progressiva. *J Med Genet* 16:147–148, 1979
14. Lutwak L: Myositis ossificans progressiva. Mineral, metabolic, and radioactive calcium studies of the effects of hormones. *Am J Med* 37:269–293, 1964
15. Moore SE, Jump AA, Smiley JD: Effect of warfarin sodium therapy on excretion of 4-carboxy-L-glutamic acid in myositis ossificans progressiva. *Arthritis Rheum* 29:344–351, 1986
16. Smith R, Russell RGG, Wood CG: Myositis ossificans progressiva. Clinical features of eight patients and their resposne to treatment. *J Bone Joint Surg* 58B:48–57, 1976
17. Lininger TE, Brown EM, Brown M: General anesthesia and fibrodysplasia ossificans progressiva. *Anesth Analg* 68:175–176, 1989

SECTION X

Nephrolithiasis

87. Nephrolithiasis

Fredric L. Coe, M.D. and Joan H. Parks, M.S.

The Renal Program, Pritzker School of Medicine, University of Chicago, Chicago, Illinois

All kidney stones are aggregates of crystals mixed with a protein matrix, and all cause disease because of obstruction of urine flow in the renal collecting system, ureters, or urethra, bleeding, or local erosion into the kidney tissue. The common stone is calcium oxalate: small, recurrent, a cause of pain from passage and obstruction, and due to metabolic disorders that mostly are treatable. Uric acid stones are uncommon (about 5% of all stones) and radiolucent but otherwise like calcium oxalate stones. Struvite stones, from infection, fill renal collecting systems, erode into the renal tissue, and cause obvious renal functional impairment. Cystine stones have only one cause, hereditary cystinuria. They grow large enough to fill the renal collecting system, begin in childhood, and can cause renal failure.

All stones need crystallographic analysis, by simple polarization microscopy or x-ray diffraction when needed. Even if a few have been, say, uric acid, the next may contain calcium oxalate or struvite. Radiographs are not helpful except that uric acid stones are lucent; the rest can look alike, although calcium oxalate stones resemble stars in the night sky, cystine stones are like eggs or staghorns and seem sculpted of a soft stone or wax, and struvite stones are mostly, rugged, ringed staghorns, that look like tree roots. We use flat plates to count stones; tomograms without prior radiocontrast injection are ideal but expensive.

Laboratory evaluation is to detect causes, so measure 24 hr urine calcium, oxalate, uric acid, citrate, pH, volume, and creatinine to estimate completeness of collection (see Chapter 17). How many urine samples is best? One is certainly minimal; we favor three, for better surety, and if we had stones, would measure four. Blood tests are for hypercalcemia; the rest is vague and unsure. Hormone measurements are never proper for initial evaluation; parathyroid hormone (PTH) is for patients who are hypercalcemic.

CALCIUM STONES

Just as bone mineral forms when a supersaturated extracellular fluid contacts an appropriate nucleation site, kidney stones form when urine or, more probably, tubule fluid becomes highly supersaturated with a calcium salt such as calcium oxalate or a calcium phosphate phase. What distinguishes the two processes are the greater levels of supersaturation in urine compared to plasma, the presence in urine and tubule fluid of powerful inhibitors of the crystallization process, and the fact that calcium oxalate is the main constituent of stones, not calcium phosphate.

The causes of calcium stones increase urine calcium or oxalate concentration; lower urine volume, so all concentrations increase; lower urine citrate, which normally forms a soluble salt with calcium and prevents crystallization; raise levels of molecules that can promote calcium oxalate nucleation, uric acid in particular; or cause abnormally high urine pH that promotes calcium phosphate crystallization or low urine pH that promotes uric acid crystallization.

Hypercalciuric States

"Idiopathic" hypercalciuria (IH) (1), the most common, occurs in families, affects both sexes equally, and has a pattern of horizontal and vertical transmission like that of a Mendelian dominant trait. About 50% of patients with calcium oxalate stone have it and are detected by a daily urine calcium excretion rate above usual normal limits of 300 mg and 250 mg for men and women, respectively; by normal serum calcium level; and by the absence of other hypercalciuric conditions such as sarcoidosis, vitamin D intoxication, immobilization, hyperthyroidism, glucocorticoid excess, rapidly progressive osteoporosis, Paget's disease, and Cushing's disease (2). Hypercalciuria raises urine calcium oxalate supersaturation (3), especially after eating.

The mechanism of the hypercalciuria is surely intestinal calcium absorption at an abnormally high rate (4), and what controversy exists concerns the cause of the high absorption rate. The most satisfactory view is that 1,25-dihydroxyvitamin D, calcitriol, levels in the serum are high as a primary defect; in eight studies, hypercalciuric patients had higher levels than normals (5–12). The high calcitriol levels can raise calcium absorption and suppress PTH secretion, leading to reduced renal tubule calcium reabsorption. After eating, calcium will enter the blood at a rapid rate compared to normal, and tubule reabsorption will be low, so serum calcium levels can remain near normal despite high absorption rates, and the calcium can be excreted rapidly into the urine. Alternative theories include a primary renal tubule leak of calcium and a primary increase in intestinal calcium absorption. Neither would explain the common pattern of low PTH (9) and high calcitriol levels, but they could account for hypercalciuria in some selected patients with high PTH levels or normal calcitriol levels.

In addition to hyperabsorption of calcium, patients conserve calcium less well than normal people when given a low calcium intake in the range of 200–500 mg daily. In balance studies, when total calcium absorption can be measured, their urine calcium clearly exceeds net calcium absorption on such diets, meaning that bone mineral is being mobilized into the urine. The reason for their labile bone mineral stores may be partly an excessive action of calcitriol. When given to normal men, this hormone promotes the same behavior as seen among infectious hepatitis patients, a loss of bone mineral during low-calcium diet (11,12). High levels of serum calcitriol are by no means universal among the patients, despite almost universal calcium hyperabsorption, suggesting that not only high serum levels but possibly also high levels of the calcitriol receptor could mediate excessive calcitriol effects. In rats bred for hypercalciuria, increased calcitriol receptor number is an established cause of increased calcitriol action (13).

Given the lability of bone mineral and the natural tendency of doctors to use low-calcium diets for treatment of hypercalciuria, one might expect reduced bone mineral density among IH patients, and to date five studies document just this (14). In particular, the patients whose hypercalciuria persists during low-calcium diet show decisively low bone mineral densities, whereas those with normal or near normal calcium retention during low-calcium diet (a minority) have normal bone mineral density. A clinical corollary of this finding must be caution concerning low-calcium diet as a treatment except among patients clearly able to respond to it with normal calcium conservation. Among patients otherwise prone to osteoporosis, low-calcium diet has an additional and obvious disadvantage. For these reasons, we favor its use in only very restricted circumstances.

Thiazide diuretic agents lower urine calcium excretion, calcium oxalate supersaturation (15), and the rate of stone production (16). Thiazide affects the connecting segment of the nephron (17), increasing calcium reabsorption rate, and presumably lowers calcium excretion in patients by a direct renal action. The drugs lower intestinal calcium absorption in patients who have severe hypercalciuria (18), but less than they lower urine calcium excretion, so calcium balance becomes more positive. Alternative treatments include low-calcium diet, sodium cellulose phosphate, and orthophosphate, all of which lower intestinal calcium absorption. The long-term effects of reduced calcium absorption, especially from low-calcium diet, may include reduced bone mineral stores, because hypercalciuric patients do not lower their urine calcium excretion rates to values as low as in normal people when both are given a very low calcium intake (9). Men who are given calcitriol in excess but at a dose that does not raise serum calcium above normal (11,12) also fail to lower urine calcium normally while eating a low-calcium diet.

Primary hyperparathyroidism causes hypercalciuria in about 5% of calcium stone formers (19); 85% have single enlarged glands, so-called adenoma, the rest have at least two enlarged glands, so-called hyperplasia (see Chapter 29). Serum calcium level is always increased, although the increase commonly is so mild that many values are needed to be sure hypercalcemia is present. Upper limits for our normal subjects are serum calcium levels of 10 mg/dl in women, and 10.1 mg/dl in men. Serum levels of at least half of our patients who have had curative surgery were all below 10.5 mg/dl (19). Urine calcium excretion is very high, despite the modest hypercalcemia, so a casual analysis can be misleading; extreme hypercalciuria and serum calcium levels of—for example—10.1 mg/dl to 10.3 mg/dl can lead one to think of idiopathic hypercalciuria, and probably accounts for misleading accounts of "normocalcemic" primary hyperparathyroidism (20–22), each of which, in retrospect, was almost certainly an instance of mild hypercalcemia.

Among patients who have had curative surgery, serum PTH levels have been elevated in between 80–100% using a carboxyl terminal assay, 60–80% with amino terminal or mild molecule assays (19), so PTH assay is more confirmatory than a structural basis of diagnosis. The best course is to establish if hypercalcemia is present, then to exclude other causes such as malignant tumors, sarcoidosis and other granulomatous diseases, vitamin D intoxication, thiazide use, lithium use, and the uncommon or rare disorders (19, and Section IV). Familial hypocalciuric hypercalcemia is a Mendelian dominant disorder, not a cause of stones, best diagnosed by family studies (19 and Chapter 32). Low PTH levels are especially valuable to detect states of primary calcitriol excess (19). Serum calcitriol is increased in most patients (23–25) as a consequence of high PTH and low serum phosphorus level, and the calcitriol stimulates intestinal calcium absorption, causing most of the hypercalciuria. Bone mineral loss into the urine also occurs.

Treatment is surgical in patients with stone disease. Stone formation is greatly reduced, as urine calcium excretion falls promptly. We follow up our patients to be sure that residual hypercalciuria is not present and that serum calcium levels remain normal.

Renal tubular acidosis (RTA) is ostensibly a cause of hypercalciuria (26), but we suspect it is as often a consequence as a cause (see Chapter 71). The defect associated with stones is reduced ability to lower urine pH; urine citrate excretion is very low, as a rule, and urine calcium is high. It is true that metabolic acidosis is a consequence of severe reductions of tubule ability to lower pH, because a pH lower than that of blood is needed to titrate urine buffers with protons and to trap ammonia as ammonium ion, for excretion. Metabolic acidosis lowers urine citrate excretion and raises urine calcium, so one is tempted to formulate the high pH, high urine calcium, and low urine pH as an expected clustering based on known physiology. However, we (27) have found that alkali treatment, which should lower urine calcium excretion, usually does not, though it may raise urine citrate excretion. Metabolic acidosis is not discernible in most patients. Early reports of RTA (28) included, as a majority, patients such as we have encountered, and labeled them as having "incomplete RTA." In families, idiopathic hypercalciuria and RTA both appear (29), and the hypercalciuria of our patients usually responds to thiazide. We are inclined to believe that the hypercalciuria comes first and that nephrocalcinosis, perhaps hypercalciuria itself, damages collecting ducts and causes the incomplete RTA.

The patients form stones composed of mainly calcium phosphate salts. High urine pH raises urine levels of dissociated phosphate, which forms brushite—calcium monohydrogen phosphate—and apatite. The stones are larger than calcium oxalate stones and grow faster, too.

Apart from sporadic and familial incomplete RTA, rare

patients have complete RTA, usually inherited as an autosomal dominant trait. They have metabolic acidosis; their urine calcium excretions fall with alkali treatment. Diamox (acetazolamide) reduces bicarbonate reabsorption by the proximal tubule and causes alkaline urine and stones. The urine is alkaline because the drug is given in multiple doses, so bicarbonate levels fall, rise between doses, and fall again as the bicarbonate is excreted. Inherited or acquired proximal RTA is a steady defect and causes neither stones nor alkaline urine. Hyperkalemic "type 4" RTA—due to obstruction, low renin or aldosterone secretion rates, or renal disease (30)—causes an acid urine pH and not stones.

Hyperoxaluric States

Primary hyperoxaluria always comes from one of two hereditary enzyme defects that raise oxalate production (31). Oxalate is an end product, excreted only by the kidneys, which filter and secrete it (32). Urine oxalate excretion is above the usual normal limit of 40 mg daily (33), in the range of 80–120 mg. The oxalate crystallizes with calcium, causing stones that begin in childhood, and tubulointerstitial nephropathy, which leads to chronic renal failure. RTA may be an early sign of nephropathy, causing an anion gap metabolic acidosis that raises serum chloride level and lowers bicarbonate level. Renal transplantation requires extensive dialytic preparation so that stored oxalate does not flood the graft and destroy it. Overproduction occurs from pyridoxine deficiency (in animals) and methoxyflurane anesthetic and occurs if one is so foolish or mistaken as to drink ethylene glycol (antifreeze) as a beverage. Treatment is with fluids, citrate (to reduce calcium ion levels), and pyridoxine, which may be helpful in low doses of 20–40 mg daily in some people. Others respond only to 300–400 mg daily, and some do not respond at all.

Enteric hyperoxaluria means that the colon absorbs oxalate excessively because small bowel malabsorption permits undigested fatty acids and bile acids to reach the colon epithelium and increase its permeability (34). Small bowel resection, intestinal bypass for obesity, and small bowel diseases such as Crohn's disease are common causes (35). Colectomy or ileostomy prevents the oxaluria. Urine oxalate is above normal, in the range of 75–150 mg daily. Urine citrate is low because of the alkali loss from the small bowel, and urine pH is low. Urine calcium usually is low, not high. Low-oxalate diet and low-fat diet reduce oxaluria; low fat reduces delivery of fatty acids to colon. Oral calcium 1–4 g, as calcium carbonate, taken with meals, crystallizes with oxalate in the gut lumen. Cholestyramine, 1–4 g with meals, adsorbs oxalate and also bile salts. The four treatments are synergistic and should be used together. Cholestyramine has important side effects of vitamin K depletion and reduced absorption of drugs.

In a way, dietary oxalate excess is an enteric oxaluria. Usual food culprits are nuts, pepper, chocolate, rhubarb, and spinach for a few devotees, and for the rest, mixtures of dark green vegetables and of fruits. Vitamin C in large doses may raise urine oxalate, and ascorbic acid itself may, in urine, break down to oxalic acid, giving a wrong impression of hyperoxaluria. Treatments are simply dietary.

Hyperuricosuric States

About 25% of calcium stone formers excrete more than 800 mg daily of uric acid (750 mg in women) and have no other apparent causes of their stones (36). Their urine pH is lower than the normal of 6.0, averaging 5.6 (37), so the uric acid can crystallize (38). Uric acid crystals can promote calcium oxalate crystallization (39) because they share structural features. Treatment with allopurinol reduced stone recurrence in a prospective, controlled trial (40), and neither allopurinol nor its metabolites affect calcium oxalate crystallization. The hyperuricosuria is due to high purine intake (41) from meats, and dietary treatment should be effective, though it has not been tested. We recommend reducing diet purine intake and reserving allopurinol for those who produce more stones, unless stone disease has been so severe that maximal certainty of treatment is desired despite the risk of drug side effects.

Low Urine Citrate

Women with stones excrete only 550 mg of citrate daily, compared to 750 mg daily for normal women (42). This decisive abnormality ought to raise risk of stones because citrate forms a soluble calcium salt, and what calcium is in the salt is not free to combine with oxalic acid. Normal men excrete no more citrate than women with stones, and men who form stones excrete about the same amount of citrate, so low urine citrate in men is not so much an abnormality as it is a trait that explains why men are four out of every five people with stones. Any oral alkali can raise urine citrate. We prefer citrate to sodium bicarbonate for its longer duration of action, and we use 25–50 mEq two or three times daily. Citrate treatment has not been tested by prospective controlled trails.

URIC ACID STONES

Mixed

About 12% of all calcium stones contain some uric acid (43), and patients who form the mixed stones form urine that is supersaturated with uric acid because its pH is below the normal level of 6.0. Hyperuricosuria is also common. The urine of mixed stone formers is like that of patients with hyperuricosuric calcium oxalate stones, and what distinguishes the two groups is simply that in one uric acid is inferred as a promoter of calcium oxalate stones and in the other the uric acid crystals are seen in the stones themselves. Probably, if all of the stones of the former group were studied, uric acid would be found in some; the distinction is not so intrinsic as it is based on accident of how patients are studied and the relative proportions of uric acid to calcium oxalate in their stones.

Treatment includes reduced diet purine for hyperuricosuria, oral alkali to raise urine pH to 6 or 6.5, and thiazide for hypercalciuria, which may occur in some patients. The hyperuricosuric calcium oxalate stone formers are defined by absence of hypercalciuria or other cause of stones, so thiazide is not usually needed or appropriate.

Pure

Only about 5% of stone formers produce pure uric acid stones. Their urine is very acid, with pH values below 5.3, which is the pK of uric acid, and frequently below 5.0. Uric acid solubility in urine is just below 100 mg/L, whereas the salts of monohydrogen urate are relatively much more soluble, so urine pH values near the pK raise uric acid supersaturation drastically by raising the fraction of the total urate that is fully protonated. For example, average normal men excrete 650 mg of uric acid in 1.2 L of urine (37), a concentration of 540 mg/L; at pK 6.0, less than 10% is undissociated, whereas at pH 5.3 50% (270 mg/L) is undissociated (2.7 times above the solubility). Uric acid stones occur in people with gout and in others with familial uric acid stones. All have low urine pH, and why the urine pH is low is unclear. Patients with ileostomy or who work in hot and dry places form scanty and acid urine, and uric acid stones. Treatment is always alkali to raise urine pH to 6 and is reduced purine intake or allopurinol for hyperuricosuria.

STRUVITE STONES

Only microorganisms that have urease enzyme can produce struvite stones, by hydrolysing urine urea to carbon dioxide and ammonia, so urinary infection is the only clinical cause of these "infection" stones. Struvite forms as the ammonia raises local pH to above 9; phosphate is fully dissociated and combines with urine magnesium and ammonium ion. Carbonate apatite is also formed from the carbonate and calcium because of high pH, so "pure" struvite stones always contain both crystals. Mixed stones also contain calcium oxalate, which is not particularly favored to form under the same circumstances as struvite and denotes the combination of metabolic and infection stone in the same patient.

Mixed

We find that about one-third of struvite stones are mixed; patients begin their stone career with passage, and their prognosis for renal function and nephrectomy is excellent. Men are nearly one-half of this group, and almost all men with struvite stones form mixed stones. Urine calcium excretion is above normal for the group in both sexes. Mean serum creatinine is normal. A few patients do have reduced creatinine clearance, which is rare among calcium stone formers (44).

Pure

Women comprise over half of this group. Stones are frequently staghorns that fill the renal collecting systems. Infection or bleeding or flank pain, rather than stone passage, calls attention to the stones. Serum creatinine levels are above normal on average, creatinine clearance is low, and hypercalciuria is not usual. Put another way, struvite stones seem to be a primary problem, not a complication of metabolic stones.

Treatment

Mixed or pure, these infected stones are treated by removal. Current practice is percutaneous nephrolithotomy, if above 2 cm in diameter, followed by extracorporeal shock wave lithotripsy (ESWL) to fragment what is left, then a second look with percutaneous nephrolithotomy to remove all debris. If stones are less than 2 cm in diameter, ESWL is an adequate monotherapy. Antibiotic agents are best used before and after removal to sterilize the urinary tract.

CYSTINE STONES

Cystine, lysine, ornithine, and citrulline share a common set of transporters in gut and kidney that can be deficient by heredity, as one of at least three autosomal recessive diseases (45). Only cystine causes disease, and only because it is insoluble enough to crystallize into stones. The stones begin in childhood, may be staghorns, and recur throughout life unless treated well.

The solubility of cystine in urine is about 1 mM/L and varies about twofold from person to person. Excretion rates in normal people are micromolar, and also in heterozygotes, so neither form cystine stones. In homozygous cystinuric people, excretion rates range from 1 to 15 mM daily, usual values being about 3–6 mM, so high fluid intake, of 3 to 6 liters daily, is adequate for most people. Nocturia is mandatory because cystine is excreted constantly. Alkaline pH increases cystine solubility, but only above pH 7.4, and to raise urine pH above serum pH requires a high dose of alkali, enough to overbalance total daily acid production. Calcium phosphate stones could be fostered. Even so, alkali is generally recommended.

If water and alkali fail to prevent stones, add a drug that forms a soluble disulfide with cysteine, such as d-penicillamine (45). Cystine is itself the cysteine disulfide and is in equilibrium with cysteine; the drug forms its own cysteine disulfide and lowers free cysteine concentration, and cystine dissociates into cysteine. All available drugs cause allergic side effects such as skin rash and serum sickness reactions and reduce smell and taste; the latter symptoms respond to zinc repletion. Thiola, long in European use, is now also available in the United States.

REFERENCES

1. Coe FL, Parks JH, Moore EM: Familial idiopathic hypercalciuria. *N Engl J Med* 300:337–340, 1979

2. Coe FL, Parks JH: Familial (Idiopathic) Hypercalciuria. In: Coe FL, Parks JH (eds), *Nephrolithiasis, Pathogenesis and Treatment, 2nd ed.* Yearbook Medical Publishers, Chicago, 108–138, 1988

3. Weber DV, Coe FL, Parks JH, et al.: Urinary saturation measurements in calcium nephrolithiasis. *Ann Intern Med* 90: 180–184, 1979

4. Coe FL, Bushinsky DA: Pathophysiology of hypercalciuria. *Am J Physiol* 247:F1–F13, 1984

5. Haussler MR, Baylink J, Hughes MR, et al.: The assay of 1,25-dihydroxy vitamin D_3: physiologic and pathologic modulation of circulating hormone levels. *Clin Endocrinol* 5:151s–165s, 1976

6. Kaplan RA, Haussler MR, Deftos LJ, et al.: The role of 1,alpha-25 dihyroxyvitamin D in the mediation of intestinal hyperabsorption of calcium in primary hyperparathyroidism and absorptive hypercalciuria. *J Clin Invest* 59:756–760, 1977

7. Gray RW, Wilz DR, Caldas AE, et al.: The importance of phosphate in regulating plasma 1,25 $(OH)_2$-vitamin D levels in humans: studies in healthy subjects, in calcium stone formers, and in patients with primary hyperparathyroidism. *J Clin Endocrinol Metab* 45:299–306, 1977

8. Shen FH, Baylink DJ, Neilsen RL: Increased serum 1,25-dihydroxyvitamin D in idiopathic hypercalciuria. *J Lab Clin Med* 90: 955–962, 1977

9. Coe FL, Favus MJ, Crockett T, et al.: Effects of low calcium diet on urine calcium excretion, parathyroid function and serum 1,25$(OH)_2D_3$ levels in patients with idiopathic hypercalciuria and in normal subjects. *Am J Med* 72:25–31, 1982

10. Broadus AE, Insogna KL, Lang R, et al.: Evidence for disordered control of 1,25-dihydroxyvitamin D production in absorptive hypercalciuria. *N Engl J Med* 311:73–80, 1984

11. Adams ND, Gray RW, Lemann J Jr: The effects of oral $CaCo_3$ loading and dietary calcium deprivation on plasma 1,25-dihydroxyvitamin D concentrations in healthy adults. *J Clin Endocrinol Metab* 48:1008–1016, 1979

12. Maierhofer WJ, Lemann J Jr, Gray RW, et al.: Dietary calcium and serum 1,25-$(OH)_2$-vitamin D concentrations as determinants of calcium balance in healthy men. *Kidney Int* 26:752–759, 1984

13. Coe L, Parks JH, Asplin JR: The pathogenesis and treatment of kidney stones, medical progress. *N Engl J Med* 327: 1141–1152, 1992

14. Li XQ, Tembe V, Horwitz GM, Bushinsky DA, Favus MJ: Increased intestinal vitamin D receptor in genetic hypercalciuric rats: A cause of intestinal calcium reabsorption. *J Clin Invest* 91:661–667, 1993

15. Weber DV, Coe FL, Parks JH, et al.: Urinary saturation measurements in calcium nephrolithiasis. *Ann Intern Med* 90: 180–184, 1979

16. Coe FL: Treated and untreated recurrent calcium nephrolithiasis in patients with idiopathic hypercalciuria, hyperuricosuria, or no metabolic disorder. *Ann Intern Med* 87:404–410, 1977

17. Costanzo LS: Localization of diuretic action in microperfused rat distal tubules: Ca and Na transport. *Am J Physiol* 248: F527–535, 1985

18. Coe FL, Parks JH, Bushinsky DA, Langman CV, Favus MJ: Chlorthalidone promotes mineral retention in patients with idiopathic hypercalciuria. *Kidney Int* 33:1140–1146, 1988

19. Coe FL, Parks JH: Primary hyperparathyroidism. In: Coe FL, Parks JH (eds.), *Nephrolithiasis: Pathogenesis and Treatment, 2nd ed.* Yearbook Medical Publishers, Chicago, 59–107, 1988

20. Johnson RD, Conn JW: Hyperparathyroidism with a prolonged period of normocalcemia. *JAMA* 210:2063–2066, 1969

21. Yendt ER, Gagne RJA: Detection of primary hyperparathyroidism, with special reference to its occurrence in hypercalciuric females with "normal" or borderline serum calcium. *Can Med Assoc J* 98:331–336, 1968

22. Wills MR, Pak CYC, Hammond WG, et al.: Normocalcemic primary hyperparathyroidism. *Am J Med* 47:384–391, 1979

23. Broadus AE, Horst RL, Lang R, et al.: The importance of circulating 1,25-dihydroxyvitamin D in the pathogenesis of hypercalciuria and renal-stone formation in primary hyperparathyroidism. *N Engl J Med* 302:421–426, 1980

24. Pak CYC, Nicar MJ, Peterson R, et al.: A lack of unique pathophysiologic background for nephrolithiasis of primary hyperparathyroidism. *J Clin Endocrinol Metab* 55:536–542, 1981

25. LoCascio V, Adami S, Galvanini G, et al.: Substrate-product relation of 1-hydroxylase activity in primary hyperparathyroidism. *N Engl J Med* 313:1123–1130, 1985

26. Transbol I, Gill JR, Lifschitz M, et al.: Intestinal absorption and renal excretion of calcium in metabolic acidosis and alkalosis. *Acta Endrocinol* 155:217, 1971 (suppl)

27. Coe FL, Parks JH: Stone disease in distal renal tubular acidosis. *Ann Intern Med* 93:60–61, 1980

28. Albright F, Burnett CH, Parson W, et al.: Osteomalacia and late ricketts: the various etiologies met in the United States with emphasis on that resulting from a specific form of renal acidosis, the therapeutic indications for each sub-group, and the relationship between osteomalacia and Milkman's syndrome. *Medicine* (Baltimore) 25:399–479, 1946

29. Buckalew VM Jr, Purvis ML, Shulman MG, et al.: Hereditary renal tubular acidosis. *Medicine* (Baltimore) 53:229–254, 1974

30. Wrong O, Davies HEF: The excretion of acid in renal disease. *Q J Med* 28:259–311, 1959

31. Williams HE, Smith LH Jr: Disorders of oxalate metabolism. *Am J Med* 45:715, 1968

32. Hagler L, Herman RH: Oxalate metabolism. *Am J Clin Nutr* (5 parts) 26:758,882,1006,1073,1242, 1973

33. Hodgkinson A, Wilkinson R: Plasma oxalate concentration and renal excretion of oxalate in man. *Clin Sci* 46:61, 1974

34. Kathpalia SC, Favus MJ, Coe FL: Evidence for size and change permselectivity of rat ascending colon: effects of ricinoleate and bile salts on oxalic acid and neutral sugar transport. *J Clin Invest* 74:805–811, 1984

35. Smith LH, Fromm H, Hoffman AF: Acquired hyperoxaluria, nephrolithiasis and intestinal disease. *N Engl J Med* 286:1371, 1972

36. Coe FL, Kavalich AG: Hypercalciuria and hyperuricosuria in patients with calcium nephrolithiasis. *N Engl J Med* 291:1344, 1974

37. Coe FL, Strauss AL, Tembe V, et al.: Uric acid saturation in calcium nephrolithiasis. *Kidney Int* 17:662–668, 1980

38. Coe FL: Uric acid and calcium oxalate nephrolithiasis. *Kidney Int* 24:392–403, 1983

39. Deganello S, Coe FL: Epitaxy between uric acid and whewellite: experimental verification. *N Jb Miner Mh Jg H* 6:270–276, 1983

40. Ettinger B, Tang A, Citron JT, et al.: Randomized trial of allopurinol in the prevention of calcium oxalate calculi. *N Engl J Med* 315:1386–1389, 1986

41. Kavalich AG, Moran E, Coe FL: Dietary purine consumption by hyperuricosuric calcium oxalate kidney stone formers and normal subjects. *J Chronic Dis* 29:745, 1976

42. Parks JH, Coe FL: A urinary calcium-citrate index for the evaluation of nephrolithiasis. *Kidney Int* 30:85–90, 1986

43. Herring LC: Observations on the analysis of ten thousand urinary calculi. *J Urol* 88:545–562, 1962

44. Kristensen C, Parks JH, Lindheimer M, Coe FL: Reduced glomerular filtration rate, hypercalciuria and clinical morbidity in primary struvite nephrolithiasis. *Kidney Int* 32:749–753, 1987

45. Segal S, Thier SO: Cystinuria. In: Stanbury JB, Wyngaarden JB, Fredrickson DS, et al. (eds.), *The Metabolic Basis of Inherited Disease, 5th ed.,* New York, McGraw-Hill, 1774–1791, 1983

SECTION XI

Appendices

i. Growth Charts for Males and Females

Robert F. Gagel, M.D.

Endocrine Section, M.D. Anderson Cancer Center, Houston, Texas

Reg. No.

Surname

Forename

Date of Birth　　　/　　/　　.
　　　　　　　　　　　　Decimal Yr.

Notes/Treatment _____

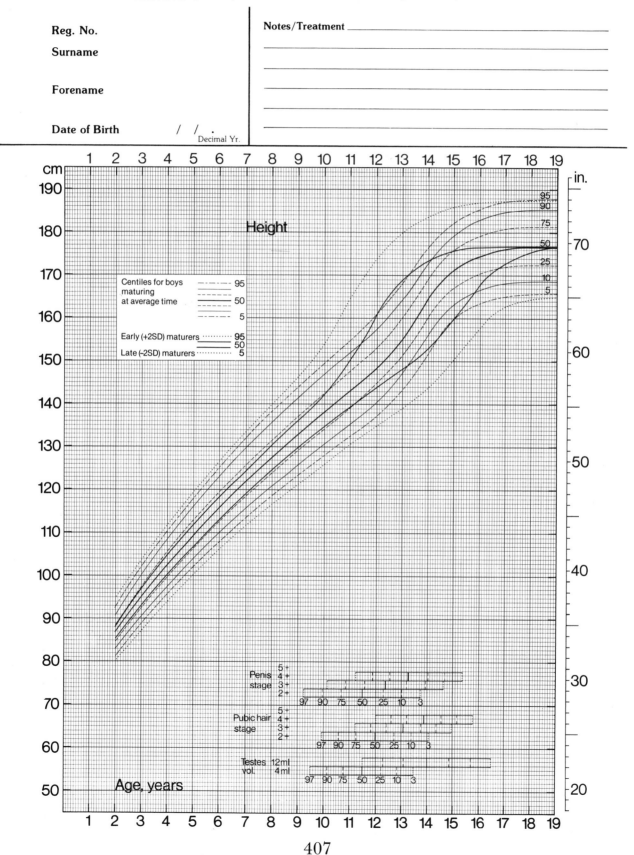

Reg. No.

Surname

Forename

Date of Birth   /   /   .
                     Decimal Yr.

Notes/Treatment

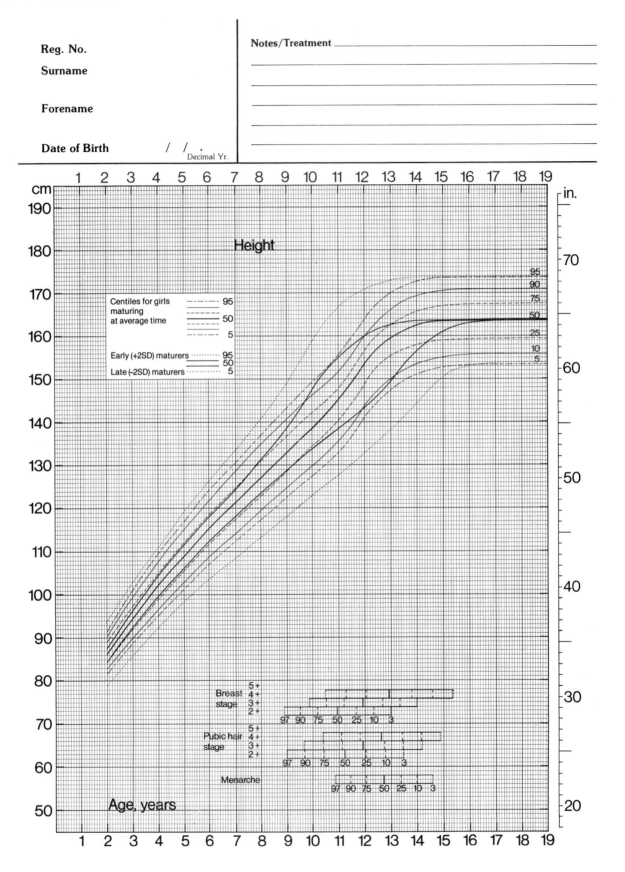

Height

Centiles for girls
maturing
at average time

         95
         50
         5

Early (+2SD) maturers ······ 95
                        50
Late (−2SD) maturers ······ 5

Breast stage   5+ 4+ 3+ 2+
            97 90 75 50 25 10 3

Pubic hair stage   5+ 4+ 3+ 2+
            97 90 75 50 25 10 3

Menarche
            97 90 75 50 25 10 3

Age, years

ii. Ossification Centers

Robert F. Gagel, M.D.

Endocrine Section, M.D. Anderson Cancer Center, Houston Texas

Age at appearance percentiles for major postnatal ossification centers[a]

| | Percentiles | | | | | |
| | Boys | | | Girls | | |
Ossification center	5th	50th	95th	5th	50th	95th
Head of humerus	37g[b]	2w	4m	37g	2w	3m3
Proximal epiphysis of tibia	34g	2w	5w	34g	1w	2w
Coracoid process of scapula	37g	2w	4m2	37g	2w	5m
Cuboid of tarsus	37g	3w	3m3	37g	3w	2m
Capitate of carpus	—	3m	7m	—	2m	7m
Hamate of carpus	2w	3m3	10m	2w	2m1	7m
Capitulum of humerus	3w	4m	13m	3w	3m	9m1
Head of femur	3w	4m1	7m3	2w	4m	7m2
Third cuneiform of tarsus	3w	5m2	19m	—	2m3	14m3
Greater tubercle of humerus	3m	10m	2y4	2m2	6m1	13m3
Primary center, middle segment of 5th toe	—	12m2	3y10	—	9m	2y1
Distal epiphysis of radius	6m2	12m1	2y4	4m3	10m	20m2
Epiphysis, distal segment of 1st toe	8m2	12m3	2y1	4m3	9m2	20m1
Epiphysis, middle segment of 4th toe	5m	14m3	2y11	5m	11m	3y
Epiphysis, proximal segment of 3rd finger	9m1	16m2	2y5	5m	10m1	19m2
Epiphysis, middle segment of 3rd toe	5m	17m	4y3	2m3	12m1	2y6
Epiphysis, proximal segment of 2nd finger	9m2	17m	2y2	5m	10m2	19m3
Epiphysis, proximal segment of 4th finger	9m3	18m	2y5	5m	11m	20m
Epiphysis, distal segment of 1st finger	9m	17m1	2y8	5m	12m	20m3
Epiphysis, proximal segment of 3rd toe	11m	19m	2y6	6m1	12m3	22m3
Epiphysis of 2nd metacarpal	11m1	19m2	2y10	7m3	13m	20m1
Epiphysis, proximal segment of 4th toe	11m2	19m3	2y8	7m2	15m	2y1
Epiphysis, proximal segment of 2nd toe	11m3	21m	2y8	7m3	14m2	2y1
Epiphysis of 3rd metacarpal	11m2	21m2	3y	8m	13m2	23m1
Epiphysis, proximal segment of 5th finger	12m	22m1	2y10	8m	14m2	2y1
Epiphysis, middle segment of 3rd finger	12m1	2y	3y4	7m3	15m2	2y4
Epiphysis of 4th metacarpal	13m	2y	3y7	9m	15m2	2y2
Epiphysis, middle segment of 2nd toe	10m3	2y1	4y1	6m	14m1	2y3
Epiphysis, middle segment of 4th finger	12m	2y1	3y3	7m3	15m	2y5
Epiphysis of 5th metacarpal	15m1	2y2	3y10	10m2	16m2	2y4
First cuneiform of tarsus	10m3	2y2	3y9	6m	17m1	2y10
Epiphysis of 1st metatarsal	16m3	2y2	3y1	11m3	19m	2y3
Epiphysis, middle segment of 2nd finger	15m3	2y2	3y4	8m	17m2	2y7
Epiphysis, proximal segment of 1st toe	17m2	2y4	3y4	10m3	18m3	2y5
Epiphysis, distal segment of 3rd finger	15m3	2y5	3y9	8m3	17m3	2y8
Triquetrium of carpus	6m	2y5	5y6	3m2	20m2	3y9
Epiphysis, distal segment of 4th finger	16m2	2y5	3y9	8m3	18m1	2y10
Epiphysis, proximal segment of 5th toe	18m2	2y6	3y8	11m3	20m3	2y8
Epiphysis of 1st metacarpal	17m2	2y7	4y4	11m	19m1	2y8
Second cuneiform of tarsus	14m2	2y8	4y3	9m3	21m3	3y
Epiphysis of 2nd metatarsal	23m1	2y10	4y4	14m3	2y2	3y5
Greater trochanter of femur	23m	3y	4y4	11m2	22m1	3y
Epiphysis, proximal segment of 1st finger	22m1	3y	4y7	11m1	20m2	2y10
Navicular of tarsus	13m2	3y	5y5	9m1	23m1	3y7
Epiphysis, distal segment of 2nd finger	21m3	3y2	5y	12m3	2y6	3y4
Epiphysis, distal segment of 5th finger	2y1	3y4	5y	12m	23m2	3y6
Epiphysis, middle segment of 5th finger	23m1	3y5	5y10	10m3	23m3	3y7
Proximal epiphysis of fibula	22m2	3y6	5y3	16mn	2y7	3y11
Epiphysis of 3rd metatarsal	2y4	3y6	5y	17m1	2y6	3y8
Epiphysis, distal segment of 5th toe	2y4	3y11	6y4	14m1	2y4	4y1

Age at appearance percentiles for major postnatal ossification centers[a] Continued.

Ossification center	Boys 5th	Boys 50th	Boys 95th	Girls 5th	Girls 50th	Girls 95th
Patella of knee	2y6	4y	6y	17m3	2y6	4y
Epiphysis of 4th metatarsal	2y11	4y	5y9	21m1	2y10	4y1
Lunate of carpus	18m2	4y1	6y9	13m	2y8	5y8
Epiphysis, distal segment of 3rd toe	3y	4y4	6y2	16m2	2y9	4y1
Epiphysis of 5th metatarsal	3y1	4y5	6y4	2y1	3y3	4y11
Epiphysis, distal segment of 4th toe	2y11	4y5	6y5	16m2	2y7	4y1
Epiphysis, distal segment of 2nd toe	3y3	4y8	6y9	18m	2y11	4y6
Capitulum of radius	3y	5y3	8y	2y3	3y11	6y3
Scaphoid of carpus	3y7	5y8	7y10	2y4	4y1	6y
Greater multangular of carpus	3y7	5y11	9y	23m1	4y1	6y4
Lesser multangular of carpus	3y1	6y3	8y6	2y5	4y2	6y
Medial epicondyle of humerus	4y3	6y3	8y5	2y1	3y5	5y1
Distal epiphysis of ulna	5y3	7y1	9y1	3y4	5y5	7y8
Epiphysis of calcaneus	5y2	7y7	9y7	3y7	5y5	7y4
Olecranon of ulna	7y9	9y8	11y11	5y8	8y	9y11
Lateral epicondyle of humerus	9y3	11y3	13y8	7y2	9y3	11y3
Tubercle of tibia	9y11	11y10	13y5	7y11	10y3	11y10
Adductor sesamoid of 1st finger	11y	12y9	14y8	8y8	10y9	12y8
Acetabulum	11y11	13y7	15y4	9y7	11y6	13y5
Acromion	12y2	13y9	15y6	10y4	11y11	13y10
Epiphysis, iliac crest of hip	12y	14y	15y11	10y10	12y10	15y4
Accessory epiphysis, coracoid process of scapula	12y9	14y4	16y4	10y5	12y3	14y5
Ischial tuberosity	13y7	15y3	17y1	11y9	13y11	16y

[a] From Garn SM, et al.: *Med Radiogr Photogr* 43:45–66, 1967.

[b] The abbreviations used include g, gestational week; w, week; m, month; y, year. The number following *m* or *y* refers to the next smaller time unit (e.g., 9y4 = 9 years 4 months).

iii. Laboratory Values of Importance for Calcium Metabolism and Metabolic Bone Disease

Robert F. Gagel, M.D.

Endocrine Section, M.D. Anderson Cancer Center, Houston, Texas

Laboratory values of importance for calcium metabolism and metabolic bone disease[a]

Test	Source of specimen	Reference Range		Reference range (International Units)
Calcium ionized	Serum or plasma		mg/dl	mmol/L
		Cord:	5.5 ± 0.3	1.37 ± 0.07
		Newborn		
		3–24 h:	4.3–5.1	1.07–1.27
		24–48 h:	4.0–4.7	1.00–1.17
		Adult:	4.48–4.92	1.12–1.23
		>60 yr		1.13–1.30
Calcium, total	Serum[b]		mg/dl	mmol/L
		Child:	8.8–10.8	2.2–2.7
		Adult:	8.4–10.2	2.1–2.55
	Urine	Ca^{2+} in diet	mg/dl	mmol/d
		Free Ca^{2+}	5–40	0.13–1.0
		Low to	50–150	1.25–3.8
		average:	100–300	2.5–7.5
		Average		
		(20 mmol/d):		
	Feces	Average: 0.64 g/d		16 mmol/d
Magnesium	Serum	1.3–2.1 mEq/L (higher in females during menses)		0.65–1.05 mmol/L
	Urine, 24 h	6.0–100 mEq/d		3.0–5.0 mmol/d
Phosphatase, acid				
Prostatic (RIA)	Serum	<3.0 ng/mL		<3.0 µg/L
Roy, Brower, and Hayden, 37 C		0.11–0.60 U/L		0.11–0.60 U/L
Phosphatase, alkaline	Serum			
			U/L	
p-nitrophenyl phosphate, carbonate buffer, 30 C		Infant:	50–165	
		Child:	20–150	
		Adult:	20–70	
		>60 yr:	30–75	
Bowers and McComb, 30 C			25–90	
IFFC, 30 C		Male:	30–90	
		Female:	20–80	
Phosphorus, inorganic	Serum		mg/dl	nmol/L
		Cord:	3.7–8.1	1.2–2.6
		Child:	4.5–5.5	1.45–1.78
		Thereafter	2.7–4.5	0.87–1.45
		>60 yr		
		Male:	2.3–3.7	0.74–1.2
		Female:	2.8–4.1	0.9–1.3
	Urine	Adult on diet containing 0.91.5 g, P and 10 mg Ca/kg: < 1.0 g/d		On diet containing 29–48 mmol P and 0.25 mmol Ca/kg: < 32 mmol/d
		Unrestricted diet: 0.4–1.3 g/d		Unrestricted diet: 13–42 mmol/d
Tubular reabsorption of phosphate	Urine, 4 h (0800–1200 h) and serum	82–95%		Fraction reabsorbed: 0.82–0.95
Vitamin A	Serum	30–65 µg/dL		1.05–2.27 µmol/L

Laboratory values of importance for calcium metabolism and metabolic bone disease[a] Continued.

Test	Source of specimen	Reference Range		Reference range (International Units)
Vitamin D₃, 25 hydroxy	Plasma	Summer: 15–80 ng/mL Winter: 14–42 ng/mL		37–200 nmol/L 35–105 nmol/L
Vitamin D₃, 1, 25 dihydroxy	Serum	25–45 pg/mL		12–46 μmol/L
Calcitonin[d]	Serum (Nichols RIA)	Basal Male Female Pentagastrin Male Female	pg/ml <36 <17 <106 <29	
	Serum (CIS 2-site IRMA)	Basal Male Female Pentagastrin Male Female	pg/ml <10 <10 <30 <30	
	Serum (Mayo Medical Lab)	Basal Male Females Pentagastrin Males Females	<19 <14 <110 <30	
Parathyroid Hormone[d]	Serum (intact, Mayo Lab)			Basal 1.0–5.0 pmol/L
	Serum (intact, Nichols Institute)	Basal	10–65 pg/ml	
	Serum (Mid-molecule, Nichols Institute)	Basal	50–330 pg/ml	
	Serum (N-terminal, Nichols Institute)	Basal	8–24 pg/ml	
Osteocalcin[d]	Serum (Nichols Institute)	Basal	1.6–9.2 ng/ml	
PTHrp[d]	Serum (intact, Nichols Institute)			Basal <0.5 pmol/L

[a] Laboratory values in this table were extracted from Wyngaarden JB, Smith LH Jr (eds): *Cecil Textbook of Medicine, 17th edition.* Philadelphia, 1985, from the section entitled "Reference Ranges and Laboratory Values of Clinical Importance" by Norbert W. Tietz. This reference provides more detailed discussion of source material and units used in this table.

[b] Divide by 2 to get mEq/L.

[c] The total serum calcium can be corrected for alterations in the serum protein concentration by the following formula: Corrected total serum calcium (mg/dl) = observed total serum calcium + [(the normal mean albumin concentration − observed albumin concentration) × 0.8]. In most situations the normal mean albumin concentration will equal 4 g/dl.

[d] The normal values listed include commercial assays. These are listed not to provide an endorsement for these assays, but because they are representative of values available for daily clinical use. It is likely that normal values in other research or commercial assays will vary to some extent.

iv. Mineral and Vitamin D RDA for Infants, Children and Adults

Robert F. Gagel, M.D.

Endocrine Section, M.D. Anderson Cancer Center, Houston, Texas

Recommended dietary allowances[a] Continues—

	Age (yr)	Weight (kg)	Weight (lbs)	Height (cm)	Height (in)	Protein (g)	Vitamin A (μg RE)[b]	Vitamin D (μg)[c]	Vitamin E (mg å TE)[d]	Vitamin C (mg)
Infants	0–0.5	6	13	60	24	kg × 2.2	420	10	3	35
	0.5–1	9	20	71	28	kg × 2.2	400	10	4	35
Children	1–3	13	29	90	35	23	400	10	5	45
	4–6	20	44	112	44	30	500	10	6	45
	7–10	28	62	132	52	34	700	10	7	45
Males	11–14	45	99	157	62	45	1,000	10	8	50
	15–18	66	145	176	69	56	1,000	10	10	60
	19–22	70	154	177	70	56	1,000	7.5	10	60
	23–50	70	154	178	70	56	1,000	5	10	60
	51+	70	154	178	70	56	1,000	5	10	60
Females	11–14	46	101	157	62	46	800	10	8	50
	15–18	55	120	163	64	46	800	10	8	60
	19–22	55	120	163	64	44	800	7.5	8	60
	23–50	55	120	163	64	44	800	5	8	60
	51+	55	120	163	64	44	800	5	8	60
Pregnant						+30	+200	+5	+2	+20
Lactating						+20	+400	+5	+3	+40

—Continues

	Water-soluble vitamins						Minerals		
	Thiamin (mg)	Riboflavin (mg)	Niacin (mg NE)[e]	Vitamin B$_6$ (mg)	Folacin (μg)[f]	Vitamin B$_{12}$ (μg)	Calcium (mg)	Phosphorus (mg)	Magnesium (mg)
Infants	0.3	0.4	6	0.3	30	0.5[g]	360	240	50
	0.5	0.6	8	0.6	45	1.5	540	360	70
Children	0.7	0.8	9	0.9	100	2.0	800	800	150
	0.9	1.0	11	1.3	200	2.5	800	800	200
	1.2	1.4	16	1.6	300	3.0	800	800	250
Males	1.4	1.6	18	1.8	400	3.0	1,200	1,200	350
	1.4	1.7	18	2.0	400	3.0	1,200	1,200	400
	1.5	1.7	19	2.2	400	3.0	800	800	350
	1.4	1.6	18	2.2	400	3.0	800	800	350
	1.2	1.4	16	2.2	400	3.0	800	800	350
Females	1.1	1.3	15	1.8	400	3.0	1,200	1,200	300
	1.1	1.3	14	2.0	400	3.0	1,200	1,200	300
	1.1	1.3	14	2.0	400	3.0	800[h]	800	300
	1.0	1.2	13	2.0	400	3.0	800	800	300
	1.0	1.2	13	2.0	400	3.0	800	800	300
Pregnant	+0.4	+0.3	+2	+0.6	+400	+1.0	+400	+400	+150
Lactating	+0.5	+0.5	+5	+0.5	+100	+1.0	+400	+400	+150

[a] Food and Nutrition Board, National Academy of Sciences/National Research Council (Revised 1980).
[b] Retinol equivalents. 1 retinol equivalent = 1 μg retinol or 6 μg β carotene.
[c] As cholecalciferol, 10 μg cholecalciferol = 400 IU vitamin D.
[d] å-tocopherol equivalents. 1 mg d-å-tocopherol = 1 å TE.
[e] One NE (niacin equivalents) is equal to 1 mg of niacin or 60 mg of dietary tryptophan.
[f] The folacin allowances refer to dietary sources as determined by *Lactobacillus casei* assay.
[g] The RDA for vitamin B$_{12}$ in infants is based on average concentration of the vitamin in human milk and other considerations such as intestinal absorption.
[h] As a result of the NIH Consensus Conference on Osteoporosis (1983), recommendations for calcium intake have been increased to 1,000 mg/day and 1,500 mg/day for pre- (after the age of 19) and postmenopausal women, respectively.

v. Formulary of Drugs Commonly Used in Treatment of Mineral Disorders

Daniel D. Bikle, M.D., Ph.D.

Department of Medicine, University of California San Francisco, and
Veterans Administration Medical Center, San Francisco, California

Formulary of drugs commonly used in treatment of mineral disorders

Drug	Application in treatment of bone and mineral disorders	Dosage (adult)	Rx Cat	Notes
Hormones and analogs				
1. Calcitonin				
Human (Cibacalcin) im or sc (0.5 mg vials)	Paget's disease	0.25–0.5 mg im or sc; q24h	Rx	Preparations for nasal administration are being tested.
Salmon (Calcimar, Miacalcin) im or sc (100, 200 IU/ml)	Paget's disease Osteoporosis	50–100 IU im or sc; qod or qd	Rx	Modestly effective and short-lived in treatment of hypercalcemia
(sc preferred)	Hypercalcemia	4–6 IU/kg im or sc; qid		
2. Estrogens				
Estinyl estradiol (Estinyl, Seminone) po (0.02, 0.05, 0.5 mg)	Postmenopausal osteoporosis	0.02–0.05 mg; qd 3/4 weeks	Rx	To reduce risk of endometrial cancer estrogens can be cycled with a progesterone during last 7–10 days or given concurrently with a progestin throughout the cycle (less break-through bleeding) 0.3 mg with calcium may also be effective
17B estradiol (Estrace) po (1, 2 mg)		1–2 mg; qd 3/4 weeks	Rx	
Conjugated estrogens (Premarin) po (0.3, 0.625, 0.9, 1.25, 2.5 mg)		0.625–1.25 mg qd 3/4 weeks	Rx	
3. Glucocorticoids				
Prednisone (Deltasone) po (2.5, 5, 10, 20, 50 mg)	Hypercalcemia due to sarcoidosis, vitamin D intoxication, and certain malignancies such as multiple myeloma and related lymphoproliferative disorders	10–60 mg; qd	Rx	Long-term use results in osteoporosis and adrenal suppression. Other glucocorticoids with minimal mineralcorticoid activity can be used.
4. Parathyroid hormone				
Human 1–34 (Parathor) iv (200 U/vial)	Diagnosis of pseudo-hypoparathyroidism	200 U; over 10 min infusion	Rx	The use of PTH to treat osteoporosis is being evaluated.
5. Progesterone				
Medroxyprogesterone (Provera) po (2.5, 10 mg)	Osteoporosis in conjunction with estrogens	10 mg; qd for final 7–10 days of cycle	Rx	The concurrent use of progesterone with estrogen may reduce some of the protective cardiovascular effects of estrogen.
Norethindrone (Micronor, Nor-QD, Norlutin) po (5 mg)		5 mg; qd for final 7–10 days of cycle	Rx	
6. Vitamin D preparations				
Cholecalciferol or D₃ po (125, 250, 400 U, often in combination with calcium)	Nutritional vitamin D deficiency Malabsorption Dietary supplement	400–1,000 U; as dietary supplement	OTC	
Ergocalciferol or D₂ (Calciferol) po (8000 U/ml drops; 25,000, 50,000 U tabs)	Hypoparathyroidism Refractory rickets	25,000–100,000 U; 3×/wk to qd	Rx, OTC	D₂ (or D₃) is not of proven value as treatment for osteoporosis.

Formulary of drugs commonly used in treatment of mineral disorders (Continued).

Drug	Application in treatment of bone and mineral disorders	Dosage (adult)	Rx Cat	Notes
Calcifediol or $250HD_3$ (Calderol)	Malabsorption Renal osteodystrophy	20–50 μg; 3×/wk to qd	Rx	$250HD_3$ may be useful in treatment for steroid-induced osteoporosis.
Calcitriol or 1,25 (20,50 μg)$(OH)_2D_3$ (Rocaltrol) po (0.25, 0.5 μg)	Renal osteodystrophy Hypoparathyroidism Refractory rickets	0.25–1.0 μg; qd to bid	Rx	Role in treatment of osteoporosis, psoriasis, and certain malignancies is being evaluated.
Dihydrotachysterol (DHT) po (0.125, 0.2, 0.4 mg)	Renal osteodystrophy Hypoparathyroidism	0.2–1.0 mg; qd	RX	
Minerals 1. Bicarbonate, sodium po (325, 527, 650 mg)	Chronic metabolic acidosis leading to bone disease	Must be titrated for each patient	Rx, OTC	
2. Calcium preparations Calcium carbonate (40% Ca) (Tums) po (500, 650 mg)	Hypocalcemia; if symptomatic should be treated iv	po; 400–2,000 mg elemental Ca in divided doses; qd	OTC	Calcium carbonate is the preferred form because it has the highest percentage of calcium and is the least expensive.
Calcium chloride (36% Ca) iv (100% solution)	Osteoporosis Rickets	iv: 2–20 ml 10% calcium gluconate over several hours		Calcium gluconate is the preferred iv form because, unlike calcium chloride, it does not burn.
Calcium bionate (6.5% Ca) (Neo-glucon) po (1.8 g/5 ml) Calcium gluconate (9% Ca) po (500, 650, 1000 mg) iv (10% solution, 0.465 mEq/ml) Calcium lactate (13% Ca) po (325, 650 mg) Calcium phosphate, dibasic (23% Ca) po (486 mg) Tricalcium phosphate (39% Ca) po (300, 600 mg)	Osteomalacia Chronic renal failure Hypoparathyroidism Malabsorption Enteric oxaluria			In normal subjects the solubility of the calcium salt has not been shown to affect its absorption from the intestine.
3. Fluoride preparations Fluoride, sodium (Luride, Fluoritab) po (2.25 mg/ml drops; 0.25, 0.5, 1.0 mg F tabs)	Dental prophylaxis in regions with nonfluoridated water	0.25–1 mg F, depending on age of child and fluoride content of water supply	Rx	Currently being investigated for treatment of osteoporosis at much higher doses Also available combined with vitamins and other minerals or for topical application to teeth
Florical (8.3 mg sodium fluoride and 364 mg calcium carbonate)	Osteoporosis	3–6 tablets/day		Not FDA approved for treatment of osteoporosis
4. Magnesium preparations Magnesium oxide (Mag-Ox, Uro-Mag) po (84.5, 241.3 mg Mg)	Hypomagnesemia	240–480 mg elemental Mg; qd	OTC	Low magnesium often coexists with low calcium in alcoholics and malabsorbers. Also found in many antacids and vitamin formulations
5. Phosphate preparations Neutra-Phos po (250 mg P, 278 mg K, 164 mg Na)	Hypophosphatemia Vitamin D resistant rickets	iv: 1.5 g over 6–8 h po: 1–3 g in divided doses; qd	Rx, OTC	IV phosphorus is seldom necessary and can be toxic if infusion is too rapid.

Formulary of drugs commonly used in treatment of mineral disorders (Continued).

Drug	Application in treatment of bone and mineral disorders	Dosage (adult)	Rx Cat	Notes
Neutra-Phos-K po (250 mg P, 556 mg K) Fleet Phospha-Soda po (815 mg P, 760 mg Na/5 ml) In Phos iv (1 g P in 40 ml) Hyper Phos-K iv (1 g P in 15 ml)	Hypercalcemia Hypercalciuria			
Diuretics				
1. Thiazides Hydrochlorothiazide (Esidrix, Hydro-Diuril) po (25, 50, 100 mg) Chlorthalidone po (25, 50 mg)	Hypercalciuria Nephrolithiasis	25–50 mg; qd or bid	Rx	Other thiazides may also be effective but are less commonly used for this purpose.
2. Loop diuretics Furosemide (Lasix) po (20, 40, 80 mg) iv (10 mg/ml)	Hypercalcemia; if symptomatic, use iv	po: 20–80 mg; q6h as necessary iv: 20–80 mg over several minutes, repeat as necessary	Rx	Ethacrynic acid may also be effective but is less commonly used for this purpose.
Miscellaneous				
1. Diphosphonates Etidronate (Didronel) po (200, 400 mg) iv (300 mg/6 ml vial)	Paget's disease Heterotopic ossification Hypercalcemia of malignancy	po: 5 mg/kg; qd for 6/12 mo for Paget's disease 20 mg/kg; qd 1 mo before to 3 mo after total hip replacement 10–20 mg/kg; qd for 3 mo after spinal cord injury iv: 7.5 mg/kg; qd for 3 d, given in 250–500 ml normal saline for hypercalcemia of malignancy	Rx Rx	Etidronate is the first-generation diphosphonate. Recent trials indicate that it is useful for osteoporosis at a dose of 400 mg qd for 2 wk every 3 mo. Pamidronate is the first of several second-generation diphosphonates approved for use in this country and abroad that show less inhibition of bone mineralization than etidronate.
Pamidronate	Hypercalcemia of malignancy	60–90 mg given as a single intravenous infusion over 24 h	Rx	Pamidronate is currently under investigation in the United States for treatment of Paget's disease of bone and osteoporosis.
2. Mitramycin or Plicamycin (Mithracin) iv (2.5 mg/vial)	Hypercalcemia of malignancy	25 μg/kg in 1 liter D5W or normal saline over 4–6 hr	Rx	Has been used in treatment of severe Paget's disease, but toxicity makes it treatment of last resort for this purpose.
3. Gallium nitrate	Hypercalcemia of malignancy	200 mg/m² qd ni D5W for 5d continuous infusion	Rx	Undergoing evaluation for use in Paget's disease

vi. Structure of Naturally Occurring Vitamin D and Synthetic Analogs

Sylvia Christakos, Ph.D.

*Departments of Biochemistry and Molecular Biology, University of
Medicine and Dentistry of New Jersey, New Jersey Medical School,
Newark, New Jersey*

Molecular weights, units, and mole equivalents for vitamin D, its metabolites, and important analogs[a]

Substance	Molecular weight	nmoles/1.00 μg	units/ 1.00 mg[b]	μg/unit[b]	nmoles/unit[b]		
					10 units	50 units	100 units
Cholecalciferol series							
D	384.3	2.60	40.0	25.0			
25(OH)D$_3$	400.3	2.49	38.4	26.0			
1,25(OH)$_2$D$_3$	416.3	2.40	36.9	27.1	0.65	3.25	6.50
24,25(OH)$_2$D$_3$	416.3	2.40	36.9	27.1			
25,26(OH)$_2$D$_3$	416.3	2.40	36.9	27.1			
1,24,25(OH)$_3$D$_3$	432.3	2.31	35.5	28.1			
Ergocalciferol series							
D$_2$	396.3	2.52	38.8	25.8			
25(OH)D$_2$	412.3	2.42	37.3	26.8			
1,25(OH)$_2$D$_2$	428.3	2.33	35.8	27.8	0.65	3.25	6.50
24,25(OH)$_2$D$_2$	428.3	2.33	35.8	27.8			
25,26(OH)$_2$D$_2$	428.3	2.33	35.8	27.8			
1,24,25(OH)$_3$D$_2$	444.3	2.25	34.6	28.9			
Analogs							
1(OH)D$_3$	400.3	2.49	38.4	26.0			
Dihydrotachysterol$_3$	385.3	2.59	39.9	25.0			
5,6-trans-D$_3$	384.3	2.60	40.0	25.0	0.65	3.25	6.5
25(OH)-5, 6-trans-D$_3$	400.3	2.49	38.4	26.0			

[a] From Norman AW: *Vitamin D: The Calcium Homeostatic Steroid Hormone.* Academic Press, New York, 462, 1979.

[b] 1.00 unit has been proposed by A. W. Norman: *J Nutr* 102, 1243 (1972) to be 65.0 pmoles for all vitamin D compounds. For vitamin D$_3$ 1.0 IU is by definition (League of Nations, 1935) 0.025 μg, which is exactly equivalent to 65.0 pmoles.

vii. Dynamic Tests

Robert F. Gagel, M.D.

Endocrine Section, M.D. Anderson Cancer Center, Houston, Texas

CALCIUM ABSORPTION TEST (1)

The calcium absorption test is useful for evaluation and classification of hypercalciuric patients (1). The test is performed by maintaining the patient on a 400 mg calcium diet for 1 wk or more prior to testing. The patient is fasted for 10–12 h prior to the start of the test except for access to distilled water. The test consists of three successive urine collections as shown in Fig. 1.

One hour before the start of the first urine collection and hourly thereafter, the patient is given 240 ml (8 oz) of distilled water. The oral calcium and milk may substitute for the distilled water at 120 min (2). The serum and urine collections are analyzed as shown in the figure. Three pieces of information can be obtained from this study. First, the calcemic response (the magnitude of the increase of serum calcium after oral calcium) can be calculated. Second, the calciuric response (increase of urinary calcium excretion) is an index of the amount of calcium absorbed by the gastrointestinal tract. Third, measurement of nephrogenous cAMP and its suppressibility by an oral calcium load is a sensitive dynamic parameter of parathyroid function. Specific calculations for each of these parameters is shown (2).

The tubular reabsorption of phosphate (TRP) is calculated from values obtained during the first urine collection using the following formula:

$$TRP = 1 - \frac{C_{Pi}}{C_{creat}} = 1 - \frac{S_{creat} \times U_{Pi}}{S_{Pi} \times U_{creat}} \text{ (all units in mg/dl)}$$

The TmP/GFR (tubular maximum of phosphate/glomerular filtration rate) is a relationship derived by Walton and Bijvoet that utilizes both the serum phosphate concentration and the tubular reabsorption of phosphate to calculate an index of phosphate clearance (3). It can be calculated from the nomogram shown in Fig. 2.*

Calcemic Response

The calcemic response equals the serum calcium (mg/dl) during the third collection period minus the serum calcium during the first urine collection period.

---

* A hypercard stack (MacIntosh computer) for computer calculation of the TmP/GF is available from L. E. Mallette, M.D., Ph.D., 2002 Holcombe Blvd. (111E), Houston, TX, 77030, and will be provided to anyone sending a blank disk and self-addressed, stamped envelope.

Calciuric Response

The calciuric response equals the calcium excretion during period three minus the calcium excretion during period one.

$$
\begin{aligned}
&\text{First urine collection} \\
&= \frac{U_{calcium} \text{ (mg/dl)}}{U_{creat} \text{ (mg/dl)}} \times S_{creat} \text{ (mg/dl)} \\[6pt]
&\text{Third urine collection} \\
&- \frac{U_{calcium} \text{ (mg/dl)}}{U_{creat} \text{ (mg/dl)}} \times S_{creat} \text{ (mg/dl)} \\[6pt]
&= \text{mg calcium per 100 mL glomerular filtrate}
\end{aligned}
$$

The upper limit of normal for the calciuric response is 0.2 mg calcium/100 mL.

Suppression of Nephrogenous cAMP

Calculation of nephrogenous cAMP requires measurement of both plasma and urinary cAMP. The nephrogenous fraction is calculated by subtracting the fraction of the total cAMP that has been contributed by clearance of cAMP from the plasma. The first step required is calculation of the total urinary cAMP:

$$
\begin{aligned}
&\text{Total urinary cAMP} \\
&= \frac{U_{cAMP} \text{ (nmol/100 mL)}}{U_{creat} \text{ (mg/dL)}} \times S_{creat} \\
&= \text{nmol/100 mL} \qquad \text{(mg/dL)}
\end{aligned}
$$

Nephrogenous cAMP (mmol/100 mL GF)

$$
\begin{aligned}
= &\text{ total cAMP} && - \text{filtered load} \\
&\text{excretion} && \text{of cAMP} \\
&\text{(nmol/100 mL GF)} && \text{(nmol/100 mL} \\
& && \text{of plasma)}
\end{aligned}
$$

THE MODIFIED ELLSWORTH-HOWARD TEST (4)

The measurement of urinary cAMP and phosphate excretion after an intravenous injection of parathyroid hormone is the preferred method for separation of hypopara-

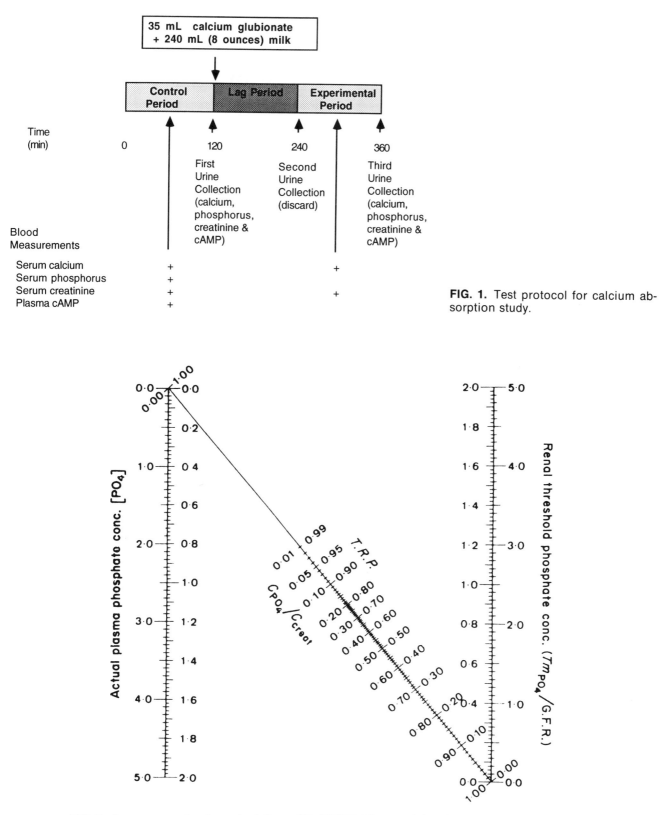

FIG. 1. Test protocol for calcium absorption study.

FIG. 2. A nomogram for the calculation of TmP/GFR. The renal threshold phosphate concentration or TmP/GFR is determined by passing a straight line through the observed serum or plasma phosphate concentration and the measured tubular reabsorption of phosphate (use equation in the text) and by reading the TmP/GFR from the rightmost axis. The data in this figure are presented as either mg/dL (left side of each axis) or mmol/L (right side of each axis). To use this nomogram all values must be expressed as a single type of unit. (From Walton RJ, Bijvoet OLM: Nomogram for derivation of renal threshold phosphate concentration. *Lancet* 2:309, 1975, with permission.)

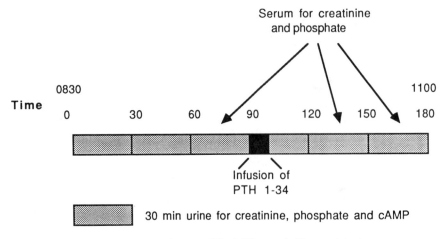

FIG. 3. Protocol for modified Ellsworth-Howard test.

thyroidism secondary to parathyroid hormone deficiency from pseudohypoparathyroidism. There have been numerous modifications of the original test protocol over the years, and the current protocol provided utilizes synthetic human parathyroid hormone-(1-34) (PTH 1-34, recently approved by the Food and Drug Administration for this purpose).

Test Protocol (5)

1. Patient should drink 200 ml of H_2O every 30 min from 0600 h to 1100 h.
2. Collect timed 30-min urine specimens from 0830 h to 1100 h for phosphate, creatinine, and cyclic AMP.
3. Draw serum samples at 0845 h, 1015 h, and 1045 h for creatinine and phosphate.
4. At approximately 0945 h, insert an indwelling catheter into a vein in the upper extremity.
5. From 1,000 h to 1,010 h infuse teriparatide acetate (Rorer Pharmaceuticals), 5 u per kg body weight (200 u maximum), intravenously at a steady rate.
6. Calculations for each parameter shown in Fig. 3 should be made for each collection and then posttreatment values compared to pretreatment values.

The formulas for calculation of response parameters are identical to those described for the calcium absorption test. Figure 4 provides an example of results utilizing this test in three patients to illustrate the differences in response in normal, pseudohypoparathyroid, and idiopathic hypoparathyroid patients.

The changes shown in Fig. 4 are illustrative of typical findings utilizing this technique but do not address the range of normal or abnormal values observed with these conditions. The reader is referred to a more complete discussion of the test for this purpose (4).

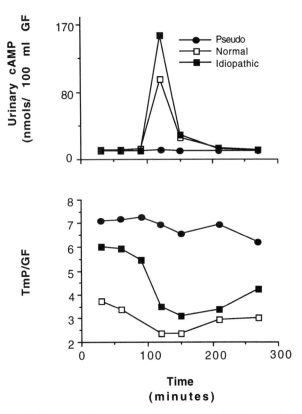

FIG. 4. Typical changes in the urinary cAMP and TmP/GF in a normal, a hypoparathyroid, and a pseudohypoparathyroid patient after an infusion of PTH 1-34 (200 u) performed by the protocol described in the text. In the normal and hypoparathyroid patients there is a prompt increase of the urinary cAMP; there is no increase in the pseudohypoparathyroid patient. The TmP/GFR is elevated in both the hypoparathyroid and pseudohypoparathyroid patients; in the hypoparathyroid patient there is a fall in the TmP/GFR after PTH 1-34 administration. (Unpublished observations of LE Mallette, JL Kirkland, RF Gagel, WM Law, and H Heath III.)

Suppression or Stimulation of Parathyroid Hormone Secretion

Suppression or stimulation of parathyroid hormone (PTH) secretion by increasing or decreasing the serum calcium concentration has been used in the past to diagnose several abnormalities of PTH secretion. The availability of sensitive and specific radioimmunoassays for intact and midregion PTH has eliminated the need for these studies in most clinical situations. Because induction of hypercalcemia or hypocalcemia may be associated with significant risk, these studies are *not* recommended outside of the research environment. References are provided for the interested reader (6, 7).

STIMULATION OF CALCITONIN SECRETION

Measurement of the basal and stimulated serum calcitonin concentration is useful for diagnosis of C-cell hyperplasia and medullary thyroid carcinoma (8). Several different protocols are currently used.

Pentagastrin Test (9)

After an overnight fast, a scalp vein needle with a three-way stopcock is placed in a large arm vein. A basal blood sample is taken, and then pentagastrin (0.5 μg/kg) is injected as a single bolus [for a 70 kg patient, 35 micrograms of pentagastrin (Peptavlon, Ayerst Corporation, 0.14 ml of a 250 μg/ml solution) are diluted in 1 ml of normal saline). Blood samples for calcitonin are taken 2, 5, 10, and 15 min after the injection.

Combined Calcium and Pentagastrin Injection (10)

Combination of a short calcium infusion prior to the pentagastrin injection has been reported to stimulate the release of calcitonin to a greater extent than either calcium or pentagastrin alone. Prior to the injection of pentagastrin, calcium gluconate (2 mg of elemental calcium/kg body weight) is infused over a 1-min period. The injection of pentagastrin follows immediately. The mean increase of the serum calcium concentration has been reported to be approximately 2.0 mg/dl.

Side Effects

Patients given pentagastrin will almost always have side effects, which can include flushing, nausea, vomiting, urge to urinate, epigastric tightness, and tingling in hands and feet. All of these symptoms subside within 2–3 min after the injection. *The patient should be warned of these side effects prior to the injection.* Although most patients consider the test to be unpleasant, family members at risk for hereditary medullary thyroid carcinoma return yearly for these studies. Pentagastrin injection has been used in children as young as 3 years of age for testing of hereditary

medullary thyroid carcinoma and is well tolerated. There have been no reports of pentagastrin stimulation of catecholamine release, a point of some potential concern in multiple endocrine neoplasia, type 2. There have been no reports that addition of calcium to the protocol results in additional side effects, although calcium may stimulate catecholamine secretion.

Normal Response

Pentagastrin stimulates a rapid release of calcitonin with peak calcitonin values observed 2–5 min after injection followed by a decline in the calcitonin concentration. Normal basal serum calcitonin values and the response to pentagastrin are generally greater in men than in women. Normal basal serum calcitonin values are generally less than 50 pg/ml (143 pmol/L), although there is considerable variation from assay to assay. After pentagastrin stimulation there may be a twofold to fourfold increase in the serum calcitonin concentration, although the normal response range varies for each assay (see Appendix iii). The response after the combined calcium/pentagastrin test is usually greater. Abnormal test results are found most commonly in patients with abnormalities of the C-cell, including medullary thyroid carcinoma and C-cell hyperplasia, but other causes should also be considered, including chronic hypercalcemia, Hashimoto's thyroiditis, and ectopic production of calcitonin by other tumors.

GLUCOCORTICOID SUPPRESSION TEST

The glucocorticoid suppression test is performed by administration of hydrocortisone (100 mg per day orally for 10 days) in a hypercalcemic patient. The serum calcium and parathyroid hormone concentrations are measured before and immediately after the completion of the course of hydrocortisone. There will frequently be a decrease of the serum calcium in patients with sarcoidosis, multiple myeloma, vitamin D intoxication, idiopathic hypercalcemia of infancy, and some malignant diseases with osseous metastases (11); if the decrease is great enough there may be a concomitant increase of the serum parathyroid hormone concentration (12). The serum calcium in primary hyperparathyroidism is generally unchanged by glucocorticoid therapy (13).

REFERENCES

1. Broadus AE, Dominguez M, Bartter FC: Pathophysiological studies in idiopathic hypercalciuria: use of an oral calcium tolerance test to characterize distinctive hypercalciuric subgroups. J Clin Endocrinol Metab 47:751–60, 1978
2. Felig P, Baxter JD, Broadus AE, Frohman LA (eds): *Endocrinology and Metabolism, 2nd Edition*. McGraw-Hill, New York, p. 1168, 1987
3. Walton RJ, Bijvoet OL: Nomogram for derivation of renal threshold phosphate concentration. *Lancet* 2:309, 1975
4. Mallette LE, Kirkland JL, Gagel RF, Law WM, Heath H III: Synthetic human parathyroid hormone-(1-34) for the study of pseudohypoparathyroidism. *J Clin Endocrinol Metab* 67: 964–972, 1988

5. Mallette LE: Synthetic human parathyroid hormone 1-34 fragment for diagnostic testing. *Ann Intern Med* 109:800–804, 1988

6. Mallette LE, Tuma SN, Berger RE, Kirkland JL: Radioimmunoassay for the middle region of human parathyroid hormone using an homologous antiserum with a carboxy-terminal fragment of bovine parathyroid hormone as radioligand. *J Clin Endocrinol Metab* 54:1017–1024, 1982

7. Gidding SS, Minciotti AL, Langman CB: Unmasking of hypoparathyroidism in familial partial DiGeorge Syndrome by challenge with disodium Edetate. *N Engl J Med* 319:1589–1591, 1988

8. Gagel RF, Tashjian AH Jr, Cummings T, Papathanasopoulos N, Kaplan MM, DeLellis RA, Wolfe HJ, Reichlin S: The clinical outcome of prospective screening for multiple endocrine neoplasia, type 2a—an 18 year experience. *N Engl J Med* 318:478–484, 1988

9. Hennessy JF, Wells SA Jr, Ontjes DA, et al.: A comparison of pentagastrin injection and calcium infusion as provocative agents for the detection of medullary carcinoma of the thyroid. *J Clin Endocrinol Metab* 39:487, 1974

10. Wells SA Jr, Baylin SB, Linehan WM, Farrell RE, Cox EB, Cooper CW: Provocative agents and the diagnosis of medullary carcinoma of the thyroid gland. *Ann Surg* 188:139–141, 1978

11. Dent CE, Watson L: Hyperparathyroidism and Sarcordosis. *Br Med J* 1:646, 1966

12. Cushard WG Jr, Simon AB, Canterbury JM, Reiss E. Parathyroid function in sarcoidosis. *N Engl J Med* 286:395–398, 1972

13. Habener JF, Potts JT. Parathyroid physiology and primary hyperparathyroidism. In: Avioli LV, Krane SM (eds), *Metabolic Bone Disease, volume II*. Academic Press, New York, 96–97, 1978

viii. Molecular Defects and Models for Disorders of Bone and Mineral Metabolism

Gilbert J. Cote, Ph.D.

Department of Medical Specialities, Section of Endocrinology,
M.D. Anderson Cancer Center, Houston, Texas

Molecular defects and models for disorders of bone and mineral metabolism[a]

Calcium homostasis		
Clinical syndrome	Molecular defect in humans	Animal models
Hypocalcemias:		
Di George syndrome (Chapter 45)	Genetic linkage to 22q11 (1)	hox-1.5 gene knockout (2)
Parathyroid hormone abnormalities	Mutations of the PTH gene (3–5)	
Pseudohypoparathyroidism (Chapter 46)	Mutations resulting in a reduction of the α subunit of stimulatory G-protein (6–8)	
X-linked hypoparathyroidism (Chapter 45)	Genetic linkage to Xq26–q27 (9)	
Hypercalcemias:		
Multiple endocrine neoplasia type 1 (Chapter 31)	Genetic linkage to chromosome 11q13 (10)	
Multiple endocrine neoplasia type 2 (Chapter 31)	Genetic linkage to centromeric chromosome 10 (11)	WAG-Rij rat model (12) Transgenic expression of *c-mos* (13)
Sporadic parathyroid adenoma (Chapter 29)	Translocation activating PRAD1 (14)	

Metabolic bone diseases		
Clinical syndrome	Molecular defect in humans	Animal models
Hypophosphatasia (Chapter 70)	Multiple missense mutations of the alkaline phosphatase gene (15, 16)	
Marfan's syndrome (Chapter 62)	*Cys* to *Ser* missense mutation of the fibrillin gene (17, 18)	Bovine model (19)
McCune-Albright syndrome (Chapter 76)	Activating mutations of the α subunit of stimulatory G-protein (20, 21)	
Osteomalacias		
Hypophosphatemic vitamin D resistant rickets (Chapter 68)	Genetic linkage to Xp22.1–22.2 (22)	Hyp mouse (23) Gy mouse (24)
Vitamin D renal hydroxylase deficiency (VDDR I) (Chapter 67)	Genetic linkage to 12q14 (25)	
Vitamin D receptor disorders (VDDR II) (Chapter 67)	Mutations of the vitamin D receptor (26, 27)	

Genetic, developmental, and dysplastic skeletal disorders		
Clinical syndrome	Molecular defect in humans	Animal models
Chondrodystrophies (Chapter 78)	Genetic linkage of the insulinlike growth factor I gene at chromosome 12q23 (28)	Transgenic mice overexpressing 15-amino acid deletion in the triple helical domain of pro alpha 1(II) collagen chain (29, 30) Japanese Quail (31)
Oteogenesis imperfecta (Chapter 77)	Several genetic defects have been observed in the collagen gene (see Chapter 72 and ref. 32)	Transgenic mice overexpressing collagen (33–35)

Molecular defects and models for disorders of bone and mineral metabolism[a] (Continued).

Clinical syndrome	Molecular defect in humans	Animal models
Osteopetrosis (Chapter 75)	*His* to *Tyr* missense mutation or an intron 5 splice acceptor mutation of the carbonic anhydrase II gene (36)	op/op mouse (37), oc/oc mouse (38), gl/gl mouse, mi/mi mouse (39), carbonic anhydrase deficient mouse (40), mib rat (41), op rat (42), ia rat (43), toothless rat (44), os/os rabbit (45), *src* gene knockout (46), *fos* gene knockout (47, 48)
Sclerosing bone disorders (Chapter 75)		Transgenic overexpression of *fos* (49)

Nephrolithiasis		
Clinical syndrome	Molecular defect in humans	Animal models
Nephrolithiasis (Chapter 87)	Genetic linkage to chromosome Xp11.22 (50)	

[a] The goal of this table is to provide an abbreviated source of information regarding a variety of metabolic bone disorders and workable animal model systems. The references provided reflect key papers, original observations, or reviews and are by no means complete. A related review of molecular genetics of mineral disorders is reference 51.

1. Scrambler P, Carey A, Wyse R: Microdeletions within 22q11 associated with sporatic and familial Di George syndrome. *Genomics* 10:201, 1991
2. Chisaka O, Capecchi M: Regionally restricted developmental defects resulting from targeted disruption of the mouse homeobox gene hox-1.5. *Nature* 350:473, 1991
3. Miric A, Levine MA: Analysis of the preproPTH gene by denaturing gradient gel electrophoresis in familial isolated hypoparathyroidism. *J Clin Endocrinol Metab* 74:509, 1992
4. Arnold A, et al.: Mutation of the signal peptide-encoding region of the preproparathyroid hormone gene in familial isolated hypoparathyroidism. *J Clin Invest* 86:1084, 1990
5. Parkinson D, Thakker R: A donor splice site mutation in the parathyroid hormone gene is associated with autosomal recessive hypoparathyroidism. *Nature Genet* 1:149, 1992
6. Weinstein LS, et al.: Mutations of the Gs alpha-subunit gene in Albright hereditary osteodystrophy detected by denaturing gradient gel electrophoresis. *Proc Natl Acad Sci USA* 87:8287, 1990
7. Spiegel AM: Albright's hereditary osteodystrophy and defective G proteins. *N Engl J Med* 322:1461, 1990
8. Patten JL, et al.: Mutation in the gene encoding the stimulatory G protein of adenylate cyclase in Albright's hereditary osteodystrophy. *N Engl J Med* 322:1412, 1990
9. Thakker R, et al.: Mapping the gene causing X-linked recessive idiopathic hypoparathyroidism to Xq26–Xq27 by linkage studies. *J Clin Invest* 86, 1990
10. Bystrom C, et al.: Localization of the MEN1 gene to a small region within chromosome 11q13 by deletion mapping in tumors. *Proc Natl Acad Sci USA* 87:1968, 1990
11. Simpson NE, et al.: Assignment of multiple endocrine neoplasia type 2A to chromosome 10 by linkage. *Nature* 328:528, 1987
12. Boorman G, van Noord M, Hollander C: Naturally occurring medullary thyroid carcinoma in the rat. *Arch Pathol* 94:35, 1972
13. Schulz N, et al.: Pheochromocytomas and C-cell thyroid neoplasms in transgenic c-mos mice a model for the human multiple endocrine neoplasia type 2 syndrome. *Cancer Res* 52:450, 1992
14. Arnold A, et al.: Molecular cloning and chromosomal mapping of DNA rearranged with the parathyroid hormone gene in a parathyroid adenoma. *J Clin Invest* 83:2034, 1989
15. Weiss MJ, et al.: A missense mutation in the human liver/bone/kidney alkaline phosphatase gene causing a lethal form of hypophosphatasia. *Proc Natl Acad Sci USA* 85:7666, 1988
16. Henthorn P, et al.: Different missense mutations at the tissue-nonspecific alkaline phosphatase gene locus in autosomal recessively inherited forms of mild and severe hypophosphatasia. *Proc Natl Acad Sci USA* 89:9924, 1992
17. Dietz HC, et al.: Marfan phenotype variability in a family segregating a missense mutation in the epidermal growth factor-like motif of the fibrillin gene. *J Clin Invest* 89:1674, 1992
18. Peltonen L, Kainulainen K: Elucidation of the gene defect in Marfan syndrome. Success by two complementary research strategies. *FEBS Lett* 307:116, 1992
19. Besser TE, et al.: An animal model of the Marfan syndrome. *Am J Med Genet* 37:159, 1990
20. Weinstein LS, et al.: Activating mutations of the stimulatory G protein in the McCune-Albright syndrome. *N Engl J Med* 325:1688, 1991
21. Schwindinger WF, Francomano CA, Levine MA: Identification of a mutation in the gene encoding the alpha subunit of the stimulatory G protein of adenylyl cyclase in McCune-Albright syndrome. *Proc Natl Acad Sci USA* 89:5152, 1992
22. Econs MJ, et al.: Multilocus mapping of the X-linked hypophosphatemic rickets gene. *J Clin Endocrinol Metab* 75:201, 1992
23. Eicher E, et al.: Hypophosphatemia: mouse model for the familial hypophosphatemia (vitamin D-resistant) rickets. *Proc Natl Acad Sci USA* 73:4667, 1976
24. Lyon M, et al.: The gy mutation: another cause of X-linked hypophosphatemia in mouse. *Proc Natl Acad Sci USA* 83:4899, 1986
25. Labuda M, Morgan K, Glorieux F: Mapping autosomal recessive vitamin D dependency type I to chromosome 12q14 by linkage analysis. *Am J Hum Genet* 47:28, 1990
26. Hughes MR, et al.: Point mutations in the human vitamin D receptor gene associated with hypocalcemic rickets. *Science* 242:1702, 1988
27. Malloy PJ, et al.: The molecular basis of hereditary 1,25-dihydroxyvitamin D3 resistant rickets in seven related families. *J Clin Invest* 86:2071, 1990
28. Mullis PE, et al.: Growth characteristics and response to growth hormone therapy in patients with hypochondroplasia: genetic linkage of the insulin-like growth factor I gene at chromosome 12q23 to the disease in a subgroup of these patients. *Clin Endocrinol* (Oxf) 34:265, 1991
29. Metsaranta M, et al.: Chondrodysplasia in transgenic mice harboring a 15-amino acid deletion in the triple helical domain of pro alpha 1(II) collagen chain. *J Cell Biol* 118:203, 1992
30. Vandenberg P, et al.: Expression of a partially deleted gene of

human type II procollagen (COL2A1) in transgenic mice produces a chondrodysplasia. *Proc Natl Acad Sci USA* 88:7640, 1991

31. Hermes JC, et al.: A new chondrodystrophy mutation in Japanese quail (Coturnix japonica). *J Hered* 81:222, 1990
32. Lee B, DAlessio M, Ramirez F: Modifications in the organization and expression of collagen genes associated with skeletal disorders. *Crit Rev Eukaryot Gene Expr* 1:173, 1991
33. Khillan JS, et al.: Transgenic mice that express a mini-gene version of the human gene for type I procollagen (COL1A1) develop a phenotype resembling a lethal form of osteogenesis imperfecta. *J Biol Chem* 266:23373, 1991
34. Bonadio J, et al.: Transgenic mouse model of the mild dominant form of osteogenesis imperfecta. *Proc Natl Acad Sci USA* 87:7145, 1990
35. Stacey A, et al.: Perinatal lethal osteogenesis imperfecta in transgenic mice bearing an engineered mutant pro-alpha 1(I) collagen gene. *Nature* 332:131, 1988
36. Roth DE, et al.: Molecular basis of human carbonic anhydrase II deficiency. *Proc Natl Acad Sci USA* 89:1804, 1992
37. Yoshida H, et al.: The murine mutation osteopetrosis is in the coding region of the macrophage colony stimulating factor gene. *Nature* 345:442, 1990
38. Seifert MF, Marks SCJ: Congenitally osteosclerotic (oc/oc) mice are resistant to cure by transplantation of bone marrow or spleen cells from normal littermates. *Tissue Cell* 19:29, 1987
39. Johnson DR, O'Higgins P: Bone surface structure in osteopetrotic grey lethal (gl/gl) and microphthalmic (mi/mi) mutant mice as revealed by scanning electron microscopy. *Bone Miner* 8:109, 1990
40. Lewis SE, et al.: N-ethyl-N-nitrosourea-induced null mutation at the mouse Car-2 locus: an animal model for human carbonic anhydrase II deficiency syndrome. *Proc Natl Acad Sci USA* 85:1962, 1988
41. Wojtowicz A, et al.: Early and transient osteopetrosis in microphthalmic MIB-rats. *Arch Ital Anat Embiol* 95:209, 1990
42. Marks SCJ, Popoff SN: Osteoclast biology in the osteopetrotic (op) rat. *Am J Anat* 186:325, 1989
43. Iizuka T, et al.: The effects of colony-stimulating factor-1 on tooth eruption in the toothless (osteopetrotic) rat in relation to the critical periods for bone resorption during tooth eruption. *Arch Oral Biol* 37:629, 1992
44. Marks SCJ, et al.: Administration of colony stimulating factor-1 corrects some macrophage, dental, and skeletal defects in an osteopetrotic mutation (toothless, tl) in the rat. *Bone* 13:89, 1992
45. Lenhard S, Popoff SN, Marks SCJ: Defective osteoclast differentiation and function in the osteopetrotic (os) rabbit. *Am J Anat* 188:438, 1990
46. Soriano P, et al.: Targeted disruption of the c-src proto-oncogene leads to osteopetrosis in mice. *Cell* 64:693, 1991
47. Johnson R, Spiegelman B, Papaioannou V: Pleiotropic effects of a null mutation in the c-fos proto-oncogene. *Cell* 71:577, 1992
48. Wang Z-Q, et al.: Bone and haematopoietic defects in mice lacking c-fos. *Nature* 360:741, 1992
49. Ruther U, et al.: Deregulated c-fos expression interferes with normal bone development in transgenic mice. *Nature* 325:412, 1987
50. Scheinman S, et al.: Localization of the gene causing X-linked recessive nephrolithiasis to the short arm of the X chromosome (Xp11.22). *J Bone Miner Res* 7:S99, 1992
51. Thakker RV: Molecular genetics of mineral metabolic disorders. *J Inherit Metab Dis* 15:592, 1992

ix. Bone Density Reference Data

Murray J. Favus, M.D.

Department of Medicine, University of Chicago, Chicago, Illinois

The reference data displayed below has been provided by the manufacturer for Hologic QDR Systems. All data, unless otherwise noted, has been obtained from Caucasian sample populations and is listed in 5 year age increments with mean ±2 standard deviations (95% confidence interval).

Table 1. Normal Bone Mineral Density (BMD) values of the AP Spine (L2-L4) in females.

AGE	BMD	DEV
20	1.051	0.110
25	1.072	0.110
30	1.079	0.110
35	1.073	0.110
40	1.056	0.110
45	1.030	0.110
50	0.997	0.110
55	0.960	0.110
60	0.920	0.110
65	0.878	0.110
70	0.840	0.110
75	0.805	0.110
80	0.775	0.110
85	0.754	0.110

Table 2. Normal Bone Mineral Density (BMD) values of the AP Spine (L2-L4) in males.

AGE	BMD	DEV
20	1.115	0.110
25	1.115	0.110
30	1.115	0.110
35	1.115	0.110
40	1.115	0.110
45	1.091	0.110
50	1.076	0.110
55	1.061	0.110
60	1.045	0.110
65	1.030	0.110
70	1.015	0.110
75	0.999	0.110
80	0.984	0.110
85	0.968	0.110

Table 3. Normal Bone Mineral Density (BMD) values of the Hip/Femoral Neck in females.

AGE	BMD	DEV
20	0.895	0.100
25	0.894	0.100
30	0.886	0.100
35	0.871	0.100
40	0.850	0.100
45	0.826	0.100
50	0.797	0.100
55	0.766	0.100
60	0.733	0.100
65	0.700	0.100
70	0.667	0.100
75	0.636	0.100
80	0.607	0.100
85	0.581	0.100

Table 4. Normal Bone Mineral Density (BMD) values of the Hip/Femoral Neck in males.

AGE	BMD	DEV
20	0.979	0.110
25	0.958	0.110
30	0.936	0.110
35	0.915	0.110
40	0.894	0.110
45	0.873	0.110
50	0.851	0.110
55	0.830	0.110
60	0.809	0.110
65	0.788	0.110
70	0.766	0.110
75	0.745	0.110
80	0.724	0.110
85	0.703	0.110

Figure 1. Sample report obtained for lumbar spine of a 47 year-old female patient.

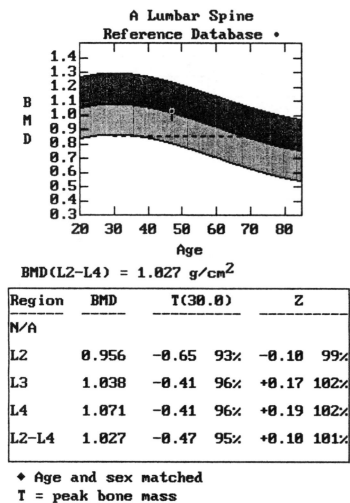

BMD(L2-L4) = 1.027 g/cm^2

Region	BMD	T(30.0)		Z	
N/A					
L2	0.956	-0.65	93%	-0.10	99%
L3	1.038	-0.41	96%	+0.17	102%
L4	1.071	-0.41	96%	+0.19	102%
L2-L4	1.027	-0.47	95%	+0.10	101%

◆ Age and sex matched
T = peak bone mass
Z = age matched   TK   10/25/91

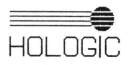

For additional information, please contact HOLOGIC, INC. 590 Lincoln St. Waltham, MA 02154.

The following reference data were supplied by the manufacturer for LUNAR DPX Scanners. All data were based on ambulatory subjects free from chronic bone diseases and not currently taking medications which may affect bone.

Figure 2. BMD values of the AP spine and femur (neck, Ward's triangle, and trochanter) in Caucasian female reference subjects.

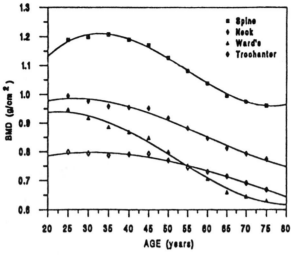

Table 5. Mean BMD values for spine L2-L4 (SD = 0.12 g/cm^2) for reference US/Europe population.

Age	FEMALE		MALE	
	n	Mean	n	Mean
20-29	467	1.188	85	1.255
30-39	499	1.207	106	1.215
40-49	716	1.170	73	1.174
50-59	969	1.081	67	1.161
60-69	476	0.995	63	1.183
70-79	105	0.960	51	1.178

Table 6. Mean female BMD values for femur regions (SD = 0.12 g/cm^2).

Age	n	Neck	Ward's	Trochanter
20-29	479	0.994	0.947	0.798
30-39	499	0.958	0.886	0.787
40-49	704	0.950	0.847	0.792
50-59	882	0.881	0.751	0.745
60-69	415	0.811	0.660	0.714
70-79	121	0.773	0.630	0.668

Table 7. Mean male BMD values for femur regions (SD = 0.12 g/cm^2).

Age	n	Neck	Ward's	Trochanter
20-29	84	1.107	1.022	0.948
30-39	95	1.038	0.922	0.900
40-49	74	1.001	0.852	0.898
50-59	73	0.985	0.809	0.920
60-69	66	0.953	0.770	0.904
70-79	46	0.872	0.685	0.841

Figure 3. Sample report obtained for AP spine of a 65 year-old female patient.

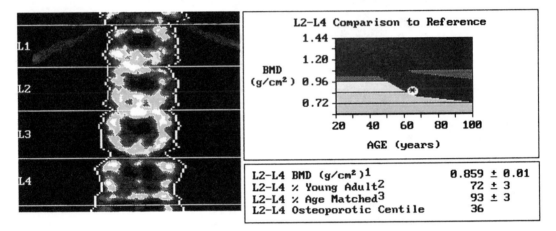

	L2-L4 BMD (g/cm^2)[1]	0.859 ± 0.01
	L2-L4 % Young Adult[2]	72 ± 3
	L2-L4 % Age Matched[3]	93 ± 3
	L2-L4 Osteoporotic Centile	36

LUNAR®   IMAGE NOT FOR DIAGNOSIS

REGION	BMD[1] g/cm^2	Young Adult[2] %	Z	Age Matched[3] %	Z
L1	0.806	71	-2.70	95	-0.36
L2	0.834	70	-3.05	91	-0.72
L3	0.912	76	-2.40	99	-0.07
L4	0.831	69	-3.08	90	-0.74
L1-L2	0.820	71	-2.75	94	-0.41
L1-L3	0.854	73	-2.63	96	-0.30
L1-L4	0.847	72	-2.77	94	-0.44
L2-L3	0.876	73	-2.70	95	-0.37
L2-L4	0.859	72	-2.84	93	-0.51
L3-L4	0.869	72	-2.76	94	-0.42

1 - Statistically 68% of repeat scans will fall within 1 SD.

2 - USA AP Spine Reference Population, Ages 20-45.

3 - Matched for Age, Weight(males 50-100kg; females 35-80kg).

For additional information, please contact LUNAR Corporation, 313 W. Beltline Highway, Madison, WI 53713.

Subject Index

431